W0043694

METHODS IN ANGIOLOGY

INSTRUMENTATION AND TECHNIQUES IN CLINICAL MEDICINE

Volume 2

Methods in Angiology:
A physical-technical introduction written for clinicians by physicians

edited by M. Verstraete

Volume 1

Data in Medicine: Collection, Processing and Presentation.
A physical-technical introduction for physicians and biologists.
edited by ROBERT S. RENEMAN and JAN STRACKEE
ISBN 90-247-2150-4

Future volumes

Otorhinolaryngology
edited by B. H. PICKARD

Nuclear Medicine
edited by K. H. EPHRAIM

Diagnostic Radiology
edited by P. P. G. KRAMER

and others

series ISBN 90-247-2349-3

METHODS IN ANGIOLOGY

A PHYSICAL-TECHNICAL INTRODUCTION
WRITTEN FOR CLINICIANS BY PHYSICIANS

Edited by

MARC VERSTRAETE, M.D.

Professor of Medicine
University of Leuven
Leuven, Belgium

Introduced by

D.E. STRANDNESS, Jr., M.D.

Professor of Surgery
University of Washington
Seattle, USA

with additional expert commentary

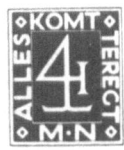

1980
MARTINUS NIJHOFF PUBLISHERS / THE HAGUE / BOSTON / LONDON

Distributors:

for the United States and Canada

Kluwer Boston, Inc.
190 Old Derby Street
Hingham, MA 02043
USA

for all other countries

Kluwer Academic Publishers Group
Distribution Center
P.O. Box 322
3300 AH Dordrecht
The Netherlands

Library of Congress Cataloging in Publication Data   CIP

Main entry under title:

Methods in angiology.

    (Instrumentation and techniques in clinical medicine; v. 2)
    Bibliography.
    Includes index.
    1. Blood-vessels − Diseases − Diagnosis. I. Verstraete, Marc. II. Series.
RC691.5.M47   616.1'3   80-16003

ISBN-13:978-94-009-8880-4   e-ISBN-13:978-94-009-8878-1
DOI: 10.1007/978-94-009-8878-1

Copyright © 1980 by Martinus Nijhoff Publishers bv, The Hague.
Softcover reprint of the hardcover 1st edition 1980

All rights reserved. No part of this publication may be reproduced, stored in a retrieval system, or transmitted in any form or by any means, mechanical, photocopying, recording, or otherwise, without the prior written permission of the publisher,
Martinus Nijhoff Publishers bv, P.O. Box 566, 2501 CN The Hague, The Netherlands.

Table of contents

List of authors

G.J. BARENDSEN, Ph.D., Laboratory of Medical Physics, University of Groningen, The Netherlands.

J.A. DORMANDY, M.D., F.R.C.S., F.R.C.S.E., Consultant Vascular Surgeon, St. James's Hospital, London, United Kingdom; Honorary Senior Lecturer in Surgery, University of London, United Kingdom.

D.E. FITZGERALD, Ph.D., M.Sc., L.R.C.P. & S.I., Director, Angiology Research Group, Irish Foundation for Human Development; Lecturer, Department of Surgery, Trinity College, Dublin, Ireland.

K.L. GOULD, M.D., Professor and Director, Division of Cardiology, Department of Medicine, University of of Texas, Medical School at Houston, Houston, Texas 77025, U.S.A.

R. GROSSE-VORHOLT, M.D., O.A., Radiological Department, Klinikum 8500 Nürnberg, West-Germany.

P. HOLSTEIN, M.D., Department of Clinical Physiology, Bispebjerg Hospital, 2400 Copenhagen N.V., Denmark.

V.V. KAKKAR, M.D., F.R.C.S., F.R.C.S.E., Professor of Surgical Science, Director Thrombosis Research Unit, King's College Hospital Medical School, London, United Kingdom.

N.A. LASSEN, M.D., Chief of the Department of Clinical Physiology, Bispebjerg Hospital, 2400 Copenhagen N.V., Denmark.

D. LAWRENCE, F.R.C.S., Research Fellow, Honorary Senior Surgical Registrar, Thrombosis Research Unit, Department of Surgery, King's College Hospital Medical School, London, United Kingdom.

R. MAYALL, M.D., Professor of Medicine, Hospital de Gambôa, Rio de Janeiro, Brasil.

D.E. STRANDNESS Jr., M.D., Professor of Surgery, Department of Surgery, University of Washington, Seattle, Washington, U.S.A.

H.J. TERRY, Ph.D., C.Eng., M.I.E.R.E., Principal Physicist, St. James's University Hospital, Leeds LS9 7TF, United Kingdom.

R. VERHAEGHE, M.D., Center for Thrombosis and Vascular Research, Department of Medical Research, University of Leuven, Belgium.

M. VERSTRAETE, M.D., F.R.C.P. (Edin.), F.A.C.P. (Hon.), Professor of Medicine, Center for Thrombosis and Vascular Research, Department of Medical Research, University of Leuven, Belgium.

D.W. WINSOR, M.D., Department of Nuclear Medicine, St. Vincent Medical Center, Los Angeles; and Co-Director, Memorial Heart Research Foundation, Inc., Los Angeles, California, U.S.A.

T. WINSOR, M.D., Clinical Professor of Medicine, University of Southern California School of Medicine; and Director of the Vascular Laboratory, St. Vincent Medical Center, Los Angeles, California, U.S.A.

E. ZEITLER, M.D., Professor, Chief of Radiology, Radiological Department, Klinikum 8500 Nürnberg, West-Germany.

List of commentators

R.W. BARNES, M.D., David M. Hume Professor of Surgery, Medical College of Virginia; Chief of Vascular Surgery, McGuire Veterans Administration Hospital, Richmond, Virginia, U.S.A.

A. BOLLINGER, M.D., Professor of Medicine (Angiology), University of Zürich, Department of Medicine, University Hospital, CH-8091 Zürich, Switzerland.

S. CHIEN, M.D., Ph.D., Professor of Physiologygy, Department of Physiology, College of Physicians and Surgeons of Columbia University, New York, New York, 10032, U.S.A.

J.D. COFFMAN, M.D., Professor of Medicine, Peripheral Vascular Section, Robert Dawson Evans Memorial Dept. of Clinical Research, University Hospital and Boston University School of Medicine, Boston, Massachusetts 02218, U.S.A.

A. CRUMMY, M.D., Professor of Radiology, Department of Radiology, University of Wisconsin Medical Center, Madison, Wisconsin 53706, U.S.A.

M. ELKE, M.D., Professor of Radiology, Department of Diagnostic Radiology, University Institute of Radiology, Kantonsspital, Basel, Switzerland.

H.L. FALSETTI, M.D., Professor of Medicine, Division of Cardiology, Department of Medicine, University of Iowa Hospitals, Iowa City, Iowa 52242, U.S.A.

J. GUNDERSEN, M.D., Ph.D., Associate Professor of Surgery, Department of Surgery, University of Lund, Central Hospital, S-29185 Kristianstad, Sweden.

H.L. NEIMAN, M.D., Associate Professor of Radiology, Director of Angiography and Sectional Imaging, Northwestern University School of Medicine/Northwestern Memorial Hospital, Chicago, Illinois 60611, U.S.A.

P. PUEL, M.D., Dean of the Faculty ,Cardiovascular surgeon, Rangueil Hospital, Toulouse, France.

V.C. ROBERTS, Ph.D., MIEE, Senior Lecturer in Bio Medical Engineering, King's College Hospital Medical School, London SE5, United Kingdom.

D.S. SUMNER, B.A., M.D., F.A.C.S., Professor of Surgery and Chief, Section of Peripheral Vascular Surgery, Southern Illinois University School of Medicine, Springfield, Illinois 62708, U.S.A.

O. THULESIUS, Professor of Clinical Physiology, Department of Clinical Physiology, Central Hospital, Växjö, Sweden.

S. UEMATSU, M.D., Assistant Professor of Neurosurgery, Department of Neurosurgery, Johns Hopkins University, School of Medicine; Director, Neurometrics Laboratory, Johns Hopkins Hospital, Baltimore, Maryland, U.S.A.

Introduction: critical appraisal of the fifteen chapters

D.E. STRANDNESS, JR.

This book brings the reader up to date on the progress in one of the most rapidly changing fields in medicine. If one simply reviews the titles of the chapters, it is clear that, with few exceptions, the topics discussed are not, in fact, of recent vintage. The major change is that the methods available are being applied on a greater scale in recent years to elucidate many of the physiological changes that occur secondary to a wide variety of peripheral vascular disease. Until recently, angiology has been largely a descriptive discipline with an insufficient amount of effort devoted to rigorously defining the pathophysiology of vascular disorders and their modification by therapy. Thus, it appears that angiology as a specialty is at long last beginning to assume its rightful place with its companion cardiology, which has approached the problems of cardiac function in a more quantitative manner.

The structure of this volume is unique in that each subject is not only presented by a qualified expert but is also subjected to an outside review by an equally competent scientist who supplied a critique of the presented material. This approach is certainly unique and might be confusing to the newcomer to the field but it tends to highlight both the areas of agreement and those which still remain a source of some confusion and disagreement. For me, reading the comments literally side by side in this chapter was a refreshing and stimulating way of reviewing a topic. It is clearly the intent of the editor to present in an open and occasionally critical, fashion honest differences that can be of great importance in assessing the proper place of the subjects. To this end, the material has in large part met this goal.

While the introduction to most texts is of a general, often philosophical nature, my role will be entirely different. Even though my bias is toward more widespread utilization of many of these methods, there is evidence that some are being misused in the study of many clinical problems. Thus, I will attempt to also be critical of those areas where it appears that such an approach is justified. The end-result for the reader will be not only a critical commentary, chapter by chapter by selected experts, but an overall assessment of the volume by me which may in some instances be in fundamental disagreement with the conclusions of the authors.

CHAPTER 1

There is little doubt that the electromagnetic flowmeter has become the most direct method of measuring velocity and volume flow in an exposed vessel. It is remarkable that this technique, which is almost 50 years old, is still undergoing modification and refinement. This method of measuring flow has been used most extensively by physiologists for both acute and chronic studies. It is, in fact, this discipline which is most familiar with its problems and limitations. While it is natural that this type of measuring system should be used by surgeons with vessels exposed at the time of operation, it is in this area where it appears that the problems have not been fully appreciated.

Unfortunately, in clinical situations, the nature of the vessel wall at the site of measurement is unpredictable in terms of wall thickness and con- stituents. Thus, the conductivity of the vessel wall remains an unknown which must be recognized. Also, the type of velocity profile present is not known, particularly when the flowmeter is used on vessels which are in close proximity to a bifurcation or atherosclerotic plaque. It is also unwise for clinicians to depend upon the manufacturer's assurance that electrical and occlusive zero are identical.

The major point to remember with this type of measurement is that the measured flow is, in fact, an approximation and that the extent of its relationship to reality remains an unknown. A suitable compromise in utilizing the electromagnetic flowmeter intelligently is to assess the per cent change in flow that occurs in response to a vasodilator such as papaverine. This, in combination with measurements of the pressure gradient across the corrected segments (where feasible), will provide some assurance that the operative procedure has been successful. However, one must recognize that this immediate flow change may not be predictive of the immediate or long term hemodynamic results. In conclusion, it is correct to state that these deceptively simple devices are probably best used for research pur- poses and by those who are prepared to familiarize themselves with the problems and pitfalls that can accompany their use.

CHAPTER 2

The plethysmograph has returned to its proper place as a method for investigating peripheral vascular dynamics. There is little doubt that it remains the best method of measuring limb blood flow. As the reader will note, the methods have been adapted and modified for purposes not originally envisioned by those who developed the technique. A point well taken is with regard to the relationship between the volume pulse amplitude and absolute levels of blood flow. While it can be shown that, in general, an increase in pulse amplitude is accompanied by a rise in blood flow, the relationship is clearly not linear. Also, those systems which are time-consuming in application, such as the water filled systems, are not useful clinically but are excellent for research purposes.

The mercury in silastic strain gauge provides an excellent compromise with regard to the other plethysmographic systems. The theoretical and practical problems with this system have been extensively evaluated and found to be solvable. Further, many of the newer systems can be calibrated electrically with the results comparing favorably with those carried out by mechanical means. This further simplifies their use since the calibration is done with the gauge on the limb. Thus, compensation for temperature changes are not as serious a problem, which can be the case when the gauge is removed from the limb for calibration.

Impedance plethysmography, on the other hand, poses more difficult problems. As rightly noted, the waveforms recorded are very similar to those obtained by other methods. However, attempts at quantitation have not been uniformly successful and this fact must be appreciated. If quantitation of flow is desired, then these systems should not be used. In spite of this obvious limitation, the impedance method has been successfully applied for the evaluation of the flow changes produced by acute deep venous thrombosis.

As properly emphasized, the analysis of the volume pulse waveform is best done in the clinical setting by visual inspection. While there is no doubt that the waveform can be quantitatively analyzed, it does not offer any advantages over simple inspection. The ability to sense the small volume changes in the digits does permit measurement of digit blood pressure and reappearance time after a reactive hyperemia test. Digit pressures are particularly useful in documenting the presence of occlusive disease in the hand in patients with cold sensitivity.

As detailed in the chapter on plethysmography, there has been voluminous work done on the blood flow in normal limbs with arterial disease under resting conditions and following some form of stress. There is nearly uniform agreement that flows at rest are not useful clinically since they are nearly always within the normal range. However, this is clearly not the case in those areas where regional ischemia may be profound, such as the forefoot and digits when ischemic rest pain is the problem. The blood flow changes brought about by chronic arterial occlusion are best determined when the circulation is called upon to increase its flow in response to some form of stress. The peak flows attained are rarely as high as in normals and the recovery time is delayed. Further, it is possible to show that the observed flow response can vary depending upon the level and extent of the arterial occlusion and the functional capacity of the collateral circulation.

CHAPTER 3

The chapter by Lassen and Holstein is a refreshing look at the continued use of isotopes since they emphasize those applications which show promise in clinical practice. As indicated, the measurements of muscle and skin flow are being used less frequently since other simpler methods of assessing the presence and degree of arterial obstruction are now available. In fact, it has been largely due to the influence of Dr. Lassen that the importance of perfusion pressure, both as an index of occlusion and prognosis, is becoming better understood and accepted by the medical profession.

The importance of the concept of skin perfusion pressure cannot be overemphasized. Many physicians might argue, of course, that it is flow and not pressure that is most critical since tissue death occurs because of inadequate perfusion, not pressure. While this is true, pressure remains the simplest, most objective method of predicting whether or not an open lesion or amputation will heal.

Also, as indicated by the authors, they are searching for other, simpler methods of measuring skin perfusion pressure. This is due to the fact that the procedure is tedious, time-consuming, and uncomfortable for the patient. Nonetheless, the concept remains a valid one which, with improvements in methodology, will become of increasing importance in clinical medicine. It is hoped that the remarkable achievements by Dr. Lassen's group will continue to the benefit of not only the patients we all serve but to those of us who are often faced with difficult therapeutic decisions in patients with threatened tissue loss.

CHAPTER 4

The chapter by FitzGerald on ultrasonic techniques presents the current state of the instrumentation and its clinical use in straightforward simple terms. While this approach will not appeal to the experienced user, this is essential background information which must be properly understood if these techniques are ever to be usefully applied in the clinical situation. The simple problems relating to probe positioning, angle and attenuation as related to frequency of the transmitted signal need to be emphasized again and again. How often does one see the inexperienced user apply the Doppler transducer at right angles to a vessel and appear perplexed when the angle is changed to 45° and not only the frequency of the return signal increases but the phasic characteristic of the velocity changes suddenly becomes more evident!

Also, the brief introduction to the differences between continuous wave and pulsed systems is important. Clearly, the devices which employ the pulsed ultrasound will never completely replace the continuous wave systems for many applications but there are areas where the use of the more sophisticated device will become indispensable. In any situation where it is important to selectively sample from either a deeply placed vessel or from some discrete point across its diameter, the pulsed method is the only possible approach.

A very practical point mentioned with regard to the 'best' audible signal obtainable becomes important when analogue recordings are made using a zero-crossing detector. If the observer cannot obtain a good audible signal, it will be nearly impossible to get a clean analogue recording which is of value. The availability of audio-spectrum analyzers will, in large part, obviate this problem. Not only can the true velocity pattern be recorded even with a poor signal to noise ratio, but it is also possible to evaluate the distribution and amplitude of the velocities recorded as related to time. Also, as properly emphasized, the phasicity of the arterial signal which is important diagnostically is related to both the nonuniform properties of the arterial wall and the peripheral resistance.

The use of pulsatility index and transit times, while of great interest, must be explored in more depth by other investigators. One reason this has been hampered is because of the need for a spectrum analyzer as well as some method of integrating the area under the curve to obtain the mean value which is necessary to make the calculation. At present the cost of such systems is prohibitively high for application in most clinical vascular laboratories.

Segmental pressures can be usefully applied to separate levels of occlusion but do have limitations related to the discrepancy between cuff width and thigh diameter. Thus, the upper thigh pressure must be interpreted with caution, taking into account those factors which may influence the measurement. It is true that the use of the wide thigh cuff is not useful in attempting to distinguish between aorto-iliac and superficial femoral disease.

The relationship between aneurysmal disease and velocity patterns demonstrated will require further documentation. While there would appear to be a rational basis for the subdivision of the degree of arterial involvement in terms of the waveforms recorded, as outlined in Fig. 16–18 in Chapter 4, the validity of such an approach will require further study in other centers. This may become a useful method of classifying arterial lesions but it remains to be proved whether it is more helpful than standard pressure and velocity recordings.

The practice of scanning the carotid bifurcation with a continuous wave Doppler should be used more frequently. The technique, while difficult to master, can be done quickly and is quite useful for detecting stenoses that reduce the arterial diameter by 50% or greater. A word of caution is urged concerning the use of a spectrum analyzer to assess turbulence with a continuous wave system. Since the entire arterial lumen is insonated, the spectral width will by definition be greater than observed with a pulsed system where the sample is taken from a discrete volume in the center of the vessel. The periorbital examination has very few false positives but is useful only if abnormal. Since it will detect only those lesions which produce a pressure and flow decrease, it will miss a significant number of stenoses that may be the source of emboli.

A very fertile area for the application of Doppler ultrasound is the assessment of aortocoronary grafts. However, I remain skeptical about the use of continuous wave ultrasound for this purpose. The pulsed systems, with or without combined B-mode imaging, are much more likely to be successful but any device designed for this purpose will probably require a considerable amount of development. To my knowledge, no such system has yet been developed but, because of the critical importance of this area, should be pursued.

As evidence accumulates regarding the usefulness of these methods, it is hoped that they will be used more widely for prospective studies. While some would argue that history and physical examination are all that is required, experience is accumulating that this is not the case. It is time that the medical profession accept this fact and proceed with more objective studies of the natural history of atherosclerosis relating both to existing risk factors and the results of intervention studies.

CHAPTER 5

Thermal techniques to estimate skin perfusion remain one of the most controversial topics in clinical medicine, particularly in relation to peripheral vascular disorders. The reasons for this are largely due to their qualitative nature and the fact that, to many observers, the methods simply confirm the obvious, i.e., the part is either warm, cold, or higher or lower in temperature than its paired part. While there is no doubt that different thermal patterns do exist in response to vascular disorders, it has been difficult to conclusively prove that these studies, in and of themselves, will, in fact, alter either the diagnostic or therapeutic approach to the patient.

With regard to extracranial arterial disease, the temperature patterns of the face on the side involved apparently change when the internal carotid is either severely narrowed or occluded. This is, of course, consistent with the known fact that, at this level of disease involvement, the blood flow to the ipsilated forehead is now dependent upon the external carotid artery instead of the internal carotid via the ophthalmic, medial frontal, and supraorbital arteries. I would argue with the contention that thermography is more accurate than any of its clinical counterparts. There are other methods which are much cheaper and can be used to accurately detect high grade stenoses or occlusions of the extracranial arteries. Further, this method does not detect those lesions which do not reduce pressure and flow and yet may be the source of emboli to the brain.

Thermography for the study of diseases of the blood supply to the arms and legs has not met with widespread acceptance. This is, again, due to the fact that other simpler and cheaper methods may be more quickly applied to arrive at the same decision relative to etiology and degree of impairment. As outlined by other authors (Chapters 3, 4, 6 and 9), many of the desired results can be more objectively assessed by a variety of techniques.

One potentially useful application of thermography is in the detection of deep venous thrombosis. Unfortunately, there have been few studies comparing the results with venography which remains the gold standard. For those interested, the best controlled study was that cited by the authors (1). Whether its usefulness will supersede other methods will depend upon comparative studies which have not yet been done.

CHAPTER 6

There is little doubt that the use of segmental blood pressures remains one of the most widely used and accepted methods of localizing and assessing the degree of arterial occlusion. Based upon intra-arterial pressure studies, there appears to be little doubt that in the leg there is gradual amplification in the systolic pressure as one proceeds distally down the limb. The problem of cuff size remains a difficult issue, particulary when measurements are made proximal to the knee. Fortunately, there are a variety of sensors available which can be used to measure the systolic pressure. The ability to estimate systolic pressure alone is not a major drawback since changes in this value occur much earlier than in the levels of either mean or diastolic pressure.

An important problem addressed by Verhaeghe is that related to patients with two-level disease (aorto-iliac and superficial femoral) in which the decision as to which lesion to correct first is often difficult. This is in those situations in which a proximal stenosis is observed but its hemo-dynamic significance is difficult to assess. As noted, it has been suggested that, by using the two narrow cuffs above the knee and high thigh, it is possible to make this assessement more accurate. It must be emphasized that this view remains very controversial with this author being skeptical as to whether this is, indeed, true. At the present time, the most reliable method assessing the hemodynamic significance of the aorto-iliac segment is by direct intra-arterial pressure measurements and their response to reactive hyperemia induced either chemically or by the cuff occlusion method. However, there is ongoing work which is very promising that suggests that the velocity patterns in the common femoral artery may be as sensitive. This would be a great help since these can be used non-invasively.

A point of great importance is the use of both the ankle/arm pressure index and absolute pressure level as a measure of the degree of perfusion to the foot. There is increasing evidence that these parameters may be helpful in predicting the outcome of sympathectomy, the ability of an open lesion to heal and the level at which an amputation may be expected to heal. Further, since pressure measurements can be made repetitively with ease, they provide the most objective method of following the natural history of the disease with or without therapy. Finally, it appears to be time that these simple measurements should be used more widely in prospective, epi-demiologic studies of peripheral arterial disease. Clinical evaluation alone should no longer be considered acceptable as the definitive endpoint upon which the effectiveness of various forms of therapy is judged.

CHAPTER 7

The chapter on the measurement of intra-arterial pressure is extremely important in detailing the problems that can arise when one is not familiar with the principles involved. In many areas of medicine today, the use of direct measurements is very common and essential for proper patient management. This is most frequently seen in intensive care units and at the time of major surgery where intra-arterial lines are a daily practice. In this setting strict attention to the details outlined by Dr. Gould are not as essential since one is simply interested in trends and not absolute accuracy. Where then do these principles become essential?

If one accepts the observation that the change in pressure, i.e., the pressure drop that occurs across a stenosis, is the most accurate method of assessing its significance, the importance of understanding the principles elucidated in this chapter becomes apparent. For example, it is now becoming commonplace to insert a needle or catheter into the femoral artery to measure the pressure in assessing the significance of the proximal arterial disease. Normally, the systolic pressure should be slightly higher than central aortic or brachial and have a prominent dicrotic wave. If the system is damped, not only will the systolic pressure measured be falsely low but the waveforms will appear rounded and abnormal. Thus, it is essential that the entire measurement system (needle, catheter, tubing, stopcock and transducer) be capable of faithfully reproducing the arterial pressure and waveform which is present. Those interested in a discussion of this problem as it relates to the peripheral arterial system should refer to ref. (2).

CHAPTER 8

The whole area of blood viscosity, particulary as it relates to clinical medicine, remains confusing and mysterious to most of us even closely related to the field. While there is no doubt that it is important, the key question which keeps arising is – How? One only needs to examine Table 3 in Chapter 8 to see that Dr. Dormandy must in part share this view as well. In examining those diseases in which hyperviscosity really appears to play a major role, they are largely conditions which are not commonly considered as being in the field of angiology. When those diseases that 'may be' in part related to hyperviscosity are listed they include venous thrombosis, intermittent claudication and Raynaud's phenomenon. I suspect that here even Dr. Dormandy would agree that evidence for the role of hyperviscosity is at best incomplete.

Nonetheless, the discussion of the rheology of blood in relationship to viscosity is admirably covered by the author and external reviewer. Thus, it should be clear that a proper understanding of the concepts involves an appreciation of the flow patterns in tubes of all sizes from the level of the major arteries down to and including the capillaries. A key point in the understanding of viscosity and its importance is the relationship between a high measured blood viscosity and circulatory insufficiency. It is also suggested that there is thus validity for measuring viscosity since this can in turn be related to one aspect of the rheological properties of blood as observed in the living circulation. The external reviewer does, however, question this conclusion to some extent.

The methods of measuring viscosity are covered in detail as well as those factors which influence it in vivo. In short, the three major factors relate to those existing in plasma, the red cell itself and the concentration of red cells in plasma. In fact, this discussion serves as the basis for the clinical classification which is used to describe the various disorders in which viscosity appears to play a role.

The major uncertainties arise in considering those conditions in which viscosity may play a role, i.e., venous thrombosis, myocardial ischemia, claudication, hypertension and Raynaud's phenomenon. While the author presents evidence for such a relationship, it appears to have been largely ignored by the medical profession. Each of the above conditions is not an implicate entity in which it is possible to implicate even a single etiologic factor, let alone viscosity. Clearly, it does not appear to be the major link in the pathogenesis of the disorders but could, of course, be a complicating factor in the pathophysiology. While it is tempting to assume that a high viscosity is important in the sequelae of the diseases, a direct relationship does not necessarily follow.

If one assumes viscosity is or may be important, the key question is how to recognize it and then correct it. A key statement relative to this problem is to suspect the problem when the degree of circulatory impairment is out of proportion to diseases of either the blood vessels or the heart. Apparently, a normal hematocrit and sedimentation rate will rule out the pure hyperviscosity states. Short of this, direct measurements of viscosity and red cell deformability are recommended in the questionable cases.

In the area of treatment, the author of the chapter might not find many allies, particularly as it relates to those conditions in which viscosity only in part contributes to the problem. While it is possible to affect all major components of the factors that contribute to viscosity, these have not as yet reached common practice.

Finally, the chapter is concluded with a brief introduction to the area of the deformability of the red blood cells and their importance, particularly in the microcirculation. This new area is of interest but must await further work not only in the methods of making the measurements but correlating the changes with observed clinical states.

CHAPTER 9

The chapter on the diagnosis of deep vein thrombosis presents a complete summary of the available modalities which can be used to detect this disorder, both prospectively and in patients suspected of having the disease. For the uninitiated, the array of tests may be confusing as to which method(s) are applicable to the particular setting in which they may be used. Fortunately, there is considerable data from good centers now available which permits firm conclusions and recommendations.

The most sensitive method is the labeled fibrinogen test which permits the detection of calf vein thrombosis at its earliest stage. There is no doubt that this method will remain the standard for prospective surveillance studies to assess not only the incidence of calf vein thrombosis but the effectiveness of prophylactic measures. However, the test does have limitations which must be recognized. The incidence of false positives has been reported to be as high as 20% in some series. Thus, a positive test must be verified by some other method which usually is contrast venography. As Dr. Kakkar indicates, contrast studies may well be negative, meaning either that it is a true false positive or the thrombi are so small that they cannot be seen. What do you do then? Repeat venography is unjustified and treatment is unnecessary unless the thrombi propagate into the tibial or popliteal veins. Continued scanning may answer this question or one of the other noninvasive tests may be used to monitor the progress of the thrombosis.

There appears to be a trend of using this test as a routine in 'high risk' patients undergoing major surgery. This is a costly venture which may be difficult to justify. For example, the study by Gallus et al. (3) has shown that, in an excellent randomized trial of 820 patients, 2.8% of control patients undergoing major general surgical procedures developed femoropopliteal thrombosis. Thus, the yield would be extremely low for thrombi that are potentially troublesome with regard to either pulmonary embolism or the postthrombotic syndrome. A key question which remains to be answered is whether this cost is justified. Further, if the patient remains at risk, i.e., in the hospital and not fully ambulatory, reinjection of the isotope will be needed if further monitoring is done.

The study from McMaster University previously cited also raises other questions with regard to surveillance as related to the other noninvasive tests. As rightly pointed out, the yield here would also be extremely low but would, of course, detect those thrombi involving the major deep veins.

The issues with regard to the symptomatic patient are now less controversial, at least when the best studies are considered. There is little doubt that Doppler ultrasound and any of the available plethysmographic systems will give comparable accuracy for major deep vein thrombosis (popliteal vein and more proximal). The major area of concern with regard to the patient with symptoms remains the calf veins. A recent report by Zielensky et al. (4), comparing impedance plethysmography (IPG) and Doppler ultrasound, showed that the IPG detected only 18% of calf vein thrombosis compared with the Doppler finding of 55% of the thrombi. It appears that any patient with suspected venous thrombosis who has either a negative or equivocal test should have a venogram performed.

It is also apparent that if the noninvasive tests are well done and positive, therapy can be given without a contrast study to verify the diagnosis. Nonetheless, the radionuclide venogram with a simultaneous perfusion lung scan does have considerable merit. It not only provides confirmatory evidence of the status of the popliteal and larger proximal veins but also gives a baseline lung scan for future comparison in case this is needed. In fact, any patient who has a perfusion scan requested should have the injection done at the foot level to also permit a scan of the major deep veins.

What of the patient with suspected deep venous thrombosis with entirely negative noninvasive tests? If there is no suggestion of pulmonary embolism, repeat noninvasive studies should be done and the patient simply followed. In this regard, it is beneficial to use Doppler ultrasound in conjunction with the plethysmographic methods since it is much more sensitive for detecting below the knee thrombi. However, it cannot be emphasized too strongly that clinical judgement and the status of the patient must be critically assessed. If the therapy is dependent upon or may be modified by the status of the deep veins, a contrast venogram *must* be ordered. This would appear to be a satisfactory approach to this small subset of patients in whom the therapeutic decision may be critical.

CHAPTER 10

There is little doubt that angiography remains the most important diagnostic study in the evaluation of many diseases which involve the arterial system. However, it must be recognized, as is evident from previous chapters, that with regard to the peripheral arterial system angiography is not necessary as a diagnostic procedure. It is no longer required to utilize this invasive technique to establish the presence of occlusive lesions supplying the lower or upper extremities. The role of angiography in this situation is to delineate the exact sites of involvement, particularly when direct arterial surgery is contemplated.

There is little doubt that the remarkable advances that have been made in this field have, in large part, been due to technological developments which have improved not only the resolution but the ability to take films in rapid sequence and thus identify in greater detail minimal changes which may be missed with single film exposure. Also, as is clearly outlined in this chapter, the techniques which are utilized must be individualized depending upon the region of the circulation to be examined and the information which is required. For example, it is now clear that single plane arteriograms are inadequate for careful evaluation of such areas as the renal arteries, the profunda femoris bifurcation in the upper thigh, and the carotid arteries in the neck. Single plane exposures in these areas will both underestimate and in some instances overestimate the degree of involvement by arterial disease. Also, I don't think it can be emphasized too strongly that the radiologist should, prior to performance of any study, consult with the referring physician to be sure that the information to be sought is agreed upon and that the most appropriate radiologic technique is employed to obtain this information. Without such collaboration, inadequate information is often obtained and can lead to incomplete information being obtained.

There is no doubt that retrograde catheter studies, particularly from the femoral or brachial route, are being employed more widely to evaluate the circulation. However, I think it should be recognized that translumbar aortography is still a very suitable and safe method of evaluating the arterial circulation to the lower extremities. Clearly, however, for any selective studies in which small amounts of contrast material are to be utilized and optimal viewing is to be achieved, this can be done only by selective placement of appropriate catheters. The comments relative to the osmolarity of the contrast media are important. Most patients who undergo arteriography find it an uncomfortable experience and any improvement which can be made to lessen this discomfort will be welcomed.

The point of continued confusion relates to the problem of allergic reactions to contrast material. There is increasing evidence that introduction of the contrast material in the arterial circulation is not associated with the same risks as when administered by the intravenous route. Complications of arteriography remain a concern for all involved. However, there is little doubt that with improvement of the techniques being utilized this is becoming less frequent. Nonetheless, it is extremely important that not only the radiologist but also the attending physician responsible for the patient's care be aware of the potential complications, particularly as related to thrombosis which may require subsequent correction by operation. From a surgical standpoint, it must be recognized that thrombosis which occurs in the presence of pre-existing atherosclerosis is much more difficult to deal with emergently than that which occurs in arteries which are normal. Thus, for patients with arteriosclerosis obliterans, it is extremely important that, prior to angiographic procedure, the status of the peripheral circulation be evaluated by one or more of the noninvasive techniques which have been so adequately covered in this volume.

While there is little doubt that a skilled radiologist may pass a catheter through an area of severe disease, this is potentially the most dangerous of all situations and must be so recognized. This point is emphasized by the author, which I think is laudable.

I would also agree with the primary reviewer that evaluation of the extracranial circulation should not be undertaken unless one is considering revascularization. While there is no doubt that the incidence of complications of this type of angiographic study is small, the results can be disastrous when they occur. I would also agree that the controversy as to priority relative to evaluation and correction of coexisting coronary artery versus extracranial arterial disease remains unsettled. Clearly, in some circumstances, the cardiac surgeons will not proceed with operations on the heart unless coexisting carotid disease is corrected first. This vexing problem and question will have to await the results of prospective studies which are not yet available. There is also no doubt that angiography with regard to any area of the arterial circulation should be performed as closely as possible to the time of contemplated surgery. While unusual, surgeons have experienced situations in which a stenotic lesion has proceeded to complete occlusion when there has been a considerable delay between the initial study and the time of operation.

With regard to the issue of acute arterial occlusion, I think the radiologists should take a dim view of any requests for studies done in patients with marked acute ischemia. This often results in delays which are totally unnecessary and further jeopardize the patient's limb. If the proper clinical evaluation along with noninvasive studies has been carried out, it is really unnecessary to utilize angiography to make the diagnosis of acute ischemia. The patient should be taken directly to the operating theater where exploration can be carried out and, if angiography is necessary, it can be done at the time of operation. This clearly enhances the chance of limb survival, particularly when the ischemia is severe.

With regard to a definition of what constitutes a hemodynamically significant stenosis, it is true that a diameter reduction of 50% or greater is generally considered to fall into that category. However, the measurement of such diameter reduction is at best an approximation because of the irregular nature of the plaque and also the fact that this may vary from one vascular bed to another and the corresponding flow rate which is present. For example, it is now known that a stenosis which reduces the diameter by less than 50% can be made significant in terms of a pressure flow decrease by adding stress, such as exercise or injection of a vasodilating agent.

With regard to the vascular disease which occurs in conjunction with diabetes mellitus, this remains a controversial issue. While there is no doubt that diabetics have more of a widespread disease involving the large and medium sized arteries, the involvement of the small unnamed arteries is not yet settled. While it is a common clinical impression that diabetics have more disease in small arteries and arterioles, this has not yet, in fact, been proved. Thus, the term diabetic angiopathy should properly be used to describe the greater incidence of large and medium sized artery involvement. The term 'microangiopathy' should be reserved to the known changes which occur in the capillaries. Also, it should be mentioned that the medial calcification is much more common in patients with diabetes mellitus although the finding of this on plane films does not imply that it is necessarily associated with the intimal lesions of atherosclerosis.

Finally, he also covers an area which has undergone a resurgence of interest and enthusiasm. That relates to the use of angiographic procedures as therapeutic modalities in a variety of situations. First, there is no question that some arterial vascular (AV) malformations and bleeding can be controlled by selective catheterization and occlusion of the offending arterial supply by a variety of measures. Obviously, this depends entirely upon the anatomic location of the problem and the consequences of introducing a foreign body or material which may produce complications. This is particularly true of AV malformations which involve the central nervous system in which it may not be feasible to carry out the same form of therapeutic maneuvers that are possible when located in the extremities.

The use of arterial dilatation as a therapeutic maneuver has been revitalized throughout the world because of the development of the Gruntzig balloon catheter. While the original prcedure was carried out either by single Teflon or coaxial Teflon catheters, introduction of the balloon method has extended the application of this method to previously untried areas. The author wisely confines his comments to those areas in which there appears to be little disagreement. While this method is also being utilized in the coronary circulation, it is far from being proven as the method of choice even for selected patients and for this reason should be considered experimental. There is little doubt that this method of relieving arterial stenoses or short occlusions can be beneficial in selected patients. No one would disagree with the author's statement that the approach is generally limited to patients in whom reconstructive arterial surgery is either not feasible or the risk is too great. However, it should also be emphasized that the use of these catheters and their success will undoubtedly be related to the careful selection of patients and the experience of the angiographer. There is little question that this technique will probably be overutilized until such time as the results become more clearly defined.

The serious concern that this author has relative to arterial dilatation even in the lower extremity is that those who developed and promoted the method have not, in fact, provided us with long-term objective evidence of its efficacy. This has led to considerable skepticism on the part of many people, and for this reason should be an item of prime concern for those who advocate its use. The results reported by Dr. Zeitler in over 2000 patients are impressive with regard to the mortality rate which to date has been zero, and only 2% required subsequent surgical intervention. This does not, of course, tell the entire story. What is really needed is evidence with regard to the durability of the procedure as it relates to the progression of the disease. Hopefully, with the utilization of some of the noninvasive techniques described in this book, the necessary information will soon become available to the medical community.

Chapter 11

Since I was the external reviewer for this chapter, few other comments are required. Nonetheless, it is important for the reader to understand that the views expressed by Dr. Lassen are the result of considerable experience not only in research studies but in their utility in the clinical situation as well. Dr. Lassen has not only the depth and breadth of experience with these methods but understands the clinical problems as well.

Chapter 12

The assessment of the hemodynamics of the venous system would almost seem superfluous in view of the clinical manifestations in the chronic stage. It is, however, a very important subject which has been given too little attention by many physicians. This attitude probably reflects the view that little useful remains to be learned and that the treatment is already standardized. This could not be further from the truth. In fact, the major problem with regard to chronic venous disease is that it has been ignored too long and it is time the field be reassessed with some of the available methods such as presented in this chapter.

Like many other areas, the use of invasive procedures, while useful, is difficult to repeat because of patient discomfort. While the use of venous pressure would appear to be simple enough, it does have the problems alluded to by the authors. It is very likely that the volumetric studies will provide a very simple method of assessing the status of the superficial and deep venous systems. The physiology involved in these areas is becoming better understood and will hopefully provide us with the type of data needed to guide the therapy in patients with deep venous thrombosis and predict which patients are most likely to go on to develop the symptoms of postthrombotic syndrome.

Chapter 13

There is no doubt concerning the value of venography for the diagnosis of venous thrombosis. The choice of technique would appear to be dependent upon the type of information desired and the experience of the radiologist. There is little doubt that if the soleal veins are to be visualized, a non-weight-bearing technique must be employed since activation of the calf muscle pump would prevent visualization of this important venous segment.

The uncertain areas are to be found in the profunda femoris vein, the iliac veins, the inferior vena cava and lastly the pelvis. Most would agree that the deep femoral vein is observed in only about 50% of the patients studied. With injections at the foot level, the major abdominal veins (iliac and inferior vena cava) are inadequately seen in 10–20% of patients. In this situation and where this segment must be seen, it may be necessary to make direct injections into the femoral vein.

The issue of complications must be raised even though most reports tend to minimize the incidence. The true incidence is really unknown since it would require a repeat study to confirm the presence of thrombi. In patients who have a normal venogram, any symptoms in the calf or thigh must be interpreted at a minimum as 'chemical phlebitis' and treated with heparin. The incidence of this may be as high as 10% but may be reduced by systemic heparinization at the time the study is done. Whether venography aggravates or extends the thrombotic process in patients with venous thrombosis is clearly unknown. This is probably because of the fact that any new symptoms may be interpreted as simple extension of the ongoing process rather than a complication of the procedure.

Cinephlebography is an interesting procedure whose value awaits the test of time. If history in a sense repeats itself, it will probably be impossible to predict the degree of disability or the subsequent clinical course from an angiographic procedure alone. Nonetheless, it certainly deserves further evaluation particulary in comparison with some of the noninvasive procedures outlined in Chapter 12.

CHAPTER 14

In the field of angiology there is probably less known about disorders of the lymphatic system than any other vascular disorder. In its most common form, it appears spontaneously without any evidence as to those factors which precipitated the problem. The treatment of lymphedema is largely supportive in minimization of the amount of swelling and prevention of secondary infections. There is little doubt that lymphedema is easily recognized and separable from other causes of limb swelling. The hallmark of lymphedema is brawny edema that not only involves the leg to varying degrees but there is invariably swelling which also involves the dorsum of the foot and the toes. This is rarely observed with other causes for leg swelling.

Lymphography is clearly the best method of describing in anatomic terms the underlying cause for the edema. Nearly without exception, there is either aplasia or obstruction of the lymphatics which leads to this irreversible process. A key question which must always be raised when patients with lymphedema are seen is to what extent a further diagnostic workup is necessary. Unfortunately, in most circumstances, lymphography cannot be considered in the same category as arteriography and phlebography. It could well be argued that, since the therapy is the same regardless of the underlying etiology, lymphography is really unnecessary. Furthermore, as outlined in this chapter, there are complications of the procedure which may further aggravate the edema. This author, for example, has seen instances where lymphography has led to a lymphangitis which further obstructs the remaining lymphatics and aggravates the pre-existing situation. As I have already indicated, the results of the lymphogram do not in the majority of cases alter the therapy or the long-term prognosis. There is, of course, one important exception to this rule and that is when a suspected neoplasm is the underlying cause of the lymphedema. If the neoplasm is not discovered by other diagnostic procedures, there are occasions in which a lymphogram may be of value.

The technique and method of visualizing the lymphatics are well described in this chapter. Also, the complications are covered thoroughly which must always be kept in mind when this diagnostic test is considered. Since our understanding of the pathophysiology of lymphedema is incomplete, it would be very helpful if lymphography could provide some clues as to the pathophysiology of the problem, but this is rarely the case.

There is little doubt that lymphography will continue to be used since it is a definitive diagnostic test with regard to those situations in which the clinical impression is not clear. However, it is very unlikely that most patients with lymphedema will ever be subjected to this procedure because of the reasons outlined above.

The comments relative to the involvement of the lymphatics in the postphlebitic syndrome are of interest. The exact role of the lymphatics in the pathogenesis of this problem has always been a subject of dispute. A fact which has never been answered with any degree of certainty is whether the described lymphatic abnormalities are primary or secondary. Clearly, from a clinical standpoint, the initial precipitating factor is obstruction of the venous system and not primary involvement of the lymphatics. An important question which needs to be answered is whether or not the abnormal lymphatic outflow is secondary to the extensive changes which occur in the skin and subcutaneous tissue of patients with this common problem. Also, the possibility that the lymphatic involvement is secondary to repeated episodes of infection is still a possibility.

One intriguing fact about lymphedema is that these patients are particularly susceptible to recurrent episodes of streptococcal infection. This is heralded by the sudden onset of chills, fever and cellulitis. Why this should be so common in patients with lymphedema remains a mystery. This intriguing association has led some investigators to postulate that, even in cases of so-called idiopathic lymphedema, the primary etiologic factor is repeated episodes of lymphangitis which may be mild but with time lead to obstruction of the lymphatics.

CHAPTER 15

The entire field of investigating the use of drugs which are developed to improve peripheral circulation has been beset with controversy, conflicting reports and confusion. It is probably correct that drugs should be classified according to their desired endpoint rather than by the all-inclusive terminology of vasodilating agents. There is little doubt that to most physicians the term vasodilation implies improvement in flow to those segments of the circulation deprived of normal arterial input. As pointed out by Dr. Verstraete it is conceivable that drugs with a beneficial effect may well do this by mechanisms other than vasodilation.

The practice of clinical testing of such drugs in the past has in many instances been very deficient, not only in the research protocol itself but in the selection of patients chosen for study. There is, of course, clear evidence that the physiologic effects of occlusion in different segments of the arterial system may, in fact, have differing responses. Early in our experience in the evaluation of lumbar sympathectomy, it became apparent that factors such as body weight and hypertension could improve walking distance and thus give spurious results which might be attributed to the procedure.

It may well be asked in reviewing the recommendations in Chapter 15 whether it is, in fact, possible to make a carefully controlled prospective trial given all the potential variables listed. Hopefully, the answer to the question is yes, but it will obviously be very difficult. Having just recently participated in such a clinical trial, it is clear that the recommendations detailed in this chapter are being followed more rigorously in the United States than they have been in the past. The time is past when a drug is simply given to the investigator who utilizes a protocol which is not only poorly designed but inadequately monitored.

Finally, it is appropriate to add to his list the necessity for close, regular monitoring of the study by not only the pharmaceutical company but ultimately by the agent responsible for licensure. This adds immeasurably to the paper work and effort but it seems to be the only answer to this difficult problem. The investigator not only has a responsibility to the patient in ensuring safety but also to the company which is paying for the study. While good studies may not always produce positive results for any particular drug, they will at least provide assurance to all parties, including the potential consumer, that the best possible evaluation has been done.

REFERENCES TO MAIN TEXT

1. Cooke ED, Pilcher MF: Deep vein thrombosis: preclinical diagnosis by thermography. Brit. J. Surg. 61: 971–978, 1974.
2. Strandness DE, Jr, Sumner DS: Hemodynamics for Surgeons, New York, Grune and Stratton, 1975, Ch. 2.
3. Gallus AS, JAMA 235: 1980, 1976.
4. Zielensky: Abst. 453, II–117, Circ. 58: 4, 1978.

1. The electromagnetic flowmeter

HUMPHREY J. TERRY

Commentary by V.C. Roberts

1. THEORY OF OPERATION

COMMENTARY

One of the most attractive features of the electromagnetic method of measurement of blood flow is the simplicity of the principle on which it works. This is known as the law of electromagnetic induction, which was postulated by Michael Faraday in 1832 (1). This law states that when an electrical conductor is moved across a magnetic field, a voltage is induced in the conductor which is proportional to the rate of movement across the magnetic field. The direction of the induced voltage is perpendicular to the direction of the magnetic field and also to the direction in which the conductor moves.

If the electrical conductor is a flowing liquid, a voltage is induced in a direction at right angles to both the magnetic field and the direction of motion, in exactly the same way. This is illustrated diagrammatically in Fig. 1. Fig. 2 shows a cross section through an electromagnetic blood flow probe which is fitted round a blood vessel. The magnet, M, sets up a magnetic field across the vessel. The flow of blood through the vessel causes a voltage to be induced across the internal diameter of the vessel, ab. Two electrodes, A and B, make contact with the outside of the blood vessel so that the voltage which appears there can be transferred to the electronic circuits in the flowmeter for amplification and processing.

With a constant, uniform magnetic field, the induced voltage is directly proportional to the diameter of the vessel and to the mean velocity of the liquid. If one ignores the effect of the vessel wall, which will be considered later, the induced voltage is also independent of the electrical conductivity and the haematocrit and viscosity of the blood. Provided the velocity profile is symmetrical about the vessel axis, the induced voltage is the same, for a given volume flow rate, whether the blood velocity is uniform across the diameter of the vessel, or is faster in the centre, and slower towards the walls of the vessel.

The voltage or e.m.f. induced by the moving conductor is equal to the vector cross-product of the velocity and the magnetic field. Thus the induced voltage is maximal when the directions are all perpendicular, deviations from the perpendicular merely serving to reduce it.

Fig. 2 appears to indicate an axial accumulation of blood cells. There is conflicting evidence for this in the literature, but as far as flow measurements are concerned such accumulation (if it occurs) is unlikely to have any effect on flowmeter sensitivity.

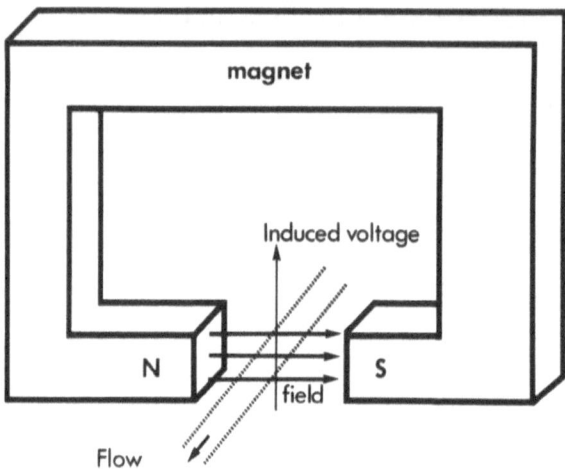

Fig. 1. The principle of the electromagnetic flowmeter.

The electromagnetic method therefore has the possibility of providing an accurate means of measurement of blood flow, without puncture of the vessel wall. The speed of response of the flowmeter enables pulsatile flow, in either direction, to be recorded, as well as the mean flow.

These theoretical advantages of the electromagnetic method encouraged research which led to great improvements in the design of flowmeters. These developments are outlined in the next section. Some of the practical problems and sources of error are considered later, in Section 4.

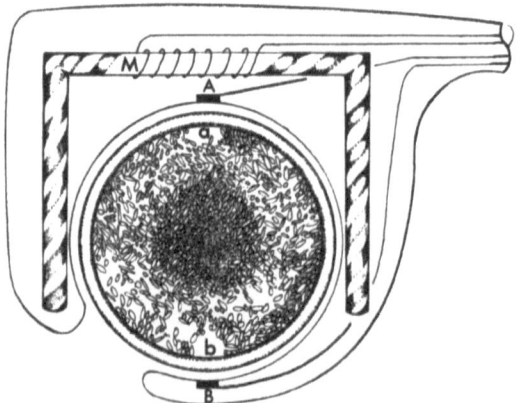

Fig. 2. Cross section through an electromagnetic probe applied to a blood vessel.

2.   DEVELOPMENT OF THE ELECTROMAGNETIC FLOWMETER

Electromagnetic flow measurements on intact arteries were obtained independently in the 1930's by Kolin (2) and Wetterer (3), using fairly similar
equipment which consisted of a permanent magnet to provide the magnetic field across the vessel, and a string galvanometer to measure the
induced voltage. The main drawback to this method was that polarisation
occurred at the electrodes causing an error voltage which was large compared with the flow-induced voltage. This eventually led to the permanent
magnets being replaced by electromagnets powered by alternating current,
so that the direction of the magnetic field, and hence the polarity of the
induced voltage, was reversed at a frequency of 60 Hz or more.

The first alternating current systems used a sinusoidal magnet current
(Fig. 3A). The use of alternating current and an electromagnet overcame
the problem of polarisation at the electrodes, but it introduced a new
difficulty, which was that the transducer acted as a transformer and a
voltage was induced in the electrode circuit by the changing magnetic field.
This problem has been largely overcome, in present-day flowmeters, by the
use of very precise methods for the construction of probes, to minimise the

Transformer, or quadrature
voltages, as they are sometimes
incorrectly called can be as much
as 1000× as big as the flow-
induced voltages and vary with
such things as probe/vessel fit,
electrode cleanliness.

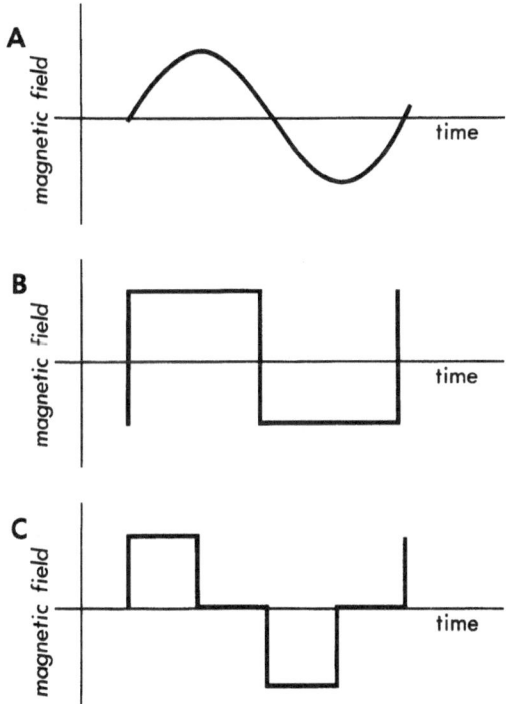

Fig. 3. Flowmeter magnet excitation waveforms: (A) sine-
wave; (B) square-wave; (C) Pulsed-field waveform.

coupling between the magnet and the electrode circuit, and by electronic circuits which cancel out the induced voltage.

Another way in which it was hoped to eliminate the 'transformer effect' was to use a different waveform for the magnetic field instead of a sine-wave. By using a rectangular waveform (Fig. 3B) it was hoped that the error voltage caused by the change in magnetic field would occupy only a very short time, each time the field was reversed, and this could be gated out electronically. Many successful 'square-wave' instruments of this type have been manufactured, although the choice of this waveform does not remove the need for careful design of the transducers and the electronics, in order to avoid errors due to the large voltage 'spikes' which are generated each time the magnetic field is reversed.

Pulsed systems work by subtracting the detected voltages during the magnet-off period (transformer voltages only) from the voltages during the magnet-on period (transformer + flow in-duced voltages). They have a markedly better baseline stability, being effectively zeroed every magnet pulse.

Various other magnet excitation waveforms have been used with the aim of eliminating the effect of the voltage produced by the transformer effect. One, which is known as the 'pulsed field' waveform, is illustrated in Fig. 3C. If the transformer effect were completely eliminated, one could assume that zero output from the flowmeter indicated zero blood flow, without the need for checking by momentary occlusion of the blood vessel. In practice, it is claimed that the zero error in some commerical instru-ments is less than 2% of the full-scale flow; however, this may still be a significant proportion of the mean flow, if one is measuring a highly pulsatile flow, in which the peak flow (and therefore the full-scale flow) is many times greater than the mean flow.

The early history of the electromagnetic blood flowmeter has been reviewed by Jochim (4) and more recent developments are summarised in a paper by Roberts (5). Although the basic principle of operation had been understood for over a hundred years, many of the theoretical aspects were not understood by the early makers and users of flowmeters. Shercliffe (6), in 1962, presented the theory of electromagnetic flowmeters, and Wyatt (7) has investigated many theoretical and practical aspects of the subject.

Many different designs of flowmeter, using sine-wave, square-wave and pulsed-field excitation, have been described in the literature (8–11) and flowmeters of all three types are now in use. The electromagnetic principle has also been applied to the construction of a catheter for the measurement of blood velocity in large vessels (12) and to the measurement of flow using a large external magnet and catheter-mounted or external electrodes (13).

3.   SELECTING A FLOWMETER FOR CLINICAL USE

3.1.   *Choice of probes (transducers)*

The choice of suitable probes is considered first for several reasons:

(a) Many users have problems with probes, whereas the electronic circuits are generally reliable and trouble-free.

(b) A substantial number of probes will be required, making the initial cost of probes greater than the cost of the electronic instrument.

(c) The cost of replacement probes can be a major part of the running costs of the system.

In general, probes can only be used with the instrument for which they have been designed, so the choice of probes is obviously linked with the choice of the electronic instrument.

3.1.1. *Number of probes required.* The number of probes which will be required depends on the range of size of vessels on which measurements are required. For a good fit on a vessel, the probe should have an internal diameter between 75 and 100% of the outside diameter of the vessel. A saphenous vein graft will therefore require probes of 3, 4 and 5 mm diameter. Surgery of the iliofemoral arteries will require probes of 6, 8, 10 and possibly 12 mm diameter. One of the most important decisions to be taken is how the probes are to be sterilised. Some manufacturers say that their probes can be sterilised by autoclaving, although there is no doubt that the high temperature and thermal stresses of autoclaving must shorten the useful life of the probe.

For a heavy clinical routine, probes must be autoclavable, but for extended life ethylene oxide should be used where possible with autoclaving used where methods are generally unsatisfactory unless nonstandard long leads are provided as shown in Fig. 4. Probes should be subjected to at least 10 autoclave cycles and testing for satisfactory working before acceptance.

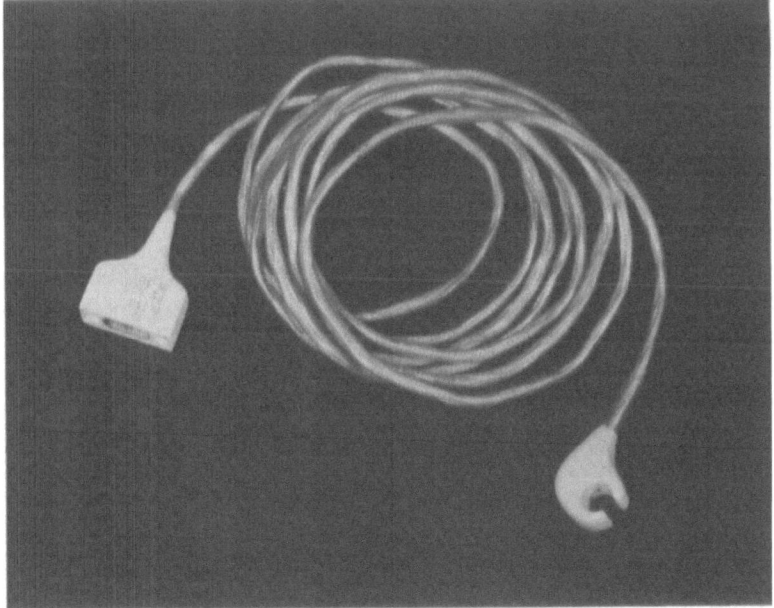

Fig. 4. Cuff-type probe, diameter 10 mm, having a permanently attached cable 1.5 m long, made by A/S Nycotron.

Sterilisation by ethylene oxide is preferable, as it does not harm the probes, but it takes longer than autoclaving, so it may be necessary to purchase several sets of probes in order to be able to make measurements while some probes are being sterilised. Other methods of sterilisation can be used, depending on local conditions, but if liquids are used, it is essential that the probe connector is kept completely clean and dry.

The use of probes with specially widened throats, or clothes-peg type probes is not recommended on diseased arteries unless the probe is calibrated in situ (see also Section 4.1).

3.1.2. *Types of probe*. Several different types of probe are available; the cuff type, which may or may not have a cover to close the gap by which the vessel is inserted into the probe, is illustrated in Fig. 4. If the surgeon requires flow measurements on vessels which are hardened by atheroma, he will need probes with a large gap for insertion of the vessel. Some probes, like that in Fig. 4, are supplied with a cable about 1.5 m long for connection to the electronic circuits; others have only a short cable attached to the probe and a connector which connects it to a longer cable. The surgeon must decide which is more convenient, bearing in mind that the pins of the connector must be kept perfectly dry at all times.

Not all manufacturers can supply catheter-mounted blood velocity probes so the availability of this type of probe should be checked, if it is likely to be required.

3.2. *Choice of the electronic instrument*

There is more agreement on the technical requirements of the electronic circuits than on the type of probes. The amplifier should have a high input impedance (about 1 MΩ or greater), a low noise level, and the ability to reject common-mode voltages (a common-mode rejection ratio at 50 or 60 Hz of at least 100,000:1, i.e., 100 dB). In order to avoid the risk of electric shock to the patient, the electrode circuit should be electrically isolated in accordance with national or international standards.

The importance of other features of the instrument will depend on the circumstances and preferences of the user. There may be a choice between battery or mains-powered systems, and between analogue and digital meters. In some flowmeters, the instrument is automatically set to the appropriate sensitivity when a probe is connected.

A calibration circuit which is connected in place of a probe, and gives a signal representing a fixed flow rate, can be very useful for checking the performance of the instrument and for deciding whether a fault is in the probe or the instrument.

If two or more probes are to be used at the same time, in close proximity, there is the possibility of interference between them unless the electronic circuits are synchronised. One should therefore decide at the outset if more than one channel will be required, and make sure that synchronisation is possible.

What might seem a fundamental difference between flowmeters, the magnet excitation waveform, is of only secondary importance, since flowmeters using at least three different waveforms (sine-wave, square-wave and pulsed-field) are all capable of giving good results.

3.3. *Evaluation*

The selection of a suitable flowmeter cannot be completed without at least one trial of the chosen system under the same conditions in which it is to be used. The following features should be checked: (a) whether the probes need to be immersed in fluid before use, to wet the electrodes, and if so, for · how long; (b) the ease of applying the probe to the vessel; (c) the noise level at the output; (d) whether any other equipment causes excessive interference and (e) the ease of operating the equipment and interpreting the output.

Our experience suggests that all probes benefit from a wetting period (whether recommended or not). This gives decreased noise and better baseline stability.

If possible, the calibration of the probes should be checked as described below in Section 4.4. Alternatively, several probes should be arranged so that each has the same flow through it so that the consistency of the flow measurements can be checked.

4. FACTORS AFFECTING SENSITIVITY

4.1. *Velocity profile*

Shercliffe has shown mathematically that the flowmeter sensitivity (the output for a certain flow rate) is constant whatever the velocity profile, provided the flow is symmetrical about the axis of the vessel (6). This is obviously an important feature in favour of this method of flow measurement, as the flow profile in arteries may vary from being parabolic in shape, with the fastest flow in the centre of the vessel, to being almost flat, with nearly all the blood travelling at about the same velocity (14).

Unfortunately, there are many circumstances when one would not expect axial symmetry of flow, such as in curved vessels or close to a bend, obstruction or irregularity in a vessel. It has been shown theoretically (6) and practically (15) that the flowmeter is very sensitive to the velocity of the fluid close to the electrodes, and errors as large as 50% or more can occur if there is a jet of rapidly-flowing blood which is off the axis of the vessel. If one suspects that the flow is asymmetric it is advisable to repeat the measurement with the probe rotated through, say 90° around the vessel in each direction to see if the flow reading remains the same.

Whenever possible, flow measurements should be made on straight vessels which are free from obstruction, and the probe should not be

The technique of placing a probe proximal to a bifurcation and then occluding each branch to determine the flow in the other by subtraction is widely used and wildly inaccurate. It is likely to lead to far greater errors (caused by changes in the peripheral resistance produced by the crossclamping) than would be expected from any flow asymmetry.

Greater errors are likely with atheroma-lined vessels. In situations of even mild disease changes in flowmeter sensitivity of as much as 50% can be produced.

placed close to branches or bends. For example, to measure internal carotid artery flow, greater accuracy may be obtained by placing a probe on the common carotid artery and closing the external carotid artery, than by placing a probe on the internal carotid artery where it would be close to the bifurcation.

4.2.   *Nature of the vessel wall*

There have been many conflicting reports on the effect of variations in the thickness or the electrical conductivity of the vessel wall. Some of the confusion in the past occurred because it was not understood that the electrical conductivity of the blood must be considered as well as the conductivity of the vessel. Wyatt (16) has shown mathematically that:

(a) if the vessel wall is very thin, its effect on the flowmeter sensitivity is very slight;

(b) if the vessel wall is thick, but its electrical conductivity is the same as the conductivity of the blood, the flowmeter sensitivity is unaffected by variation of the thickness. This is not as surprising as it might at first seem, when one realises that the flowmeter accuracy is unchanged if the velocity profile changes so that there is rapid flow in the centre of the vessel and no flow at the vessel wall;

(c) for a vessel wall the thickness of a normal artery, the flowmeter sensitivity will depend on the ratio between the conductivity of the vessel and the blood.

If one knew the electrical conductivity of the blood and the vessel wall, and the thickness of the latter, a correction factor could be calculated for each reading. Unfortunately, it has been found that the normal procedures of dissecting and handling a vessel during surgery cause its conductivity to increase, possibly by a factor of two or more (17). Its conductivity may become similar to that of blood, which would explain why it was found that placing one length of artery inside another to double the effective wall thickness, did not alter the flowmeter sensitivity (18).

In practice, one can expect the presence of an artery to cause the flowmeter sensitivity to be up to 10% greater than if no vessel were present. Calibration on porous prosthetic arteries indicates that the sensitivity may be increased by up to 16% compared with human veins or canine arteries, because of the lower conductivity of the prosthetic material.

4.3.   *Blood conductivity and haematocrit*

Some flowmeters in the past had a rather low input impedance, and this made their accuracy dependent on the conductivity of the fluid, even when using a cannulating probe, in which there was no vessel wall to affect the sensitivity. With most modern flowmeters variation in fluid conductivity, relative to the conductivity of the wall, alters the sensitivity as described in Section 4.2 above. The conductivity of blood increases as the proportion of plasma in the blood rises and the haematocrit falls, giving a higher flowmeter reading for the same flow. With normal arteries the variation in haematocrit which may occur at operation is likely to give errors of up to 10%.

4.4. Calibration of probes

That accurate calibration is not easy, can be deduced from the extra charge which some manufacturers make for factory calibration of probes.

Many different methods have been tried, using human, animal and synthetic vessels or no vessel at all and various kinds of blood or other fluids. From Sections 4.2 and 4.3 above, it will be seen that a calibration using excised vessels and saline has very little value except for comparing one probe with another, because of the importance of the conductivity of the vessel and the fluid.

One of the best methods of in vitro calibration is to construct a cuff probe with an integral tube so that it can be calibrated during manufacture as if it were a cannulating transducer (19). This removes the need for any kind of vessel inside the probe and makes the calibration virtually independent of the fluid. After calibration, the unwanted tubular extension at each side of the probe is machined away and the gap is cut to form a cuff probe. The same result could be obtained by making a smooth, watertight joint between a cuff probe and a tube of the same internal diameter, but it is not easy to do this and achieve symmetrical streamline flow through the probe.

Any method of in vivo calibrations must ensure that the flow is at a rate which is large enough to make baseline errors negligible, and jets of rapid flow, caused by injecting through an intra-arterial needle, must be avoided. Fig. 5 shows one calibration procedure which has been found to work well when a vein has been inserted as an arterial bypass graft. A small branch of the vein is used to connect a 50 ml syringe via a short, wide-bore tube. The blood flow measurement is integrated as the syringe fills under the arterial pressure. A number of probes can be calibrated in quick succession by repeating the process with probes of different diameter at different positions on the vein graft, or on proximal arteries, any intervening branches being temporarily occluded.

Once a probe has been satisfactorily calibrated, there is no reason why its sensitivity should change, so there is no need to repeat the calibration at regular intervals.

This is only partly true. The sensitivity of the probe is unlikely to change. However, the sensitivity of the probe/vessel combination will change every time the probe is used. Between a normal vein or artery the likely change is of the order of 10%, but if the probe is used on diseased vessels some estimate of the sensitivity change must be made.

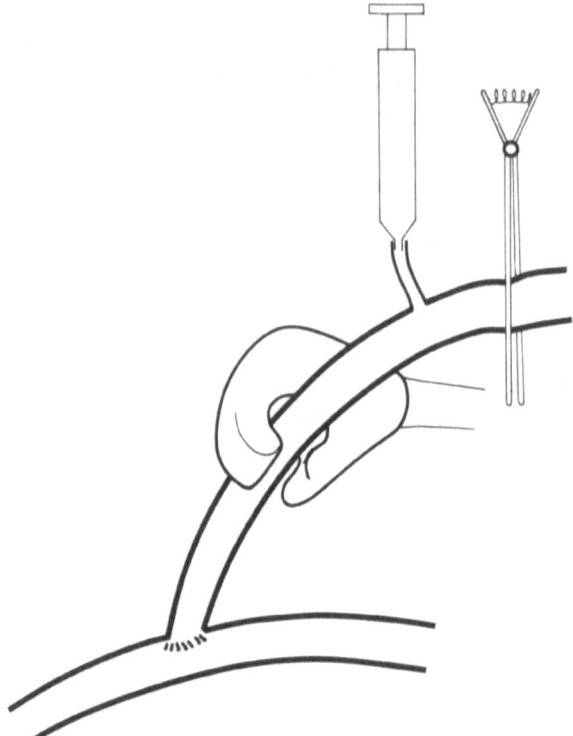

Fig. 5. Calibration of flowmeter at operation. The flowmeter output is integrated while the 50 ml syringe fills with blood.

5. Procedure for clinical measurements

When a measurement is required, a suitable position on a vessel is chosen, preferably on a straight, uniform vessel for the reasons given in Section 4.1 above. The external diameter of the vessel is measured with calipers, and a probe is selected having a diameter up to 25% less than this.

See previous comments on Section 3.3.

Some manufacturers recommend that the probe be immersed in alcohol or saline before use, in order to 'wet' the electrodes. This may not be necessary if the flow signal is large and an increased noise level is acceptable.

As soon as the probe has been fitted to the vessel, the magnet excitation is switched on and the polarity of the flowmeter is changed, if necessary, to take account of the direction of flow through the probe. The flowmeter sensitivity is adjusted to match the calibration factor of the probe, unless this is done automatically.

Occlusion of the vessel should be done as far from the probe as possible ($> 5 \times$ probe diameter) to avoid disturbing the electrical fields. If possible a non-metallic occluder should be used to avoid disturbing the magnetic field. In general, all surgical instruments should be kept well away > 10 cm from the probe, during measurement.

As soon as it is confirmed that the flowmeter is working, the vessel is closed for a few seconds, distal to the probe, so that the zero can be checked and adjusted if necessary. Provided the occlusion is not prolonged, any resulting reactive hyperaemia lasts for only a few seconds.

6. CLINICAL APPLICATIONS

6.1. *Carotid arteries*

The main value of flow measurements during carotid arterial surgery is that the surgeon can check that there is no major obstruction to the internal or external carotid arteries caused, for example, by an unseen embolus. The most convenient means of measurement during operations on the bifurcation of the common carotid artery is to place the probe on the common carotid artery, and to close the internal and external carotid arteries, one at a time, for a few seconds, to determine the flow in each artery.

Some surgeons insert a plastic tube as a shunt to supply blood to the internal carotid artery during the endarterectomy, in order to minimise the time for which the internal carotid artery flow is interrupted. It is not possible to measure flow in the shunt by applying a cuff-type probe to the tube or to an artery in which the tube is inserted, because the plastic does not conduct electricity. If a flow measurement is required with the shunt in position, the surgeon must choose between applying a cuff probe to a part of the artery which does not contain the shunt, or incorporating a cannulating probe in the shunt.

It might be assumed that one could predict the normal blood flow in the internal carotid artery, because of the autoregulation of cerebral blood flow. It has been found, however, that blood flow at operation varies with the arterial pressure (20) and with the concentration of CO_2 in the blood. A typical value at operation is about 250 ml min^{-1} (21).

6.2. *Microsurgery*

Electromagnetic measurement of blood flow in vessels of less than 2 mm diameter is possible, but the measurement becomes less easy, and less reliable, in small vessels, particularly if the flow is low. Intra-operative measurements have been made to determine the flow through microsurgical anastomoses between the superficial temporal artery and an intracranial artery (22). If the main purpose of the measurement is simply to indicate the patency of the anastomosis, it may be more convenient to use a Doppler ultrasonic blood flow detector (23).

6.3. *Cardiac surgery*

One of the earliest clinical applications of the electromagnetic flowmeter was the measurement of aortic regurgitation after aortic valve surgery (24) although little has been published on this subject in recent years. Although the ascending aorta is not an ideal site for flow measurements because of the curvature of the vessel and the proximity of the aortic valve, the flowmeter can give a reliable indication of the presence of reverse flow during diastole.

In recent years there has been some interest in the measurement of flow in aortocoronary grafts and it has been suggested that the flow on completion of a satisfactory graft should exceed 20 ml min^{-1} (25). If there is a serious obstruction to flow, it is likely to be at the distal anastomosis, or in the smaller distal vessels, so it will not be evident from a lack of pressure or pulsation in the graft, and the electromagnetic flowmeter provides a relatively simple and convenient method of checking the adequacy of the reconstruction.

There is, as yet, no convenient way of measuring coronary bypass flow postoperatively. It is possible, however, to apply an extractable probe to the aorta during surgery, and to release and withdraw it subsequently without further surgery (26).

6.4.   Peripheral arterial surgery

There have been numerous reports of flow measurements during reconstructive operations, mainly involving the femoral and popliteal arteries, from 1963 onwards (27, 28). There has been general agreement on the value of flow measurements for indicating the presence of a major obstruction to flow (29) and for demonstrating the immediate effect of procedures such as lumbar sympathectomy (30) blood transfusions (31) or the injection of a drug (21).

Resting volume flow rate offers little indication of likely success or failure. However, flows measured followed the injection of a vasodilator will indicate whether a previously significant stenosis has been removed. Differential pressure measurements across the reconstructed site will be of additional benefit. There is now some evidence that flow velocity rather than volume flow rate may be of greater prognostic value.

There has, however, been considerable debate on the value of flow measurements for predicting the success of an arterial reconstruction. One might expect that a major arterial obstruction, which was sufficient to cause intermittent claudication, would cause a reduction in the resting blood flow. If this were so, a patient with intermittent claudication would have a reduced blood flow at the start of a reconstructive operation, and the success of the operation could be judged from the increase in flow which occurred when the obstruction was removed. That this is not the case, was shown by Gaskell in 1956 using venous occlusion plethysmography to measure limb blood flow before and after arterial surgery (32). He found that blood flow at rest varied widely from patient to patient, and was not reduced in patients who suffered from intermittent claudication.

If one wishes to detect the effect of a stenosis which does not reduce the resting blood flow, but which restricts the flow when a large flow of blood is required, as is the case during vigorous exercise, then the logical move is to reduce the peripheral resistance when measuring the flow. This is most conveniently done by the intra-arterial injection of a vasodilator.

In general, one finds that surgeons who have reduced the peripheral resistance at operation by vasodilators, generous replacement of fluid loss or lumbar sympathectomy, have found that a high flow at operation indicates a greater probability of a successful reconstruction, while other surgeons, who report lower flows at operation, find that there is no correlation between flow and success rate.

6.5. *Other flow measurements*

The measurement of flow in most major arteries of the body has been reported, including arteriovenous fistulae for renal dialysis (33), branches of the coeliac axis during compression of that artery (34), and the measurement of femoral artery flow as an indicator of peripheral perfusion following cardiac surgery (35).

The measurement of flow in veins is not easy because the low pressure and the thin vessel wall make it difficult to achieve a good fit between the lumen of the probe and the surface of the vessel. The influence of intermittently inflated leggings on femoral vein flow has been demonstrated by Roberts and Cotton (36).

7.   INTERPRETATION OF THE ARTERIAL FLOW WAVEFORM

Almost all flowmeters have an upper-frequency limit which is above 20 Hz and they are therefore able to give a faithful indication of the pulsatile blood flow waveform. However, most users have ignored the shape of the flow waveform and have considered only the mean flow, being unaware that an arterial obstruction can cause a significant change in the flow waveform while having a negligible effect on the mean flow.

In 1951, Dornhorst suggested that an arterial obstruction acts as a low-pass filter; that is, it filters out the high-frequency components in the flow waveform, making the rising and falling parts of the waveform less steep (37). This results in a smaller peak for the same mean value, and the waveform is described as 'damped' or 'smoothed'. This process is illustrated in Fig. 6–8.

Fig. 6 shows a normal arterial flow waveform. Fig. 7 shows the arterial flow waveform, distal to an arterial stenosis, in the same patient. For comparison, the waveform in Fig. 8 was obtained by passing the normal flow waveform (Fig. 6) through a simple electronic filter. Although the last two figures are not identical, it is easily seen that both have a diminished rate of rise and fall, and reduced pulsatility when compared with Fig. 6.

A stenosis causes the flow in that part of the artery, and distally, to be

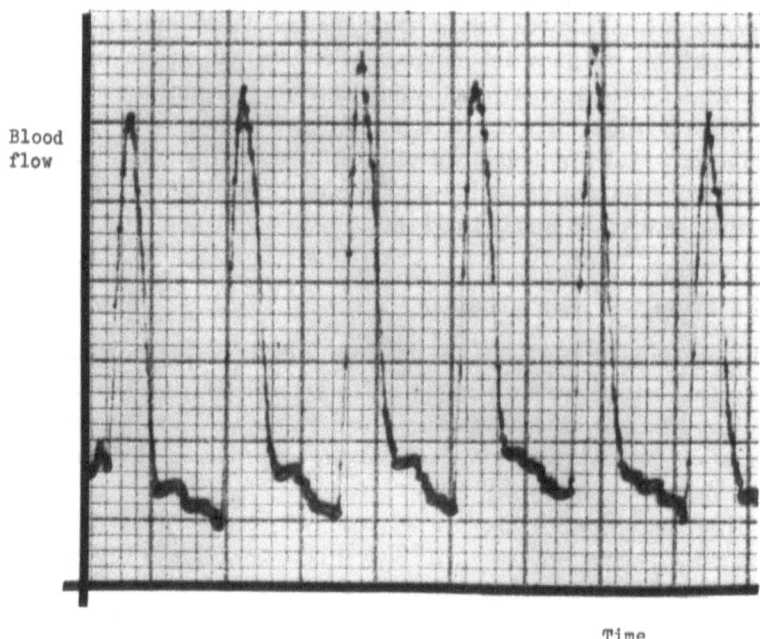

Fig. 6. Normal arterial flow waveform.

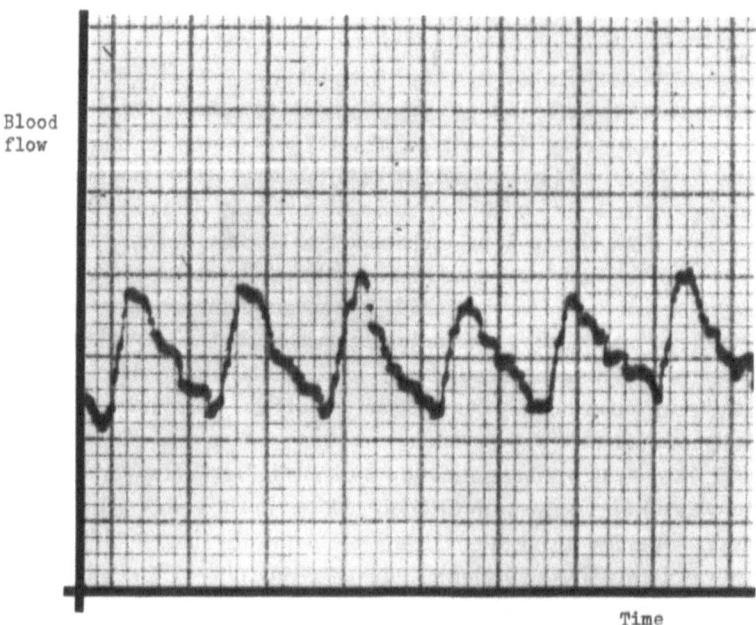

Fig. 7. 'Damped' arterial flow waveform, distal to a stenosis.

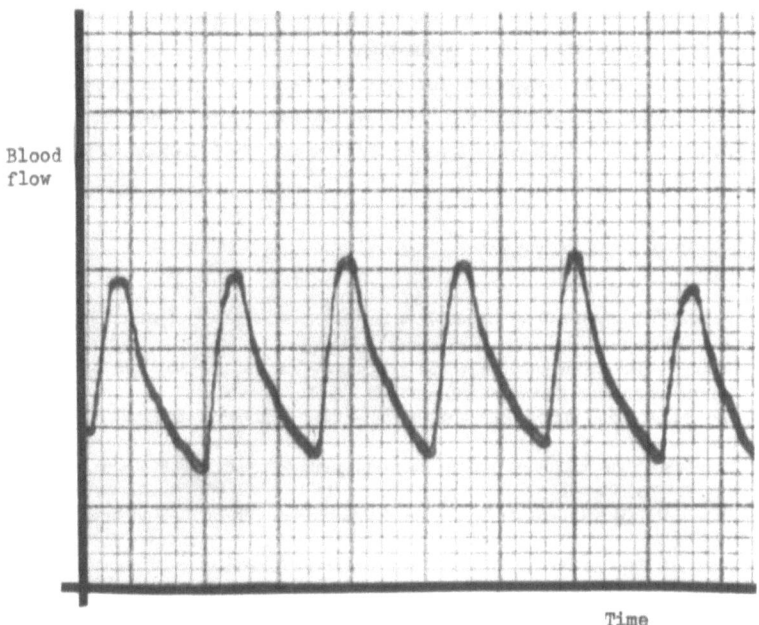

Blood
flow

Time

Fig. 8. 'Damped' waveform obtained by passing waveform in Fig. 6 through a low-pass electronic filter.

'damped' but the effect diminishes as one moves proximally away from the stenosis, so it is advisable to make measurements on the distal, rather than the proximal, side of a reconstruction if that is possible. For example, an unintended constriction at the distal anastomosis of a bypass graft can be detected by making the measurement near the distal end of the graft, whereas it may not be apparent from a measurement at the proximal end.

8.   PROSPECTS FOR FUTURE DEVELOPMENTS

Recent developments in electromagnetic flowmeters have made them easier to use, and continuing research is likely to lead to flowmeters which are less affected by asymmetric flow profiles. It is inevitable that electromagnetic probes will continue to be expensive to produce, and one is unlikely to see a large expansion in the number of flowmeters in use.

The strongest competitor of the electromagnetic flowmeter is the ultrasonic instrument using the Doppler effect. Under appropriate conditions, it can give velocity measurements of comparable accuracy (38), and if the internal diameter of the vessel is known the flow rate can be calculated. The Doppler system has two advantages: there is no uncertainty about the zero level, and simple systems can be relatively cheap.

In future, one can expect to see improved, but expensive, electromagnetic flowmeters being used, mainly for research, by those who are prepared to devote the necessary time and effort to their measurements, while the ultrasonic instruments are likely to become popular for the routine checking of arterial reconstructions and the speedy detection of stenoses or emboli.

REFERENCES TO MAIN TEXT

1. Faraday M: Experimental researches in electricity, 2nd series; 5, Terrestrial magneto-electric induction. Phil Trans. 122: 163–177, 1832.
2. Kolin A: An electromagnetic flowmeter; principle of method and its application to blood flow measurements. Proc. Soc. exp. Biol. (N.Y.) 35: 53, 1936.
3. Wetterer E: A new method of measuring blood flow in unopened vessels. Z. Biol. 98: 26, 1937.
4. Jochim KE: The development of the electromagnetic flowmeter. I.R.E. Trans. biol. med. Eng. 9: 228–235, 1962.
5. Roberts VC: Measurement of flow in intact blood vessels. CRC. Crit. Rev. Bioeng. 1: 419, 1973.
6. Shercliffe JA: The Theory of Electromagnetic Flow Measurement, Cambridge, Cambridge University Press, 1962.
7. Wyatt DG: Electromagnetic blood flow measurements. In: I.E.E. Medical Electronics Monographs 1-6. London, Peter Peregrinus. 1971. p 181.
8. Wyatt DG: Electromagnetic flowmeter for use with intact vessels. J. Physiol. (Lond.) 173: 8P, 1964.
9. Denison AB, Spencer MP, Green HD: A square wave electromagnetic flowmeter for application to intact blood vessels. Circulat. Res. 3: 39, 1955.
10. Hognestad H: Square-wave electromagnetic flowmeter with improved baseline stability. Med. res. Eng. 5: 28, 1966.
11. Westersten AS: Apparatus and process for measuring fluid flow. U.S. Patent 3316762, 1967.
12. Mills CJ: A catheter tip electromagnetic velocity probe. Phys. med. Biol. 11: 323, 1966.
13. Kolin A: A new approach to electromagnetic blood flow determination by means of catheter in an external magnetic field. Proc. nat. Acad. Sci. (Wash.) 65: 521, 1970.
14. McDonald DA: Blood Flow in Arteries, London, Edward Arnold, 1974, p 101.
15. Goldman, SC, Marple NB, Scholnik WL: Effect of flow profile on electromagnetic flowmeter accuracy. J. appl. Physiol. 18: 652, 1963.
16. Wyatt DG: Dependence of electromagnetic flowmeter sensitivity upon encircled media. Phys. med. Biol. 13: 529–534, 1968.
17. Ferguson DJ, Landahl HD: Magnetic meters: Effects of electrical resistance in tissues on flow measurements and an improved calibration for square-wave circuits. Circulat. Res. 19: 917, 1966.
18. Spencer MP, Denison AB: Square-wave electromagnetic flowmeter for surgical and experimental application. Methods med. Res. 8: 321–341, 1960.
19. Clark DM, Wyatt DG: An improved perivascular electromagnetic flowmeter. Med. Bio-Eng. 7: 185, 1969.
20. Tindall GT, Craddock A, Greenfield JC: Effects of the sitting position on blood flow in the internal carotid artery of man during general anaesthesia. J. Neurosurg. 26: 383, 1967.
21. Terry HJ: The electromagnetic measurement of blood flow during arterial surgery. Biomed. Eng. 7: 466, 1972.
22. Chater N: Surgical results and measurements of intraoperative flow in microneurosurgical anastomoses. In: Microneurosurgical Anastomoses for Cerebral Ischaemia, Springfield, Ill., Thomas, 1976, p. 295.

23. Mozersky DJ, Summer DS, Barnes RW, Strandness DE: Intraoperative use of a sterile ultrasonic flow probe. Surg. Gynecol. Obstet 136: 79, 1973.

24. Delin NA, Ekestrom S, Johansson L: Measurement of aortic regurgitation at operation. Acta chir. scand. Suppl. 356B: 44–50, 1966.

25. Kayser KL, Johnson WD: Patency of coronary bypass grafts (letter). J. thor. cardiovasc. Surg. 73: 321, 1977.

26. Williams BT, Sancho-Fornos S, Clarke DB, Abrams LD, Schenk, WG: Continuous measurement of cardiac output after open heart surgery. In: Blood Flow Measurement, London, Sector Publishing, 1972, p 119.

27. Cappelen C, Hall KV: Electromagnetic Blood Flowmetry in Clinical Surgery. Acta. chir. scand. Suppl. 356B: 129–133, 1967.

28. Terry HJ, Taylor GW: Quantitation of flow in femoropopliteal grafts. Surg. Clin. North Amer. 54: 85–94, 1974.

29. Cotton LT, Roberts VC, Cave FD: Value of the electromagnetic blood flowmeter in arterial reconstruction. In: Blood Flow Measurement, London, Sector Publishing, 1972, p 107.

30. Terry HJ, Allan JS, Taylor GW: The effect of adding lumbar sympathectomy to reconstructive arterial surgery in the lower limb. Brit. J. Surg. 57: 51–55, 1970.

31. Cronestrand R: Blood flow after reconstruction of the carotid, subclavian, renal and leg arteries. In: Blood Flow Measurement, London, Sector Publishing, 1972, p 111.

32. Gaskell P: The rate of blood flow in the foot and calf before and after reconstruction by arterial grafting of an occluded main artery to the lower limb. Clin. Sci. 15: 259–269, 1956.

33. Anderson CB, Etheredge EE, Harter HR, Codd JE, Graff RJ, Newton WT: Blood flow measurements in arteriovenous dialysis fistulas. Surgery 81: 459, 1977.

34. Edwards AJ, Hamilton JD, Nichol WD, Taylor GW, Dawson AM: Experience with the coeliac axis compression syndrome. Brit. med. J. 1: 342–345, 1970.

35. Aksnes EG, Cappelen C, Hall KV: Cardiac output and regional (femoral) blood flow in the early postoperative period after heart surgery. Acta. chir. scand. Suppl. 357: 299, 1966.

36. Roberts VC, Cotton LT: Positive pressure circulatory-assist devices for the leg. In: Blood Flow Measurement, London, Sector Publishing, 1972, p 115.

37. Edholm OG, Howarth S, Sharpey-Schafer EP: Resting blood flow and blood pressure in limbs with arterial obstruction. (With a note on pulse pressure changes by A.C. Dornhorst.) Clin. Sci. 10: 361, 1951.

38. Reneman RS, Clarke HF, Simmons N, Spencer MP: *In vivo* comparison of electromagnetic and Doppler flowmeters: with special attention to the processing of the analogue Doppler flow signal. Cardiovasc. Res. 7: 557, 1973.

2. Plethysmography

GERHARDES J. BARENDSEN

Commentary by A. Bollinger

1. INTRODUCTION

The word plethysmograph is derived from the Greek words 'plethynein' (to increase) and 'graphein' (to write). It indicates an instrument which records an increase of a volume. The word is commonly used for instruments which noninvasively measure the blood flow in peripheral vascular beds (primarily in the extremities), starting from volume variations.

With the continuing development of reconstructive vascular surgery the noninvasive measurement of extremity blood flow is becoming increasingly important for the diagnosis and the evaluation of the functional significance of peripheral arterial disease, and the postoperative follow-up.

In Section 2 of this chapter the various types of plethysmographs are described which can be used for the recording of the heart synchronous volume pulses. Pulse pick-ups and oscillographs, although not purely plethysmographic methods, are included because these are also used for the diagnosis of peripheral arterial disease. Attention is paid to the convenience of application in clinical study, the calibration of the plethysmographs and the influence of the measuring methods on the blood flow.

Venous occlusion plethysmography is one of the oldest methods to measure the blood flow in extremities. Section 3 discusses in detail to what extent this method can be used, which conditions must be fulfilled and which kinds of errors should be avoided. In the last section various procedures for blood flow studies in the lower leg are described. Values of the blood flow in normal subjects and in patients with arterial disease are given.

2. PLETHYSMOGRAPHIC METHODS FOR PULSE RECORDING AND BLOOD FLOW MEASUREMENTS

2.1. *Pulse pick-ups*

Palpation of the arteries plays an important role in the clinical examination of patients with arterial disease. In normal subjects the great arteries can be palpated without difficulty on the places where these arteries are close to the skin (1, 2).

To record the arterial pulsations, various kinds of pulse pick-ups are developed; a feeler being placed on the skin above the artery instead of the finger.

Generally the pick-ups for recording the pulsations of the great arteries may be divided into two groups.

(a) The feeler exerts only a slight force on the underlying artery, so the displacements of the arterial wall are monitored. The artery almost maintains the round form. Fig. 1 gives a scheme of this type of pick-up. A relatively long leaf spring with a feeler at the free end is fixed in a holder which is fastened to the skin with a bandage, at some distance from the artery. The bending of the spring is measured with a strain-gauge and measuring bridge (3) or a piezo-electric crystal (4).

(b) The feeler exerts a relatively great force on the arterial wall, so that the artery is partially deformed. The displacement of the feeler is slight, so that it is mainly the varying blood pressure exerting some force on the feeler which is measured. Fig. 2 gives a scheme of this pick-up. The main frame is pressed firmly upon the skin on both sides of the artery, the feeler being connected with a stiff spring mounted on both sides in the frame. The bending of the spring is measured by strain-gauges (5), piezo-electric crystals (6), capacitive or inductive elements (7).

To record the arterial pulsations reliably, the pulse pick-ups should have

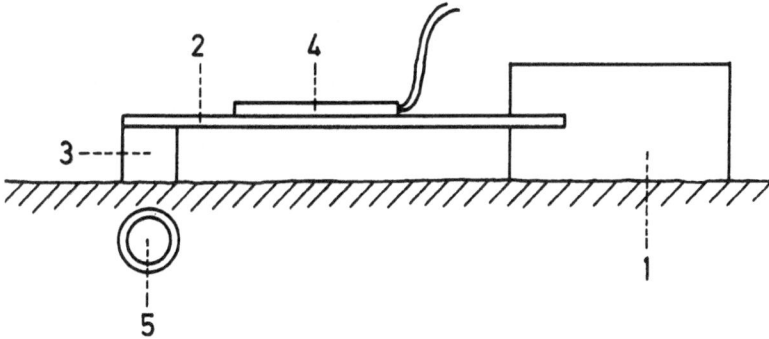

Fig. 1. Scheme of pulse pick-up exerting a slight pressure on the artery. I: holder, 2: leaf spring, 3: feeler, 4: strain gauge, 5: artery.

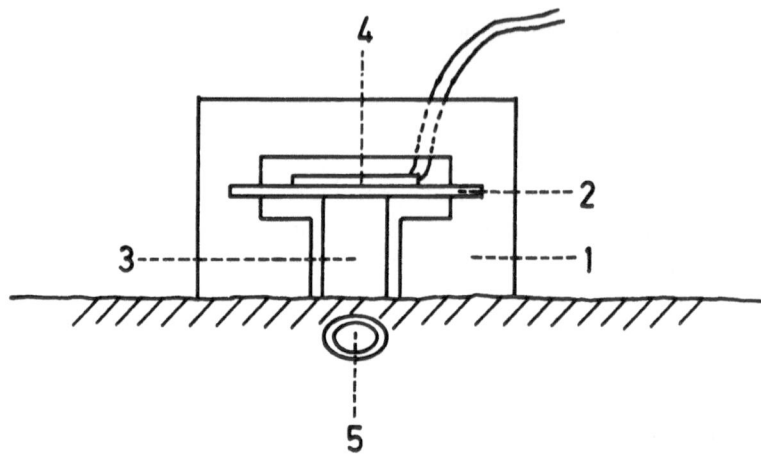

Fig. 2. Scheme of pulse pick-up exerting a great pressure on the artery. 1: main frame, 2: stiff spring, 3: feeler, 4: strain-gauge, 5: artery.

COMMENTARY

Pulse pick-up systems provide useful qualitative information. However, the curves cannot be used as a quantitative measure of blood flow.

a flat frequency response of 0.1 Hz to 20 Hz, which a good construction of the instrument makes feasible.

Pulse pick-ups with a sensitive element in contact with the skin are developed to record the pulsations in the small arteries of the fingers and the toes. Brecht and Boucke (8) used a condenser microphone (infraton) with a flat frequency response from 0.3 to 150 Hz. An improved design was used by Kappert (1), the frequency response being flat from 0.03 to 1200 Hz for what he calls 'acral oscillography'.

However, the interpretation of physiological events recorded with mechanical transducers gives rise to some difficulties. The 'volume pulse' as recorded with the pick-up described under the first group, showed the same shape as the arterial pressure pulse recorded intra-arterially with a needle and pressure transducer (4).

In Fig. 3 recordings are given of the pulsation of the radial artery produced by a pick-up described under the second group, together with a photo-electric plethysmogram of the thumb of the same limb (see also Section 2.3). While the photo-electric plethysmogram is assumed to record volume pulsations, it is obvious that both recordings have the same shape. Because healthy arteries expand almost linearly in the normal physiological pressure range, pressure and volume pulses will have identical shapes, so the question whether volume or pressure pulses are recorded is not relevant in this case. If a diseased artery expands nonlinearly, however, the recorded pulses will be an ill-defined mixture of pressure and volume pulses which are difficult to interpret (9). In addition, the recordings will also reflect the mechanical properties of the tissues surrounding the artery and the skin above the artery.

2.2. Oscillography

Oscillography is a method to record volume pulsations in a segment of an extremity by means of an air-filled cuff. The cuff is applied to the thigh, the calf or the ankle and inflated to various pressures. The volume pulsations in the extremity segment cause volume changes in the cuff. Because the air in the cuff is compressible, the volume changes can be detected as pressure changes, provided that the temperature in the cuff is nearly constant. The pressure pulsations are recorded with mechanical or electrical pressure transducers.

With most commercial oscillographs two cuffs can be applied simultaneously on symmetrical sites upon the extremities of a supine subject. The cuffs are inflated to 33.3 kPa (250 mm Hg) and during 4–5 heart beats the pulsations are recorded. Next the pressure in the cuffs is decreased in steps of 3.33 kPa (25 mm Hg) and after each step the pulsations are recorded. The whole procedure must be performed rapidly because, after reaching the systolic blood pressure, blood is collected in the venous system distal to the cuffs and venous pressure rises.

Maximal oscillations (oscillometric index) are usually obtained at approximately the mean blood pressure of the subject. The absolute values of the oscillations depend on the way in which the cuffs are applied and on the individual systolic and diastolic blood pressures and limb volumes of the subject, so 'normal' values cannot be given (2, 10).

In patients with muscular atrophy of one limb, for example, there may be reduced amplitudes of oscillation on the diseased side without evidence of arterial occlusive disease.

The oscillograph of Gesenius (11) is a mechanical instrument which consists of two cuffs, a balloon pump and a pressure meter to inflate the cuffs to various pressures, two pressure transducers and an ink-writing recorder (Fig. 4). The cuffs are inflated simultaneously, after inflation each cuff is connected with its own pressure transducer. Due to the low sensitivity of the mechanical recording system and the low paper speed of the

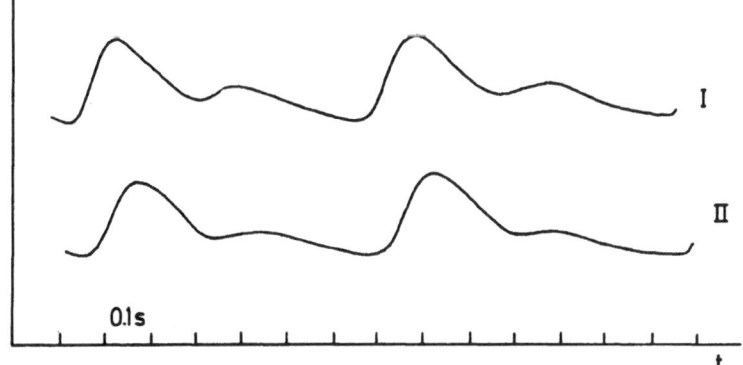

Fig. 3. Records of (I) the pulsations of the radial artery with a pulse pick-up and (II) the photo-electric plethysmogram of the thumb of the same limb.

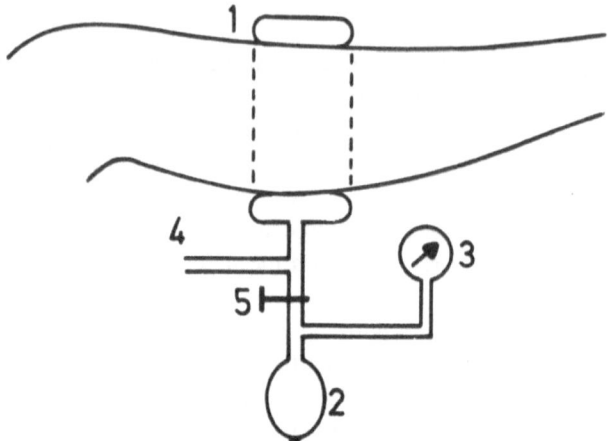

Fig. 4. Principle of the mechanical oscillograph (only 1 cuff is drawn). 1: cuff, 2: balloon, 3: pressure meter, 4: connection to pressure transducer, 5: stop cock.

recorder the shape of the volume pulsations cannot be analyzed, and only the following parameters are considered: (a) the ratio of the maximal amplitudes on the left and right limb; (b) the pressure in the cuffs when the amplitudes are maximal; (c) the ratio of the maximal amplitudes from the upper leg and the lower leg (2).

Fig. 5 gives oscillograms from the calves of a normal subject made with this instrument.

With electrical pressure transducers the pressure pulsations in the cuffs can be accurately recorded with high sensitivity, so that with these instruments the shape of the pulsations can be analyzed when a recorder with a paper speed of 25 or 50 mm/sec is used. Also the pulsations of the fingers and toes can be measured in this way. By introducing a known amount of air in each cuff the amplitudes of the oscillations can be calibrated. Brecht and Boucke (8) described such a system.

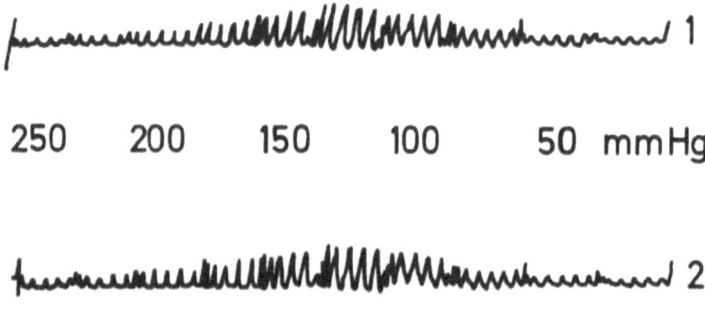

Fig. 5. Oscillograms of the calves of a normal subject made with a mechanical oscillograph. 1: right leg, 2: left leg (from ref (74) with permission).

2.3. · Photo-electric plethysmography

2.3.1. Principle. Photo-electric plethysmography is based on the fact that tissue is more transparent to red and near-infrared light than whole blood. Thus the attenuation of light passing through tissue indicates the blood content of this tissue.

A photo-electric plethysmograph consists of a light source and a photosensor. The electrical signal from the photosensor is amplified and recorded.

Two different methods may be used: (a) The light source and the photosensor are placed opposite each other with the transilluminated tissue between them (Fig. 6). Variations in the amount of blood in the tissue cause variations in the amount of light reaching the sensor: when the blood volume increases a smaller amount of light will reach the sensor, when the blood volume decreases the opposite takes place (12). Because a measurable amount of light has to reach the sensor, the application of transillumination is limited to the fingers, toes, ear-lobes, nose and skin folds.

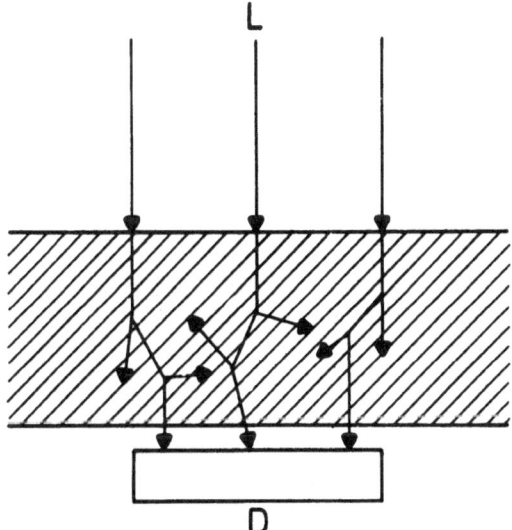

Fig. 6. Transillumination photo-electric plethysmography.
L: incident light, D: detector, hatched area: tissue.

(b) The light source and the sensor are placed on the same side of the tissue (Fig. 7). The sensor monitors the reflected and multiple scattered light. An increase of the amount of blood results in a decrease of the light received by the sensor and vice versa (13–16). The reflection photoplethysmograph can be applied to virtually every part of the body (14, 17).

The physiological events recorded by a photoplethysmograph are the

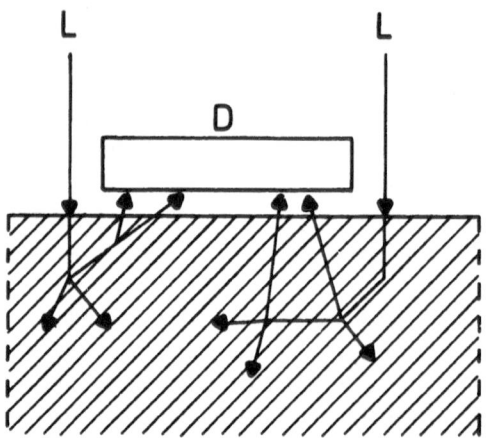

Fig. 7. Reflection photo-electric plethysmography. L: incident light, D: detector, hatched area: tissue.

blood volume pulse caused by the heart action and blood volume variations caused by respiration and vasomotor activity in the vascular bed of
the skin.

2.3.2. *Design of the instrument.*   When choosing a suitable photosensor,
the following criteria must be considered (18).

(a) High sensitivity. Only about 1% of the incident light is transmitted or
backscattered from the tissue, and the volume pulsations cause variations
of only about 1% of that light. The advantage of using red or near-infrared
light is that the amount of transmitted or backscattered light is not significantly influenced by the degree of hemoglobin saturation of the blood.

(b) Adequate frequency response. To display the blood volume pulse
faithfully, a flat frequency response to about 20 Hz is necessary.

(c) Long-term stability for the study of slow events.

(d) Small size in order to be easily attachable to the skin.

In commercially available photo-electric plethysmographs various pho-
tosensors are used: cadmium sulfide photoresistors (14, 15, 19), cadmium
selenide photoresistors (18, 20), silicon solar cells (16, 19) and photo-
transistors (17, 21).

Incandescent lamps (14, 15, 19) and light emitting diodes (LED) are
used as light sources (21, 22). The advantage of using the LED is that
heating of the skin does not occur, which may be a problem with incandescent lamps. To avoid heating of the skin (which may influence the
blood flow at the site of the probe), incandescent lamps are used on a
voltage lower than normal; also fiber optics light guides may be used
(20). In Fig. 3 pulsations of the thumb are compared with the pulsation
recorded by a mechanical pick-up on the radial artery.

If the photosensor is sensitive to the normal lighting of the room, it has to be covered with a dark cloth.

The photoplethysmograph may be attached to the skin with adhesive tape or with bandages. The maximal amplitude of the pulsations is recorded with a contact pressure of 0.7 kPa (5 mm Hg) to 5.3 kPa (40 mm Hg) between the plethysmograph and the skin (14). Within this pressure range the shape and amplitude of the pulsations did not change significantly, while above 5.3 kPa (40 mm Hg) the amplitude of the pulsations decreased.

2.4.   *Volume displacement plethysmographs*

2.4.1. *Water-filled plethysmograph.*   In its simplest form this plethysmograph consists of a rigid water-filled chamber which encloses a limb segment. A funnel is mounted on the top of the chamber and volume changes of the enclosed limb cause corresponding changes in the water level in the funnel (Fig. 8). The displaced quantity of water can be measured with methods described below.

A technical problem concerns the seal of the plethysmograph on the extremity. The seal has to be watertight, but the pressure exerted on the extremity should be as low as possible so that the superficial veins are not compressed and the blood flow in the skin is not affected. Most often thin

The cumbersome sealing of water plethysmographs is the main reason that this accurate instrument is rarely used in clinical medicine.

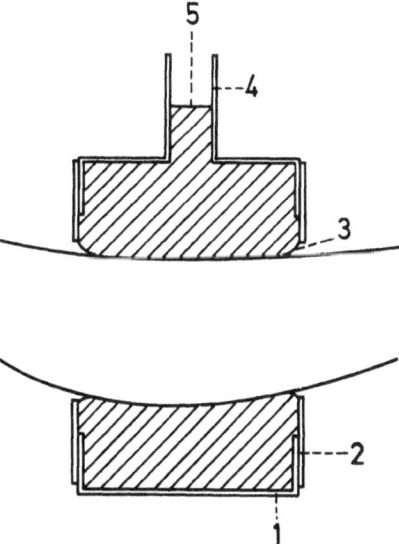

Fig. 8. Scheme of a water-filled plethysmograph.
1: plethysmograph chamber, 2: rigid rings, 3: thin rubber diaphragms, 4: funnel, 5: water level.

rubber diaphragms (23) or thin rubber sleeves which enclose the whole extremity segment in the plethysmograph are used (24, 25).

To avoid an outward bending of the thin rubber when the hydrostatic pressure in the plethysmograph increases due to the increase of limb volume, rigid perspex or metal rings or iris diaphragms which fit the limb accurately are mounted at each end of the plethysmograph (23–26). It is necessary to have a number of these rings available to accommodate the individual limb segments.

Because the temperature of the water surrounding the limb segment has a great influence on the blood flow, in the plethysmograph a system for maintaning a constant water temperature should be included. Double-walled metal plethysmographs have been described by Greenfield (26) and Abrahamson (23), double-walled plexiglass plethysmographs by Wood (24) and Nielsen and Paulev (25). A heating element with a sensitive thermostat and a stirring device are necessary parts of the plethysmograph for maintaining a constant temperature. Various methods can be used to measure the water displacement.

(a) The position of the free water surface in the transparent funnel is projected on a moving film (27).

(b) Optical sensing of the water surface with a lamp and a photodetector (28). The arrangement is such that only the light refracted by the water in the glass funnel reaches the photodetector (Fig. 9).

(c) Conductance measurement. Two vertical metal wires (29) or carbon rods (30) are mounted in the funnel (Fig. 10). The electrical conductance between the two electrodes varies with the level of the water in the funnel and can be measured with a Wheatstone bridge.

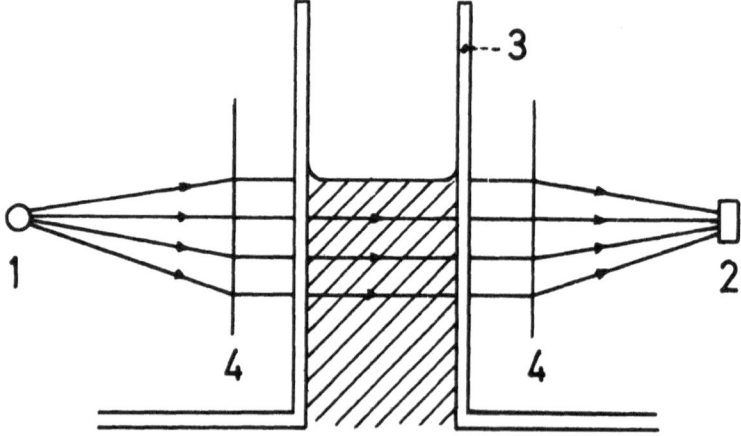

Fig. 9. Optical sensing of the water level in a transparent funnel. 1: light source, 2: photodetector, 3: transparent funnel, 4: lenses.

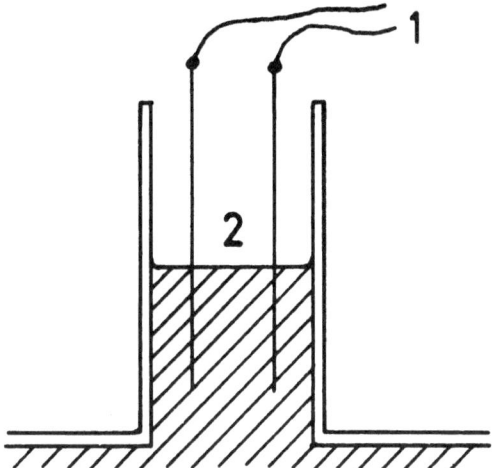

Fig. 10. Sensing of the water level with two metal wires. 1: electrical leads to measuring bridge, 2: metal wires.

(d) Capacitance measurement. A pair of concentric cylindrical electrodes, of which the outer one is grounded and the inner one has an insulating layer, is mounted vertically in the funnel, forming a capacitor The capacity varies with the level of the water in the funnel and the capacity changes can be measured with a high-frequency measuring bridge (31).

(e) Hydrostatic pressure measurement. The hydrostatic pressure at a fixed point in the funnel beneath the water surface changes in accordance with the rising of the water column above that point. These pressure variations can be measured with a dip-tube and an appropriate pressure transducer (Fig. 11) (32).

The adhesion between the water and the funnel or electrodes may be a cause of hysteresis and nonlinearity. These effects can be reduced by adding some wetting agent to the water in the plethysmograph.

With the above methods the pressure on the water surface in the funnel is atmospheric. With the following methods the plethysmograph is closed and the changes in the volume or the pressure of the air above the water surface is measured.

(f) The displacement of the air above the water is measured with a Brodie-bellows (Fig. 12) (23, 24). On the bellows an ink-writing pen is mounted. Thoren (33) used pistons with angled writing pens. These mechanical systems are relatively slow (natural frequency about 2 Hz) so the pulse wave cannot be recorded with fidelity. However, these systems can be used for blood flow recording with venous occlusion (see Section 3).

(g) The displacement of the air above the water can be measured with a pneumotachograph (see air-filled plethysmographs).

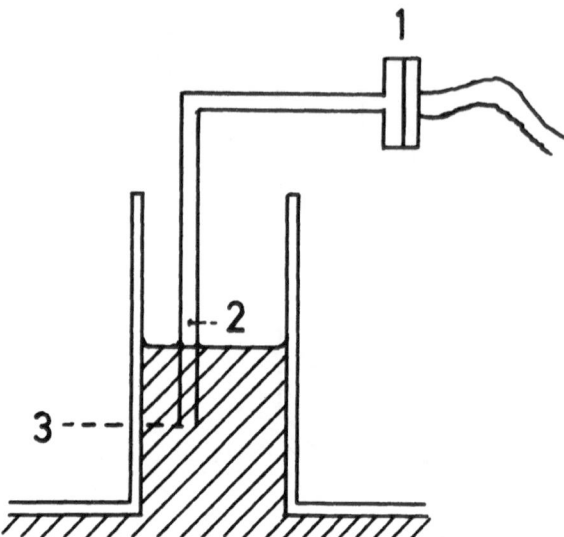

Fig. 11. Measurement of the hydrostatic pressure at the tip of a tube.
1: pressure transducer, 2: tube, 3: level of pressure measurement.

(h) Pressure measurement. Pressure changes of the air above the water
can be measured with sensitive pressure transducers (34–36).

The advantage of using the water-filled plethysmograph is that the
displacement of water is directly related to the volume changes of the
extremity segment; it is, therefore, the most accurate instrument for blood
flow measurement with venous occlusion. Calibration is easy to perform
by the injection of a known volume of water into the plethysmograph with

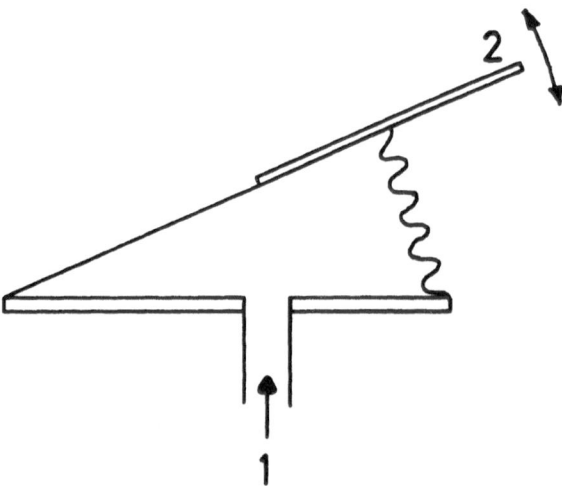

Fig. 12. Scheme of a Brodie bellows. 1: air inlet, 2: writing pen.

a syringe. Serious drawbacks, however, are as follows. (a) The instrument is heavy and cumbersome, and the application on the limb is time-consuming. (b) Any movement of the extremity will cause serious artifacts on the recording. (c) The hydrostatic pressure exerted by the water on the upper part of the limb differs from that on the lower part; this may affect the blood flow in the limb. (d) The temperature of the water influences the blood flow. Barcroft and Edholm (37) investigated this influence in the forearm and they concluded that a temperature of 34 °C was optimal.

As far as the present author knows, water-filled plethysmographs are not commercially available; they are only built in research laboratories, where the greatest possible accuracy is required.

2.4.2. *Air-filled plethysmographs.* With this plethysmograph, the displacement of air is measured instead of the displacement of water. When the same construction is used as in the case of the water-filled plethysmograph, the problems with the seal are greater because a leakage of the seal is not so easily detected. Changes in the temperature of the air within the plethysmograph have a strong influence on the readings.

Dahn et al. (38) described a plethysmograph which consisted of a rigid acrylic cylinder with a sealing diaphragm on both sides. The diaphragms were constructed of thin rigid plastic plates which were layered partly covering each other. Together the plates formed a cone with an adjustable opening. The plates were enclosed in a wrapping sleeve of soft latex foil, airtight and glued to the edge of the cylinder. When the wrapping sleeve was evacuated a rigid sealing diaphragm was formed. The extension of the wrapping was fastened to the limb with adhesive tape. With a pneumotachograph the displacement of the air in and out of the plethysmograph was measured (Fig. 13) (38, 39). As the pneumotachograph measures a pressure drop that depends linearly on the air flow, the pressure signal is integrated electronically with respect to time to provide the volume changes of the limb. The frequency response of their plethysmograph was flat to 25 Hz when the flowmeter system was optimally damped by the adjustment of needles valves on both sides of the transducer. A similar construction was used to measure the limb blood flow in newborn infants (40).

The problems with the seal can be avoided with the cuff-plethysmograph described by Dohn (41). The plethysmograph consists of a rubber cuff (Fig. 14) with a thin inner wall of soft rubber and a stiff rubber outer wall, connected by soft rubber folds. The cuff encloses a 5 cm segment of the extremity and is filled with air to a pressure of 390 Pa (40 mm H_2O) to ensure a tight fit around the extremity.

The pressure changes resulting from the volume changes of the extremity are between 10 and 100 Pa (about 1–10 mm H_2O), so the total

The possibility of water temperature control may be an advantage when the response of blood vessels to local cooling is examined. Exaggerated reaction to local cold is found, for example, in Raynaud's disease.

The air-filled plethysmographs of Dohn and Barbey are relatively easy to handle and useful in clinical medicine.

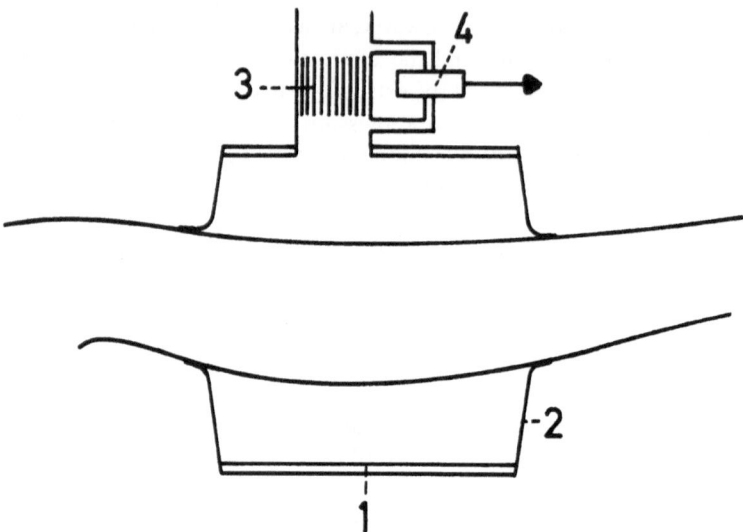

Fig. 13. Scheme of a rigid air-filled plethysmograph. 1: plethysmograph chamber, 2: sealing diaphragms, 3: pneumotachograph, 4: pressure transducer.

pressure exerted by the cuff is lower than 500 Pa (50 mm H_2O).

For measurements on the hand or foot, double-walled gloves or bags can be made (41, 42).

Calibration of this plethysmograph can be performed by injection (or withdrawal) of a known volume of air into or from the cuff.

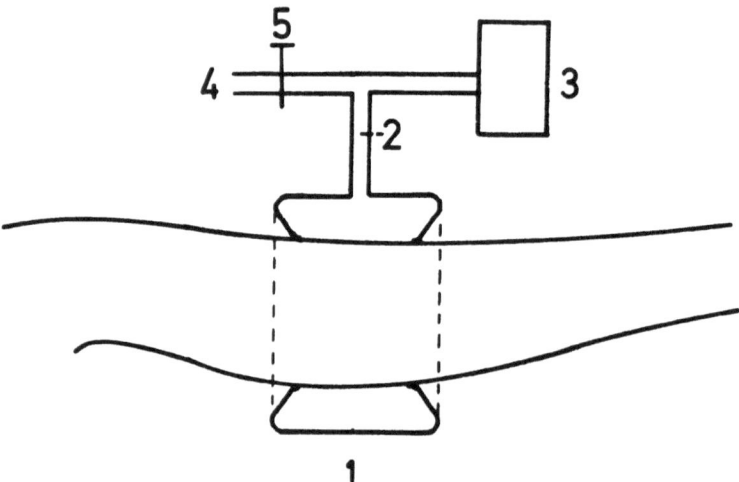

Fig. 14. Scheme of a cuff plethysmograph. 1: cuff, 2: connection to pressure transducer, 3: pressure transducer, 4: connection to air supply system, 5: stop cock.

Due to the small pressure range, there exists a linear relation between the pressure changes measured with a sensitive differential pressure transducer and the volume changes of the air within the cuff.

Instead of the specially constructed Dohn-cuffs, Barbey and Barbey (43) used 5 cm wide blood pressure cuffs which can be wrapped around the limb. Usually these cuffs are inflated to 1.3–2.6 kPa (10–20 mm Hg); the rubber balloon does not surround the limb segment entirely. To reduce the influence of temperature changes the cuff is connected with an air-filled reservoir with copper gauze or brass partitions functioning as a heat sink (36, 43), so that the base line shift and overshoot are reduced as much as possible.

2.4.3. *Capacitance plethysmograph.*   The capacitance plethysmograph, first described by Figar (44), consists of an electrode which surrounds a limb segment (Fig. 15). This electrode forms one plate of a condenser, the skin of the limb forms the other plate. The capacitance of the condenser changes in accordance with the change of the distance between the plates as a result of volume variations of the limb. The capacitance changes can be measured with a high-frequency measuring bridge. As the capacitance changes are only small, it is of essential importance to surround the plethysmograph with an earthed screen.

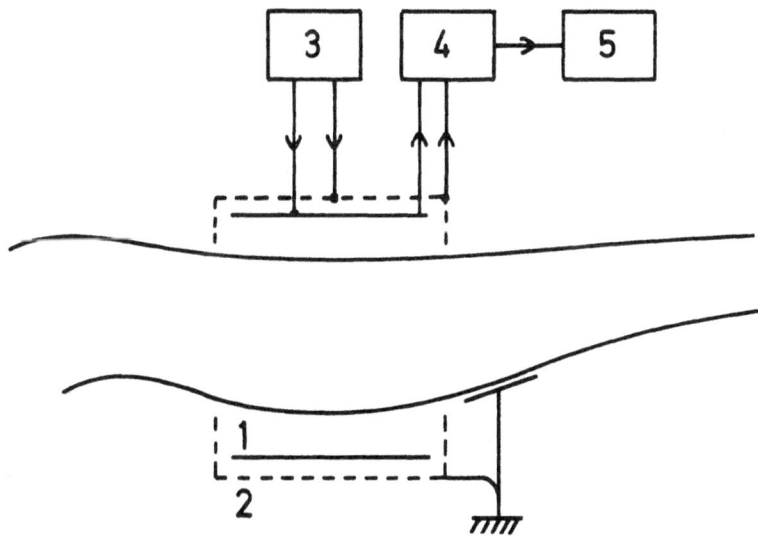

Fig. 15. Scheme of a capacitance plethysmograph. 1: outer electrode, 2: hot shield, 3: generator, 4: amplifier–detector, 5: recorder.

The outer electrode can be constructed as a metal capsule to be placed around the finger (44), as a loosely woven shield of insulated hook-up wire (45) or as a contoured metal cylinder made from molds of the lower arm or leg (46). Wood and Hyman (47) described a cuff that consists of a flexible copper wire cloth screen separated from the arm or the leg at a constant spacing by a layer of polyurethane filter foam; this cuff is wrapped around the arm or the leg. A 'hot shield' separated from the active screen by another layer of foam is maintained at the same potential as the active screen.

Ideally there should be a linear relationship between the change in capacitance ΔC and the relative increase in limb volume, i.e.

$$\frac{\Delta V}{V} = k \cdot \Delta C.$$

with k a calibration factor. A theoretical analysis (48) shows that the method may produce considerable errors, because the spacing between the electrodes is not always uniform (the limb is not cylindrical and the volume increase is not uniform along the length of the limb).

A serious disadvantage of the capacitance plethysmograph is the problem of the calibration, i.e., the determination of the relationship between capacitance change and volume increase. Wood and Hyman (47) used a standard calibration cone to calibrate each cuff, of which the crosssectional area could be increased by a known percentage. Hyman et al. (45) used a flat watertight balloon placed against the skin underneath the screen. With the injection of a known amount of saline into the balloon the 'apparent volume' of the limb increases, which changes the output of the instrument.

The capacitance plethysmograph has several advantages: the limb is not enclosed in an air- or watertight chamber, so the plethysmograph does not exert any pressure on the limb and heat exchange with the environment is made possible.

2.5.   *Strain-gauge plethysmograph*

The strain-gauge plethysmograph was first described by Whitney (49); it consists of a thin silastic tube filled with mercury. At both ends the tube is closed with metal electrodes which guarantee a good electrical contact with the mercury thread. The electrical resistance of the mercury thread can be measured with a Wheatstone bridge.

The silastic tube is stretched around the extremity so that changes in the circumference cause changes in the length of the mercury thread. From the resulting electrical resistance changes the volume variations of the limb segment can be calculated.

The resistance, R, of the mercury thread is given by:

$$R = \rho \frac{l}{a} \tag{1}$$

with ρ = specific electrical resistance of mercury,
            l = length of the mercury thread,
            a = cross-sectional area of the mercury thread.

The mercury enclosed in the silastic tube has a constant volume, v:

$$v = a \cdot l \tag{2}$$

thus $$R = \frac{\rho}{v} \cdot l^2 \tag{3}$$

By differentiation follows:

$$\frac{dR}{R} = 2\frac{dl}{l} \tag{4}$$

When the gauge is stretched around a cylinder with cross-sectional area, A, and circumference, l, then:

$$l = b\sqrt{A} \tag{5}$$

with b = a constant that depends on the form of the cross-section of the cylinder.
Substitution gives:

$$R = \frac{\rho b^2}{v} \cdot A \tag{6}$$

When the cylinder has a volume, V, and length, L, then it follows that:

$$R = \frac{\rho b^2}{v \cdot L} \cdot V \tag{7}$$

If L is a constant and the form of the cross-section does not change during expansion or contraction (so b is a constant), then:

$$\frac{dR}{R} = \frac{dV}{V}. \tag{8}$$

So the relative resistance change is equal to the relative volume change of the cylinder.

Relation (4) may be verified by measuring the relative elongation of the gauge on a measuring bench with a micromanipulator and simultaneously measuring the relative resistance change. In this way a mechanical calibration of the electrical output of the instrument may be performed.

The gauges are constructed of silastic tube with a small bore (between

0.2 and 0.5 mm) and a relatively thick wall (between 0.2 and 0.6 mm) to prevent a flattening of the tube when stretched around a limb segment.

However, in the application of the strain-gauge to the limb several error sources result in deviations from the ideal relation (equation 8); these will be discussed briefly.

The gauges are mounted on the limb with some tension to ascertain a tight fit to the skin and to prevent shifting during movements of the limb. By this tension the skin and underlying tissues are compressed to some degree, so that the measured value of the volume increase with the strain-gauge may differ from the real volume increase without the strain-gauge (49–52). Thus the elastic properties of the gauges, the skin and the underlying tissue play an important role in determining the volume increase from the measured resistance changes. The influence of the tissue elasticity can be reduced by the insertion of small plastic blocks between the gauge and the skin (53). However, this measure to spread the pressure has only minor results (54).

Despite of these possible sources of error, Whitney strain-gauges are of great use in the evaluation of peripheral arterial disease. They offer the possibility to combine measurements of blood flow and systolic blood pressure in digits.

The mounting of the plethysmograph may be another source of error. The simplest type of gauge consists of a single strand which is held in its position on the limb with adhesive tape (55). The connecting leads are also taped to the skin to prevent a pull on the gauge (Fig. 16). The mercury thread encircles the limb completely,.but the tension with which the gauge is stretched around the limb cannot easily be adjusted.

Whitney (49) used a double-strand plethysmograph with a mounting that permitted mechanical calibration with the gauge on the limb (Fig. 17). In this mounting the electrodes are fastened in a terminal block, a semicircular groove in another block accommodates the looped end of the gauge. The distance between the two blocks can be changed by an adjustment screw, enabling mechanical calibration of the electrical output of the gauge by stretching the gauge by a known amount.

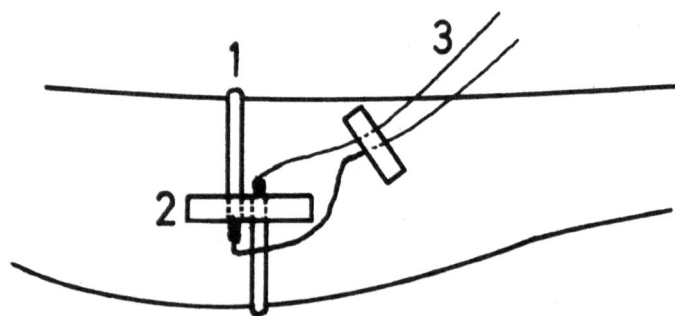

Fig. 16. Mercury-in-rubber strain-gauge plethysmograph. 1: single strand strain-gauge, 2: adhesive tape, 3: electrical leads to measuring bridge.

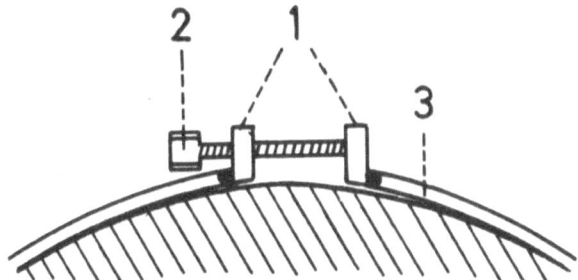

Fig. 17. Mounting of mercury strain-gauge for mechanical calibration on the limb as described by Whitney (49). 1: terminal blocks, 2: adjusting screw, 3: mercury strand.

The mounting described by Brakkee and Vendrik (50) is much simpler but it cannot be used for mechanical calibration (Fig. 18). With their type of mounting the gauge does not encircle the limb entirely, but there is a gap between the ends of the mercury thread, resulting in a systematic error. This type of mounting cannot be used conveniently on fingers and toes.

Mechanical calibration with a Whitney-type mounting is correct even when there is a compression of the tissues by the gauge. However, when the gauge mounting is touched displacements of the gauge resulting in calibration errors can hardly be avoided (50).

Electrical calibration of the gauges is much easier to perform (50, 51, 56, 57). A calibration resistance is switched into one of the ratio arms of the

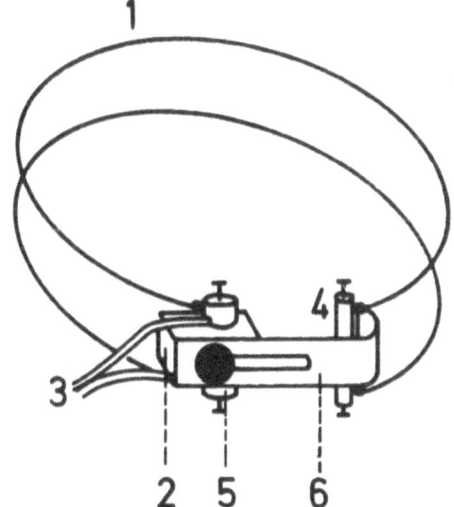

Fig. 18. Mounting of double strand strain gauge as described by Brakkee and Vendrik (50). 1: mercury strands, 2: terminal block, 3: wiring, 4: metal end bar, 5: clamping screw, 6: adjustable slide.

Wheatstone bridge, the strain-gauge and a low-value resistance forming the other arms (Fig. 19). The calibration signal obtained by a temporary increase of the resistance of 1% is the same as that which would be obtained if the resistance of the strain-gauge arm was increased with 1%. However, the resistance of the leads between the gauge and the bridge input is part of the total resistance of the arm with the strain-gauge. The lead resistance should be kept small in comparison with the strain-gauge resistance, or the lead resistance should be eliminated by using a four terminal resistance measuring technique (57).

As the temperature coefficient of resistivity of mercury is relatively high, Whitney included a temperature compensation in the measuring circuit. However, even without this no significant errors occur when the gauge has reached a thermal equilibrium after application to the limb and when the environmental temperature does not change much during the measurement (58).

2.6.   Electrical impedance plethysmography

In impedance plethysmography the volume changes of a limb segment are

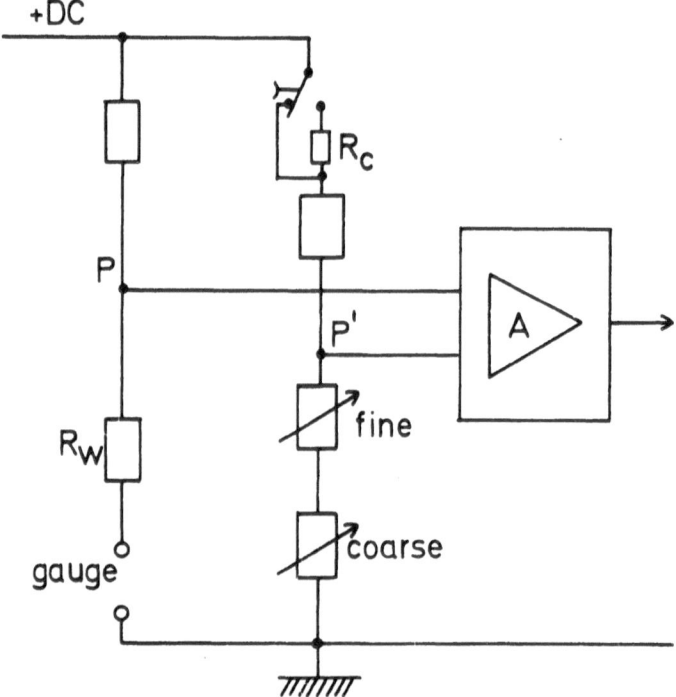

Fig. 19. Scheme of measuring bridge with calibration resistance. R_w: resistance of the leads from the gauge to the bridge. R_e: calibration resistance.

deduced from the changes in the electrical impedance of the segment. The method was first suggested and used by Nijboer (59), and the technique has been widely used in recent years, not only for the examination of the arterial and venous flow in limbs but also for the measurement of cardiac output. The method is also called rheography (60).

Two outer circumferential band electrodes (Fig. 20) are used to supply a constant alternating current to the limb. Because the frequency of the current is usually in the range from 60 kHz to 200 kHz, the current tends to spread homogeneously through the tissue. Two inner circumferential band electrodes are used to measure the voltage across the segment situated between them.

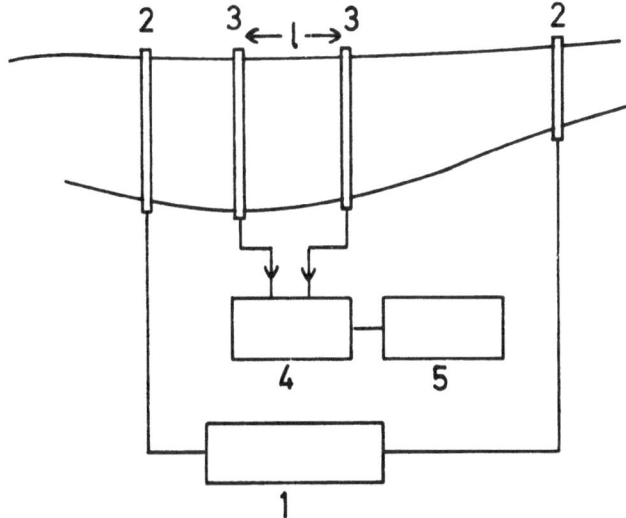

Fig. 20. Scheme of an electrical impedance plethysmograph. 1: constant current source, 2: current electrodes, 3: voltage measuring electrodes, 4: amplifier-detector, 5: recorder.

If the limb segment is considered as a homogeneous conductor, and if changes in the impedance are assumed only to be caused by volume changes, a relationship can be derived between the impedance and the volume.

As the impedance is measured at a fixed frequency, a complex conductivity is not considered and the impedance of a volume conductor can be written as:

$$Z = \rho \cdot \frac{l}{A} \qquad (9)$$

with ρ = specific resistance,
        l = length,
        A = cross-sectional area of the conductor.

The volume, V, of the conductor is:

$$V = l \cdot A \tag{10}$$

thus $$Z = \rho \frac{l^2}{V}. \tag{11}$$

If the length of the conductor is constant, the change in impedance, ΔZ, is proportional to the change in volume, ΔV:

$$\Delta Z = \rho l^2 \left(\frac{l}{V_1} - \frac{l}{V_2} \right) = -\rho l^2 \frac{\Delta V}{V_1 V_2} \tag{12}$$

If the volume changes are small, then $V_1 \simeq V_2 \simeq V$, so:

$$\Delta Z = -\rho l^2 \frac{\Delta V}{V^2} = -Z \cdot \frac{\Delta V}{V} \tag{13}$$

or

$$\frac{\Delta Z}{Z} = -\frac{\Delta V}{V}. \tag{14}$$

With equation (3) this formula can be rewritten:

$$\Delta V = -\frac{\Delta Z}{Z} \cdot V = -\frac{\Delta Z}{Z} \cdot \rho \cdot \frac{l^2}{Z} \tag{15}$$

which is the formula given by Bonjer (61) and Van den Berg and Alberts (62).

If the conductor has a circular cross-section, formula (15) can be written as:

$$\Delta V = \frac{C^2 l}{4\pi l Z} \cdot \Delta Z \tag{16}$$

with C = circumference of the conductor. This formula is used by Kubicek et al. (63).

The changes in impedance, in the frequency range used, are in the order of 0.1 Ω or 0.1% of the basic impedance of the limb segment. Therefore, it is necessary to use a real current source in order to provide a constant current and an amplifier with a very high input impedance for the measurement of the voltage changes.

In 1967 Hill et al. (64) claimed that changes in impedance could not be measured in accordance with volume changes of the limb, but that the impedance changes were only due to electrode artifacts as a result of pressure to the electrodes. The method was defended by Kinnen (65) and Gessert et al. (66), who validated the relation $Z = \rho \cdot l/A$ by measuring the basal impedance of leg segments with varying lengths. They concluded that since Z is a linear function of both l and l/A, the impedance changes cannot be caused by electrode pressure artifacts.

There is an excellent agreement between the pulse records with impedance plethysmography and mechanical air-filled plethysmographs (62), strain-gauge plethysmography (67) and the arterial flow velocity obtained with an ultrasonic Doppler instrument (68). However, there is a considerable amount of evidence that factors other than volume changes contribute to the impedance changes measured: changes in tissue resistivity due to changes in blood distribution in the segment and changes in velocity of the blood in the arteries during the cardiac cycle. Moving blood has a different impedance from static blood because the blood cells are not spherically symmetrical and can align themselves in the direction of the flow (68, 69). Model experiments with whole blood have shown that in rigid tubes there is a rise in conductivity in the longitudinal direction and a decrease in the radial direction; these are flow dependent (70, 71).

In view of the foregoing, it should be contended that the impedance plethysmograph can only be calibrated accurately with reference to some other technique (72).

2.7.   Clinical applications of pulse wave recording

2.7.1. Analysis of the pulse wave form.   A reliable recording of the pulses is a prerequisite for the analysis of the pulse wave forms. Therefore, it is of essential importance that the instruments used (plethysmograph–amplifier–recorder) have a flat frequency response up to about 20 Hz and that the recorded pulse curve has a sufficient amplitude so that its characteristic features can be distinguished. The paper speed of the recorder should be in the order of 25 mm/sec to 50 mm/sec.

In this context the mechanical oscillograph (11) appears to be unsuitable for the analysis of the pulse curves. Water-filled plethysmographs have a frequency response up to about 2Hz and are cumbersome in clinical routine measurements.

Usually the clinical application of pulse wave recording is limited to the fingers and the toes. Most suitable for this purpose are the photo-electric plethysmograph (73, 74), the strain-gauge plethysmograph (75), the infraton pulse pick-up (1) and the impedance plethysmograph (60, 76). In general, these methods give virtually identical results.

Because cold causes vasoconstriction of the peripheral vessels, particularly in the skin, it is essentially important that the hands and feet of the subject are comfortably warm while recordings of the pulse wave are made. Indirect warming of the arms and legs may be brought about by a 'hot box' during ca. 30 min to reach skin temperatures of about 36 °C (74).

Qualitative analysis. The pulse curve of a normal subject has a steep up-

---

If pulse recordings with electrical impedance are used as qualitative examination, there is no objection. Because of factors other than blood volume changes which influence the readings attempts of quantitation seem questionable.

Segmental recordings of pulse curves may be performed by pneumatic cuffs applied to thigh, calf and foot. They help the physician for the approximative localization of arterial occlusive lesions. Pathological curves on all the levels examined, for example, speak in favor of iliac artery obstruction. The comparison with pulse palpation and auscultatory findings yields the best results.

From cold fingers and toes it is often impossible to get any suitable pulse curve. Direct (water bath) and indirect warming are useful to eliminate cold induced vasospasm. If no pulsations are recorded with warm feet, the presence of severe arterial occlusive disease is suggested.

Amplitude ratios, crest and inclination time help to describe the form of the pulse waves, but cannot be used as quantitative indices for blood flow. Most accurate is an experienced eye.

slope, a sharp peak and a concave down-slope with or without a dicrotic wave. In older normal subjects the dicrotic wave is mostly absent.

In patients with arteriosclerotic obstructive disease the up-slope is less steep, the peak is less sharp and the down-slope is straight or convex without a dicrotic wave (74).

In our experience, the form of the down-slope is one of the most important criteria in the diagnosis of arterial obstructive disease.

In Fig. 21, an example is given of the pulse curves of the great toes of a patient with an occlusion of the superficial femoral artery in the left leg. The curves are made simultaneously with photo-electric plethysmographs. The abovementioned features can clearly be distinguished.

Using photo-electric plethysmography on the big toes, Hylkema (74) gives the following criteria: (a) concave down-slope: obliteration very unlikely; (b) straight down-slope; obliteration likely; (c) convex down-slope: obliteration practically certain; (d) no pulsations: obliteration certain.

Quantitative analysis. The following parameters may be used to quantify the shape of the pulse curve (Fig. 22):

(a) The ratio of the amplitudes from the left and right side.

(b) The propagation time: the time between the commencement of the QRS-complex of the e.c.g. (or the R-top) and the beginning of the up-slope of the pulse curve.

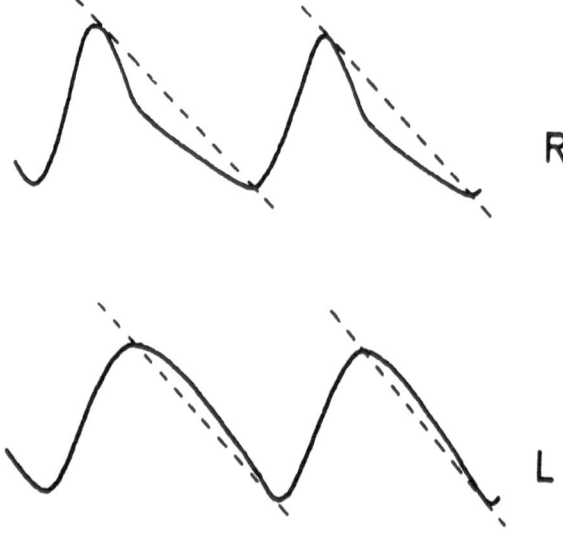

Fig. 21. Photo-electric plethysmograms of the great toes of a patient with an occlusion of the superficial femoral artery of the left leg. R: right leg, L: left leg.

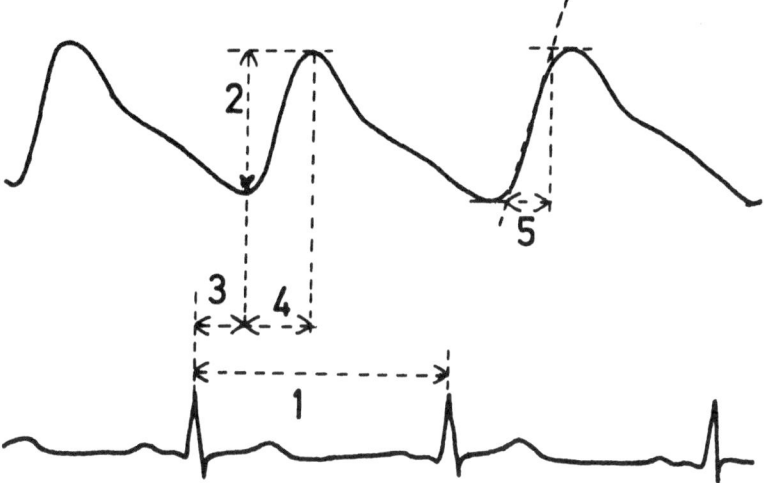

Fig. 22. Photo-electric plethysmogram of the big toe of a normal subject. Lower trace: electrocardiogram. 1: R-R-interval, 2: amplitude, 3: propagation time, 4: crest time, 5: inclination time.

(c) The crest time: the time between the commencement of the up-slope and the top of the curve.

(d) The inclination time: the time between the commencement of the up-stroke and the intersection of the tangent to the up-slope and a horizontal line through the top of the curve (1).

Hylkema (74) gives the following values (times in seconds):

amplitude ratio:	between 0.5 and 2.0	not conclusive,
	<0.5 or >2.0	obliteration likely.
propagation time:	<0.35	not conclusive,
	0.35 – 0.37	obliteration likely,
	>0.37	obliteration practically certain.
crest time:	<0.27	not conclusive,
	0.27 – 0.29	obliteration likely,
	>0.29	obliteration practically certain.

Kappert (1) gives an upper limit of the normal value of the inclination time: 0.2 sec. The upper limits for the other parameters given by Kappert correspond with those given by Hylkema.

Wave form analysis. Strandness (75) used Fourier-analysis to quantify the harmonic content of digit pulses recorded with a strain gauge in normal subjects and in patients with arteriosclerosis obliterans, assuming a regular periodicity of the heart rate. This method, however, is not suitable for clinical routine measurements.

2.7.2. *Pulse reappearance time.* In addition to pulse wave recording on

The propagation time is relatively long in young subjects with elastic arteries and shortened in elder patients with stiff large vessels. In the latter, a delay due to arterial occlusive disease is compensated in part by the increase in pulse wave velocity in the central arteries.

the toes with the subject at rest, a simple test can be performed to evaluate limb blood supply and to determine the functional circulatory reserve capacity in patients with arteriosclerotic disease.

A cuff around the distal thigh is used to occlude the arterial flow to the leg during a fixed period. Then the cuff is suddenly deflated and the reappearance of the pulse waves is recorded continually. The time delay between the deflation of the cuff and the reappearance of the pulse waves indicates the absence or presence of hemodynamically important impediments of the blood stream. Fig. 23 gives representative curves of the measurements in a normal subject and in a patient with an obstruction of the superficial femoral artery.

Hylkema (74) gives the following criteria:

pulse reappearance time   <12 sec: no conclusions can be drawn.
                          12–16 sec: obliteration likely.
                          >16 sec: obliteration practically certain.

Fronek et al. (77) use an arterial occlusion period of 4 min with a cuff around the calf (below knee) and a mercury-in-rubber strain-gauge around the toe. In 22 control subjects the reappearance time (PRT) was less than 1 sec. They also measured the time needed to reach 50% of the

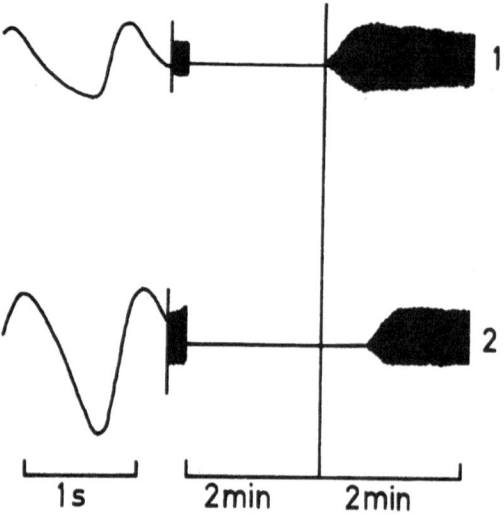

Fig. 23. Photo-electric plethysmogram of the big toe of a normal subject (1) and a patient with an obstruction of the superficial femoral artery (2) before, during and after 2 min arterial occlusion. Left part: enlarged plethysmogram at rest (paper speed 25 mm/sec). Middle part: 2 min arterial occlusion (paper speed 15 mm/min). Right part: reappearance of the pulsations (paper speed 15 mm/min). (From ref. (74).)

preocclusion amplitude, (PRT/2), which was 3.4 ± 0.8 sec in the control group. A significant delay of the PRT and especially of the PRT/2 was found in 60 patients with angiographically documented ischemic disease of the lower extremities, ranging from 10 to more than 120 sec.

2.7.3. *Other applications of pulse recording: Pulse wave velocity measurements.* Mechanical pulse pick-up and photoplethysmographs are used to measure the velocity of the pulse wave between various points of the arterial tree (3, 4, 6, 9). From these measurements data on vessel wall properties as a function of age, sex and blood pressure have been obtained.

Pulse curve of the fingers in patients with Raynaud's Phenomenon. Pulse recording of the fingers of patients with Raynaud's Phenomenon in a water bath of various temperatures is used to assess the severity of the disease (78). The measurements may be performed with photoplethysmographs or strain-gauge plethysmographs.

Supraorbital plethysmography. To record the flow dynamics in the frontal and supraorbital arteries a photo-electric plethysmograph may be used as a routine screening and a follow-up procedure in symptomatic patients with cerebrovascular ischemia (21).

Cardiac output measurements. Impedance plethysmography is widely used to measure changes in cardiac output noninvasively (63, 79, 80, 81).

Blood pressure measurements in the limbs. Photo-electric plethysmography and strain-gauge plethysmographs are used to measure the systolic pressure in the limbs (see Chapter 6).

In patients with vasospastic Raynaud's disease the descending limb of the pulse contour is often intersected by small waves.

3. VENOUS OCCLUSION PLETHYSMOGRAPHY

3.1. *Principle of the method*

Venous occlusion plethysmography was first described by Brodie and Russel (82). The method is based on the principle that a cuff around an extremity can be inflated to such a pressure that the draining veins are completely occluded while the inflow of blood through the arterial system is not impeded. The venous drainage of blood from the distal part of the extremity is thus prevented. The increase of the volume of the extremity during venous occlusion is determined with a plethysmograph; from this increase, as a function of time, the blood flow can be calculated.

The occlusion cuff is mostly applied to the upper arm or the thigh as close as possible to the elbow or the knee (Fig. 24). To determine the flow in the hand or foot, the cuff is applied to the wrist or the ankle. Specially constructed small cuffs are applied to the base of the digits to measure digital blood flow.

At first sight venous occlusion plethysmography seems to be an easy method to perform. A lot of meaningful details, however, are important. They require skill and experience.

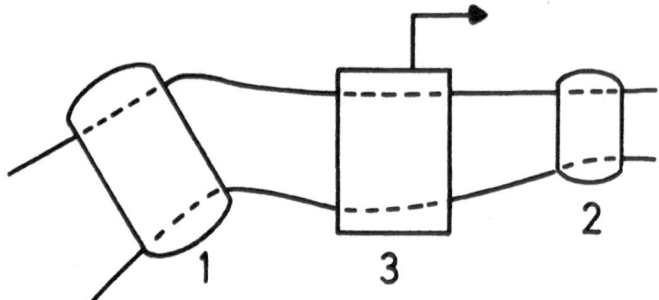

Fig. 24. Venous occlusion plethysmography. 1: cuff around the thigh, 2: cuff around the ankle, 3: plethysmograph.

The above-described principle implies that several conditions must be fulfilled to obtain reliable quantitative flow measurements. These conditions are discussed below.

3.2. Cuff pressure for venous occlusion

The first condition is that the veins are entirely occluded during the time that the cuff is inflated. However, the pressure exerted on the deep veins does not equal the pressure in the cuff because there exists a pressure gradient in the tissue beneath the cuff.

Landowne and Katz (83) measured the tissue pressure within the calf muscles at various depths beneath a 9 cm wide cuff. They concluded that a cuff pressure of 6.65 kPa (50 mm Hg) would be sufficient to occlude the veins in the calf.

Ludbrook and Collins (84) measured the pressure gradients in forearm subcutaneous tissue and muscle beneath and at the edges of a pressurized plethysmograph. The subcutaneous pressure was virtually constant at 1 cm from the edge, the intramuscular pressure at 4 cm from the edge (Fig. 25). From these measurements the conclusion can be drawn that the occluding cuff should have at least a width of 8 cm.

Bethge et al. (85) compared the measured flow values with occluding cuffs of 5 cm width pressurized to 10.6 kPa (80 mm Hg) and 12 cm width pressurized to 6.6 kPa (50 mm Hg). They concluded that for each individual an optimal cuff pressure should be selected in relation to the extremity circumference and blood pressure.

The present author uses a cuff around the thigh with a width of 12 cm. Blood flow measurements in the calf of subjects at rest with cuff pressures between 1.33 kPa and 13.3 kPa (10 mm Hg and 100 mm Hg) have indicated that a cuff pressure of 6.6 kPa (50 mm Hg) is sufficient to occlude the veins in the thigh of normal subjects at rest (54), if one assumes that the pressure in the venous system distal to the cuff does not increase significantly.

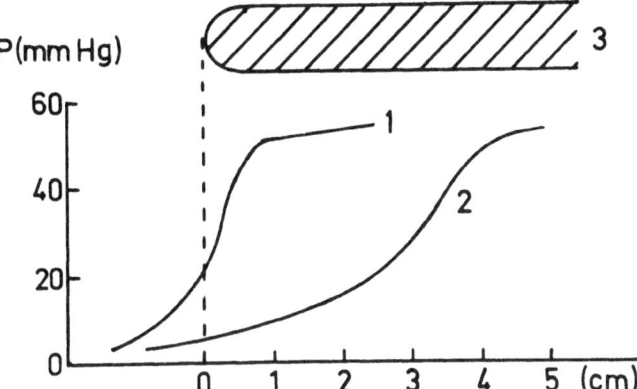

Fig. 25. Pressure at the edge of a cuff inflated to 8.0 kPa (60 mm Hg). 1: subcutaneous pressure, 2: intramuscular pressure. (From ref. (54).)

The second condition is that the arterial inflow to the limb segment distal to the cuff is not impeded. There is general agreement that in a normal subject at rest a pressure in the occluding cuff between 5.3 kPa (40 mm Hg) and 9.3 kPa (70 mm Hg) does not impede the arterial inflow (23, 86).

However, various authors have shown (87, 88, 89) that the blood pressure in the supplying arteries in previously occluded tissues is decreased immediately following a period of 5 min arterial occlusion, and that an occluding pressure of 9.2 kPa can impede the arterial supply so that the flow readings become too low. Therefore the occluding pressure should be chosen to be as low as possible. This also applies to patients with arterial obstructive disease in whom, for instance, distally from an obstruction, the arterial pressure may be low.

3.3. Position of the extremity

The third condition is that during venous occlusion the venous pressure distal to the cuff does not increase too much. It has been shown that the apparent rate of inflow is scarcely affected with venous engorgement up to 2% (90), but a considerable increase in venous pressure influences the blood flow by decreasing the perfusion pressure. Moreover, the complete occlusion of the veins beneath the cuff may be hampered.

To fulfill this condition the venous system must be as empty as possible at the start of the venous occlusion, so the venous vessels must have collapsed. The pressure/volume relation of a vein segment may illustrate this (Fig. 26). With negative transmural pressure the vein segment is collapsed and the volume is very small. The volume can increase without a significant increase in pressure until the cross-section of the vein segment

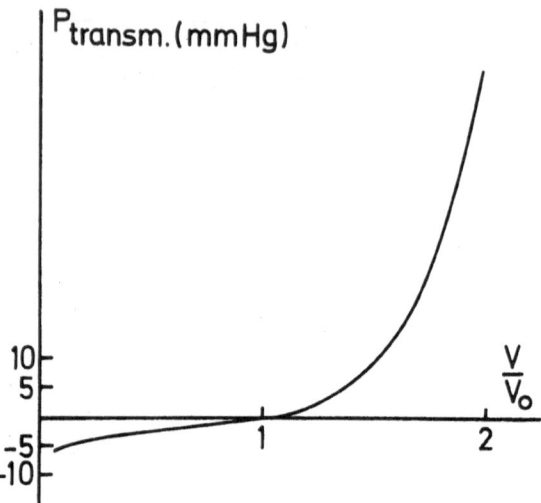

Fig. 26. Pressure–volume relation of a vein segment. V_0: volume of the vein segment when the cross-section is circular at zero transmural pressure.

is circular. If the volume increases to a greater extent the transmural pressure increases very rapidly.

Thus the measuring site must lie above heart level (5–15 cm) and the extremity segment under investigation must have a small angle (about 15°) with the horizontal plane (Fig. 27). This position also facilitates the rapid emptying of the venous system at the end of the occlusion. The muscles of the extremity should be thoroughly relaxed, so that the venous volume capacity is not reduced by the contraction of the muscles. These measures are especially important at a high arterial inflow, as after exercise of arterial occlusion (reactive hyperemia).

With high flow rates the linear volume increase after venous occlusion may last for one pulsation only. The accuracy of measurements in this situation is decreased. It is difficult to draw a correct line to characterize the maximal ascending slope. This problem becomes particularly evident in fingers with their low venous capacity.

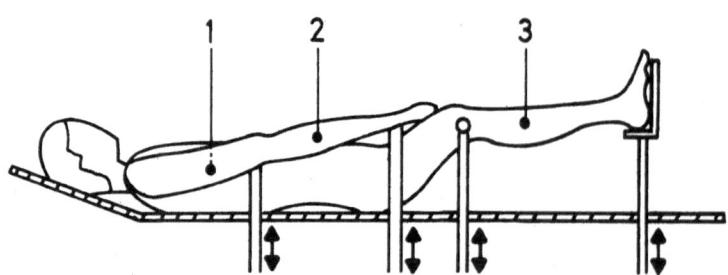

Fig. 27. Scheme of the supports of extremities. 1: heart level, 2: measuring site on forearm, 3: measuring site on calf.

3.4. *Duration of venous occlusion*

The duration of each venous occlusion is directly related to the amount of blood that can be collected in the venous system without a significant increase in pressure and to the rate of blood flow to the limb segment under investigation.

In normal subjects, the mean venous volume capacity of the calf at 0 kPa (0 mm Hg), i.e., the difference between the venous volume at this pressure and the volume in the collapsed state, is about 1.2 ml/100 ml tissue and at 1.6 kPa (12 mm Hg) about 2.0 ml/100 ml tissue (91).

In normal subjects and in patients with arterial obstructive disease, the blood flow at rest varies between 0.5 and 5 ml/100 ml.min, so starting with collapsed veins the duration of venous occlusion at the thigh can be at least 20 sec. However, when the blood flow is 30 ml/100 ml.min, for instance during reactive hyperemia, the occlusion can last only 4 sec without the venous pressure increasing to more than 1.6 kPa (12 mm Hg).

As an illustration in Fig. 28, two records are given of the volume increases of the calf in a normal subject, measured with a strain-gauge plethysmograph during venous occlusion with a cuff pressure of 6.6 kPa (50 mm Hg). Record 1 was made with the subject at rest; record 2 was made during reactive hyperemia. In the initial part of both curves the volume change is linear and the flow can be calculated from the slope of these parts. When the distal venous pressure increases the flow is gradually reduced and the curve deviates from the straight line. After some time the distal venous pressure reaches the occluding pressure and draining starts, until the inflow becomes equal to the outflow and the curve becomes a nearly horizontal line.

With high flow rates the linear volume increase after venous occlusion may last for one pulsation only. The accuracy of measurements in this situation is decreased. It is difficult to draw a correct line to characterize the maximal ascending slope. This problem becomes particularly evident in fingers with their low venous capacity.

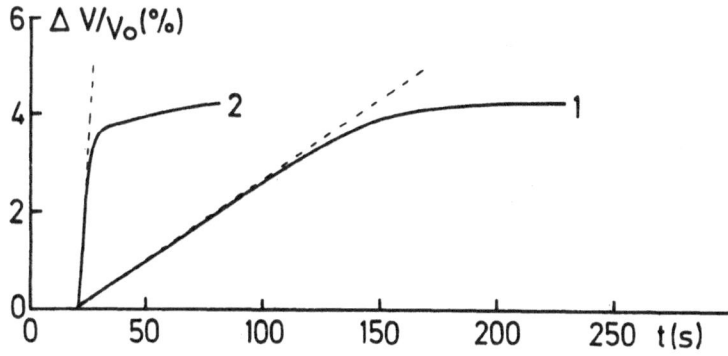

Fig. 28. Records of the volume increase of the calf during venous occlusion. 1: when the flow is low (at rest), 2: when the flow is high (during reactive hyperemia).

In patients with arterial occlusive disease it is always preferable to use distal venous occlusion.

3.5. The use of a distal cuff

To determine the flow in a segment of the forearm or the calf a second cuff is sometimes used distal to the plethysmograph (Fig. 24). By this cuff the flow towards and from the hand or foot is prevented to contribute to the volume increase of the arm or calf respectively.

The distal cuff can be used in two ways: (a) for arterial occlusion and (b) for venous occlusion.

In (a) the distal cuff is inflated to suprasystolic level to prevent arterial inflow and venous outflow from the hand or foot. The disadvantage of this method is that the arterial occlusion necessarily changes the hemo-dynamics of that part of the extremity which is proximal to the cuff. After about 1 min the situation has become stabilized, but the systolic pressure has been increased 5–10%, the diastolic pressure about 2–3% by reflec-tions at the occlusion site (92). During the first 1–2 min after the applica-tion of distal arterial occlusion the flow in the forearm or calf increases. Obviously the distal arterial occlusion must be interrupted after about 10 min (dependent on the pain felt by the patient) so this method cannot be used for prolonged experiments.

In (b) the distal cuff is inflated to the same pressure as that for venous occlusion so that only the venous return from the hand or foot is pre-vented. With this method the disadvantage of hemodynamic changes is removed. The venous occlusion cannot be of the same duration as the arterial occlusion, for the increasing venous pressure in the hand or foot causes leakage underneath the cuff. However, when the distal cuff is inflated synchronously with the proximal cuff, the measurements can be repeated as often as necessary.

The results of various authors (54, 92, 93) show that a distal cuff must be used for reliable measurements of segmental blood flow in subjects at rest. However, when the flow is measured during reactive hyperemia or exercise hyperemia (see Section 4), the contribution of the hand or foot flow is negligibly small and the use of a distal cuff is not necessary (93).

3.6. Calculation of the volume flow values

As has been stated briefly in Section 3.1, the flow to a segment of an extremity can be calculated from the curves recorded during venous oc-clusion. For this purpose a line is drawn through the lowest points of a number of successive volume pulsations. In the ideal case, this is a straight line.

The mean flow, q, during a time, Δt, is defined by:

$$q = \frac{\Delta V}{\Delta t_m} \tag{17}$$

with ΔV = volume increase of the extremity,

          Δt_m = measuring time, see Fig. 30.

Now ΔV = y/z

with y = deflection of the recorder pen during the measuring time,

and z = calibration pulse (deflection per unit volume change).

Thus:

$$q = \frac{y/z}{\Delta t_m}.$$ (18)

Usually the flow is given in ml/100 ml tissue.min. With the strain-gauge plethysmograph relative volume changes are recorded (ml/100 ml tissue). With other types of plethysmographs, the volume increase and the calibration pulse are recorded in ml, so the volume of the segment under study must be measured and the value of y/z has to be divided by this volume (in units of 100 ml tissue). When Δt_m is measured in seconds, the value of q must be multiplied by 60 to obtain the flow in ml/100 ml.min.

Occasionally the inflation of the cuff produces an abrupt rise (jump) in the record (Fig. 29). This artefact is caused by movements of the extremity or by squeezing of blood from beneath the cuff in the segment of the extremity in the plethysmograph. These artefacts can almost always be prevented by rearranging the cuff or the position of the extremity.

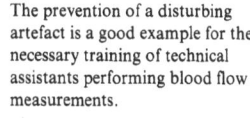

The prevention of a disturbing artefact is a good example for the necessary training of technical assistants performing blood flow measurements.

An accurate determination of the slope of the line through the lowest points of the pulsations requires a rather high paper speed of the recorder (between 2.5 and 5 mm/sec). Though special ruler systems have been described to simplify and to speed up the calculations (46, 94) the procedure is time-consuming. Therefore, automation of the procedure is very attractive in cases of prolonged experiments.

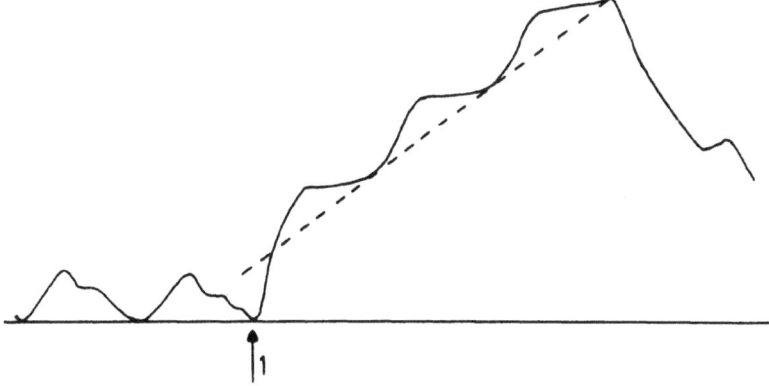

Fig. 29. Record of volume pulsations before and during venous occlusion. Cuff inflation (1) produces a 'jump' in the record.

3.7. *Automation of the measurements*

Inflation and deflation of the occluding cuff should be very rapid. If commercially available blood pressure cuffs are used, the resistance to the airflow can be diminished by replacing the tubes by plastic or metal connections with an inner diameter of about 8 mm. With two short rubber tubes the cuff is connected with a wide-bore tube (about 3 cm). The cuff is connected with the air reservoir by means of wide-bore electromagnetic valves. With this set-up, the pressure in the cuff reaches 90% of the reservoir pressure within 0.1 sec.

With the electromagnetic valves, the inflation and deflation of the cuff can be performed automatically, the valves being energized with the aid of a timer. However, the venous occlusions start and finish at arbitrary moments during the heartcycle (Fig. 30). The occlusion time can be diminished when each occlusion is made to start and to finish at the moment when the volume pulsations have reached their lowest points (Fig. 31). This can be attained by triggering the valves by means of impulses derived from the R-top of the electrocardiogram. Then the occlusion time becomes equal to the measuring time, and the occlusion can be shortened to 2 or 3 heartbeats. With the aid of special amplifiers the flow can be read directly from the recorder. A complete description of the system has been given earlier by the present author (54, 95).

Automatic outprint of results in ml/100 ml.min shortens considerably the time of evaluation. A visual control of the plethysmographic curves, however, should not be omitted in order to recognize technical errors. Some of the tracings are unsuited for automation of measurements.

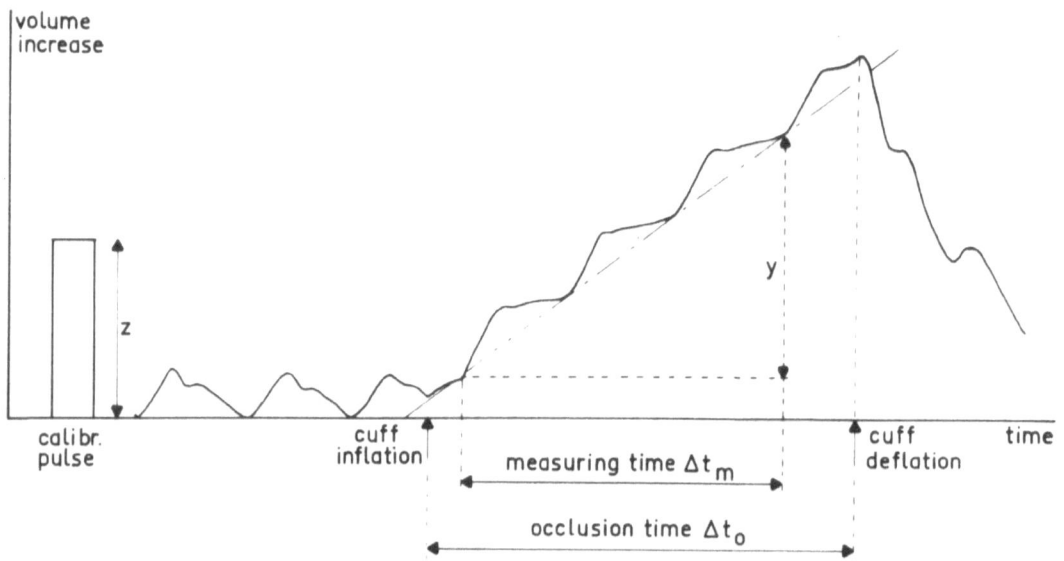

Fig. 30. Calculation of the flow from the volume increase during venous occlusion. The mean occlusion time is one heart period longer than the measuring time.

3.8. Clinical applications

3.8.1. *Blood flow measurements in the calf.* Blood flow measurement in the calf is the most important clinical application of venous occlusion plethysmography. In patients with peripheral arterial disease the complaints are caused mainly by stenoses or obstructions of the large supplying arteries. Therefore, a quantitative determination of the maximal blood flow still admitted through the arterial system to the leg is important in evaluating the functional significance of the disease, in indicating arteriography and in following up patients after therapeutic measures (see also Section 4).

Quantitative flow measurements can be made with the various types of plethysmographs described in Sections 2.4 and 2.5.

The water-filled plethysmograph is rarely used in clinical routine nowadays because of the drawbacks mentioned in Section 2.4.1, although it is the most accurate method for blood flow measurements.

The rigid air-filled plethysmograph and the capacitance plethysmograph have partly the same drawbacks and are not generally applied, as far as the author knows.

The Dohn air-filled cuff plethysmograph and the strain-gauge plethysmograph are easy to handle, they cause the patient little discomfort and can be kept in position during changes in posture, exercise and other

Simultaneous measurements in calf and foot with two-channel plethysmographs allow a more detailed analysis of peripheral hemodynamics. During maximal reactive hyperemia in the calf region foot blood flow remains low or is not measurable (phenomenon of blood flow diversion or hemometakinesia). When calf blood flow begins to decrease reactive hyperemia develops in the distal foot area.

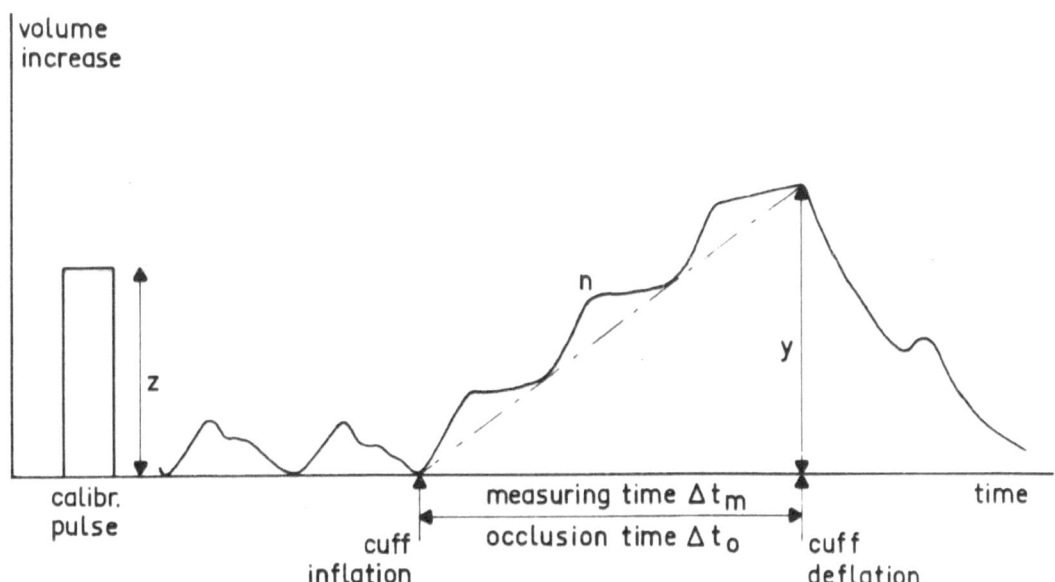

Fig. 31. Calculation of the flow when the occlusion is triggered by impulses derived from the R-top of the electrocardiogram. The occlusion time is equal to the measuring time. n: occlusion during n heart periods.

functional states. Therefore they are the methods of choice for clinical routine measurements.

The cuff plethysmograph described by Barbey and Barbey (43) exerts a relatively high pressure on the tissue, which tends to oppose the accumulation of blood in the limb segment beneath the cuff and to encourage accumulation in the limb segments distal and proximal of the cuff.

Several workers have compared the results from various types of plethysmographs.

Whitney (49) performed simultaneous measurements on the forearm with a water-filled plethysmograph and with the strain-gauge plethysmograph. He found considerable differences between the results of the two types. Dahn and Hallböök (96) and Paulev et al. (56), however, concluded that there were no systematic differences in absolute blood flow values, provided that the strain-gauge is applied to the muscular middle part of the forearm. Moreover Paulev et al. (56) ascertained that there was a great and similar intrinsic accuracy in the water-filled and in the strain-gauge plethysmographs.

Fewings and Whelan (46) compared the capacitance with the rigid air-filled and water-filled plethysmographs. They found a general agreement between the results of the capacitance and air-filled plethysmographs, but the results of both these methods differed significantly from those obtained with the water-filled plethysmograph, probably due to the hydrostatic pressure of the water.

Englund et al. (97) perfunded human limbs with a heart–lung machine and simultaneously measured the flow with a strain-gauge plethysmograph around the calf. They found a linear relationship between the values and concluded that strain-gauge plethysmography is a valid method.

Mulz and König (53) compared the strain-gauge plethysmograph with an air-filled cuff plethysmograph (initial pressure 0.8 kPa, 6 mm Hg) and an impedance plethysmograph. Measurements were performed with subjects at rest. They concluded that only the strain-gauge plethysmograph gave exact, linear results immediately after the application of venous occlusion. The flow values obtained from the linear parts of both curves did not differ significantly. The results from the impedance plethysmograph deviated largely, however.

3.8.2. *Venous diseases.*   Plethysmography is widely used in the evaluation of venous diseases. The methods of study and clinical application are discussed in Chapter 9.

3.8.3. *Capillary filtration.*   After the inflation of the occluding cuff the volume of the distal leg segment increases rapidly until the pressure in the distal veins reaches the level of the occluding pressure. Then the veins beneath the cuff open up again and venous drainage starts until venous outflow equals the arterial inflow. When the inflation of the cuff is sustained, gradually the volume of the limb increases further (Fig. 32) due to filtration of fluid through the capillary wall (98, 99). Celander and Marild (100) have shown that about 80% of the venous pressure increase is transmitted to the capillaries.

From the slope of the curve a capillary filtration coefficient (CFC) can be determined (52):

$$\text{CFC} = \frac{Q}{V_0 \, \Delta P_{cap}} \quad \text{(ml/100 ml.min kPa)}.$$

with

Q = volume increase per minute

V = reference volume

ΔP_{cap} = capillary pressure

Filtration studies can give information about capillary lesions, and the influence of the treatment of venous oedema on the capillary filtration can be studied (99).

Normal values of CFC are about 0.0007 ml/100 ml.min. kPa for the adult and 0.0015 ml/100 ml.min. kPa for the infant.

4.   BLOOD FLOW IN THE LOWER LEG

4.1.   *Blood flow at rest*

It is very important to standardize the methods and conditions in order to obtain reliable and comparable results. The subject or patient is supine and

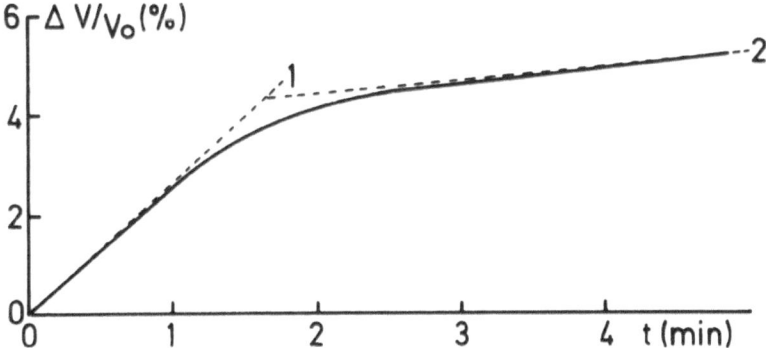

Fig. 32. Volume increase of the calf during prolonged venous occlusion. 1: increase due to arterial inflow, 2: increase due to capillary filtration.

relaxed on an examination table in a quiet room. The leg is supported above heart level (see Section 3.2) and the calf muscles are entirely relaxed. The ambient temperature is about 24 °C. The subject is allowed to rest at least 15 min before measurements are performed.

The flow in the calf at rest varies spontaneously as a result of various control mechanisms. Therefore a series of 10–15 measurements should be made to determine the mean value (54, 101). The coefficient of variation in a series is of the order of 10%.

Great differences exist between the mean values measured on different days, although the measuring conditions are standardized. The coefficient of variation of the means is of the order of 15% (54).

In contrast to calf blood flow at rest, foot and finger blood flow are often decreased in severely ischemic limbs (rest pain or beginning gangrene).

Interindividually the mean flow values differ widely, the coefficient of variation being 30% or more. Table 1 gives the mean flow values reported by several authors. From these results it is obvious that there are no significant differences between the flow values in normal subjects and patients with obstructive arterial disease, therefore the measurement of the flow at rest cannot contribute to the diagnosis of this disease.

Table 1. Blood flow at rest (ml/100 ml.min), with standard deviation, in the calves of normal subjects and patients with obstructive arterial disease.

Author	Mean flow		Plethysmograph
	Normals	Patients	
Hillestad (102)	3.6 ± 1.3	3.4 ± 1.0	water-filled
Strandell et al. (103	3.6 ± 1.2	4.5 ± 1.6	air-filled
Dahn (104, 105)	3.0 ± 1.3	3.4 ± 1.4	water-filled
Gottstein (106)	2.2 ± 1.0	2.4 ± 1.0	air-filled cuff
Hallböök (107)	3.2 ± 0.2		strain-gauge
Barendsen (54)	3.5 ± 1.1	2.5 ± 1.3	strain-gauge
Lorentsen (108)	2.2 ± 0.3	2.4 ± 0.3	air-filled cuff

4.2.   *Reactive (postocclusion) hyperemia*

Because the blood flow at rest does not allow a differentiation between normal subjects and patients with obstructive arterial disease, information about the functional capabilities of the arterial system can only be obtained from measurements during a period of increased flow. For this purpose a period of arterial occlusion is widely used, the flow being measured during the postocclusive hyperemia. Exercise of the muscle groups concerned is another method for increasing the blood flow (see Section 4.3).

4.2.1. Period of arterial occlusion.   For the determination of the capabilities of the arterial system the period of arterial occlusion should necessarily be chosen long enough so that the vasodilatation of the occluded segment is nearly maximal. On the other hand, for clinical practice the occlusion period should be as short as possible, so that the occlusion does not give too much discomfort to the patient.

Fig. 33 is an original record of flow measurements after 5 min arterial occlusion with triggered venous occlusion (strain-gauge plethysmograph). From the original records the flow can be calculated and plotted as a function of time.

Several authors have measured the maximal flow in the calf after different periods of arterial occlusion. Fig. 34 gives the maximal flow in the calf of 5 normal subjects. The maximal flow does not increase very much when the occlusion period lasts longer than 5 min. Our results are in general agreement with those of Hillestad (109), Dahn (104) and Bollinger (101). It appears, however, that the maximal dilatation is not yet obtained after 20 min of circulatory arrest (109).

Some authors use an occlusion period of 3 min (105, 106, 107, 110, 111), others of 5 min (54, 102, 103, 108, 112). Patients with serious intermittent claudication can generally endure 5 min arterial occlusion without serious objections, therefore this period is the most suitable for clinical studies (54, 102).

The authors preferring occlusion periods of 3 min state that patients with advanced arterial occlusive disease may develop considerable pain during an occlusion lasting 5 min. When patient groups with different degrees of ischemia are compared it may be preferable to use 3 min.

4.2.2. *Cuff pressure for arterial and venous occlusion.* The cuff pressure for arterial occlusion should be about 6.6 kPa (50 mm Hg) above the individual systolic pressure. Incomplete arterial occlusion can be detected

In patients with ischemia a cuff pressure of 40 mm Hg is recommended. Even this pressure may be too high, especially in the foot region, where a pressure drop to values below 40 mm Hg is frequently observed during reactive hyperemia.

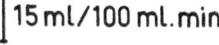

15 ml/100 ml.min

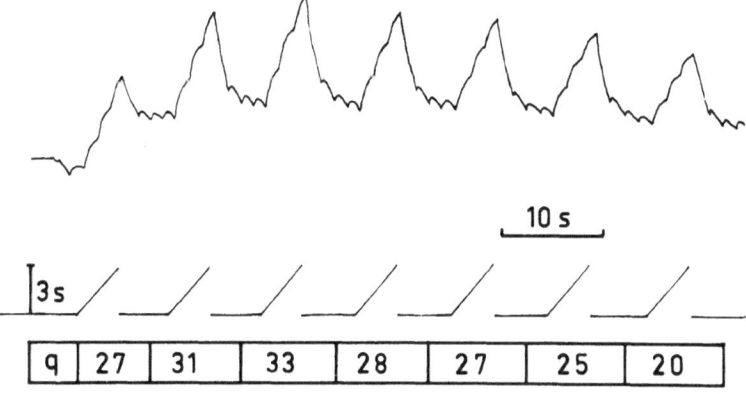

Fig. 33. Record of flow measurements after 5 min artial occlusion. Upper trace: signal of strain-gauge plethysmograph. Lower trace: the height of the ramps indicate the occlusion times. The calculated flow values are also given.

by an increase of the volume of the distal leg segment during the occlusion.

During arterial occlusion the blood pressure in the occluded segment decreases to nearly zero (89). During the first phase of the reactive hyperemia the blood pressure is also lower than normal. As has been stated in Section 3.2, the venous occlusion can impede the arterial inflow in this phase of reactive hyperemia. In Fig. 35 typical flow curves of a normal subject after 5 min arterial occlusion, measured with different venous occluding pressures, are given. The cuff width was 12 cm. With a cuff

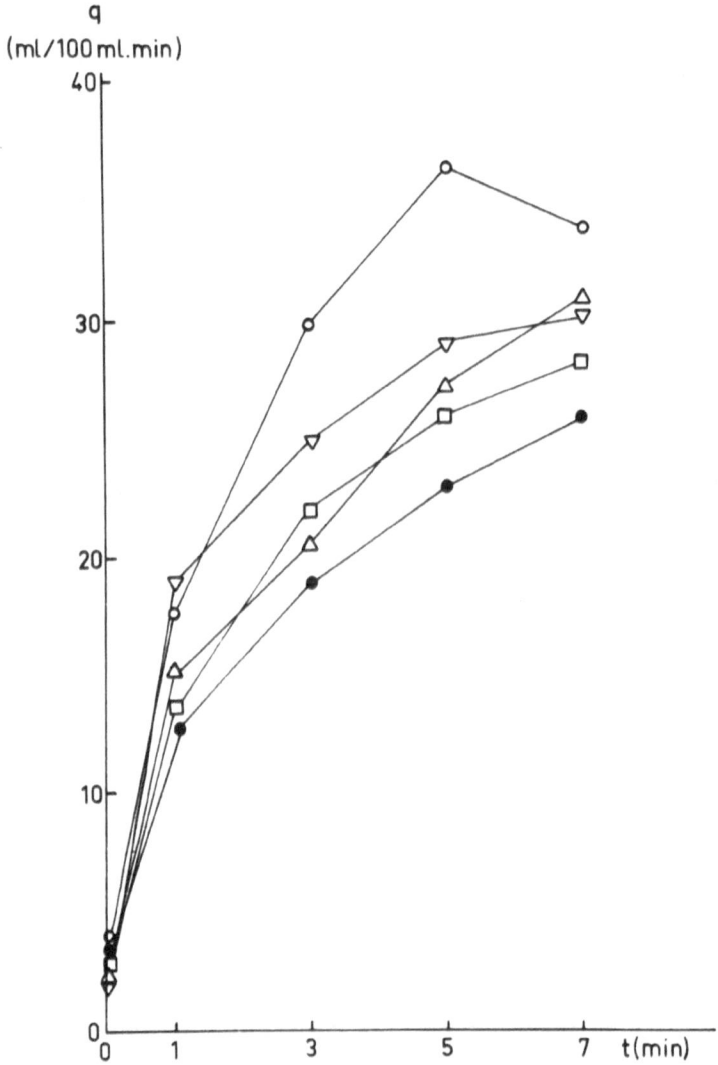

Fig. 34. Maximal flow in the calf of 5 normal subjects after different periods of arterial occlusion. (From ref. (54).)

pressure of 9.3 kPa (70 mm Hg) the arterial inflow was impeded. For studies on normal subjects a pressure of 6.6 kPa (50 mm Hg) in a cuff of 12 cm width is most suitable for venous occlusion. In patients with arterial disease this pressure may be too high, however (74).

4.2.3. *Maximal flow and time of maximal flow.*   The maximal flow is the most important parameter which is used to characterize the hyperemic

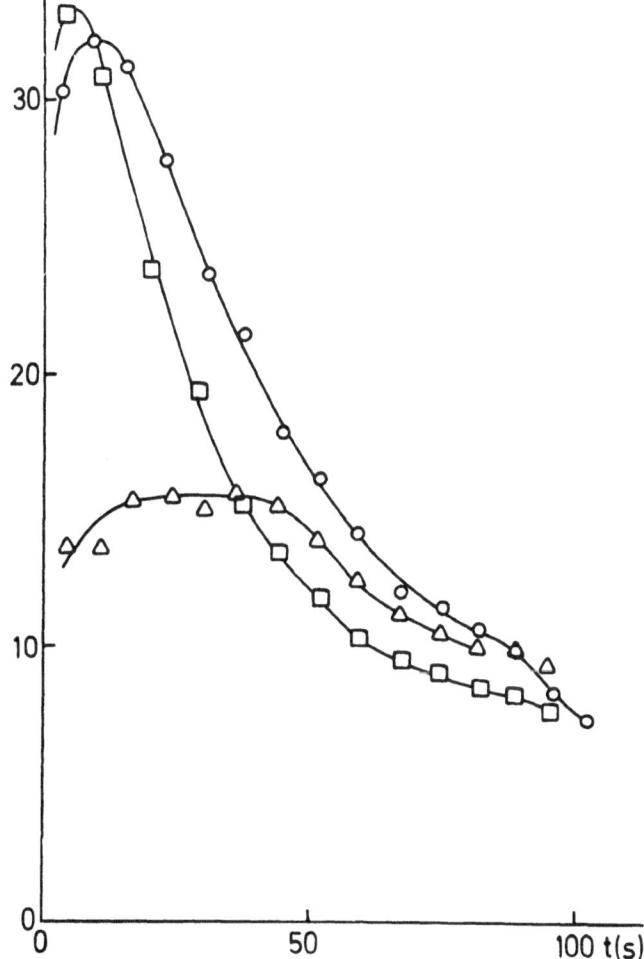

Fig. 35. Maximal flow in the calf of a normal subject after 5 min arterial occlusion with different venous occluding pressures. (From ref. (54).) □: $P_{cuff} = 6.6$. kPa (50 mm Hg). ○: $P_{cuff} = 8.0$ kPa (60 mm Hg). △: $P_{cuff} = 9.3$ kPa (70 mm Hg).

response. The reproducibility of the maximal flow value with repeated measurements in the same subject on the same day is quite good. Fig. 36 gives an example. The maximal flows after the second and third occlusion are slightly increased, while the duration of the hyperemia is decreased. Eichna and Wilkens (87) already described this phenomenon (augmenta-

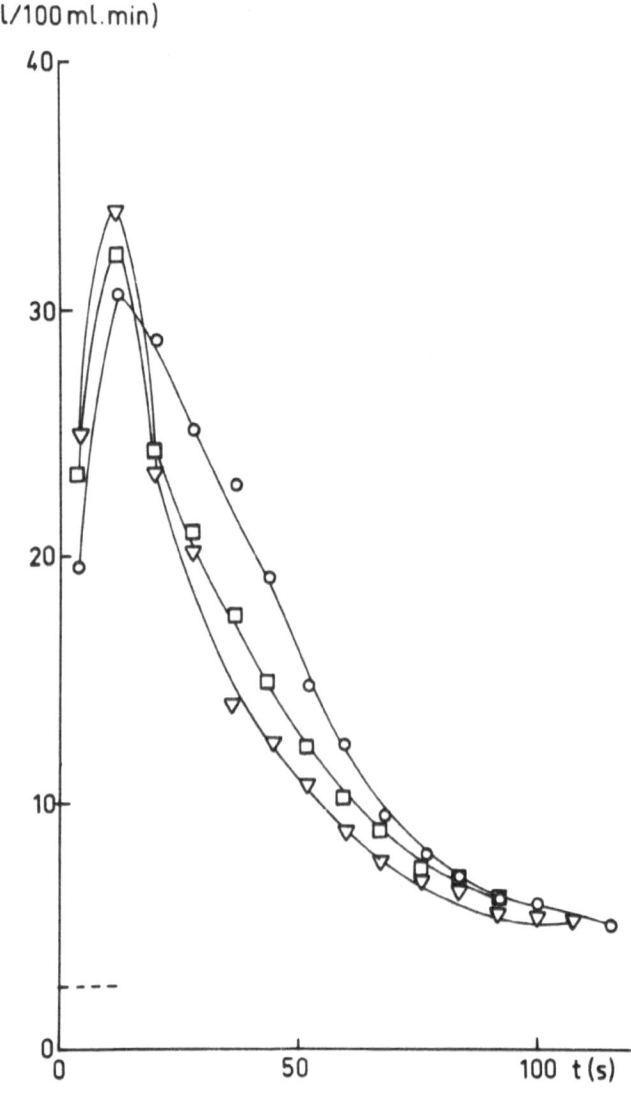

Fig. 36. Representative measurements of the blood flow in the calf of a normal subject after 5 min arterial occlusion with intervals of 10 min between the occlusions. – – –: flow at rest, ○: first occlusion, □: second occlusion, ∇: third occlusion. (From ref. (54).)

tion). However, the differences are only about 5% of the mean value. When the measurements are repeated on different days the reproducibility is less good, due to physiological variations of the subject. The coefficient of variation was found to be about 12% (54).

Table 2 gives some reported values of the maximal flow after 5 min arterial occlusion. From these results it is obvious that the interindividual variations are rather great.

The time interval between the onset of symptoms and the measurement is important. After acute and subacute limb artery occlusions a spontaneous increase of peak reactive hyperemia is to be expected during the first year corresponding to collateral development. The mean increase is about 100%. In chronic isolated occlusions of the iliac arteries the hyperemic response in the calf segment is better than in patients with chronic obstructions of the superficial femoral artery.

Table 2. Maximal flow (with s.d.) after 5 min arterial occlusion in normal subjects.

Author	Max. flow (ml/100 ml.min)	Number of legs	Plethysmograph
Strandell (103)	36.3±7.2	10	Dohn-cuff
Hillestad (109)	28.2±7.6	48	Water-filled
Ehringer (93)	29.7±7.5	95	Water-filled
Lorentsen (108)	25.2±2.9	6	Cuff
Barendsen (54)	28.9±5.4	10	Strain-gauge

The time of maximal flow (Fig. 37) is a parameter which characterizes the profile of the hyperemic flow curve. In normal subjects the maximal flow is reached within 20 sec after the end of the arterial occlusion (74, 93).

Fig. 37 also gives an example of the hyperemic flow in the calf of a patient with intermittent claudication due to an obstruction of the common iliac artery. The maximal flow is only 9 ml/100 ml.min and the time of maximal flow is about 25 sec. In patients the maximal flow and the time of maximal flow vary widely, due to differences in the seriousness of the disease, the localization of obstructions, the number and caliber of collateral vessels etc. This is reflected in the values of the maximal flow reported by several authors (see Table 3).

Table 3. Some reported values of the maximal flow (with s.d.) after 5 min arterial occlusion in patients with peripheral arterial disease.

Author	Maximal flow (ml/100 ml.min)	Number of legs	Seriousness and location of disease	Plethysmograph
Strandell (103)	19.1±7.9	7	one leg affected	Dohn-cuff
i.d.	12.8±6.9	8	both legs affected	i.d.
Hillestad (102)	9.5±4.4	34	no advanced disease	Water-filled
Siggaard-Andersen (128)	18.7±5.2	28	only sclerosis	Dohn-cuff
i.d.	5.7±3.8	72	obst.a.fem.sup.	i.d.
i.d.	4.0±1.8	26	obst.a.iliaca	i.d.
Ehringer (129)	10.0±4.0	20	obst.a.fem.sup.	Water-filled
i.d.	12.6±5.3	10	aorto-iliac	i.d.
Barendsen (54)	11.3±4.4	10	obst.a.fem.sup. or a.iliaca	Strain-gauge
Hylkema (74)	7.7±3.0	45	obst.a.fem.sup.	Strain-gauge
i.d.	10.3±4.0	27	obst.aorto-iliac	i.d.

4.3. *Postexercise hyperemia*

Contracting skeletal muscles need much more oxygen and metabolic substrates than muscles at rest. To satisfy the heightened needs the flow in the muscles must increase greatly. Various regulatory mechanisms come into operation, which cause a strong local vasodilatation in the exercising muscles and general cardiovascular readjustments: the cardiac output and blood pressure increase and the blood supply to the various vascular beds is readjusted.

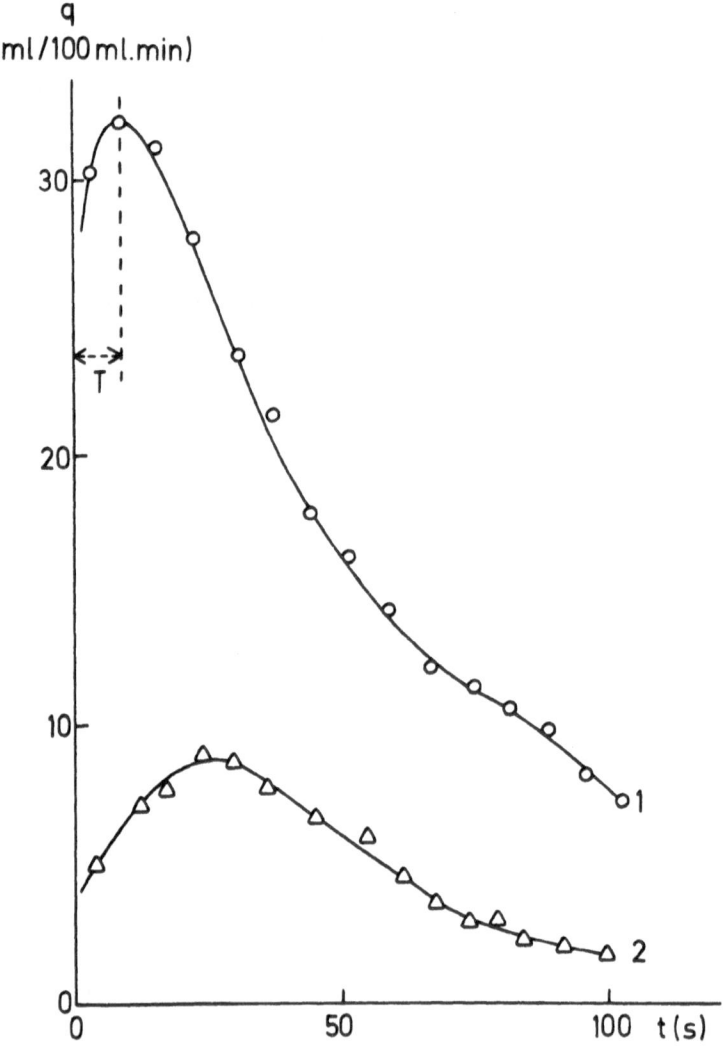

Fig. 37. Flow in the calf of a normal subject (1) and a patient with an obstruction of the common iliac artery (2).

During strong contractions the flow in the muscles is reduced because the blood vessels are compressed by the intramuscular pressure. After a contraction the flow is increased (exercise hyperemia). Thus the flow varies greatly during rhythmical exercise.

Measurements of the flow during contractions cannot be performed simply with venous occlusion plethysmography because the muscles move strongly and the volume (or girth) changes during the contractions; moreover the increased intramuscular pressure expels blood beneath the cuff (113). Therefore measurements during exercise are made with invasive techniques, for instance the ^{133}Xenon clearance method (116, 117, 118), the dye dilution method (119) or the thermodilution method (120, 121).

Measurements of postexercise hyperemia can be performed technically simply, but the extremity has to be supported above heart level; therefore the subject has to be in the supine position. Various workers have described ergometers for exercising the calf muscles (54, 109, 113, 117, 122) which are based on the principle that the foot treads a pedal which rotates on an axis. The pedal lifts a weight over some vertical distance or is loaded by springs.

A scheme of the ergometer, developed by Lubbers and van den Berg, and used by the present author is given in Fig. 38. The torque M exerted by the foot on the pedal is measured with strain-gauges on a measuring arm. The angle of rotation ϕ is measured with a potentiometer on the axis of rotation. The angular velocity $\dot\phi$ is calculated electronically, as is also the total work over the working phase $\int M \, d\phi$. The load consists of roll springs which exert a constant force on the weight arm. By changing the springs and/or the point of application on the weight arm the load can be varied.

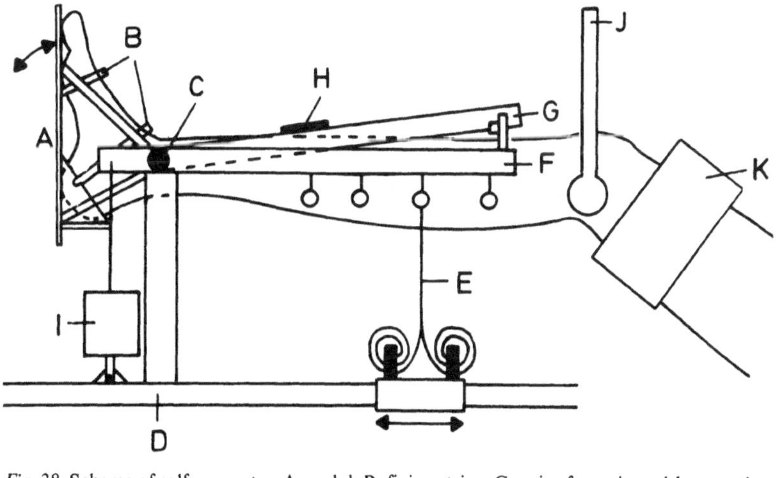

Treadmill exercise provokes higher and longer lasting increases in calf blood flow. A trained observer is ready for the first measurement in supine position 1 min after the end of the performance. This is sufficient in most instances to get the peak flow in patients with ischemic disease, in whom the blood flow response may be extremely delayed (up to 30–40 min).

Fig. 38. Scheme of calfergometer. A: pedal, B: fixing strips, C: axis of rotation with potentiometer, D: frame, E: springs, F: load arm, G: measuring arm, H: strain-gauges, I: brake cylinder, J: knee supports, K: cuff. (From ref. (54).)

4.3.1. *Isometric contractions*.   Sustained isometric contractions, mainly of the forearm muscles, have been widely used to study their cardio-vascular effects, central and peripheral (123–125). A review of these effects have been given by Hudlická (126).

The contraction strength is nearly always expressed as a percentage of the maximal voluntary contraction force (M.V.C.) of the muscle groups concerned. The M.V.C. differs widely between subjects.

It was found that cardiac output, oxygen uptake, heart rate and arterial blood pressure all increased in response to sustained isometric contractions.

Almost instantaneously after a contraction the flow reaches a maximal value that depends on the strength and time of the contraction. The flow decreases rapidly to the level at rest. The maximal flow differs widely between individuals, therefore normal values cannot be given with a reasonable degree of accuracy. Sustained isometric contractions have not been used to evaluate the seriousness of arterial disease.

4.3.2.   *Rhythmic exercise*.   Rhythmic exercise cannot be standardized easily because there are many variables: the load, the period of exercise, the rhythm of the contractions and the ratio of the duration of the contraction and the time between contractions.

Fig. 29 is an example of flow measurements with a strain-gauge plethysmograph after min light exercise (load 3 W, 30 contractions per minute) on the calfergometer. The large deflections at the beginning of the record are caused by the muscle contractions during the exercise. Immediately

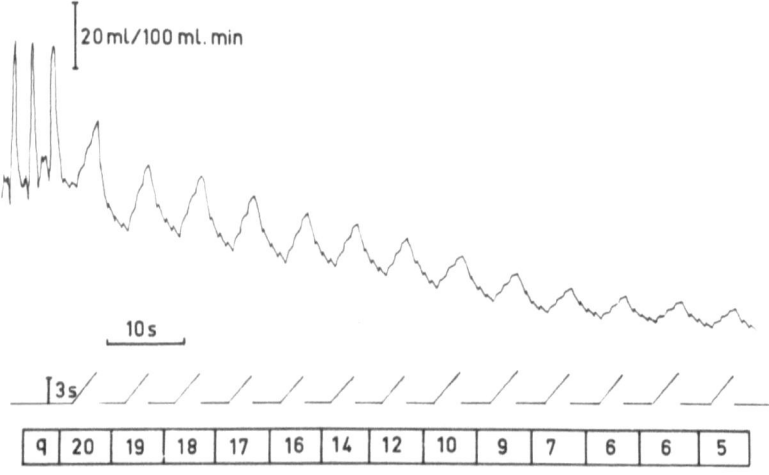

Fig. 39. Example of flow measurements after 1 min exercise on the calf ergometer with triggered venous occlusion plethysmography. Load: 3.0 W. Lower trace: the height of the ramps indicates the occlusion time. (From ref. (54).)

after the exercise the flow is highest, then the flow decreases rapidly to the level at rest.

An example of exercise hyperemia in the calf of a normal subject after 3 min exercise with a low, medium and high load is given in Fig. 40. The flow after 5 min arterial occlusion is also given. Obviously the flow pattern after the exercise is not the same as that after the arterial occlusion. During exercise the blood pressure in the calf does not decrease as is the case during arterial occlusion, and during exercise a continuous adaption of the cardiac output takes place; therefore the increased flow can be supplied easily. Generally the maximal flow after heavy exercise is greater than after 5 min arterial occlusion.

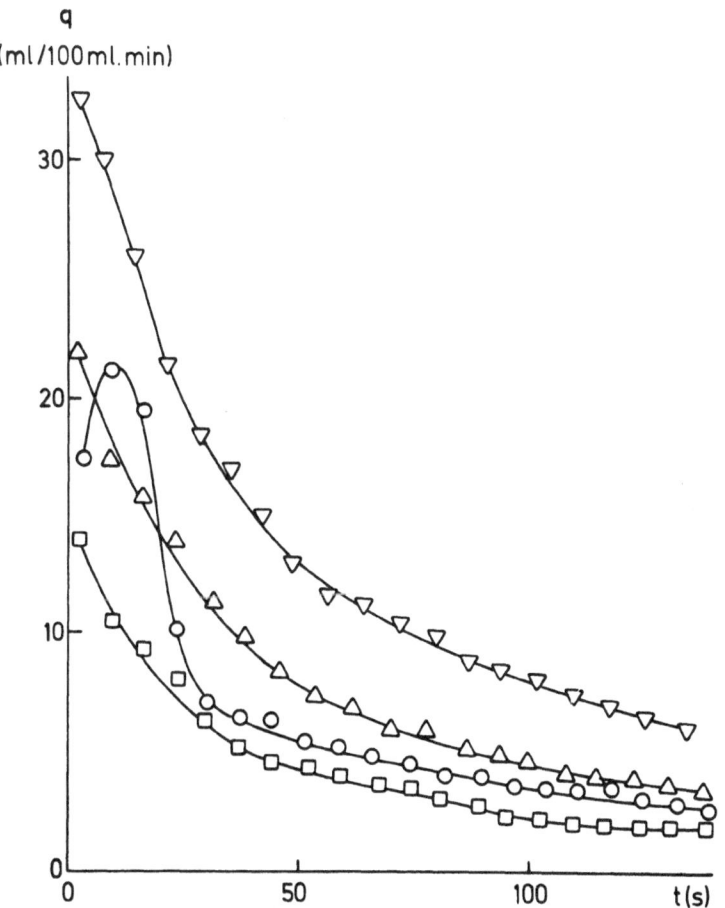

Fig. 40. Example of exercise hyperemia in the calf of a normal subject after 3 min exercise with different loads. Reactive hyperemia after 5 min arterial occlusion is also given. ○: reactive hyperemia, □: load 4,3 W, △: load 6 W, ▽: load 7.6 W.

Fig. 41 gives an example of the results in a patient with intermittent claudication due to an obstruction of the superficial femoral artery after 5 min arterial occlusion and after exercise until claudication (3 min exercise, load 3 W). The maximal flow is low and the hyperemia lasts very long.

Table 4 gives the results of several workers obtained from normal subjects and patients with intermittent claudication. The results differ quite strongly, probably due to the differences in the exercise procedures. In normal subjects the amount of work that can be performed maximally depends on the physical fitness and endurance of the individual subjects. In patients with peripheral arterial disease it is limited by the onset of claudication pain, and depends on the seriousness of the disease. However, the pain threshold is not the same in each patient.

4.3.3. *Ischemic rhythmic exercise.*   The intention of ischemic rhythmic exercise is that the blood flow in the calf is increased to the maximal possible value. Ischemia is produced by the inflation of a cuff around the thigh to a suprasystolic pressure. During the ischemic period exercise is performed until the subject is not able to exercise any more.

This method has not been used widely for the evaluation of peripheral arterial disease. In normal subjects the maximal flow after the ischemic exercise period is greater than after the same exercise without ischemia (127). In patients Shepherd (127) found no differences between the flow after exercise and after ischemic exercise. However, Jacobs and Reich (115) found a mean flow of 13.3 (s.d. 4.7) ml/100 ml.min in 19 patients after exercise and a mean flow of 18.0 (s.d. 10.9) ml/100 ml.min after ischemic exercise. Hillestad (109) found a mean flow of 29.8 (s.d. 6.0) ml/100 ml.min in 32 normal subjects and a mean flow of 12.4 (s.d. 5.5) ml/100 ml.min in 16 patients with intermittent claudication. However, the exercise was not continued until claudication.

In the author's opinion ischemic rhythmic exercise cannot contribute substantially to the evaluation of peripheral arterial disease. Moreover, the method is very uncomfortable to normal subjects and patients.

There is perhaps one exception where maximal blood flow yields additional information. During physical training of patients with intermittent claudication submaximal flow rates decrease, but maximal flow increases. This behavior is probably explained by alterations in the metabolic capacity of skeletal muscles. A maximal stimulus for vasodilation is required to demonstrate increased blood flow capacity.

4.4.   *Flow measurements without venous occlusion*

Flow measurements in the calf can be performed by changing the position of the leg (74, 91). When the leg of a supine subject is tilted above heart level (with the center of the calf 30 cm above heart level, the lower leg with an upward slope of about 20° and the knee bent slightly) the veins in the calf empty rapidly. When the leg is laid down again (with the center of the calf about 10 cm below heart level) the veins refill as a result of arterial inflow if the venous valves are competent. During the first phase of refilling there is no venous outflow; this can be proved by an interpolated venous

Table 4. Maximal flow (with s.d.) in the calf of normal subjects and patients after exercise. Patients exercised until claudication.

Author	Exercise	Plethysmograph	Normal subjects		Patients		Remarks
			Number of legs	Max. flow (ml/100 ml.min)	Number of legs	Max. flow (ml/100 ml.min)	
Barcroft (113)	Weight on pedal 60 strokes/min during 6 min	Air-filled	6 6	9 kg: 19.0 15 kg: 31.8	—	—	Values without corrections introduced by the author
Strandell (103)	Weight on pedal: 6 kg 60 strokes/min	Air-filled cuff	10 10	Sub. max work: 19.5±4.9 Max. work: 27.0±4.8	10	8.7±5.3	
Hillestad (109)	Weight on pedal: 4.5 kg 30 strokes/min during 1 min	Water-filled	22	Submax. work: 12.0±3.8	16	9.4±3.2	
Tonnesen (114)	Weight on pedal: 3–15 kg 20–55 strokes/min during 6 min	Strain-gauge	24	Max. work: 45.2±12.4	35	11.2±7.2	
Barendsen (54)	Calf ergometer 30 strokes/min	Strain-gauge	5 5	Submax. work: 31.5±5.0 Max. work: 40 ±12	5	17 ±4	Patients without very serious complaints
Jacobs (115)	Weight on pedal: 5.5 kg 24 strokes/min	Strain-gauge	—	—	24	12.5±4.7	

occlusion. Thus the arterial inflow can be calculated from the slope of the curve (91).

Fig. 42 gives an example of flow measurements with this method in a patient with intermittent claudication after a period of exercise.

With this method the flow cannot be measured in as rapid a sequence as with venous occlusion, and only with a plethysmograph which permits movements of the leg.

The method has not yet been fully evaluated, but seems to be an alternative examination in cases of low arterial pressure at the level of the thigh or in the case of patients who have undergone an operation of the femoropopliteal arteries recently. The method showed that in a number of patients with low thigh pressure venous occlusion with a cuff pressure of 6.6 kPa (50 mm Hg) impeded the arterial inflow (74).

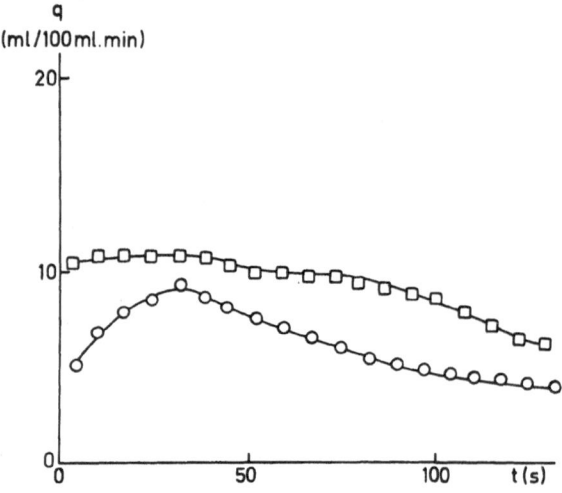

Fig. 41. Exercise hyperemia in the calf of a patient with intermittent claudication (□) and reactive hyperemia after 5 min arterial occlusion (○).

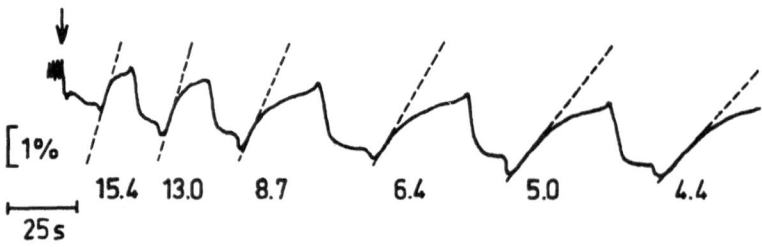

Fig. 42. Example of flow measurements with the 'tilting-laying down' method after exercise. (From ref. (74) with permission.)

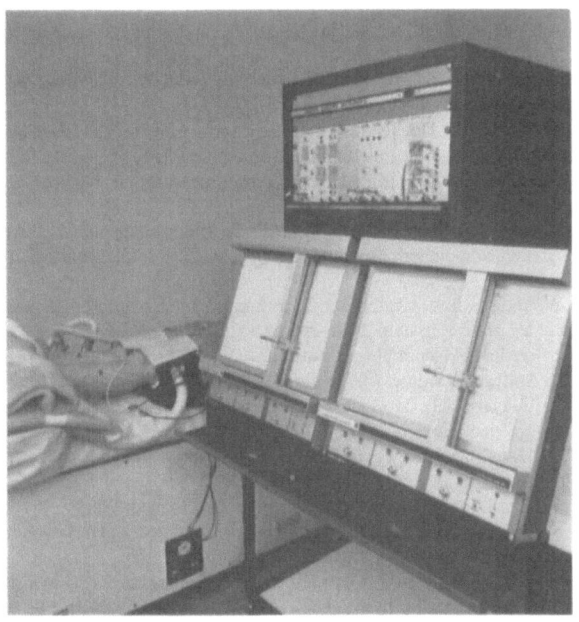

Fig. 43. JSI-PERIFLOW SU-4, Janssen Scientific Instruments.

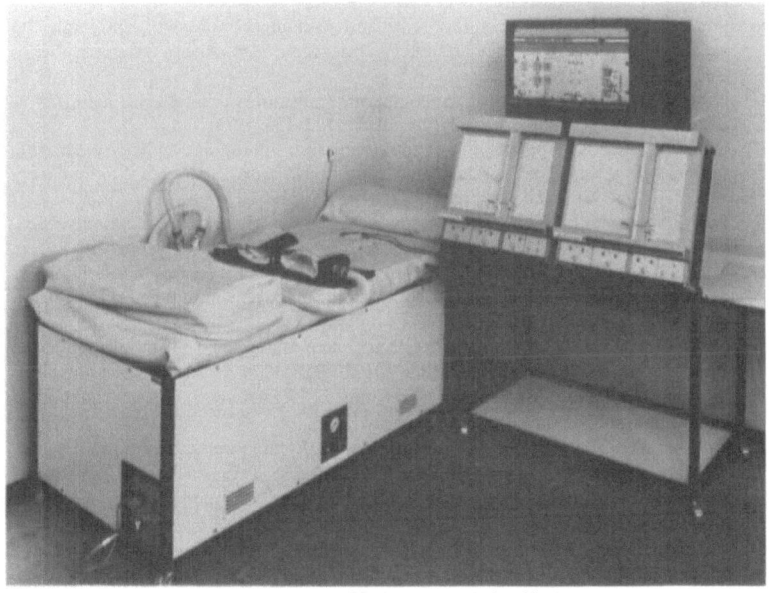

Fig. 44. JSI-PERIFLOW SU-4, Janssen Scientific Instruments.

REFERENCES TO MAIN TEXT

1. Kappert A: Oscillometry, oscillography and sphygmography. In: Diagnosis of Peripheral Vascular Diseases, Bern, Huber, 1971, p. 34–46.

2. Rau G: Allgemeine diagnostische Verfahren. In: Angiologie, Stuttgart, G. Thieme, 1974, p. 207–226.
3. David E: Eine Methode zur fortlaufenden differentiellen Registrierung der Puls-wellengeschwindigkeit am Menschen. Z. Biol. 115: 118–133, 1967.
4. De Monchy C, Van der Hoeven GMA: Pulse wave transmission times in central aorta and peripheral arteries in normal children. Blood Vessels 13: 129–138, 1976.
5. Pressman GL, Newgard PM, Eige JJ: Direct force measuring transducer used in blood pressure research. Med biol. Eng. 5: 195, 1967.
6. Zangeneh M, Nassereslami H: Das Verhalten der Pulswellengeschwindigkeit im Bein in Abhängigkeit von Lebensalter und Geschlecht. Z. Kreislaufforsch. 56: 368–374, 1967.
7. Busse R, Wetterer E, Bauer RD, Pasch Th, Summa Y: The genesis of the pulse contours of the distal leg arteries in man. Pflügers Arch. ges. Physiol. 360: 63–79, 1975.
8. Brecht K, Boucke H: Neues elektrostatisches Tiefton-Mikrophon und seine Anwen-dung in der Sphygmographie. Pflügers Arch ges. Physiol. 256: 43–54, 1952.
9. Weinman J, Hayat A, Raviv G: Reflection photoplethysmography of arterial blood volume pulses. Med. biol. eng. Comput. 15: 22–31, 1977.
10. Cranley JJ, Mahalingam K, Ferris EB: Extending the vascular examination by non-invasive means. Amer. J. Surg. 134: 179–182, 1977.
11. Gesenius H: Oszillographie und Arteriographie. Dtsch. med. Wsch. 74: 1–14, 1949.
12. Matthes K: Untersuchungen über die Sauerstoffsättigung des menschlichen Arterien-blutes. Arch. exp. path. Pharmak. 179: 698–705, 1935.
13. Hertzman AB: The blood supply of various skin areas as estimated by photoelectric plethysmography. Amer. J. Physiol. 124: 328–340, 1938.
14. De Pater L, Van den Berg JW, Bueno AA: A very sensitive photoplethysmograph using scattered light and a photosensitive resistance. Acta physiol. pharm. neerl. 10: 378–390, 1962.
15. Van den Berg, Jw, Vafi A: A very sensitive two-channel photoplethysmograph, the vasotest, for peripheral vascular surgery. Proc. Kon. Ned. Akad. Wetensch. (Series C66) 30–36: 1963.
16. Uretzky G, Palti Y: A method for comparing transmitted and reflected light photo-electric plethysmography. J. appl. Physiol. 31: 132–135, 1971.
17. Omura Y, Lee K: Applications of ultra-miniature photoelectric plethysmographic sensors with a very short response time to the non-traumatic study of the circulatory system. Trans. Amer. Soc. art. Organs 17: 392–404, 1971.
18. Fine S, Weinman J: The use of photoconductive cells in photoplethysmography. Med. biol. Eng. 11: 455–462, 1973.
19. Muir JFK, Fox RH, Stranc WE, Stewart FS: The measurement of blood flow by a photoelectric technique and its application to the management of tubed skin pedicles. Brit. J. plast. Surg. 21: 14–31, 1968.
20. Challoner AVJ, Ramsay CA: A photoelectric plethysmograph for the measurement of cutaneous blood flow. Phys. med. Biol. 19: 317–328, 1974.
21. Barnes RW, Clayton JM, Bone GE, Slaymaker EE, Remertson J: Supraorbital photo-plethysmography. J. surg. Res. 22: 319–327, 1977.
22. Webster MHC, Patterson J: The photoelectric plethysmograph as a monitor of micro-vascular anastomoses. Brit. J. plast. Surg. 29: 182–185, 1976.
23. Abrahamson DI: Circulation in the Extremities, New York and London, Academic Press, 1967.
24. Wood JE: The Veins, Boston, Little, Brown, 1965.
25. Nielsen SL, Paulev PE: A simple water plethysmograph with standardized sleeves. Scand. J. clin. Lab. Invest. 29: 159–161, 1972.
26. Greenfield ADM: A simple water-filled plethysmograph for the hand or forearm with temperature control. J. Physiol. (Lond.) 123: 62–64P, 1954.
27. Bauer M, Ioannovich J, Schlögl R: Eine neue Apparatur zur Finger-Venenverschlusz-plethysmographie. Kritik des Verfahrens und diagnostische Möglichkeiten. Z. Kar-diol. 64: 647–660, 1975.
28. Stolinski C, Sirs JA, Ardill BL, Fentem PH: A photoelectric volume transducer for use with a water-filled plethysmograph. J. appl. Physiol. 22: 1161–1164, 1967.

29. Cooper KE, Kerslake DM: An electrical volume recorder for use with plethysmographs. J. Physiol. (Lond.) 114: 1–2P, 1951.
30. Jewell BR, Wilkie DR: A simple transducer system for use in plethysmography. J. Physiol. (Lond.) 85: 3–5P, 1966.
31. Sigdell JE: A Plethysmographic System with a Capacitive Displacement Transducer and Automatic Reset, (Rep. 1:68 Res. Lab. med. Electronics), Göteborg, Chalmers University of Technology, 1968.
32. Hyman C, Winsor T: An electric volume transducer for plethysmographic recording. J. appl. Physiol. 21: 1403–1404, 1966.
33. Thoren O: Blood flow patterns of the forearm of critically ill post-traumatic patients. A plethysmographic study. Acta chir. scand. Suppl. 443, 1974.
34. Vanhuyse VJ, Raman ER: Interpretation of pressure changes in plethysmography. Phys. med. Biol. 16: 111–117, 1971.
35. Vanhuyse VJ, Raman ER: Temperature dependence of pressure changes in plethysmography. Phys. med. Biol. 17: 288–292, 1972.
36. Vanggaard L, Østergaard J: Thermal problems in plethysmography and pressure/volume recording. Aviat. Space environ. Med. 48: 308–310, 1977.
37. Barcroft H, Edholm OG: The effect of temperature on blood flow and deep temperature in the human forearm. J. Physiol. (Lond.) 102: 5–20, 1943.
38. Dahn I, Johnson B, Nilsen R: A plethysmographic method for determination of flow and volume pulsations in a limb. J. appl. Physiol. 28: 333–336, 1970.
39. Nilsen R: On the clinical use of pulse plethysmography of the calf. Scand. J. clin. Lab. Invest. 25: 391–412, 1970.
40. Kleinberg F, Newmann LL, Dong L, Phibbs RH: A volume displacement plethysmograph to measure limb blood flow in the newborn infant. Mayo Clin. Proc. 51: 430–432, 1976.
41. Dohn K: Plethysmographs usable during functional states recording volume changes in ml per 100 ml of extremity. Rep. Steno Mem. Hosp. (Copenh.) 147–168, 1956.
42. Graf K, Westersen A: Untersuchungen über Eigenschaften und Verwendungsmöglichkeiten eines flexibelen Extremitätenplethysmographen. Acta physiol. scand. 46: 1–18, 1959.
43. Barbey K, Barbey P: Ein neuer Plethysmograph zur Messung der Extremitätendurchblutung. Z. Kreislaufforsch. 52: 1129–1140, 1963.
44. Figar S: Some basic deficiencies of the plethysmographic method and possibilities of avoiding them. Angiology 10: 120–125, 1959.
45. Hyman C, Burnap D, Figar S: Bilateral differences in forearm blood flow as measured with capacitance plethysmograph. J. appl. Physiol. 18: 997–1002, 1963.
46. Fewings JD, Whelan RF: Differences in forearm blood flow measured by capacitance and volume plethysmography. J. appl. Physiol. 21: 334–340, 1966.
47. Wood JR, Hyman C: A direct reading capacitance plethysmograph. Med. biol. Eng. 8: 59–70, 1970.
48. Sigdell JE: A theoretical study of capacitance plethysmography, Med. biol. Eng. 9: 447–457, 1971.
49. Whitney RJ: The measurement of volume changes in human limbs. J. Physiol. (Lond.) 121: 1–27, 1953.
50. Brakkee AJM, Vendrik AJH: Strain gauge plethysmography; theoretical and practical notes on a new design. J. appl. Physiol. 21: 701–704, 1966.
51. Hallböök T, Mausson B, Nilsén R: Strain gauge plethysmograph with electrical calibration. Scand. J. clin. Lab. Invest. 25: 413–418, 1970.
52. Sigdell JE: Venous occlusion plethysmography, part 2. Biomed. Eng. 10: 342–345, 1975.
53. Mulz D, König E: Vergleichende plethysmographische Untersuchungen mit Luftplethysmographie, Quecksilber-plethysmographie und Venenverschluszrheographie. Z. Kardiol. 63: 358–374, 1974.
54. Barendsen GJ: Blood Flow in Human Extremities at Rest, After Arterial Occlusion and After Exercise, Thesis, University of Groningen, 1973.
55. Needham TN: The measurement of blood flow: strain gauge plethysmography. Biomed. Eng. 7: 266–269, 1972.

56. Paulev P, Nielsén SL, Neumann F, Keiding N: Strain gauge versus water plethysmography. Description of simplified systems and analysis of differences and accuracy. Med. biol. Eng. 12: 437–445, 1974.
57. Hokanson DE, Sumner DS, Strandness DE: An electrically calibrated plethysmograph for direct measurement of limb blood flow. I.E.E.E. Trans. biomed. Eng. 22: 25–29, 1975.
58. Youdin M, Reich T: Mercury in rubber (Whitney) strain gauge. Temperature compensation and analysis of error caused by temperature drift. Ann. biomed. Eng. 4: 220–231, 1976.
59. Nyboer J: Electrical Impedance Plethysmography, Springfield, Ill., Thomas. 1970.
60. Kaindl F, Polzer K, Schuhfried F: Rheographie, eine Methode zur Beurteilung peripherer Gefäsze, Darmstadt, Steinkopff, 1967.
61. Bonjer FH: Circulatieonderzoek door Impedantiemeting, Thesis, Groningen, Oppenheim, 1950.
62. Van den Berg Jw, Alberts AJ: Limitations of electric impedance plethysmography. Circulat. Res. 11: 333–339, 1954.
63. Kubicek, WG, Kottke FJ, Ramos MU, Patterson RP, Witsoe DA, Labree JW, Remole W, Layman TE, Schoening H, Garamela JT: The Minnesota impedance cardiograph-theory and applications. Biomed. Eng. 9: 410–416, 1974.
64. Hill RV, Jansen JC, Fling JL: Electric impedance plethysmography: a critical analysis. J. appl. Physiol. 22: 161–168, 1967.
65. Kinnen E: A defence of electrical impedance plethysmography. Med. res. Eng. 8: 6–8, 1969.
66. Gessert WL, Reid KA, Nyboer J: Reliability of tetrapolar electrical impedance plethysmography. Biomed. Sci., Instr. 5: 143–152, 1969.
67. Schreibman JG, Mott D, Naylor GP, Charlesworth D: Comparison of impedance and strain gauge plethysmography in the measurement of blood flow in the lower limb. Brit. J. Surg. 62: 909–912, 1975.
68. Brown BH, Pryce WIJ, Baumber D, Clarke RG: Impedance plethysmography: can it measure changes in limb blood flow? Med. biol. Eng. 13: 674–682, 1975.
69. Schreinicke G: Ein Beitrag zur Entstehung der Impedanzpulscurve (Rheogramm). Elektromedizin 13: 216–221, 1968.
70. Visser KR, Lamberts R, Korsten HHM, Zijlstra WG: Observations on blood flow related electrical impedance changes in rigid tubes. Pflügers Arch. ges. Physiol. 366: 289–291, 1976.
71. Visser KR, Lamberts R, Poelmann AM, Zijlstra WG: Origin of the impedance cardiogram investigated in the dog by exchange transfusion with a stroma-free haemoglobin solution. Pflügers Arch. ges. Physiol. 368: 169–171, 1977.
72 Woodcock JP: Plethysmography. Biomed. Eng. 9: 406–409, 1974.
73. Elings HS: Fotoelectrische Plethysmografie met Behulp van Diffuus Gereflecteerd Licht, Thesis, Groningen, V.R.B., 1959.
74. Hylkema BS: Tussen Polspalpatie en Aortografie, Thesis, Groningen, V.R.B., 1975.
75. Strandness DE: Peripheral Arterial Disease, London, Churchill, 1969.
76. Montgomery LD, Moody DL, Williams BA: An electrode system for tetrapolar electrical impedance plethysmography of the finger. I.E.E.E. Trans. biomed. Eng. 24: 385–386, 1977.
77. Fronek A, Coel M, Bernstein EF: The pulse-reappearance time: an index of overall blood flow impairment in the ischemic extremity. Surgery 81: 376–381, 1977.
78. Wouda AA: Raynaud's Phenomenon. Photoelectric plethysmography of the fingers of persons with and without Raynaud's Phenomenon during cooling and warming up. Acta med. scand. 201: 519–523, 1977.
79. Yamakoshi K, Togawa T, Ito H: Evaluation of the theory of cardiac output computation from transthoracic impedance plethysmogram. Med. biol. eng. Comp. 15: 479–488, 1977.
80. Secher NJ, Thomson A, Arusbo P: Measurement of rapid changes in cardiac stroke volume. An evaluation of the impedance cardiographic method. Acta anaesthesiol. scand. 21: 353–358, 1977.

81. Betz R, Bastanier CK, Mocellin R: Die Impedanzkardiographie als Methode zur quantitativen Bestimmung des Herzzeitvolumens? Vergleichende Messungen mit dem Fikschen Prinzip. Basic res. Card. 72: 46–56, 1977.

82. Brodie TG, Russel AE: On the determination of the rate of blood flow through an organ. J. Physiol. (Lond.) 32: 47–48P, 1905.

83. Landowne M, Katz LN: A critique of the plethysmographic method of measuring blood flow in the extremities of man. Amer. Heart J. 23: 644–675, 1942.

84. Ludbrook J, Collins GM: Venous occlusion pressure plethysmography in the human upper limb. Circulat. Res. 21: 139–147, 1967.

85. Bethge KP, de Caleya D, Barbey K: Methodische Aspekte zur pneumatischen Segmentplethysmographie. II: Das Problem der Staumanschettenbreite und des Staumanchettendrucks. Z. Kardiol. 64: 636–646, 1975.

86. Graf K, Rosell S: Der Effekt plethysmografischer Füllungsdrucke bis 20 cm H_2O auf die lokale Extremitätendurchblutung. Acta physiol. scand. 62: 323–335, 1964.

87. Eichna LW, Wilkins RW: Blood flow to the forearm and calf. II: Reactive hyperemia: Factors influencing the blood flow during vasodilation following ischemia. Bull. Johns Hopk. Hosp. 68: 450–458, 1941.

88. Patterson GC, Whelan RF: Reactive hyperemia in the human forearm. Clin. Sci. 14: 197–209, 1955.

89. Bollinger A, Barras JP, Mahler F: Measurement of foot artery blood pressure by micromanometry in normal subjects and in patients with arterial occlusive disease. Circulation 53: 506–512, 1976.

90. Greenflield ADM, Patterson GC: The effect of small degrees of venous distension on the apparent rate of blood flow to the forearm. J. Physiol. (Lond.) 125: 525–533, 1954.

91. Barendsen GJ, Van den Berg Jw: Venous pressure–volume relation and calf blood flow determined by changes in posture. Cardiovasc. Res. 10: 206–213, 1976.

92. Graf K: Zur Methodik der venösen Okklusionsplethysmographie. Die Wirkung distaler Gefaszokklusion auf die Durchblutung im Unterarm. Acta physiol. scand. 60: 70–89, 1964.

93. Ehringer H: Die reaktive Hyperämie nach arterieller Sperre. In: Messmethoden bei arteriellen Durchblutungsstörungen, Berlin, Huber, 1971, p. 20–33.

94. Greenfield ADM, Whitney RJ, Mowbary JD: Methods for the investigation of peripheral blood flow. Brit. med. Bull. 19: 101–109, 1963.

95. Barendsen GJ, Venema H, Van den Berg Jw: Semicontinuous blood flow measurements by triggered venous occlusion plethysmography. J. appl. Physiol. 31: 288–291, 1971.

96. Dahn I, Hallböök T: Simultaneous blood flow measurement by water and strain gauge plethysmography. Scand. J. clin. Lab. Invest. 25: 419–428, 1970.

97. Englund N, Hallböök T, Ling G: The validity of strain gauge plethysmography. Scand. J. clin. Lab. Invest. 29: 155–158, 1972.

98. Kitchin AH: Peripheral blood flow and capillary filtration rates. Brit. Med. Bull. 19: 155–160, 1963.

99. Van Schalm T: Plethysmographic Studies on Peripheral Circulation and Capillary Filtration of the Human Lower Leg. Thesis, Nijmegen, Giesbers, Haarsma, Tissen, 1973.

100. Celander O, Marild K: Regional circulation and capillary filtration in relation to capillary exchange in the foot and calf of newborn infants. Acta paediatr. 51: 385–400, 1962.

101. Bollinger A: Durchblutungsmessungen in der klinischen Angiologie. Bern, Huber, 1969.

102. Hillestad LK: The peripheral blood flow in intermittent claudication. Acta med. scand. 174: 23–45, 1963.

103. Strandell T, Wahren J: Circulation in the calf at rest, after arterial occlusion and after exercise in normal subjects and in patients with intermittent claudication. Acta med. scand. 173: 99–105, 1963.

104. Dahn I: On clinical use of venous occlusion plethysmography of calf. I: Methods and controls. Acta chir. scand. 130: 42–60, 1965.

105. Dahn I: On clinical use of venous occlusion plethysmography of calf. II: Results in patients with arterial disease. Acta chir. scand. 130: 61–75, 1975.

106. Gottstein K, Sedlmeyer I, Schöttler M: Quantitative Messungen der Unterschenkeldurchblutung von Gesunden und von Kranken mit peripheren Zirkulationsstörungen. Z. Kreislaufforsch. 58: 332–344, 1969.

107. Hallböök T: Blood flow measurements with strain gauge plethysmography in early postoperative course after reconstructive arterial surgery of lower limb. Acta chir. scand. 137: 233–242, 1971.

108. Lorentsen E: Blood pressure and flow in the calf in relation to claudication distance. Scand. J. clin. Lab. Invest. 31: 141–146, 1973.

109. Hillestad LK: The peripheral blood flow in intermittent claudication. VI: Plethysmographic studies. The blood flow response to exercise with arrested and with free circulation. Acta med. scand. 174: 671–685, 1963.

110. Isacsson SO: Venous occlusion plethysmography in 55-year-old men. A population study in Malmö, Sweden. Acta med. scand. Suppl. 537, 1972.

111. Mörl H: The special hemodynamics and metabolism in severe disturbances of peripheral blood flow and their treatment. Atherosclerosis 26: 617–627, 1977.

112. Romanovska L, Prerovsky I, Stribrna I: Blood flow and vascular resistance in lower limbs in hypertensives at rest and at reactive hyperemia. Cor Vasa 19: 61–65, 1977.

113. Barcroft H, Dornhorst AC: The blood flow through the human calf during rhythmic exercise J. Physiol. (Lond.) 109: 402–411, 1949.

114. Tonnesen KH: Muscle blood flow during exercise in intermittent claudication. Circulation 37: 402–410, 1968.

115. Jacobs S, Reich T: Calf blood flow in intermittent claudication, Arch. Surg. 110: 1465–1468, 1975.

116. Lassen NA, Kampp M: Calf muscle blood flow during walking studied by the Xe^{133} method in normals and in patients with intermittent claudication. Scand. J. clin. Lab. Invest. 17: 447–453, 1965.

117. Tonnesen KH: Blood flow through muscle during rhythmic contraction measured by [133]Xenon. Scand. J. clin. Lab. Invest. 16: 646–654, 1964.

118. Clausen JP, Lassen NA: Muscle blood flow during exercise in normal man studied by the [133]Xenon clearance method. Cardiovasc. Res. 5: 245–254, 1971.

119. Wahren J, Jorfeldt L: Determination of leg blood flow during exercise in man: an indicator-dilution technique based on femoral venous dye infusion. Clin. Sci. molec. Med. 45: 135–146, 1973.

120. Hlavová A, Linhart J, Prerovsky I, Ganz V, Fronek A: Leg blood flow at rest during and after exercise in normal subjects and in patients with femoral artery occlusion. Clin. Sci. 29: 555–564, 1965.

121. Sorlie D, Myhre K: Determination of lower leg blood flow in man by thermodilution. Scand. J. clin. Lab. Invest. 37: 117–124, 1977.

122. Folkow B, Haglund U, Jodel M, Lundgren O: Blood flow in calf muscle of man during heavy rhythmic exercise. Acta physiol. scand. 81: 157–163, 1971.

123. Bonde-Petersen F, Mork AL, Nielsen E: Local muscle blood flow and sustained contraction of human arm and back muscles. Europ. J. appl. Physiol. 34: 43–50, 1975.

124. Kilbom A, Brundin T: Circulatory effects of isometric muscle contractions, performed separately and in combination with dynamic exercise. Europ. J. appl. Physiol. 36: 7–17, 1976.

125. Riendl AM, Gotshall RW, Reinke JA, Smith JJ: Cardiovascular response of human subjects to isometric contraction of large and small muscle groups. Proc. Soc. exp. biol. Med. 154: 171–174, 1977.

126. Hudlicka O: Muscle Blood Flow. Its Relation to Muscle Metabolism and Function, Amsterdam, Swets and Zeitlinger, 1973.

127. Shepherd JT: The blood flow through the calf after exercise in subjects with arteriosclerosis and claudication. Clin. Sci. 9: 49–58, 1950.

128. Siggaard-Andersen J: Obliterative vascular disease. Classification by means of a Dahn plethysmograph. Acta chir. scand. 130: 190–198, 1965.

129. Ehringer, Denck H, Deutch E: Quantitative Durchblutungsmessung zur Objektivierung des Therapie-erfolges nach Gefäszoperationen. Dtsch. med. Wschr. 92: 600–608, 1967.

3. Isotope techniques

N.A. LASSEN AND P. HOLSTEIN

Commentary by P. Puel

1. INTRODUCTION

Radioisotopes have been used routinely for the evaluation of patients with occlusive arterial disease in our hospital for many years. The tests employed, i.e., mainly measurement of muscle blood flow, skin blood flow and skin perfusion pressure are based upon Kety's 'local clearance method' (1). This principle is based upon the use of tracers that diffuse so freely between the tissue and the capillary blood that the washout of the tracer is determined by the local blood flow. Tracers such as the inert gas ^{133}xenon and antipyrine labeled with ^{125}iodine or ^{131}iodine can 'follow' even high rates of blood flow (flow limitated tracers). Other tracers such as ^{24}sodium and ^{99m}technetium (e.g., as pertechnetate) pass more slowly across the capillary membrane (partially diffusion-limited tracers), but they may still be useful at the lower blood flow rates which exist in low tissues (see below).

During the last years, measurement of muscle blood flow and skin blood flow by radioisotopes has been used only occasionally (see Chapter 11). These tests arc now replaced by measurement of ankle and toe blood pressure by the strain gauge technique. It is the skin perfusion pressure (SPP), or skin blood pressure, that we now measure by radioactive tracers. This parameter is used practically exclusively for the determination of the safe level of major leg amputation.

2. THE TECHNIQUE OF DETERMINING THE SKIN PERFUSION PRESSURE

The principle introduced in 1967 (2, 3) is the local clearance method in disguise. The SPP is determined as the external pressure which just suffices to arrest the washout of a locally injected tracer.

We use ^{99m}pertechnetate, ^{131}iodine, or 4-iodo-antipyrine labeled with

COMMENTARY

This technique must be carried out strictly according to the recommended protocol in order to minimize the possibility of undesirable and often uncontrollable effects on the local blood flow, which include the following: (a) injection puncture traumatism. (b) Changes in vasoconstrictor tonicity, especially in the distal parts of the limb and which can be caused by any physical changes or emotional upset. (c) Venous return flow which reacts to the slightest changes in position. (d) The filling of subcutaneous tissue (gravitational edema) or dehydration brought on by the diuretic drugs or denutrition.

[131]iodine or [125]iodine dissolved in sterile water at a concentration of about 0.1–0.2 mCi/ml. Histamine is always mixed with the radioactive solution so that the injectate contains $50\mu g/0.1$ ml. This results in vasodilatation of the skin and minimizes the influence of temperature-induced spontaneous variations in skin blood flow. [133]Xenon is not practical owing to diffusion of this tracer into the subcutaneous adipose tissue, in which it has a high solubility.

About 0.1 ml of the tracer–histamine mixture is injected intradermally so that a small weal is raised. Counterpressure is obtained by placing a conventional arm blood pressure cuff so that it covers the depot. In order to measure the local pressure over the injected skin area even more precisely, we employ in addition a 12 cm × 12 cm (inflatable part 11 cm by 11 cm) thin-walled plastic bag that is interposed between the depot and the blood pressure cuff. The bag is filled with a small amount of air and connected to a manometer (Fig. 1). It is this manometer and none connected to the outer cuff that we employ. The small plastic bag overlies the

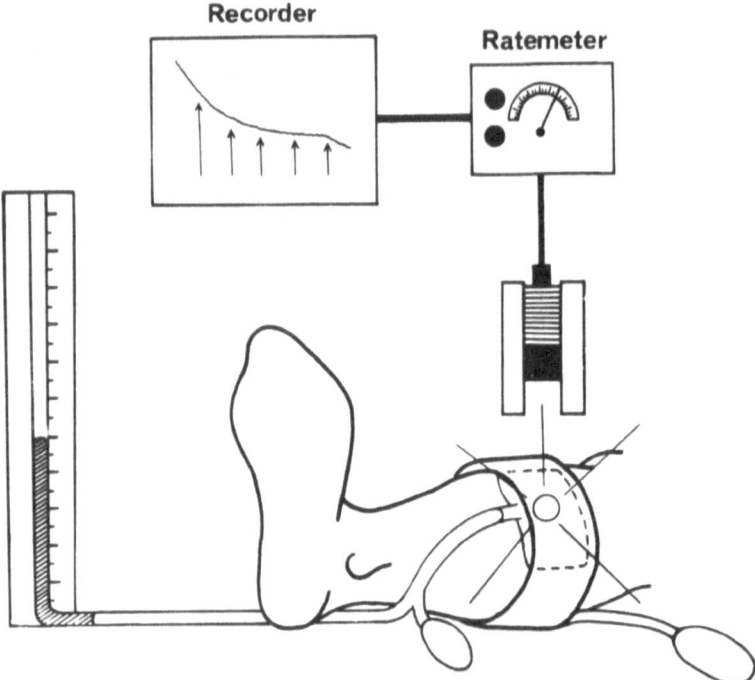

Fig. 1. Measurement of skin perfusion pressure (SPP) on the calf by washout cessation external pressure. The local clearance from an intradermal isotope–histamine depot is recorded by conventional equipment. External pressure to the labeled skin is applied with a blood pressure cuff and measured with an air-filled plastic cushion between the skin and the cuff coupled to a mercury manometer.

injected skin area smoothly (without wrinkles) even where the surface is irregular, as on the foot.

A scintillation detector is placed over the blood pressure cuff at a distance of about 10 cm from the depot, and the clearance is recorded semilogarithmically. When a constant clearance (a descending straight line) has been observed for about 3 min with no counterpressure applied, then this pressure is raised stepwise, resulting in a stepwise decrease in isotope washout rate (Fig. 2). In order to determine the pressure at which the clearance stops, it is necessary at the highest pressure steps (made at intervals of 5 mm Hg) to observe the curve for about 5 min at each step. The SPP is taken to be the pressure midway between the highest pressure at which flow still can be discerned and the pressure level above this at which flow cessation is observed.

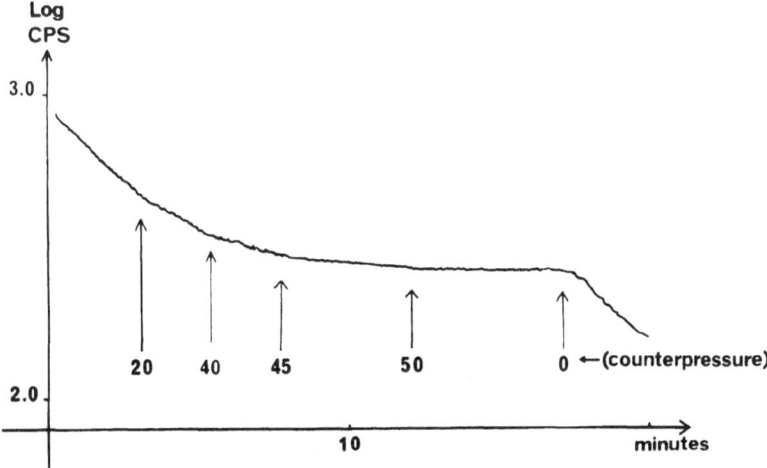

Fig. 2. The local washout from an intradermal depot of ^{131}I-antipyrine mixed with histamine during stepwise increasing external counter pressure. Washout cessation occurs at an external pressure of 50 mm Hg. Skin perfusion pressure = 48 mm Hg.

The most important source of error is movement artifact. The leg must be kept immobile at a constant distance from the detector, and this demands proper fixation of the leg. We use sandbags and analgetics, which in practically all cases are given intravenously (Demerol 35 mg in repeated doses). Another source of error that is related to movement artifact is seen when the skin is edematous. Then the external compression, by displacing the tissue fluid, will cause the skin to move away from the detector. Therefore, in case of edema, the swelling should be squeezed away by applying a pressure of about 40–80 mm Hg for some 5 min prior to the study.

The room temperature should be 'thermoneutral' (about 25 °C), so that the patient feels comfortable with light clothing and the skin temperature is warm (about 28–32 °C). Arm blood pressure should always be taken simultaneously. We block the thyroid by 0.5 g of potassium iodide before injecting iodine-containing tracers.

The sites of measurements, i.e., where the isotope–histamine depot is injected intracutaneously, have been standardized. For evaluating the circulation of the foot, we inject the solution on the dorsal surface, approximately midway between the base of the digits and the ankle joint. In determining the level of major leg amputations, the depot is injected on the anterolateral part of the calf 10 cm distal to the knee joint, i.e., just superficial to the proximal attachment of the anterior tibial muscle. If the result of this measurement demonstrates that a distal or a blow-knee amputation cannot be performed, we measure the SPP on the thigh on the anterolateral surface. Sometimes measurements are made at more than one level, e.g., 10, 20, and 30 cm above the knee joint.

However, in most cases the situation is sufficiently elucidated by one measurement, i.e., at the standard site 10 cm below the knee. A total mapping out of the limb is only occasionally required.

In the event that amputation of the extremity of the foot is considered, one would be wise to measure blood flow in the sole, from which the covering strip will be created.

This measurement is of utmost importance, since the result is pivotal in deciding whether the amputation is to be above or below the knee.

3. CLINICAL USE OF SKIN PERFUSION PRESSURE

In normal individuals, the external pressure on the skin that results in flow cessation lies just slightly above the diastolic blood pressure (4) when measured at heart level (Fig. 3). In patients with occlusive arterial disease, the SPP decreases if the arterial narrowing is severe enough to cause a decrease in the local diastolic blood pressure. In many claudicants, when measured at rest only, the systolic peak is reduced distal to the arterial lesion, whereas the diastolic blood pressure remains practically unchanged. This implies that measurement of the SPP cannot be employed as a diagnostic test. It is primarily a method of measuring the local circulatory condition in the most severe cases, that is, cases of manifest or impending gangrene. The clinical value of the SPP is that healing of wounds in ischemic areas is closely related to this parameter (5, 6).

Is it the mean flow pressure, or the residual pressure below the point of blockage?

In a series of 60 below-knee amputations (Fig. 4) this correlation is apparent (7). Out of 8 cases with SPP below 20 mm Hg, no less than 6 (75%) failed to heal, requiring reamputation at above-knee level. Out of 12 cases with SPP between 20 and 30 mm Hg, 4 cases (33%) failed to heal and out of 40 cases with SPP above 30 mm Hg, only 4 cases (10%) failed to heal. The difference in failure rate is highly significant ($p < 0.01$). Also, in the 30 nondiabetic cases the differences in healing rates were significantly correlated to the level of SPP ($p < 0.05$), but in the 30 diabetic cases no correlation to the SPP was found (see Fig. 4), and there were only 4

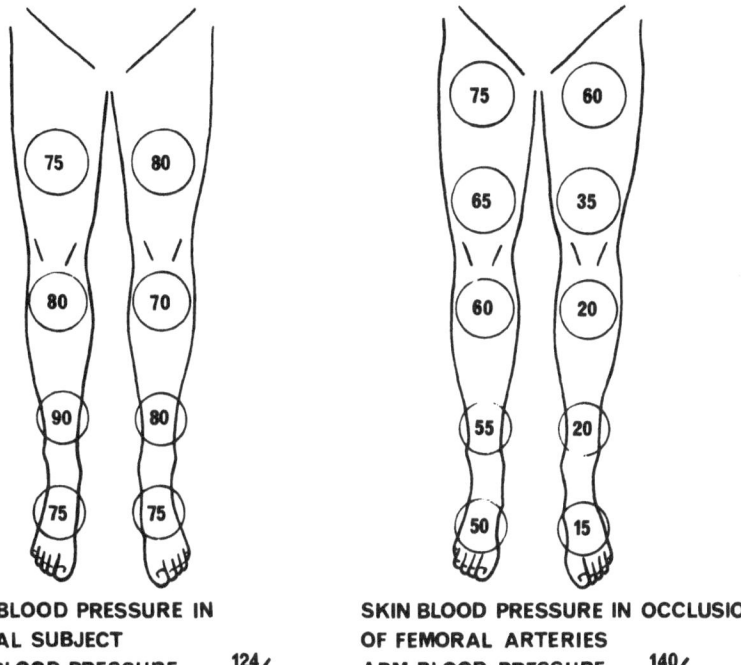

SKIN BLOOD PRESSURE IN NORMAL SUBJECT
ARM BLOOD PRESSURE $^{124}/_{74}$

SKIN BLOOD PRESSURE IN OCCLUSION OF FEMORAL ARTERIES
ARM BLOOD PRESSURE $^{140}/_{75}$

Fig. 3. Skin perfusion pressure (skin blood pressure) measured on both legs in a normal subject at various levels (left) and in a patient with arterial occlusive disease (right). In the patient's right leg there is an occlusion of the superficial femoral artery. In the left leg, there is an occlusion of both the superficial and the deep femoral arteries. Gangrene of the toes on the left leg was present.

failures in this group compared to 10 failures in the nondiabetic group $(0.05 < p < 0.10)$. These findings should be seen against the difference in distribution of SPP in the two groups. The SPP averaged 33.7 mm Hg (range 8–68 mm Hg) in the nondiabetic group and 56.7 mm Hg (range 18–93 mm Hg) in the diabetic group $(p < 0.001)$, and there were only 6 cases in the diabetic group with a SPP of below 30 mm Hg.

In the majority of these cases the amputation was carried out with the conventional technique using an anterior and a posterior flap. Recent experiences with the sagittal technique, as well as the technique where a long posterior flap is employed, have shown the same correlation.

It should be emphasized that an adequate SPP is by no means a guarantee against failures. Infection and hematoma may destroy the result even if the perfusion pressure is normal. Extensive skin necroses may be caused by infection without the presence of major arterial occlusion. This situation is often misjudged, because ischemic skin necrosis is so frequent in amputation surgery. Measurement of the SPP is very valuable in this

Can't the difference between the average SPP values of the 2 groups be explained by the topography of the lesions? Don't diabetic patients tend to have blockage of the vessels distally? Lumbar sympathectomy may have an effect on the SPP; in which way?

situation because the prognosis of the stump can be determined when minor wound necrosis appears. Of course, extreme efforts to eliminate edema must be undertaken before injection of the tracer solution. Occasionally, the measurement should be the usual 10 cm distal to the knee joint. If measurements are performed more proximally, for example at the level of the knee joint, the pressure values will not be representative of the prognosis of the below-knee stump.

We have presented the preoperative measurements of SPP that yield a fairly good prognostic index; but we are well aware that variations in SPP may occur along the line of a planned amputation. In low pressure regions, the trauma of operation and especially that of tight bandages may cause

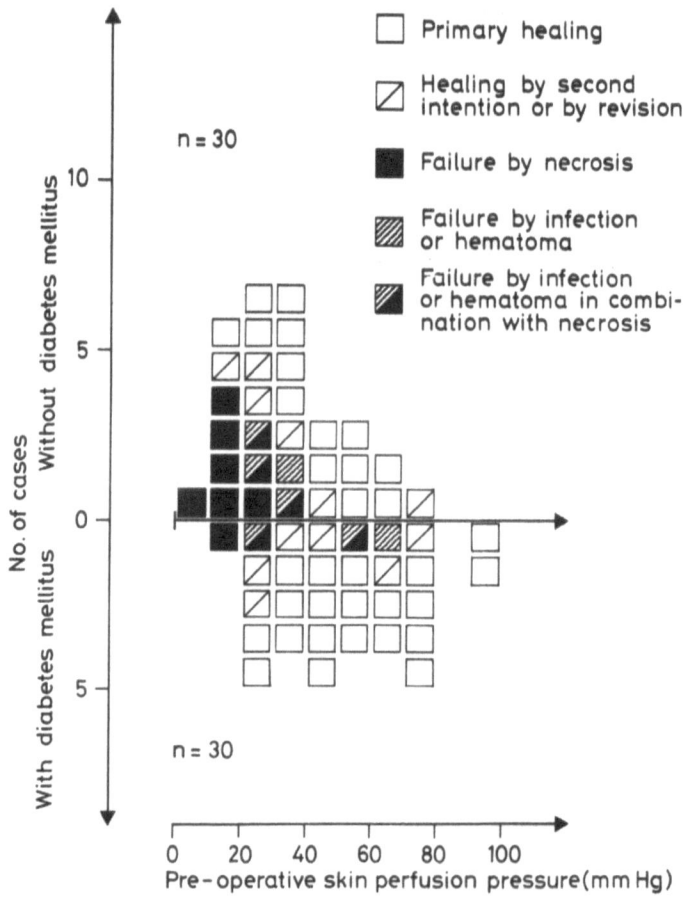

Fig. 4. Results in 60 below-knee amputations correlated to the skin perfusion pressure.

necrosis of extensive areas of skin. But postoperative measurements have also shown that the SPP may increase. Such an amelioration may be caused by an increase in systemic blood pressure or by an improvement of the arterial pathway. Such phenomena are difficult to anticipate. Moreover, an increase in the distal blood pressure may also be due to the hemodynamic effect of the amputation itself. According to simple physical principles (Poiseuille), an elimination of a major part of the low pressure area will result in an increase of the driving pressure distal to the arterial narrowing. As shown in Fig. 5 this increase in pressure, however, takes place in most cases when the SPP is above 20 mm Hg, i.e., when the prognosis is already good. This effect does not subsequently influence the chance of healing significantly. It should also be noted that the standard technique of measuring pressure with radioisotopes entails an element of

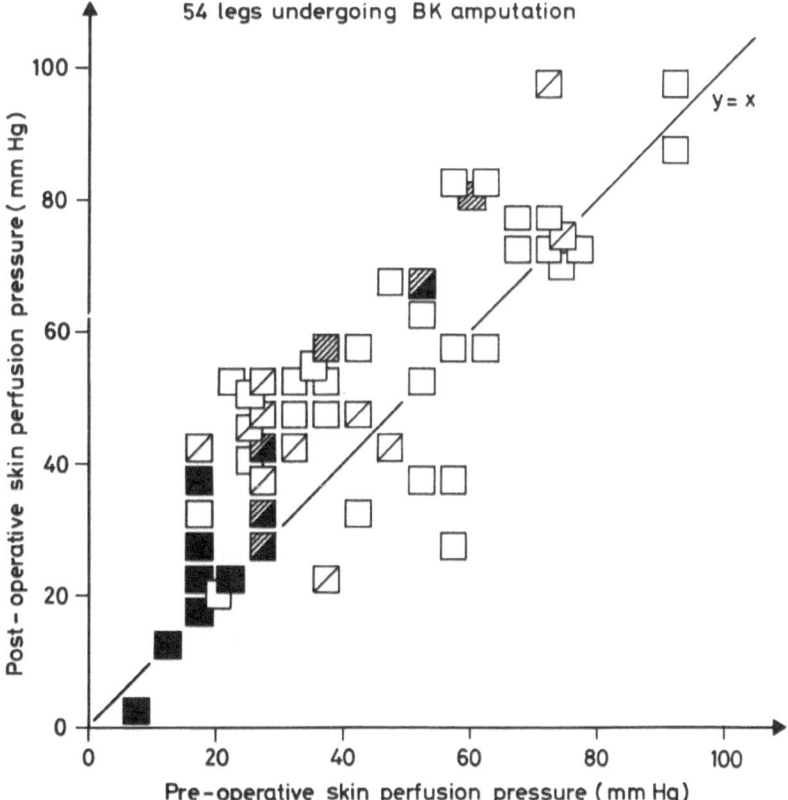

Fig. 5. The preoperative skin perfusion pressure compared to the postoperative skin perfusion pressure measured 4–8 weeks after surgery in 54 legs undergoing below-knee amputation.

pseudoamputation, because the cuff encircling the limb reduces the flow.

The prognostic figures as outlined for below-knee amputations are similar in above-knee amputations in which a preoperative SPP of below 30 Hg is predictive of ischemic wound complications (8). The consequences of such complications are, however, different from the reamputation necessary in the ischemic below-knee stump. In the above-knee stump the ischemic ulcer may heal over perhaps several months because the vast amount of soft tissues allows diminution of ischemic wounds by scar retraction. On the other hand the ischemia may also show as a major breakdown of the stump, a life-threatening condition in a weak patient.

In minor distal amputations the SPP measured on the dorsal side of the foot is of prognostic value. However, one must take into account that, especially on the foot, infections may destroy the tissues in spite of adequate circulation. On the other hand spontaneous remissions in circular condition may be even dramatic on the foot (9), and thus a low SPP may change to an adequate SPP over a period of a few months. This will influence the prognosis of skin lesions such as amputation wounds.

4.   WHY USE RADIOISOTOPES?

As mentioned previously, we use radioisotopes practically only in the determination of the safe level of amputation. Strain gauges for distal blood pressure recording are used for assessing the diagnosis and the prognosis of the leg (10) and the pre- and postoperative control of vascular arterial reconstruction (11), as well as to control the results of medical therapy (10). Having discovered the simplicity, accuracy and efficacy of this method, it is cumbersome to go on with a slow method such as the isotope washout technique. Both methods were, however, at hand when we started studies on amputation. However, strain gauge measurements on the calf for determining amputation level were soon given up, because good plethysmographic curves could not be obtained at low pressures and because sclerosis of the arteries occasionally caused the measured pressures to be extremely high, viz., the cuff pressure was not transmitted properly to the interior of the arteries.

We are eager to abandon the isotope washout technique. Local injections in low pressure tissues are not attractive and the lengthy time of compression causes pain and discomfort. Photo-electric recording of skin perfusion pressure is rapid, but it cannot be applied to all patients and a very careful selection of the skin area studied is necessary (12). At the present time, other methods, such as Doppler ultrasound and skin blood flow measurement, by heat clearance or isotopes, are being investigated

(13–16) and comparative studies must decide which method is the best. Our preliminary experience with some of these methods has not been encouraging. Transcutaneous oxygen tension measurements appear at the moment most promising. Other principles may be employed and we here make a plea to medicotechnicians to develop rapid and sensitive non-invasive techniques to measure the circulation in the skin at levels close to zero. Meanwhile we continue with the somewhat tedious isotope method. To be without skin perfusion pressure measurements is not acceptable in clinical routine.

REFERENCES TO MAIN TEXT

1. Kety SA: Measurement of regional circulation by the local clearance of radioactive sodium. Amer. Heart. J. 38: 321, 1949.
2. Dahn I, Lassen NA, Westling H: Blood flow in human muscles during external pressure or venous stasis. Clin. Sci. 32: 467, 1967.
3. Nilsén R, Dahn I, Lassen NA, Westling H: On the estimation of local effective perfusion pressure in patients with obliterative arterial disease by means of external compression over a Xenon-133 depot. Scand. J. clin. Lab. Invest. 19 (Suppl. 99): 29, 1967.
4. Holstein P, Lund P, Larsen B, Schomacker T: Skin perfusion pressure measured as the external pressure required to stop isotope washout. Methodological considerations and normal values on the legs. Scand. J. clin. Lab. Invest. 37: 649, 1977.
5. Holstein P, Lassen NA: Assessment of safe level of amputation by measurement of skin blood pressure. In: Vascular Surgery, Philadelphia, London, Toronto, Saunders, 1977, p 105.
6. Lassen NA, Holstein P: Use of radio-isotopes in assessment of distal blood flow and distal blood pressure in arterial insufficiency. Surg. Clin. N. Amer. 54: 39, 1974.
7. Holstein P, Sager P, Lassen NA: Wound healing in below knee amputations in relation to skin perfusion pressure. Acta orthop. scand., submitted for publication.
8. Holstein P, Dovey H, Lassen NA: Wound healing in above knee amputations in relation to skin perfusion pressure. Acta orthop. scand., submitted for publication.
9. Holstein P, Lassen NA: Transitory ischemia of the lower limbs. Surgery, submitted for publication.
10. Holstein P, Krähenbühl B, Lassen NA: Induzierte Hypertonie in der Behandlung peripherer arterieller Krankheit. In: Hypertonie. Risikofaktor in der Angiologie, Baden-Baden, Brüssel, Köln, Witzstroch, 1976, p 157.
11. Noer I, Tønnesen KH, Sager P: Preoperative estimation of run-off in patients with multiple level arterial obstructions as a guide to partial reconstructive surgery. Arch. Surg., accepted for publication.
12. Holstein P, Nielsen PE, Barras J-P: Blood flow cessation at external pressure in the skin in normal human limbs. Photoelectric recordings compared to isotope washout and to local intra-arterial blood pressure. Microvasc. Res., accepted for publication.
13. Barnes RW, Shanik GD, Slaymaker EE: An index of healing in below-knee amputation: Leg blood pressure by Doppler ultrasound. Surgery 79: 13, 1976.
14. Kostuik JP, Wood D, Hornby R, Feingold S, Mathews V: The measurement of skin blood flow in peripheral vascular disease by epicutaneous application of Xenon^{133}. J. Bone Jt. Surg. 58-A: 833, 1976.
15. Moore WS: Determination of amputation level. Measurement of skin blood flow with Xenon^{133}. Arch. Surg. 107: 798, 1973.
16. Raines JK, Darling RC, Buth J, Brewster DC, Austen WG: Vascular laboratory criteria for the management of peripheral vascular disease of the lower extremities. Surgery 79: 21, 1976.

4. Doppler ultrasound arterial scanning

DERMOT E. FITZGERALD

Commentary by R.W. Barnes

1. INTRODUCTION

The purpose of this chapter is to describe some of the information which can be obtained by using continuous-wave Doppler ultrasound to examine the peripheral arteries in man. The use of these instruments in the examination of peripheral veins and the measurement of segmental blood pressure in the limbs is described in other chapters. In this chapter some space is given to description of clinical techniques of examination to assist those to whom the methods may be unfamiliar and also to point out some of the sources of error which may produce poor results when using Doppler ultrasound. There is a growing ill-informed opinion that Doppler ultrasound instruments are simply rather sophisticated acoustical instruments with greater sensitivity than the traditional clinical stethescope. This opinion is manifestly incorrect and can only be expressed as a result of a lack of knowledge. The descriptions which follow below attempt to show the type and range of information that is available from Doppler ultrasound scanning from the clinician's point of view. Undoubtedly the instrumentation and the techniques are in the relatively early stages of development and as interest in this area builds up much refinement will occur. The Doppler system has been the Cinderella of clinical ultrasound.

2. BASIC PHYSICS

Sound is a mechanical energy form which travels as a wave through a material by means of physical vibration of the particles of that material (Fig. 1). The speed at which the sound travels depends on the characteristics of the material only. A sound wave may be generated with a piezoelectric crystal. When an alternating voltage is placed between the opposite faces of a disc of such a crystal, its thickness is caused to vary in step with the voltage as shown in Fig. 2. The vibration of the crystal causes the particles of the material in contact with it to vibrate and in this way the sound wave is created.

The frequency of the sound is determined by the frequency of the alternating voltage used to generate it. Frequencies in the range from 15

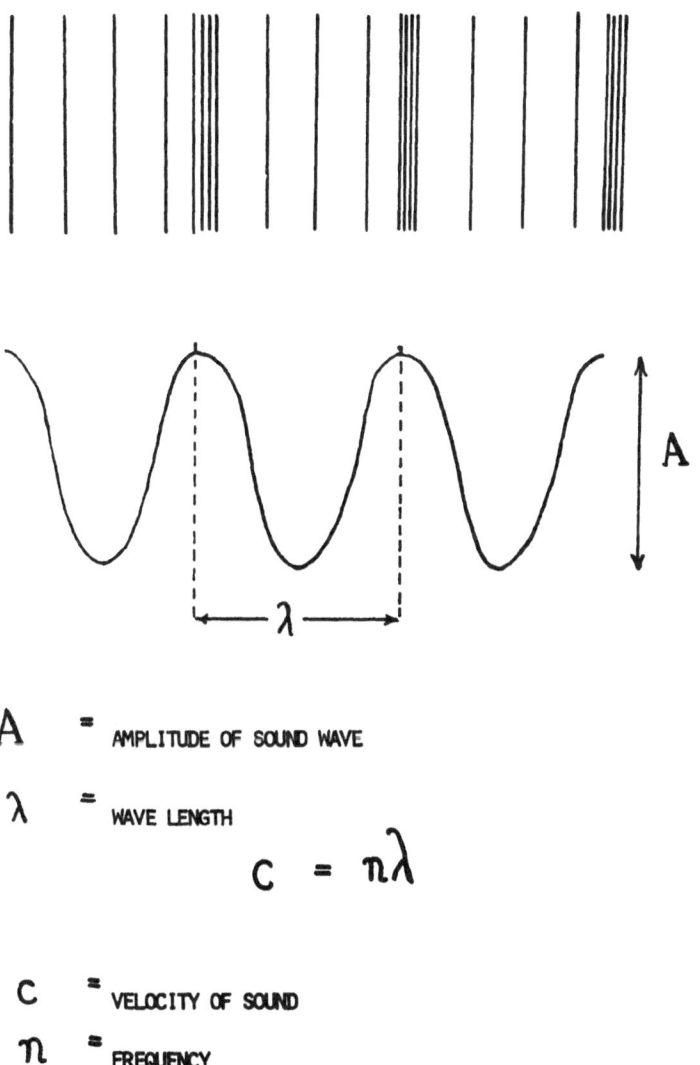

A $=$ AMPLITUDE OF SOUND WAVE

λ $=$ WAVE LENGTH

$$C = n\lambda$$

C $=$ VELOCITY OF SOUND

n $=$ FREQUENCY

Fig. 1. Definition of ultrasound.

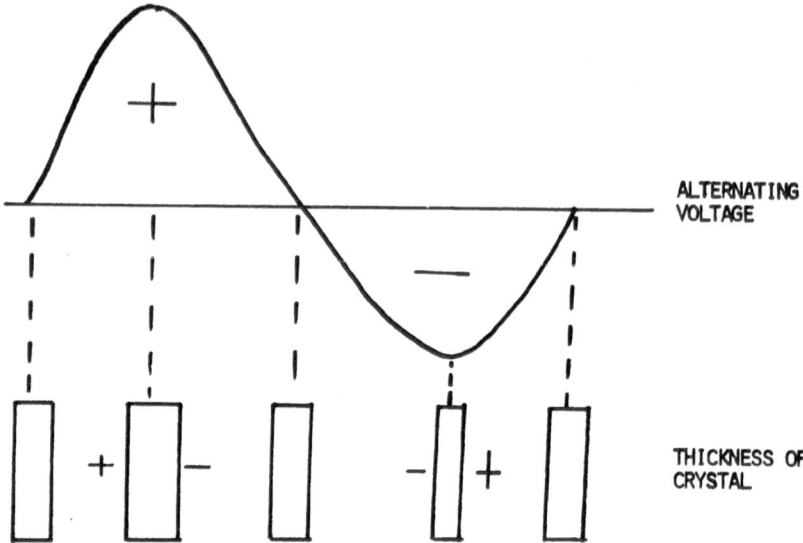

Fig. 2. The piezo-electric effect.

Hz to 20 kHz are audible to the human ear. Sound of frequency greater than 20 kHz is referred to as ultrasound. Clinical ultrasound techniques use frequencies mainly in the range 1–10 MHz.

Diagnostic ultrasound is divided into two separate techniques based on two fundamentally different principles: pulse echo imaging and Doppler shift motion detection (Fig. 3).

The pulse echo techniques are based, like sonar, on measuring the time delay between transmission of a brief pulse of sound and reception of an echo reflected from some remote structure (Fig. 4). The time delay is a measure of the distance to the echoing structure; A-, time/position-, B- and real-time B-scanning are all different modes of display of pulse echo time delay data.

Doppler shift methods are based on the fact that if the reflecting object is moving along the same direction as the beam of ultrasound, the frequency of the reflected wave is shifted from the frequency originally transmitted (Fig. 5). The magnitude of this frequency shift (Δf) is proportional to the velocity of the moving object (v) thus:

$$\Delta f = \pm \frac{2fv \cos \theta}{c}$$

where c is the velocity of propagation of ultrasound and θ is the angle between the direction of travel of the ultrasound beam and the direction of movement of the reflecting structure.

The instrument used most often for clinical Doppler shift studies is

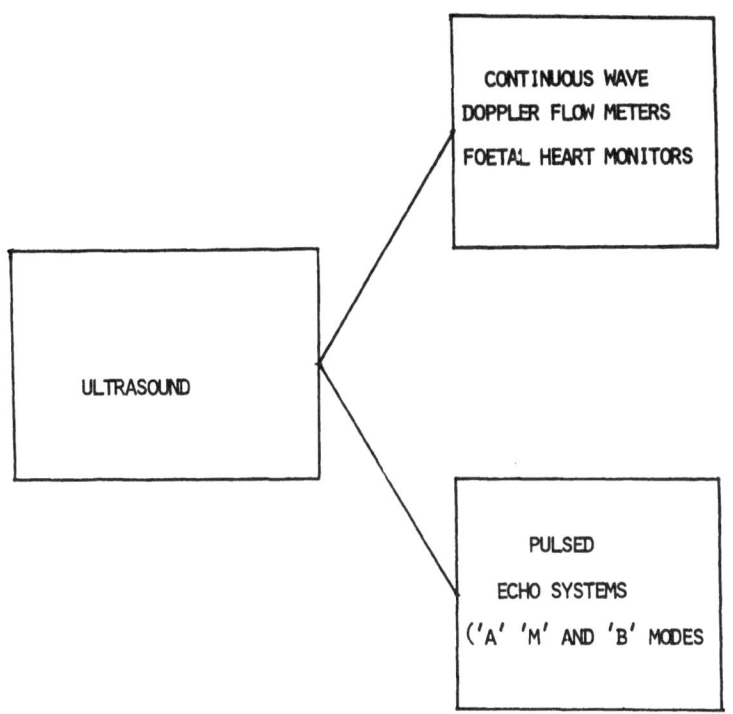

Fig. 3. Clinical ultrasound systems.

shown schematically in Fig. 5. The probe consists of two piezo-electric crystals, one serving as transmitter and the other as receiver. There are many different designs of probe incorporating a variety of geometrical arrangements (1).

In operation the transmitter is continuously driven at a constant frequency by an alternating voltage generated by the oscillator. Reflected ultrasound is accepted by the receiver crystal and converted to electrical voltage. The receiver circuiting in the instrument operates on this electrical voltage to extract from it any components of frequencies different from the original transmitted frequency. Electrical signals are thus generated of frequencies equal to the Doppler shift.

Thus, if the reflecting structure were moving with constant velocity, v, in the ultrasound beam, there would be a single Doppler shift frequency and the output signal would be a pure tone, i.e., single frequency. But if the reflecting structures possess a variety of velocities then the output signal will consist of a mixture of tones. This is the case when the reflecting objects are the red blood cells. The actual mixture of tones – the frequencies present as well as their relative strengths – is dependent on the distribution

COMMENTARY

The diagram of Fig. 5 portrays the Doppler ultrasound beam intercepting the blood vessel at nearly right angles to the path of blood flow. In practice the optimal Doppler frequency shift resulting from blood flow occurs when the sound beam intercepts the blood vessel at approximately 45° with the axis of flow. Obviously the greatest frequency shift theoretically occurs when the Doppler ultrasound beam is in the axis of blood flow. However, to achieve such conditions the Doppler probe would be nearly parallel with the skin and the great distance from the point of skin contact to the point of interception of the blood vessel would result in marked attenuation of ultrasound by the tissues. In clinical practice an angle of the Doppler probe with the skin of approximately 45° provides the optimal frequency shift, although an angle of 30–60° is satisfactory.

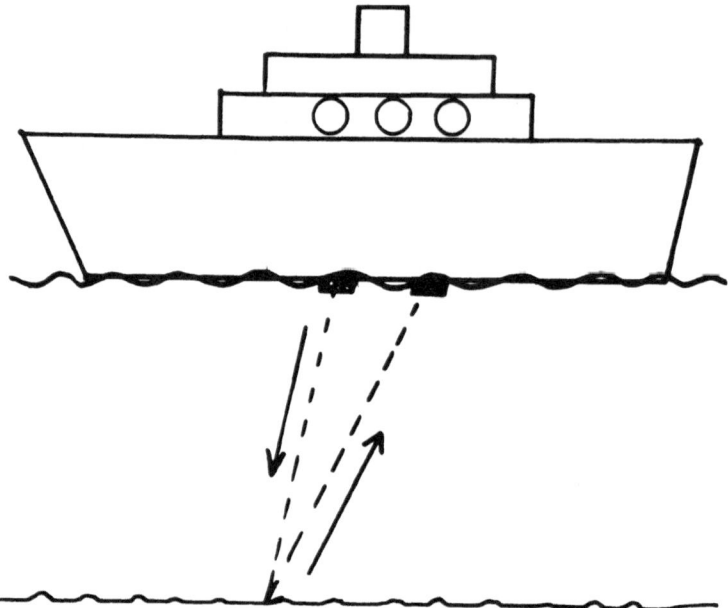

Fig. 4. Sonar depth sounding: a pulse ultrasound beam is transmitted from the ship and reflected from the sea bed back to the ship. The time taken for this to occur indicates the distance between the ship and the sea bed.

of red blood cell velocities present in the ultrasound beam and determines the quality of the output signal. When the transmitted frequency is 5 MHz or 10 MHz the range of Doppler shift frequencies obtained from the blood in the human circulation falls in the audible range of frequencies. Thus the output signal (Fig. 6) is very commonly applied to earphones or loud-speakers for auditory analysis. It may also be quite conveniently tape-recorded for later examination and detailed analysis.

The most thorough analysis of this signal now possible is a spectrum analysis: the decomposition of the signal into the pure frequency components and the measurement of the strengths of those components. If the Doppler shift signals originate from blood flow in the circulation, these components vary throughout the cardiac cycle. From each instant in the cycle to the next, the spectrum will vary.

Conventionally the Doppler shift spectrum is displayed on the 'sonagram' (Fig. 7) where the x-axis is the time axis, along the y-axis is plotted the Doppler shift frequency and the optical density of the display is proportional to the strength of the tone at each instant. Thus the 'sonagram' gives a qualitative spectrum analysis of the blood flow Doppler shift signal.

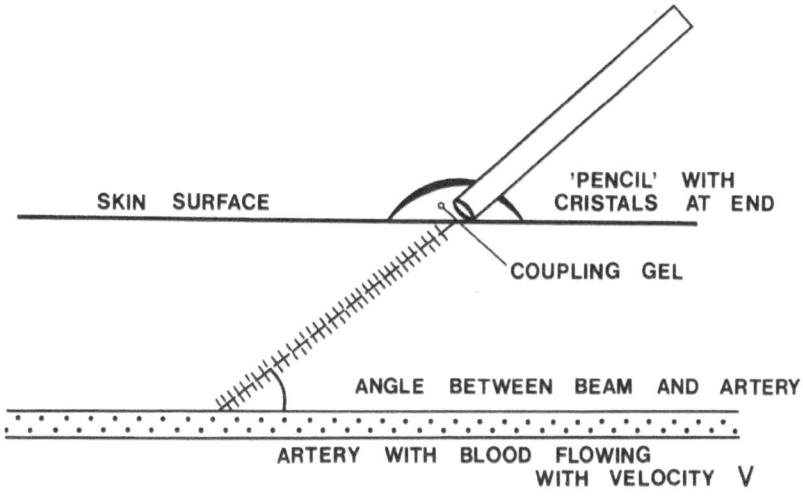

SKIN   SURFACE

'PENCIL'   WITH
CRISTALS   AT   END

COUPLING   GEL

ANGLE   BETWEEN   BEAM   AND   ARTERY

ARTERY   WITH   BLOOD   FLOWING
WITH   VELOCITY   V

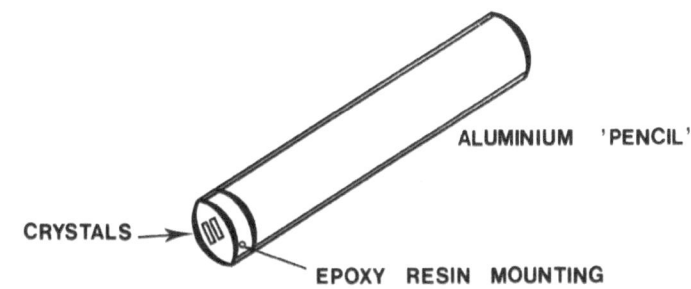

ALUMINIUM   'PENCIL'

CRYSTALS

EPOXY   RESIN   MOUNTING

Fig. 5. Diagrammatic representation of the Doppler ultrasound system (see text).

The 'sonagram' is most usually derived from tape-recorded signals and so might be more accurately described as a pseudo-real time spectrum analysis. All of the 'sonagrams' used in this chapter were obtained in this way. Real time spectrum analysis is also possible but the instrumentation required is more expensive. Often the full spectrum analysis is not required but only the maximum Doppler shift frequency at each instant during the cardiac cycle. i.e., the envelope of the 'sonagram'. Circuits to measure and temporarily hold the maximum Doppler shift frequency are usually incorporated into the Doppler instrument. The most common such circuit is the zero crossing detector. Such circuits can give erroneous results due to the electronic noise and interference and therefore phase-lock loop detectors are coming more into use for this application. The output from such a circuit would be as shown (Fig. 8). During the cardiac cycle there is an initial period of predominantly forward flow, followed by predominantly reverse flow. Some Doppler shift instruments are not capable of dis-

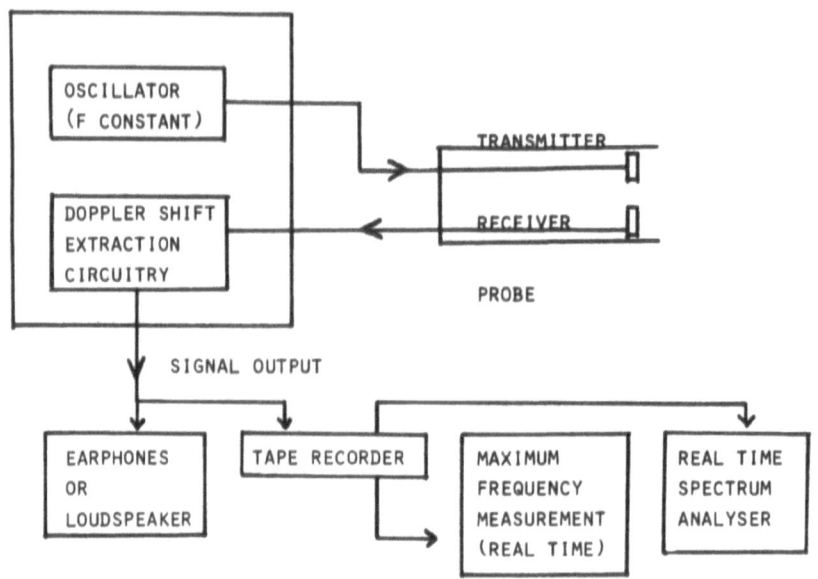

Fig. 6. Block diagram of the Doppler ultrasound system including alternative ways of processing the signal output.

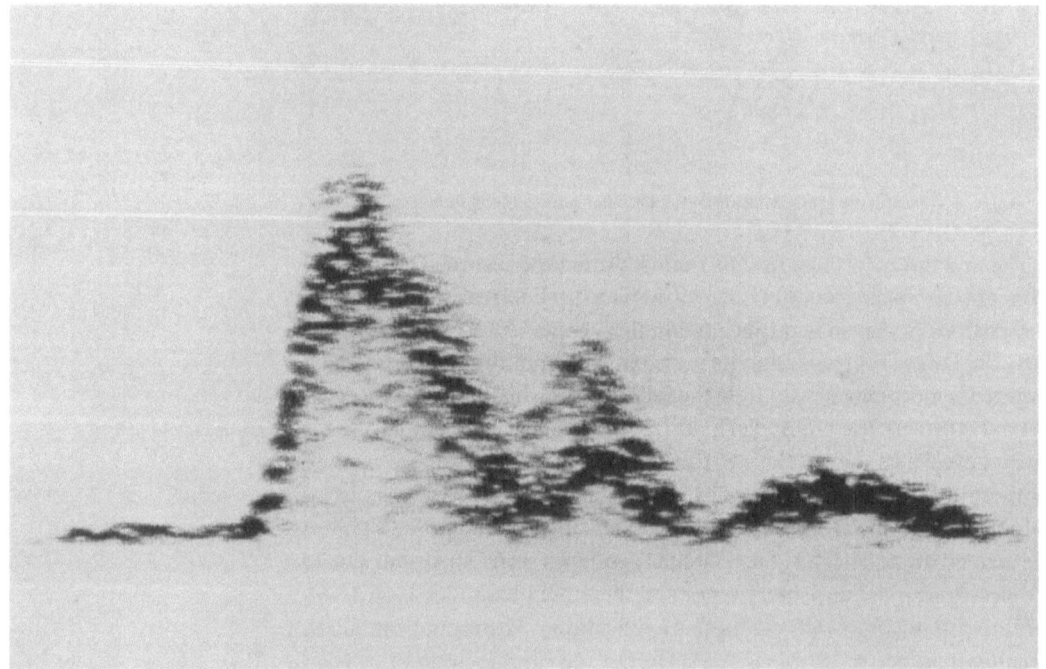

Fig. 7. A normal femoral artery sonagram, time is along the x-axis and Doppler shift frequency is in the y-axis. The optical density of the display is proportional to the strength of the signal tone at each instant.

tinguishing reverse from forward flow and the output from such non-directional instruments would be as shown in Fig. 8. In this diagram, the second hump would be due to predominantly reverse flow.

Any moving structures in the beam, regardless of their depth, which reflect ultrasound to the receiver crystal will result in Doppler shift signals. Thus the continuous-wave Doppler instrument is range insensitive. In an attempt to overcome this drawback, pulsed Doppler instruments have been developed. In this case a brief pulse of transmitter frequency ultrasound is sent out and the Doppler shifted echo pulses are range-gated, i.e., Doppler shifted echoes only from structures at fixed depths into the tissues are received and analysed. By varying the depth in the range of interest, Doppler shift signals may, in principle, be analysed from a series of points across the diameter of a blood vessel. Such instruments are not yet in widespread clinical use but do promise major advances in the diagnostic capability of Doppler shift ultrasound.

3.   HANDLING THE PROBE

The application of the ultrasound probe to the patient would seem to be the most simple clinical procedure and yet it is probably one of the most common sources of error and artifact. The skills required are not difficult to learn, but do require concentration and some attention to detail. There are two basic designs of probe in clinical use, pencil shaped, and flat. Both designs have advantages and disadvantages. The flat probe is easier to hold in position on the skin when the appropriate signal has been located, but its shape makes it awkward to manipulate if angulation is required to obtain the 'best signal'. If a period of continuous monitoring is required then a flat probe is more suitable for fixing in position with adhesive tape or bandage. If the examiner has a tremor in the hand then this can produce artifacts in the signal. This may be produced by causing the probe to rub against the skin in the area of examination, or occasionally if a large quantity of acoustic jelly has been used the movement may create a stirring movement in the jelly, causing artifact. If bubbles or particles of dust get into the jelly this can also cause disturbance of the signal.

One of the most common errors made, particularly when learning the techniques, is to press into the tissues with the probe. One can have some sympathy with the beginner who may have difficulty in locating a particular arterial pulse, then with some relief locates a blood flow signal and responds with the intention of transfixing the vessel with the probe for fear that the signal may go away, or perhaps even become louder if the probe is forced closer. The beginner must remember that the ultrasound beam extends for several centimeters beyond the end of the probe and that,

It is true that excessive pressure with the probe must be avoided, particularly when assessing arteries or veins on the foot. However, it is important to realize that Doppler instruments operating at higher frequencies, such as 10 MHz, suffer significant attenuation of the ultrasound beam when assessing vessels deeper than 3 or 4 cm. When using such instruments it may be necessary to use moderate pressure when evaluating arterial signals in the thigh or at the groin.

A useful technique to stabilize the probe, particularly during recording of Doppler arterial velocity signals, is the use of a mechanical probe holder to maintain a fixed position and angle of the probe relative to the vessel being examined. An excellent device is one which employs a magnetic base and an arm of flexible segments which can be made rigid by a simple internal cable mechanism (Enco Manufacturing Company, Chicago, Illinois 60639).

provided there is no gas or bone in the way, then the signal will travel through the tissues adequately. These errors may arise more often when using a pencil probe. This shape of probe has the advantage of being easier to aim and direct, but is open to artifact interference if there is tremor in the examiner's hand. This probe should be held like a pencil, and the heel of the examiner's hand should rest steadily on the patient, while the fingers remain in a relaxed gentle grip on the probe. In some instances it may be

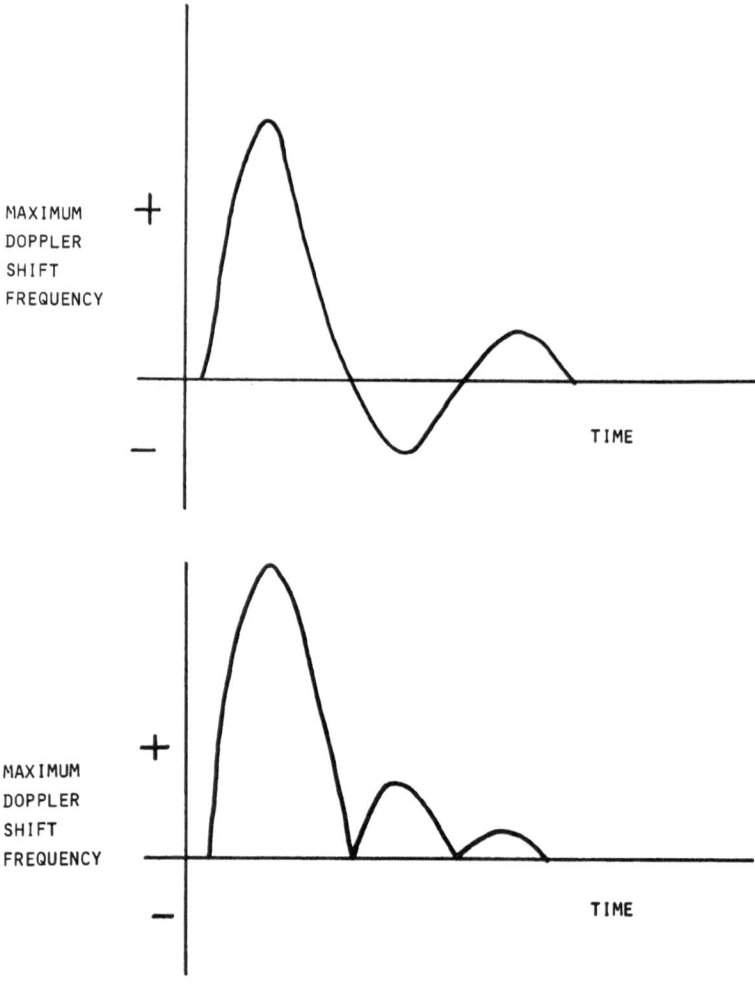

Fig. 8. These wave shapes are typical systemic arterial Doppler signal outputs, the upper diagram represents a bidirectional output with reverse flow shown below the zero line. The lower diagram represents a unidirectional output, where reverse flow is displayed above the zero line. A sonagram even from a directional instrument is usually displayed like the lower waveform.

necessary to steady the probe even further by applying the fingers of the examiner's other hand gently around the probe and resting them on the patient. This forms a type of tripod arrangement between the probe and both hands of the examiner laid on the patient. In many instances a very low flow pulse in the foot can be detected and recorded in this fashion when it would otherwise be recorded as absent. The difference in application between the two basic types of probe is shown in Fig. 9. In using the pencil

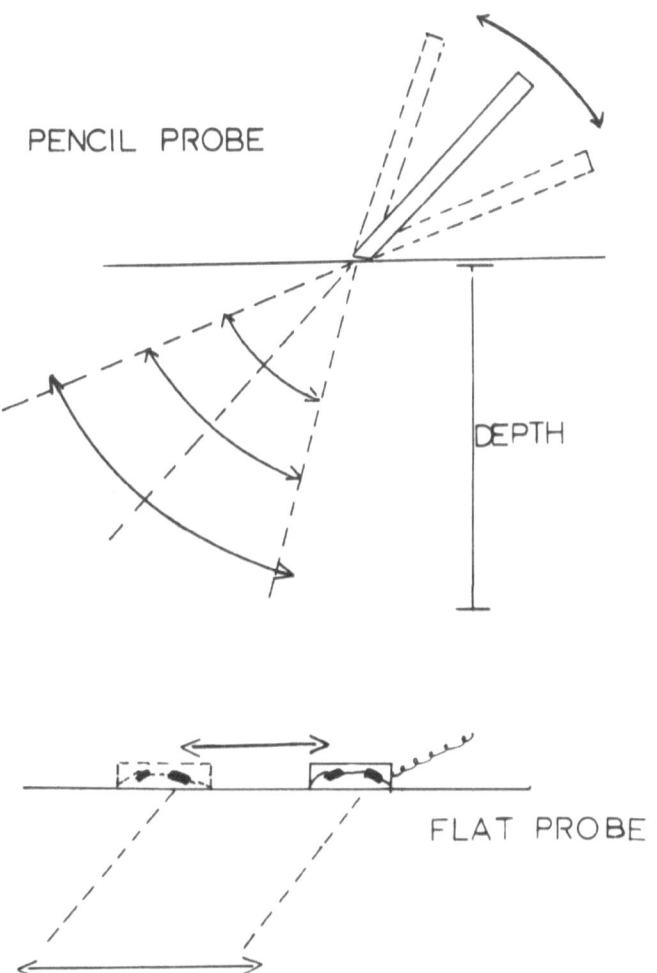

Fig. 9. The two basic designs of Doppler probe are pencil shaped or flat. The pencil probe can be manipulated to sweep the tissues with the ultrasound beam. The flat probe can be held in situ more easily.

probe it can be seen that slight changes in angle of the probe produce quite wide sweeps of the ultrasound beam through the tissues. This contrasts with the flat probe which can be made to slide over the surface of the skin at a more or less fixed angle. This should be remembered when recording weak pulses, for example, in an elderly patient who might move slightly at the time of recording, or when the inflating of a blood pressure cuff causes the limb to move slightly. If a pencil probe is being used, the examiner must hold the probe so that it is 'fixed' to the patient. Although the pencil shape probe has disadvantages for the beginner, these are outweighed by the advantage of sweeping the beam through the tissues. These sweeping movements can be made in X or Y planes or in semicircular patterns. The examiner must now remember that it is a blind search and careful concentrated listening may be required, depending on the area being examined. In the lower limb this searching may be required in the popliteal or the femoral region in order to locate a number of vessels and so isolate one from another. The sweeping movement must be made slowly and steadily and time must be allowed for a flow signal to occur, particularly in situations where the pulse signal may be poor. This type of examination is best done with examiner waring headphones. If difficulty is being experienced in locating the vessel, extraneous noises in the room can be most distracting. The examiner has to try to build an image in his mind of the sweeps being made through the tissues by the methodical angulation of the probe. The use of a loudspeaker system is valuable for demonstration but is not adequate for the method of examination just described.

This leads on to the problem of obtaining a 'good' signal. This is sometimes the most difficult skill to teach. Some individuals are quick to 'tune-in' to a radio station accurately, while others are satisfied to listen without adjusting the radio accurately so long as they can hear something. The same is very much the situation when using a Doppler probe to detect blood flow. Most people can learn to 'tune-in' to a radio station if they are interested, and the same applies to a Doppler ultrasound examination of peripheral arteries. The first objective when sweeping the tissues with the ultrasound beam is to locate a position where there is a blood flow signal. The sweeping movements then are reduced to very slow and slight changes of position until the 'best' signal is obtained (Figs. 10 and 11). This usually means moving the ultrasound beam in and out of the area of the pulse signal in both X and Y directions until a 'good' signal quality is obtained or the 'best' signal from that site. If the artery is diseased the volume setting of the apparatus should perhaps be kept constant during this procedure (keeping box volume setting constant). This approach to hunting the tissues with the ultrasound beam is of considerable practical importance. Quite often when the probe is placed on the patient, a pulse is detected very quickly. In areas such as the common femoral artery the first vessel

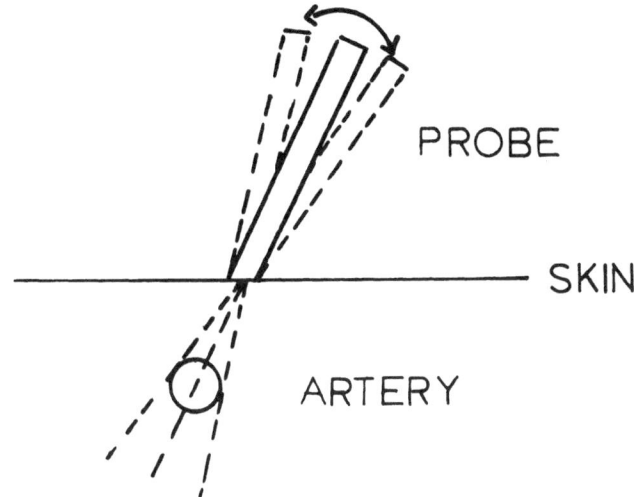

Fig. 10. Fine movements of the pencil probe are required to 'tune-in' to the arterial flow.

detected may be a branch, or it may be the superficial or deep femoral artery. A certain amount of intelligent hunting of the tissues will separate small vessels with higher pitch sounds from larger vessels. A degree of practice is necessary to become familiar with sounds of large and small arteries. The beginner should learn from listening to normal vessels comparing, digital, radial, femoral and carotid arteries. If the Doppler ultrasound equipment is being used simply as an acoustical instrument for hearing pulses, then much of the description above will be more or less irrelevant. However, if serious application of the equipment is planned then reliable collection of signals for analysis is very important.

4.   DOPPLER ULTRASOUND ARTERIAL PULSE WAVEFORMS

The signal obtained from Doppler ultrasound examination is different from other noninvasive vascular measurement methods in that the signal is derived from a specific vessel. It is possible to examine a number of different anatomical sites simultaneously or to record at a number of different sites along the same vessel simultaneously using a number of probes.

The classical arterial pulse waveform is shown in Fig. 12. This can be divided into a number of parts: an ascending slope, which is related to the acceleration of blood cells through the ultrasound beam, that occurs with contraction of the left ventricle of the heart; and a descending slope which develops as the blood cells decelerate after ventricular systole. There may

Arterial velocity events in diastole truly reflect changes in peripheral vascular resistance. This reviewer has shown in animal model studies that the ratio of diastolic reverse flow velocity to peak systolic flow velocity is linearly related to the limb peripheral vascular resistance as determined by comparing Doppler waveforms with electromagnetic blood flow and pressure studies.

then be a period of reverse flow followed by a small secondary burst of forward flow before the next cardiac contraction. Simple observation of these parts of the waveform can give information about the artery under examination. An easy way to demonstrate this is to place a probe over the radial artery, and then clench the fist tightly for about 2 min and then relax the hand. The changes in the arterial pulse can be clearly heard as the resistance to flow into the hand is increased during clenching, and then reduced during relaxation. If the signals are recorded, the changes are bound to occur in the parts of the waveform following the ascending slope. Thus it can be seen that this portion of the waveform reflects circulatory conditions distal to the site of measurement. The rising slope of the waveform is related to the rate of increase of blood velocity leaving the left ventricle and so is associated with the contractility of the myocardium. If

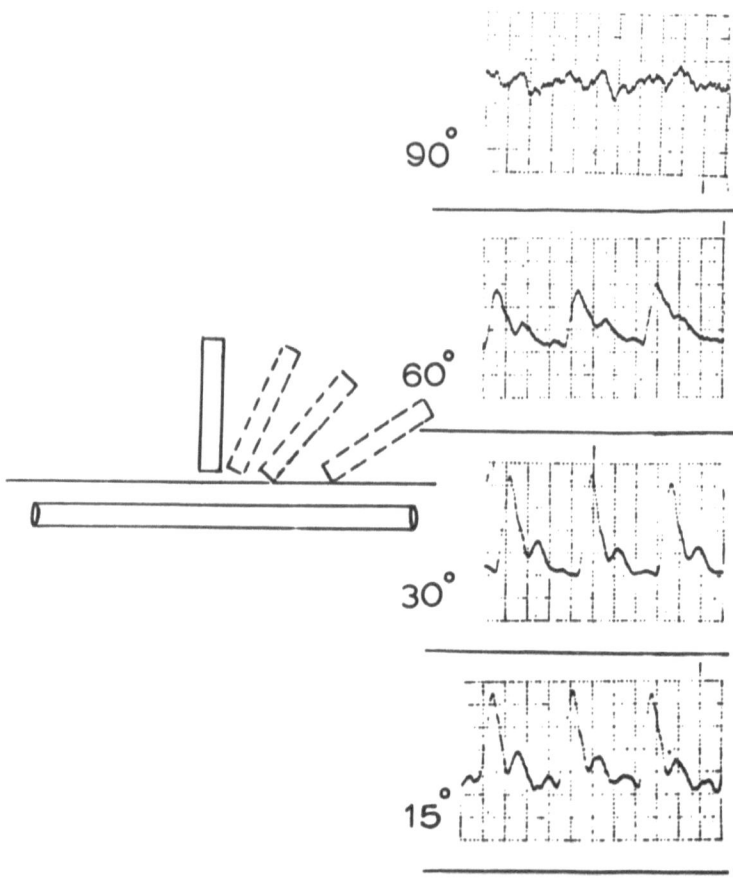

Fig. 11. The effect of angulation of the probe to the line of the artery on the signal output.

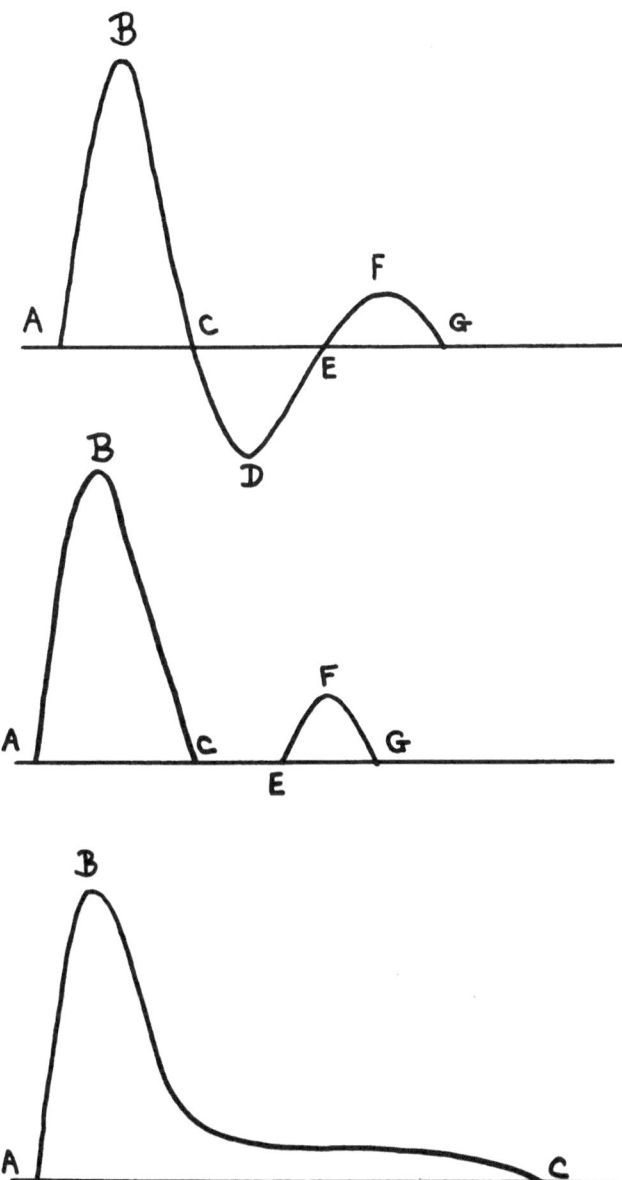

Fig. 12. The arterial waveshape may be divided into parts: A–B is the
ascending slope which is the acceleration of blood occurring with ventricular contraction; B–C is the descending slope which is the deceleration
of blood after ventricular contraction; C–D–E is the reverse flow element
reflected from the periphery; E–F–G is the secondary forward flow. In the
middle diagram reverse flow does not occur, but is marked by a pause in
blood movement. In the lower diagram peripheral resistance is lowered
and some degree of continuous flow is present.

the pulse of the brachial artery is recorded during exercise, then as the blood pressure and heart rate increase so does the steepness of the rising slope of the Doppler pulse waveform in association with the increase in acceleration of the blood. Special equipment has been designed to study this in the arch of the aorta (2). In simultaneous recording from the brachial and femoral artery the same extent of change in the ascending slope has been observed. However, in the presence of disease in the artery there may be a degree of dissipation of energy and a loss of acceleration resulting in a slower rise and a lower peak in the waveform.

The rate of deceleration is related to the resistance to flow distal to the site of measurement. Dynamic changes in this parameter can be measured with a fixed probe attached over a selected pulse site. The simple test of clenching and relaxing the fist while recording the radial artery demonstrates this. A set of radial artery pulse recordings are shown (Fig. 13) which were recorded while the subject placed the hand in a water bath. The temperature of the water was changed and the resulting change in the blood velocity waveform recorded. The change in the descending slope is clearly seen as vasodilation occurs. In this way a relative index of change for a particular set of circumstances can be monitored for a particular arterial bed. Similar types of change have been observed in the posterior tibial artery during whole body tilting, feet downwards, where there is an increase in peripheral resistance in the foot induced by the change from horizontal to near vertical posture. Such a measure of change in peripheral resistance could be of interest to physiologists and pharmacologists.

There are variations in the waveform shape from different anatomical arterial sites, and these are due mainly to characteristics associated with the vascular bed being supplied by the vessel. Organs with low blood flow resistance have a waveform shape with a flat descending slope and no reverse flow component, for example the renal artery. The common carotid artery is another site with characteristic shape.

In a peripheral artery in the arm or leg the descending part of the wave will usually reach the zero flow baseline, unless there is hyperaemia with continuous forward flow present (Fig. 12). Occasionally reverse flow may seem to commence before the end of the last part of the descending slope has reached the zero level. When this occurs there is simultaneous forward and reverse flow occurring. Occasionally in a radial artery forward–reverse–forward flow elements are seperated from each other by periods of no flow within the one cardiac cycle. This is presumably associated with a degree of balance between resistance in the periphery and constriction in the main feeding artery.

Apart from these observations, which can be made about the waveform shape and refer to physiological events, further analysis and classification is possible, which is useful in detecting obstructive arterial disease. A

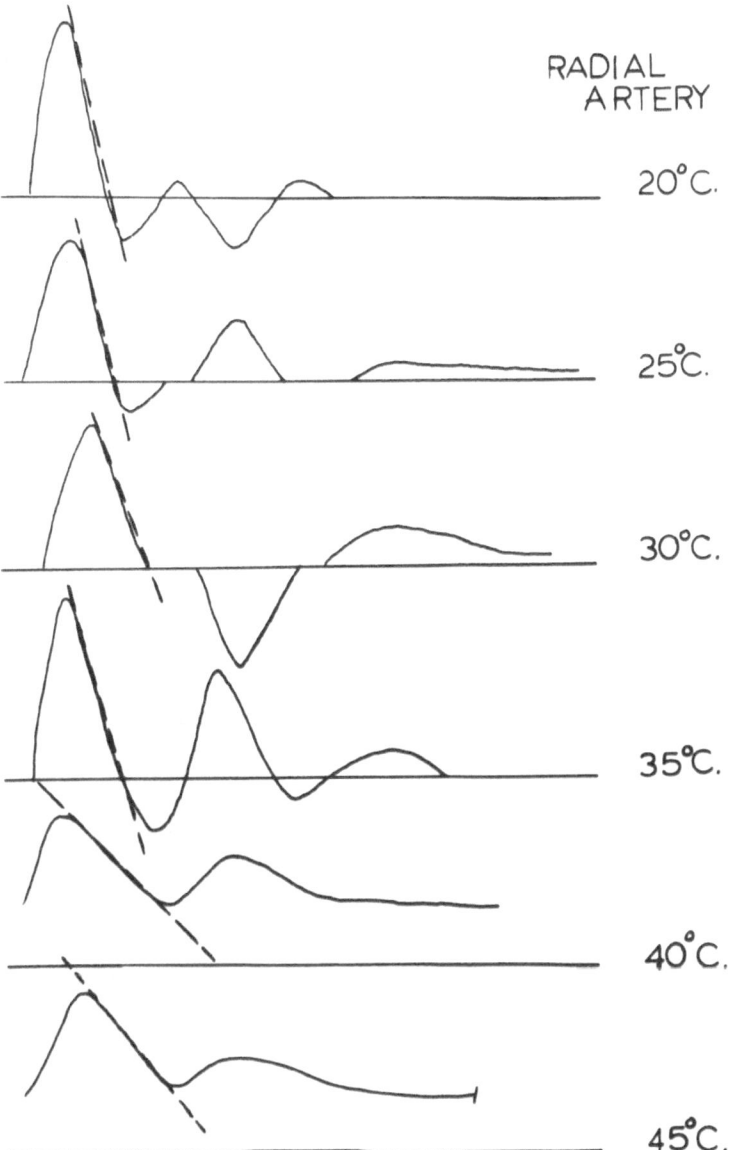

RADIAL
ARTERY

20°C.

25°C.

30°C.

35°C.

40°C.

45°C.

Fig. 13. The changes in waveshape which occur in the radial artery while changing the temperature of the hand. The descending slope B–C gradually opens out, the reverse flow element gives way to continuous forward flow as hyperaemia develops with peripheral dilatation and reduced resistance. At the cold temperature there are two reverse flow elements and secondary forward flow elements.

Although the pulsatility index, damping factor and transient time are useful quantitative indices of abnormalities of arterial flow velocity, these techniques generally do not provide much more clinical information than that possible by qualitative assessment of audio signals, analogue (zero crossing detector) waveforms and quantitative measurement of segmental limb blood pressures. This reviewer feels that Doppler signal analysis is most valuable in the femoral and carotid arteries, where real time sound spectrum analysis may eventually provide the most sensitive indices of early atherosclerosis. In addition to pulsatility indices, the analogue recording may be further characterised by measurements of such indices as acceleration time, deceleration time and other measurements on the waveform as described by Fronek et al. (1).

particular waveform shape can be characterised and given a numerical value, this has been called pulsatility index (PI) which is defined as the sum of the maximum energy of the Fourier harmonics divided by the mean energy term (3). Another method of obtaining this index is by using a planimeter to obtain the integral of the pulse waveform displayed on a sonagraph, thus:

$$PI = (P/P)\bar{V} \text{ where } \bar{V} = o \int Vdvt = A/_T.$$

Therefore $PI = (P/PXT)/A$ where P/P is the peak height of the forward flow, if present, in cm/sec, and A is the integral of the pulse velocity waveform over one pulse length in sq. cm/sec, and T is the pulse length in seconds. If a series of pulse waveforms are recorded at two points along the length of an artery the distal pulse waveform should be as pulsatile as the proximal one, or even more pulsatile. However if there is a loss of energy due to the work required to pass through a diseased artery then there will be a reduction in the pulsatile shape and the ratio of the proximal and distal pulsatility indexes gives a damping factor. Physiological changes can produce marked alteration in the waveform as has been shown, and it is therefore valuable to relate to pulses along the same arterial segment by the damping factor (DF) as most changes will be common to both pulse waves unless the length of segment chosen is very long, such as the common femoral to posterior tibial artery. Small local changes could occur in the foot, that would not necessarily be reflected in the main supply artery at the inguinal ligament.

Another valuable measure is the pulse pressure transit time along a segment of artery and this is measured in milliseconds. Transit time (TT) is directly related to length of artery being measured, and to pressure of blood and stiffness of the arterial wall. If these parameters are measured over a segment of artery, and the systolic blood pressure in the segment is also included, then it is possible to make an accurate classification of the condition of the artery and state whether it is patent, stenosed or obstructed.

5.   LOWER LIMB DOPPLER SCAN

The measurement of transient time requires a Doppler instrument with two transducers for simultaneous signal recordings from two sites on the limb. Unfortunately, most available Doppler units provide only a single probe attachment.

To make a Doppler scan of the arterial system in this area, the pulse sites usually recorded include the abdominal aorta, common femoral popliteal, posterior tibial, dorsalis pedis and peroneal arteries. Samples of arterial pulses are recorded from each of these sites seperately, and then the procedure is repeated using two probes, one on the proximal pulse, and the other on the distal site to obtain transit time over each arterial segment. After this systolic blood pressure is measured in the limb, above and below the knee and at the ankle. When seeking the abdominal aorta difficulty may occur if gas filled bowel is in the way, or if the patient is excessively obese. Firm pressure with one hand as if palpating the abdomen, may move the bowel sufficiently to give an acoustic window for the Doppler beam on to the aorta.

Normal ranges of values for pulsatility index, damping factor and transit time have been assembled from a large number of scans of normal healthy people, the range is as shown in Fig. 14. The usual diagnostic scan uses the pulse sites listed, however in some circumstances it may be desirable to follow an artery at short intervals along its length. Pulsatility index and damping factor can be calculated for each of these, but transit time cannot be measured reliably over lengths of less than 10–12 cm.

The results obtained from a typical scan of a patient with intermittent claudication due to obstruction of the left superficial femoral artery are shown in Fig. 15. There is a marked lengthening of transit time and a reduced pulsatility of the popliteal pulse with a large damping factor for this segment. Although there is further loss of pulsatility at the posterior

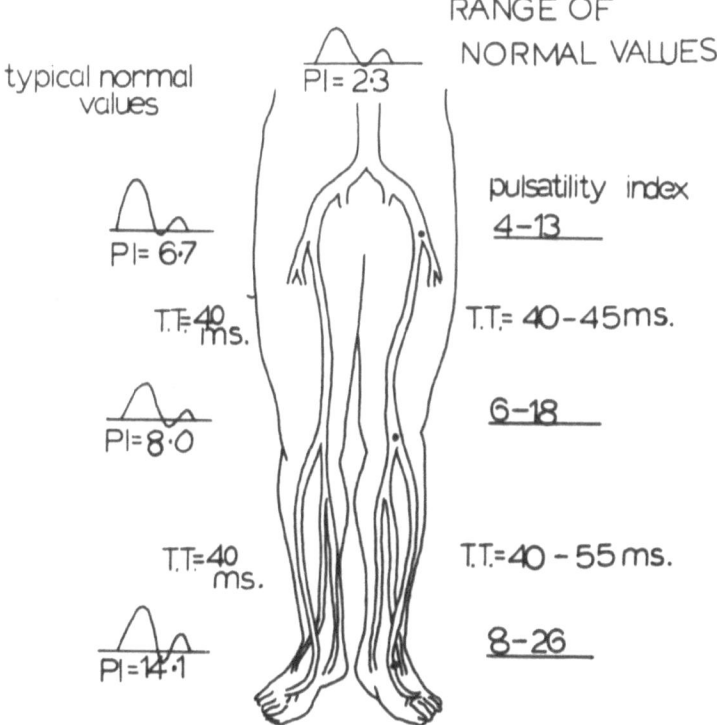

Fig. 14. A typical set of normal values, and the normal range of value of pulsatility index (PI) and transit time (TT) for the lower limb arteries.

tibial artery the transit time in this segment is normal which indicates an adequate 'run-off' in the lower leg. On the right side there is a normal transit time in each segment but also a progressive lowering of pulsatility at the popliteal and posterior tibial pulses, indicating distributed disease without complete occlusion. Blood pressure measurements in the leg further support these findings. On exercise testing there is the expected

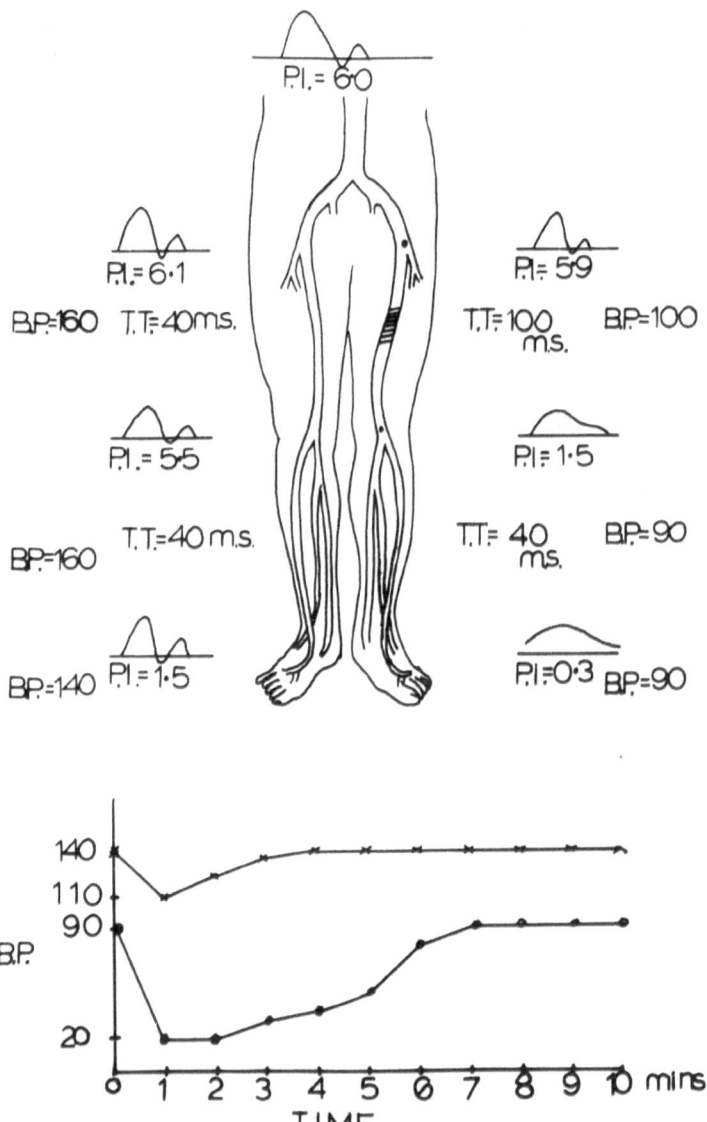

Fig. 15 documents the fact that segmental limb blood pressures, which are generally much more easily obtained than velocity recordings, are useful to detect the presence of arterial disease, even that mild enough to only result in abnormalities during stress. Greater differentation of inflow (aorta-iliac) disease from superficial femoral artery occlusive disease might have been possible if two thigh pressure measurements (proximal and distal) had been made using somewhat narrower cuffs (12 × 40 cm bladder). When thigh pressure measurements are made using the conventional wide (19 × 40 cm) cuff, a low value may reflect either aorta-iliac or superficial femoral artery disease, or both. With two thigh pressure measurements, a normal proximal thigh pressure signifies a normal inflow while a low proximal thigh pressure signifies aorto-iliac disease.

Fig. 15. The results of a Doppler scan showing the identification of a femoral artery obstruction, and mild disease in the opposite leg.

drop in pressure in the left leg, but also some drop in pressure in the right leg indicating the presence of a stenotic lesion which becomes haemo-dynamically apparent on demand for increased blood flow.

By using these parameters a method of grouping for the purpose of clinical classification has been assembled (Figs. 16–18). To test the reli-ability of this method of scanning and classification a study was carried out comparing the results with arteriography. The patients were admitted to the Vascular Surgical Service for routine work-up which included arteriog-raphy. A Doppler scan was also performed by separate personnel. At the end of a number of months the data was assembled and presented to the radiologist for comparison with the arteriogram and reports. Out of 267 arterial segments examined in this way, 265 correct groupings by Doppler scanning were confirmed by arteriography (Table 1) (4). The two errors occurred where a severe stenosis showed the passage of some contrast medium in the arteriogram, but on scanning the results indicated obstruc-tion. It could be argued that the stenosis was haemodynamically effective as a complete obstruction but for the purpose of the study arteriography was being used as the standard.

6. ARTERIAL ANEURYSM DETECTION

The detection of arterial aneurysms is also possible with Doppler ultra-sound scanning (5). During the course of routine scanning and analysis of sonagrams it was observed that a rippling high frequency sound following

This reviewer is interested in this documentation of a biphasic systolic velocity waveform distal to aneurysmal disease. The reviewer has no direct experience with this technique. Inasmuch as most laboratories record Doppler signals using the zero crossing detector, it would be important to know if such 'saw-tooth' abnormalities also are detected routinely by such analogue recordings.

Group		$P.I._1$	$P.I._2$	D.F.	T.T.	B.P.
1A	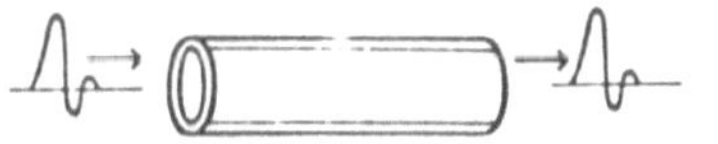	N	N	<1,0	N	N
1B	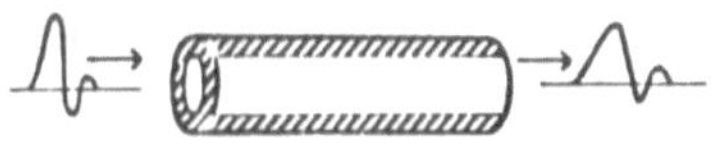	N	≈N	<1,0	N	N
1C	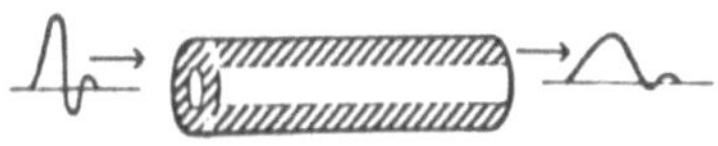	≈N	≈N	<1,0	<N	≈N

Fig. 16. Doppler scan classification of arteries. Group 1: no obstruction but changes in the arterial wall.

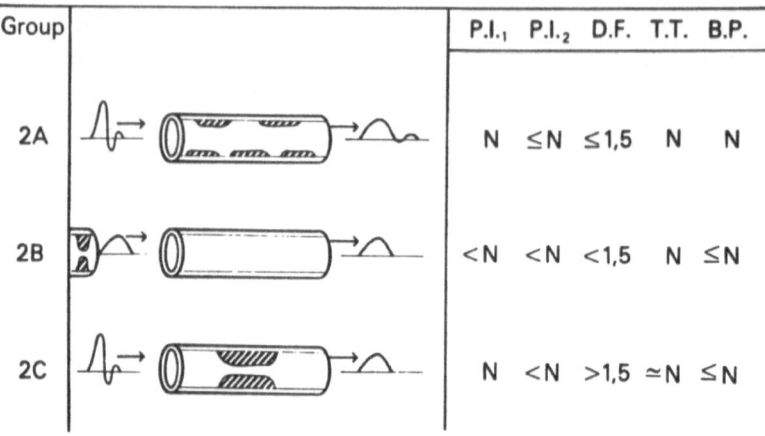

Group		P.I.$_1$	P.I.$_2$	D.F.	T.T.	B.P.
2A		N	≤N	≤1,5	N	N
2B		<N	<N	<1,5	N	≤N
2C		N	<N	>1,5	≈N	≤N

Fig. 17. Classification Group 2: various arrangements of distributed plaques and partial obstructions.

rapidly after the initial forward flow peak was associated with a 'saw-tooth' disturbance of the sonagram maximum frequency envelope (Fig. 19). In a study involving a series of 19 patients with aneurysms this type of signal was observed. The following illustrations (Figs. 20 and 21) show an arteriogram with an aortic aneurysm measuring 4 cm × 4.5 cm together with the sonagrams recorded from the aorta above the lesion and from the femoral arteries. The unusual femoral artery waveform is characteristic of the aneurysmal signal. This patient was successfully operated upon and one month after reconstructive surgery the femoral artery sonagrams did not show the aneurysm signal.

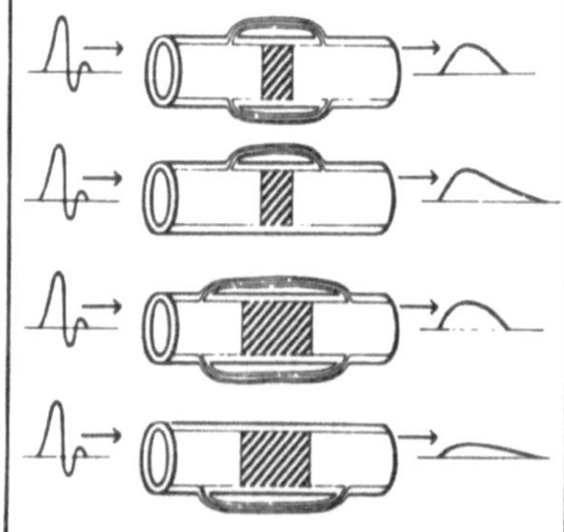

Group		P.I.$_1$	P.I.$_2$	D.F.	T.T.	B.P.
3A		≈N	<N	<1,5	>N <70	<N
3B		≈N	<N	>1,5	>N <70	<N
3C		≈N	<N	<1,5	>70	<N
3D		≈N	<N	>1,5	>70	<N

Fig. 18. Classification of Group 3: obstruction with various degrees of collateral development.

Table 1. Single blind comparison of Doppler ultrasound arterial segment diagnosis compared with arteriography.

Arterial segment	Exam.	Gp. 1	X-ray	Gp. 2	X-ray	Gp. 3	X-ray
Aorto–fem	80	41	41	26	25	13	14
Fem–pop	80	13	13	27	27	40	40
Pop–posttib	80	17	17	23	22	40	41
Pop–dors.ped	27	4	4	9	9	14	24
Total	267	75	75	85	83	107	109

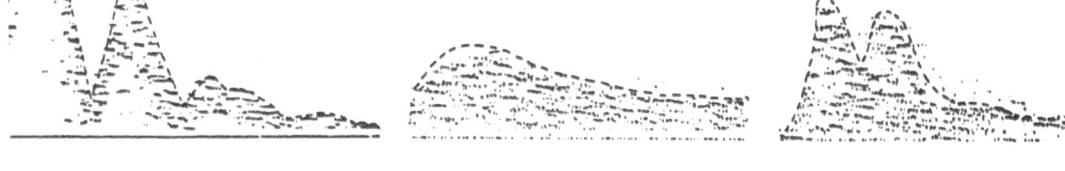

normal   obstructive   aneurysmal

Fig. 19. Sonagrams showing a normal femoral artery signal, a femoral artery signal with obstruction in the aorto-iliac segment, and a femoral artery signal with an aortic aneurysm.

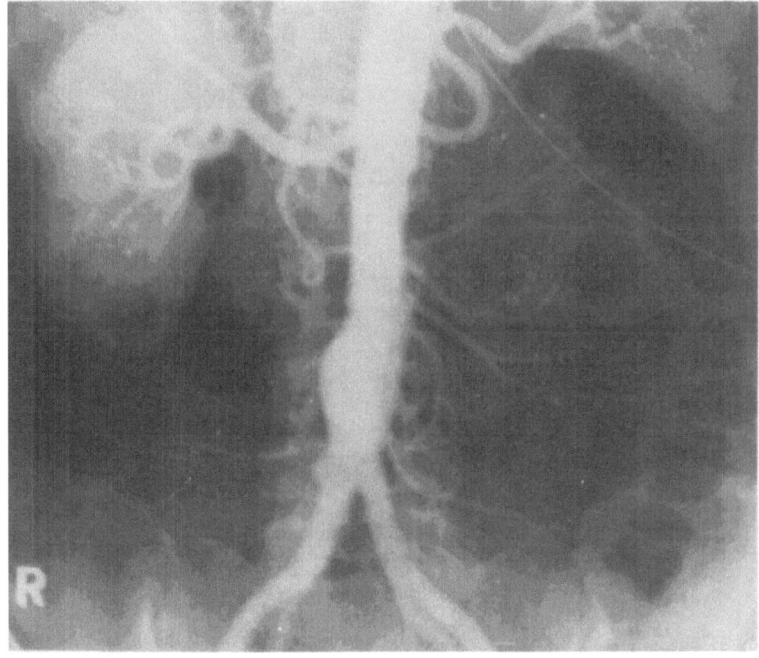

Fig. 20. The aortic aneurysm which was first identified by Doppler scanning.

The example (Fig. 22) shows a sonagram from a femoral artery 4 months after an aortofemoral reconstruction. The pulse is damped and there is continuous flow present. The same patient was examined two years later and found to have a femoral aneurysm at the lower end of the arterial reconstruction. The sonagrams show the shape of the pulse waveform above, over, and below the lesion. There is a marked change in the waveform shape which is poststenotic in character before reconstructive surgery, and then becomes 'saw-tooth' shape with the development of the

BEFORE SURGERY

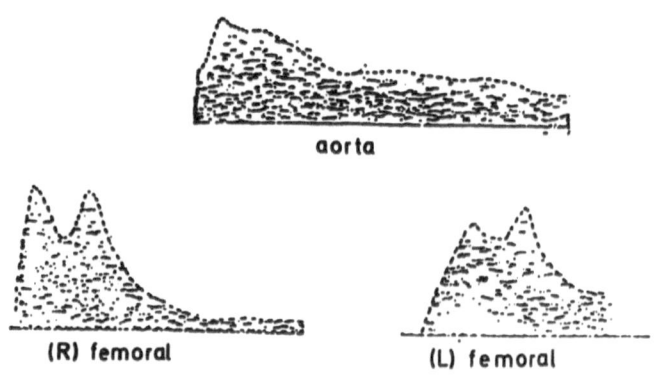

AFTER SURGERY

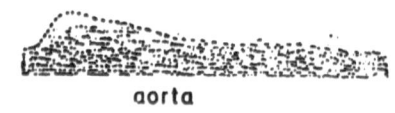

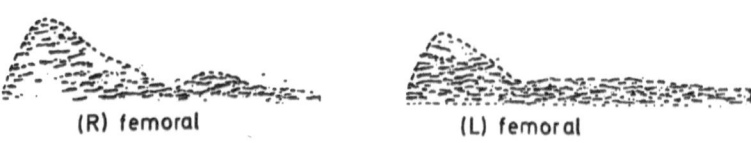

Fig. 21. Sonagrams obtained before and after reconstructive surgery for the aneurysm shown in Fig. 20.

aneurysm. The cause of the velocity pattern observed in these situations is not clear. It may be due to turbulence set-up in the aneurysm, or perhaps more likely the aneurysm wall itself may impart secondary waves to the blood after the initial systolic surge. It has been noticed when scanning large abdominal aortic aneurysms that laterally traversing the lesion the 'aneurysm signal' may not be present in each place examined. This may be due to the presence of thrombus in parts of the aneurysmal sac preventing wall movement of the type that causes the typical signal.

7.   SCANNING OF THE HEAD AND NECK ARTERIES

Scanning of the vessels in the head and neck requires some more skill from the examiner and some modification of the techniques. The lengths of artery to be examined are shorter and so transit time measurements are of less importance. The conditions that one is looking for more commonly belong to classification group 1 and 2 and seldom involve obstruction and

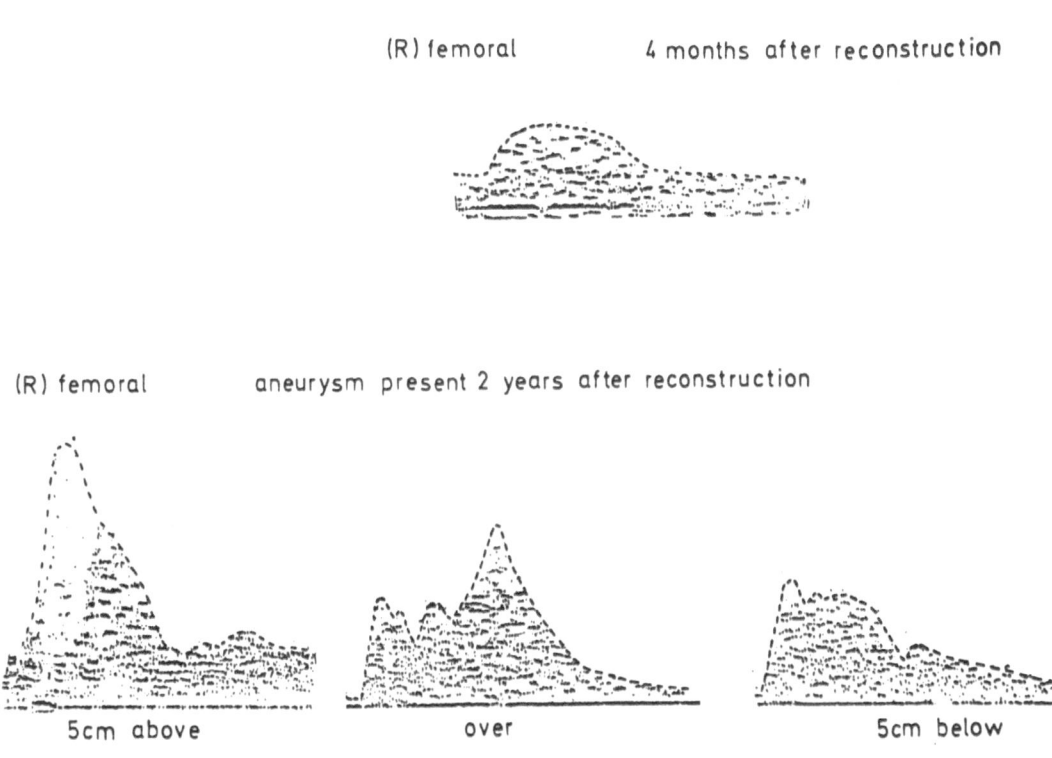

Fig. 22. Sonagrams from a femoral artery before reconstructive arterial surgery and two years after surgery when an aneurysm had developed at the anastamosis site.

Assessment of carotid artery flow velocity in the neck by Doppler is a more challenging procedure than periorbital Doppler examination. However, examination of the common carotid artery and its branches provides the most sensitive detection of disease at the carotid bifurcation, particularly if sound spectral analysis techniques are employed. However, such velocity assessment is most readily carried out with pulse Doppler imaging systems in which visualization of the arterial branches may be carried out in order to ascertain the location of detected flow velocity signals. Using conventional continuous-wave Doppler instruments, information may be obtained when the examiner becomes sophisticated in audibly interpreting the differences of velocity signals in the branches of the carotid artery. The external carotid artery carries flow to the relatively high resistance vascular bed of the face. Thus, the signal may have a prominent systolic component and one or more diastolic sounds with relatively low flow during diastole, unless the face is markedly vasodilated. In contrast, the normal internal carotid artery supplies blood to the brain which has a relatively low vascular resistance. Thus, the systolic velocity will be higher pitched and there will be a higher diastolic flow velocity with less discrete diastolic sounds. Stenosis of the internal carotid artery will result in an abnormal 'gruff' signal or a 'bubbling' signal. At the site of stenosis the velocity may be very high pitched with a 'hissing' characteristic. Unfortunately, calcification at the diseased carotid bifurcation frequently inhibits ultrasound transmission so that there may be acoustically silent areas in the area of such calcification. By analysing the sound spectrum of signals

collateral circulation. The shape of the sonagram waveform is important and it has been shown (6) that the ratio of the first and second peak of the common carotid pulse wave is of value in assessing the presence of disease in the system (Fig. 23). There is an increase in the height of the second hump in the waveform and this may also be associated with a reduction in the height of the first peak which will cause a reduction in the ratio of the two heights.

Apart from this calculation, observation of the signal for evidence of turbulence or damping that would indicate the presence of a lesion proximal to the point of measurement is of great importance. It is for this reason that skill in handling the probe, detecting the appropriate artery and obtaining the 'best' signal is all-important. Scanning of the carotid system can be performed with the patient either sitting upright, or lying down. Some investigators prefer the sitting position, particularly when locating the internal carotid branch. Scanning should commence at the lower end of the common carotid artery, just above the clavicle. It will be necessary to 'sweep' the tissues and find the main artery and not some of its branches. There may be difficulty with signals coming from the jugular vein, particu-

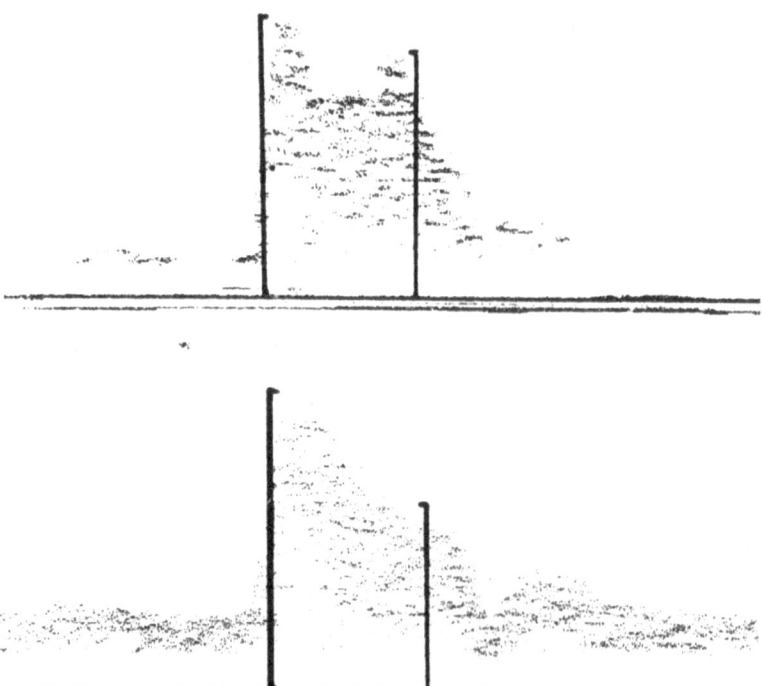

Fig. 23. Sonagrams from the carotid artery showing the relationship of the first and second peak in a normal and an abnormal. The ratio of the height of the first and second peak is reduced in the abnormal sonagram.

larly on the right side of the patient as these will often carry a pulsatile modulation conducted up from the heart. By careful 'sweeping' and 'hunting' of the tissues an appropriate line on to the artery can be found. To begin with, the inexperience examiner may lose confidence or patience or both. The artery may be followed at intervals along its length up to the bifurcation. The probe should then be moved along the external branch and recordings made. From this point the angle of the probe is pivoted inwards, upwards, and slightly backwards under the jaw bone to detect the internal carotid branch. This signal often has a different tone and the point at which this artery bends over before entering the skull is often the area from which the Doppler signal is obtained. To complete the examination, signals should be collected from the vertebral artery either at the root of the neck or from the back of the neck between the cervical vertebrae. This latter approach is carried out with the patient sitting, and the head bent forward to open the spaces between the vertebrae. The probe is placed to the side of the midline, facing slightly inwards. This is one of the very few occasions when pressure may be applied to the probe with some advantage as the vessel is protected by its pathway through the vertebrae. Examination of these vessels is important if vertebral artery steal is suspected, but a Doppler instrument with bidirectional characteristics will be required. Examination of the supraorbital artery and the occlusion of the superficial temporal artery is a useful and established test to illicit patency of the intracranial part of the internal carotid artery (7, 8).

8.   CLINICAL INFORMATION AVAILABLE FROM DOPPLER ULTRASOUND SCANNING OF ARTERIES

From what has been described above, the clinician can obtain the following diagnostic information from Doppler scanning of peripheral arteries:

(1) The presence of 'patent' arterial segments.
(2) The presence of 'stenosis or distributed plaques'.
(3) The presence of arterial obstruction.
(4) The classification of collateral circulation.
(5) The identification of arterial aneurysm.
(6) The presence of good or bad 'run-off'.

The reliability of the scanning technique has been shown to compare favourably with arteriography, and it can be applied to arteries in the arms and legs, and also the neck. Studies are being made at present to further extend the range of application, and preliminary information is available from investigations of the coronary circulation, and also of human foetal circulation.

obtained distal to calcified segments, the degree of carotid stenosis may be estimated. Lesions narrowing the lumen by 25–50% will result in abnormal spectral broadening during systole with increased amplitude of the Doppler signal in the low frequency range. Between 50 and 75% stenosis, distal velocity signals reveal abnormal low-frequency spectral broadening in both systole and diastole. Distal to a stenosis of 75% or greater, there is loss of the normal waveform with marked spectral broadening and a more continuous signal.

The periorbital Doppler examination is useful to detect significant carotid stenosis or occlusion from the origin of the internal carotid artery to the level of the ophthalmic artery within the skull. This reviewer feels that most examiners will find greater accuracy in assessing carotid occlusive disease by means of periorbital Doppler examination than by examining the carotid artery in the neck. The advantage of periorbital examination is the fact that no recordings are required, inasmuch as the direction of ophthalmic artery flow and the effect of compression manoeuvers of branches of the external carotid artery and each common artery provide assessment of carotid patency and the source of collateral circulation.

Although subclavian steal may be inferred by abnormal systolic pressure in the affected arm, correct assessment of vertebral artery flow direction is fallible and the discrimination of vertebral artery flow from other possible collateral arteries in the neck is difficult.

9. DOPPLER ULTRASOUND SCANNING OF CORONARY ARTERIES

This reviewer is skeptical of the clinical feasibility of routinely assessing coronary artery blood flow or flow in coronary bypass grafts using conventional continuous-wave Doppler instruments. Although timing of diastolic flow relative to the electrocardiogram may document detected flow in the coronary circuit, the clinical fallibility of this technique and the difficulty in its performance detract from its potential as a routine screening procedure.

It is possible to monitor arterial blood flow signals across the chest wall in the area of the heart. This has been used in patients that have undergone surgical reconstruction with either venous by-pass or internal mammarian artery anastamoses to the coronary artery (9). The mammarian artery is relatively easy to locate in the rib spaces on either side of the sternum. The intercostal vessels are usually shielded by rib bone. Again this is one of the few occasions that the examiner may use pressure with the probe. A directional Doppler instrument is valuable because if there is doubt in identifying mammarian or intercostal arteries, then angulation of the probe will show if the flow direction is following the line of the rib or the line of the sternum. In those situations where this artery has been used to anastamose to the left anterior descending coronary artery the comparison of the two sides of the chest is very useful (Fig. 24). A directional Doppler will assist in determining the direction of flow in the reconstruction and of course will indicate the presence or absence of flow. The problem of absent flow can be reduced considerably by mapping the course of these vessels between rib spaces on both sides of the chest.

There are difficulties in making this examination. It requires experience and concentration particularly when attempting to locate the coronary vessels. The patient with a large chest, either muscular or obese, or the presence of large lung fields may make the examination very difficult. Some of these problems can be reduced by positioning the patient so that the heart may be brought nearer to the rib cage, either sitting, leaning forward, or lying on one side.

The left anterior descending branch of the left coronary artery is the most accessible vessel. This can often be traced in two or three rib spaces. The right marginal branch of the right coronary artery can be located by beaming medially and posteriorly from the right side of the sternum when the patient lies over on that side. In each of these examinations the probe must be used to sweep the tissues and hunt for the signal required. The caridac movement sounds will be loud and in the lower frequency range. Mammarian arteries have typical systemic artery sounds similar to a radial artery. The coronary artery pulse waves are quite different (Fig. 25). There is evidence of flow occurring before ventricular contraction. This is reduced sharply as contraction occurs, and as diastole develops flow starts again in a succession of peaks. Recordings of the flow pattern have been made in the mammarian artery during surgery which show the changes that occur on joining that artery to the coronary circulation (Figs. 26 and 27). It can be seen that the systolic peak of the normal systemic artery is greatly reduced after anastomosis, and a large diastolic flow occurs instead. Further studies and developments in this area of examination are presently being conducted.

10. MONITORING FOETAL CIRCULATION

A technique is being developed using Doppler ultrasound to locate and
monitor blood flow signals in the umbilical cord (10). This method consists
of using the echo B scan to locate the umbilical cord and to give the relative
position for directing the Doppler beam. Signals from the vein and arteries
in the cord are detectable (Fig. 28). The method is quite easy to apply and
offers interesting possibilities for further research in this area. It is also
possible to locate foetal arteries and record from them as well. The only

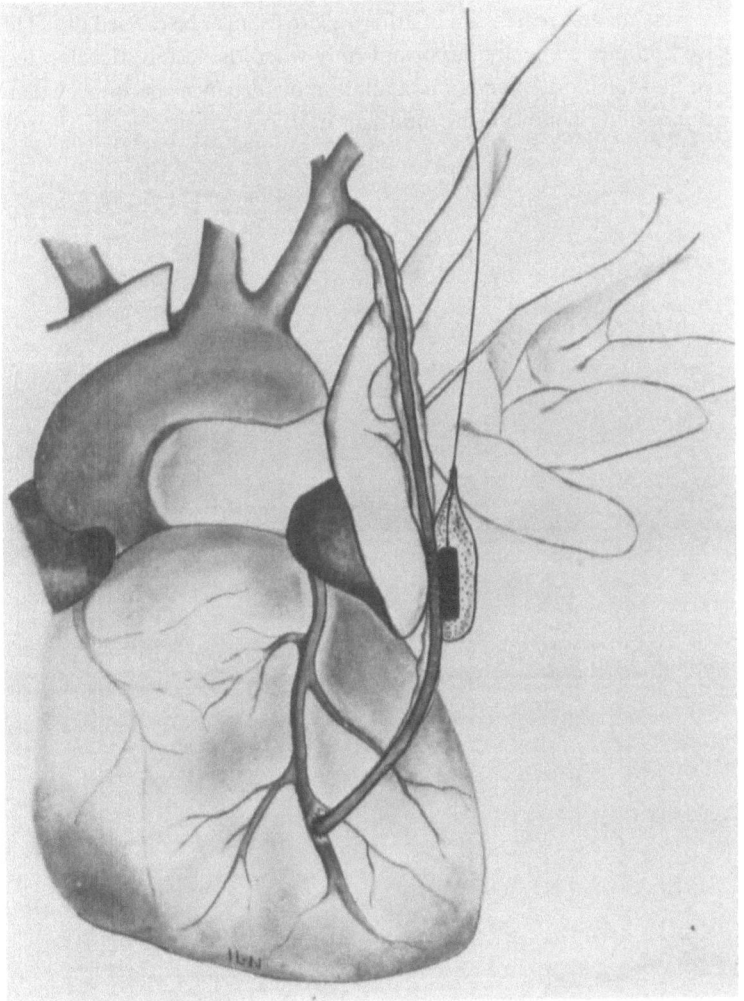

Fig. 24. A diagram showing the anastomosis of the internal mammarian artery to the left
anterior descending coronary artery being monitored with a flat Doppler probe.

difficulty experienced with this method so far is when the foetus is unusually active and moves in position. It is possible to record for quite long periods of time and also te repeat recordings intermittently if required.

11.   HEALTH CARE POTENTIAL

This reviewer agrees that many of these newer noninvasive screening techniques may provide valuable epidemiologic information about the prevalence and natural history of atherosclerotic vascular disease and the influence of various prophylactic and therapeutic interventions. However, it must be shown that the variance associated with repeated measurements does not encroach upon the alterations that may occur in the course of progression or regression of arterial disease.

The applications discussed so far relate to arterial system investigations in the presence of disease which is frequently clinically evident. The sensitivity of Doppler ultrasound scanning increases the potential value of the method so that early detection of disease, and the study of such problems as progression and regression of atherosclerosis, may be carried out. This disease becomes clinically important only when the lesions develop to a degree that haemodynamic or coagulation disturbances become evident. The causes of the condition are multifactorial covering practically all areas

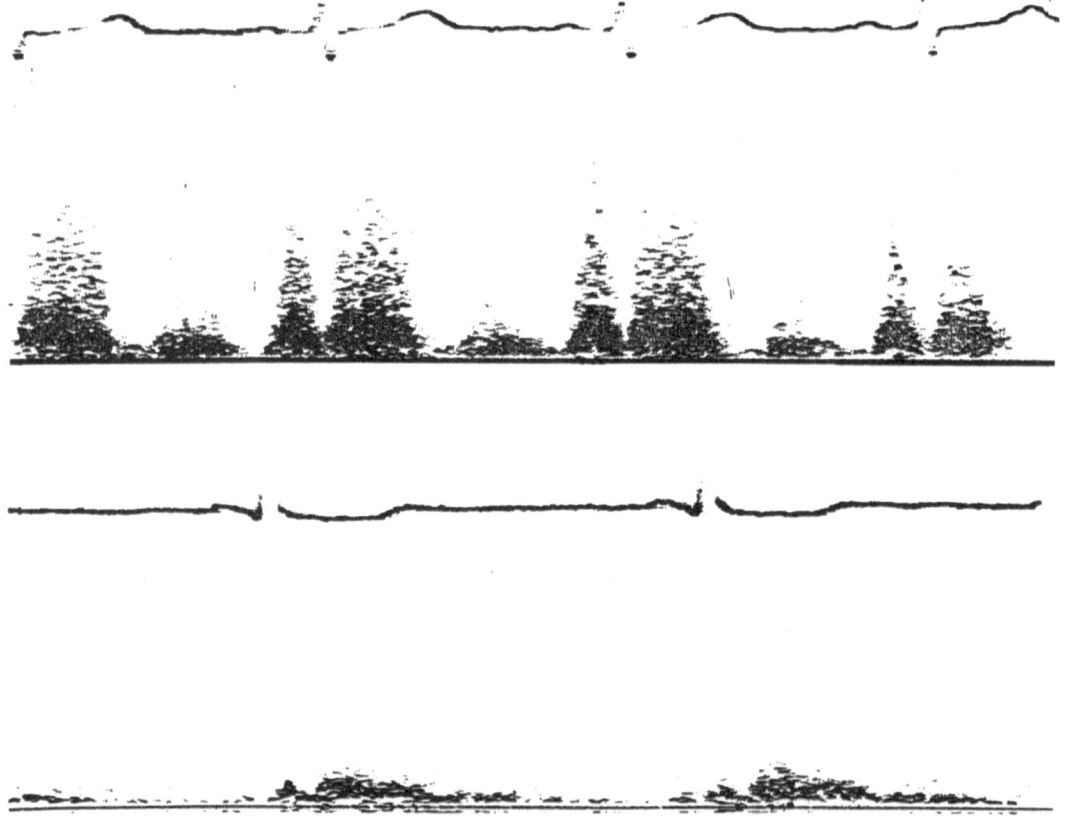

Fig. 25. The upper sonagram is from a normal coronary artery (LAD) recorded transcutaneously.
The lower sonagram is from a patient with an obstructive coronary artery (LAD) disease and severe angina pectoris.

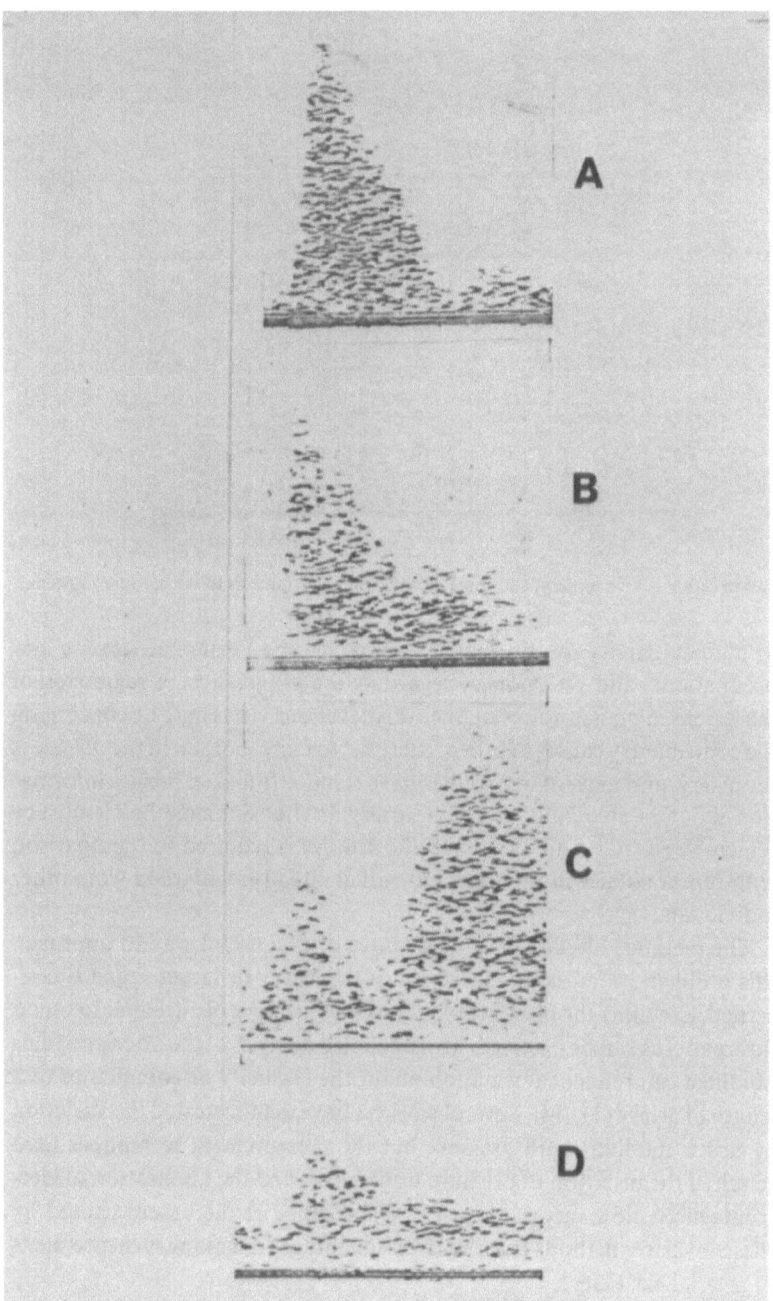

Fig. 26. Sonagrams of the mammarian artery recorded from outside the chest (A), from inside the chest (B), after anastomosis (C) and a week after surgery (D).

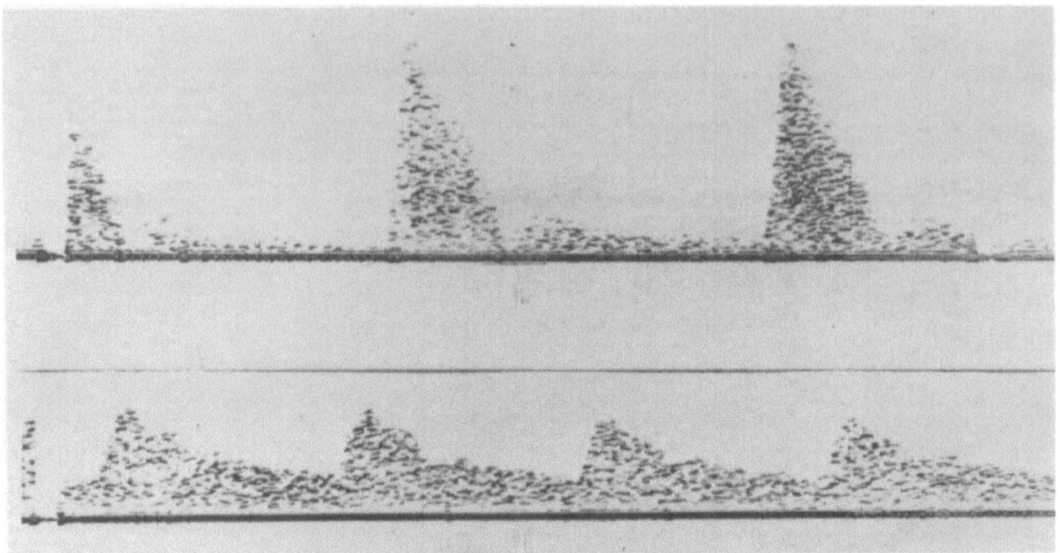

Fig. 27. Sonagrams of the mammarian artery before surgery, and three months after anastamosis to the coronary system.

of human activity, psychological, metabolic and hormonal, genetic and occupational and yet evidence regarding the progression or regression of the lesions in man is not available. Whatever our views may be concerning the contributary causes of atherosclerosis, the target organ of the disease is the artery, and most of our studies have singularly lacked precise information about the changing state of the artery. In choosing a method it must be remembered that data about specific arteries is required for comparison with repeat studies in the same individual and also with data from other individuals.

The methods already described above offer a useful way to approach this problem so far as measurement of the artery or target organ is concerned. Certainly the presence of lesions that produce disturbance to blood flow patterns can be detected. More detailed analysis of the arterial signals obtained can render information about the elasticity or compliance of a length of artery (11–14). Several workers have demonstrated the variation in elastic modulus with pressure but the measurement techniques used required the insertion of pressure transducers and the application of electromagnetic flow meters (15). The disturbance of the tissues caused by these invasive methods is a major disadvantage to making measurements of arterial elasticity.

The elasticity or compliance of a vessel can be calculated by relating the blood pressure and pulse wave velocity or transit time along a length of blood vessel (11, 14). It has been shown that stiffness of the femoral artery increases with age (11). Blood pressure can be altered by whole body tilting and measurements made in peripheral arteries at different degrees of tilt to produce a curve of elasticity values. The body tilting procedure can be either feet downwards or head downwards in order to increase or decrease the local pressure in the limbs (14). This type of approach offers very interesting possibilities for studying early changes in the physical characteristics of the arterial wall. The carotid arteries and femoral arteries are among the most common locations for the development of atherosclerosis and this method of approach is suitable for studying these anatomical areas. One of the problems in studying atherosclerosis in humans has been the difficulty in obtaining data about the target organ, the artery. Now there are ways of approaching the vessels safely and in a clinically acceptable way. There will be further development in both apparatus and techniques but even at this time it is possible to obtain valuable data which should be included in future studies of atherosclerosis.

12. CONCLUSION

In most clinical centres dealing with peripheral arterial conditions the sole method of investigation used is arteriography. There is an increasing

The reviewer agrees with the author that the medical community must increase its sophistication in the use of non-invasive screening techniques to assess the peripheral circulation. It is true that Doppler ultrasound may be the most versatile and accurate method to enhance our understanding of vascular disease. However, the reviewer urges caution in extending some of the sophisticated techniques in this chapter to routine clinical surveillance by practicing clinicians. It is the feeling of this reviewer that more simple qualitative methods to assess the Doppler signal, including simple audio analysis and possibly recording with zero crossing detectors, provide the most inexpensive and practical method to introduce some of these concepts into routine clinical practice. Finally, the merits of quantitation of peripheral vascular disease by means of segmental leg pressure measurements should bring the greatest accuracy and sensitivity to the clinician with the least expense and challenge to his traditional concepts of vascular disease.

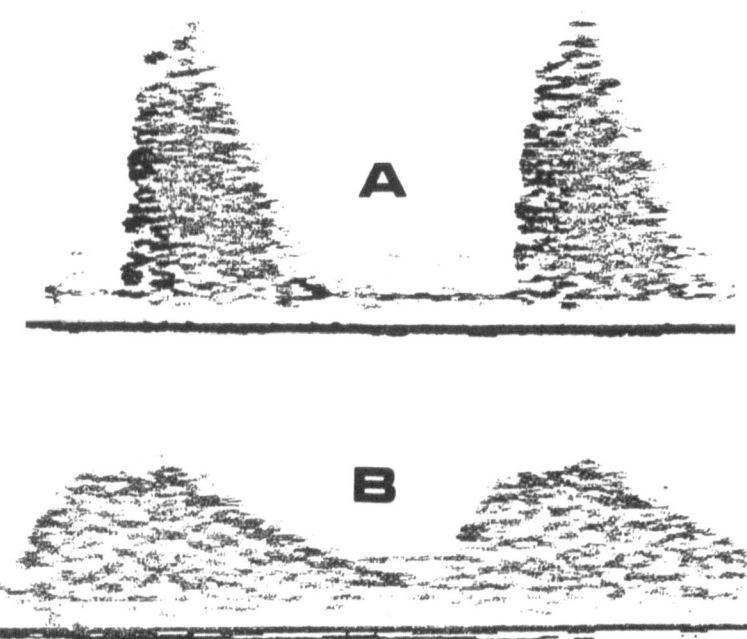

Fig. 28. Sonagrams of the umbilical artery (A) and vein (B), obtained transcutaneously using pulsed echo scanning to locate the umbilical cord.

awareness of the value of noninvasive techniques and so the time is at hand for the practice of routine arteriography to be re-appraised. Undoubtedly angiography is necessary for the surgeon to plan reconstructive proce- dures; however, it is not uncommon to have this diagnostic investigation performed simply when confirmation of the presence of obstructive arte- rial disease is required, or even when limb amputation is the form of treatment contemplated. A more rational approach to the assessment of peripheral arterial disease should be considered and a selection of the appropriate noninvasive methods used to screen patients, thus saving arteriography for the ones that can be seriously considered suitable for surgical reconstruction. This approach is particularly important in the assessment of the elderly patient. Because Doppler ultrasound scanning gives information about specific arteries which compares favourably with arteriography the method deserves serious consideration for inclusion in routine clinical evaluation of patients. The attitude that Doppler ultra- sound is merely a method of listening to pulses, which only reveals evi- dence as to the presence or absence of blood flow in a vessel, has delayed the introduction of the method into clinical practice in a wider and more comprehensive manner. Some of the data processing techniques referred to in this chapter would require a routine clinical establishment to invest in rather unusual equipment such as tape recorders and audiofrequency analysers, however this is not really a drawback when the type of data made available is considered. As interest develops at the clinical level, automatic data processing methods will become more readily available. The use of Doppler scanning for the early detection of arterial disease, and the monitoring of the progression or regression of arterial disease, offers possibilities which have not been available to us in the past, and which the medical profession as a whole should give careful consideration to in the future.

ACKNOWLEDGEMENTS

I wish to express my gratitude to all of those who have assisted me in the studies described, including secretarial and technical staff, and the many clinical and science colleagues, most of whom are named in the references.

REFERENCES TO MAIN TEXT

1. Wells PNT: Ultrasonic Doppler probes. In: Cardiovascular Applications of Ultrasound, Amsterdam, North Holland Publishing Company, 1974, p 125–131.
2. Light LH: Initial evaluation of transcutaneous aortovelography – a new non-invasive technique for haemodynamic measurements in the major thoracic vessels. In: Cardiovascular Applications of Ultrasound, Amsterdam, North Holland Publishing Company, 1974, p 325–360.
3. FitzGerald DE, Gosling RG, Woodcock JP: Grading dynamic capability of arterial collateral circulation. Lancet 66–67, 1971.
4. FitzGerald DE, Carr J: Peripheral arterial disease: assessment by arteriography and alternative non-invasive measurements. Amer. J. Roentgenol. 128: 385–388, 1977.
5. FitzGerald DE, Brew WKM, Fortesque-Webb CM, Donnelly C: Detection of arterial aneurysms with Doppler ultrasound. J. I. Coll. Phys. Surg. 5: 11–14, 1975.
6. Mol JMF, Rijcken: Doppler haematotachographic investigation in cerebral circulation disturbances. In: Cardiovascular Applications of Ultrasound, Amsterdam, North Holland Publishing Company, 1974, p 305–314.
7. Barnes RW, Garrett WV, Slaymaker EE, Reinertson JE: Doppler ultrasound and supra-orbital photoplethysmography for non-invasive screening of carotid occlusive disease. Amer. J. Surg. 134: 183–186, 1977.
8. Bone GE, Slaymaker EE, Barnes RW: Non-invasive assessment of collateral blood flow of the cerebral hemispheres by Doppler ultrasound. Surg. Gynaecol. Obstet. 145: 873–876, 1977.
9. FitzGerald DE, Fortesque-Webb CM, Ekestrom S, Liljeqvist, Nordhus O: Monitoring coronary artery blood flow by Doppler shift ultrasound. Scand. J. thor. cardiovasc. Surg. 11: 119–123, 1977.
10. FitzGerald DE, Drumm JE: Non-invasive measurement of human fetal circulation using ultrasound: a new method. Brit. med. J. 2: 1450–1451, 1977.
11. Gosling RG, King DH: Continuous wave ultrasound as an alternative and complement to X-rays in vascular examinations. In: Cardiovascular Applications of Ultrasound, Amsterdam, North Holland Publishing Company, 1974, p 266–282.
12. McCormack PD, FitzGerald DE: The visco-elastic arterial flow model and the ultrasound Doppler probe. J. Inst. Maths. Applics. 16: 361–370, 1975.
13. McCormack P, Brew WK, Fortesque-Webb CM, FitzGerald DE: Visco-elastic arterial flow model using the ultrasound Doppler flowmeter. In: Clinical Blood Flow Measurement, London, Sector Publishing, 1976, p 48–52.
14. Brew WKM, FitzGerald DE: Transcutaneous assessment of arterial elasticity. Ultrasound Med. Biol. 2: 263–270, 1976.
15. Gow BS: The influence of smooth muscle on the viscoelastic properties of blood vessels. In: Cardiovascular Fluid Dynamics. New York, Academic Press, 1972.

REFERENCE TO COMMENTARY

1. Fronek et al: Noninvasive physiologic tests in the diagnosis and characterization of peripheral arterial occlusive disease. Am. J. Surg. 1973, 126: 205–214.

5. Thermography

TRAVIS WINSOR AND DAVID WILEY WINSOR

Commentary by S. Uematsu

1. INTRODUCTION

Thermography is a scanning technique which gives a photographic display of temperature differences of the surface of the body or inanimate objects. The thermograph measures the heat emission in the infrared portion of the electromagnetic spectrum in contrast to radiography which measures the energy of X-rays and gamma rays of the same electromagnetic spectrum. The achievement of a satisfactory translation of the natural, invisible, infrared emission of the human body to a visible representation has resulted in the discipline of medical thermography.

2. HISTORY

About 400 B.C. Hippocrates studied the temperature of the human body as related to disease. In his teachings at Cos he presented an early observation that acute disease was characterized by an increased temperature (1–3). Around 1595 Galileo developed the first clinical thermometer; however it was Santorius who applied the use of the thermometer to human disease (1–3). In 1800 Sir William Herschel, an English astronomer (Fig. 1) discovered that the sun's spectrum contained electromagnetic energy of longer wavelengths than the red light seen by using a prism (4). In 1830 Edwards summarized the relationship between temperature recordings in health and disease (2). In 1835 Becquerel and Breschet observed that the temperature of inflamed parts was higher than that of healthy ones and established that the mean normal body temperature was 37 °C (3). In 1840 Sir F.W. Herschel, son of Sir William, recorded invisible wavelengths on paper and called the display a 'thermograph' (5). In 1837 Wunderlich established the principles of thermometry and their relation to disease and brought universal acceptance of the clinical thermometer (1–3). In 1834,

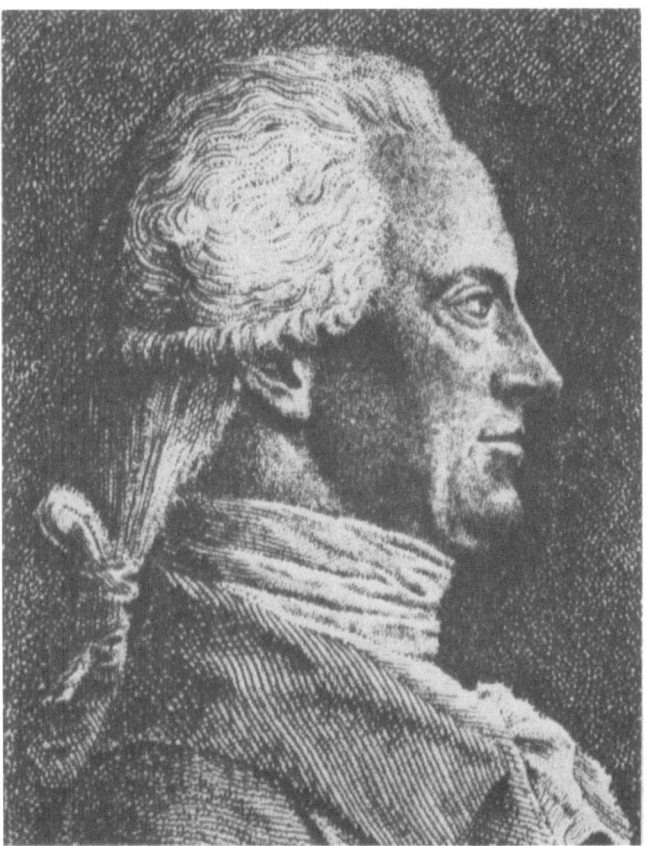

Fig. 1. Sir William Herschel in 1800 discovered that the sun's spectrum contained energy of longer wavelengths than those of red light.

Hardy described the emissivity from human skin of infrared wavelengths greater than 4 μm and demonstrated that living human bodies emit radiations in the long wavelength infrared band as if living human beings were 'black bodies' (6). In 1959 Astheimer and Wormser described an infrared camera which utilized a scanning mirror and a sensitive thermistor heat detector and rotating chopper. The incoming infrared energy was compared 200 times/sec with the energy being emitted by a constant temperature reference black body. The energy variations were displayed on photographic film as a series of varying gray densities (7). In 1957, R.H. Lawson of the Royal Victoria Hospital in Montreal pioneered and established the field of medical thermography. He observed in two cases of breast cancer that the skin overlying the affected area was hotter than the surrounding normal skin (8). From this observation the Barnes scanner was developed and made available in about 1957. In 1960 Lloyd Williams et al. reported on infrared studies among 100 patients with lumps in their breasts (9). In April of 1962, Dr. Gershon-Cohen at the Albert Einstein Medical Center in Philadelphia initiated cooperative studies to explore the overall potential of thermography as a diagnostic tool (2). In 1963 R.H. Lawson published the first paper suggesting that there was a correlation between the amount of temperature rise and the degree of malignancy in breast cancer (2).

Since 1963 the thermographic technique has been applied in almost every field of medicine, the major areas of interest being soft tissue abnormalities, the arthritis, synovitis, trauma, venous thrombosis, malignancies of skin, bone and breast and other tissues, cerebral vascular insufficiency, sprains, strains and whiplash injuries of the back and neck. Also the effect of drugs, vasomotion, smoking, pregnancy, A-V fistulae, causalgia, cervical ribs, frostbite, burns and many other conditions influencing the skin or its adjacent tissues have been investigated.

3. PHYSIOLOGY AND PHYSICAL PRINCIPLES

The skin temperature represents a balance between the heat transferred from the underlying tissues to the skin and the heat lost from the skin to the environment.

Thermal energy transport may be discussed in terms of three processes. These are conduction, radiation and convection. Normally, conduction occurs within the body from the tissues to the skin while radiation and convection cause the transfer of heat from the skin to the environment. The heat loss from the skin is divided roughly 50% by radiation loss and 50% by convective loss. The radiation of man is in a wavelength range of 3–18 μm with a maximum value of 9–10 μm. Evaporative cooling is negligible for patients who have been equilibrated in the proper clinical environment. In order to accurately measure human body radiation and make comparisons from time to time, it is necessary to have the room temperature as constant as possible, usually 70 °F. The air flow over the patient should be uniform. The amount of heat loss is directly proportional to the temperature of the environment.

The skin is the major medium by which the regulation of body temperature takes place. Temperature regulation is necessary to maintain a constant internal environment of the organs essential to life processes. A constant internal body temperature (core temperature) is accomplished by changes in heat production of the internal body organs and muscles and by changes in the isolating capacity of the skin. The skin temperature varies as it responds to the physical laws of heat exchange, adapting itself to the internal temperature of the body. Love has suggested that the temperature

70°F corresponds to 21°C.

of the avascular skin minus the temperature of the room divided by the temperature of the core of the body, which is assumed to be an oral temperature of $37 + 1\,°C$ or $38\,°C$, minus the temperature over a vein is proportional to the blood flow (10).

Also, Burton has developed a thermal circulation index which is an index of blood flow under special circumstances (11). The formula states that the relationship of the external *physical* drop in temperature, that is from skin to environment, divided by the internal *physiological* drop of temperature, that is from rectum to skin, is an index of the blood circulation in the skin. The external physical factors which must be known or kept constant are environmental temperature, sweat loss with evaporation and humidity. The physiologic gradient depends on where the skin temperature measurement is made, whether over subcutaneous fat or muscles, and blood flow. Since blood flow is the only factor which changes rapidly, the skin temperature may be measured. The nomogram (Fig. 2) utilises this formula to reveal changes in blood circulation of the part being measured. For example, if the room temperature is $23\,°C$ and the rectal temperature $37\,°C$, then a skin temperature of $30\,°C$ would give an index of 1. If the temperature rises to $33\,°C$, the index becomes 2 which means that the blood circulation is twice as great at the higher skin temperature compared with the lower one. When working at different room temperatures, a

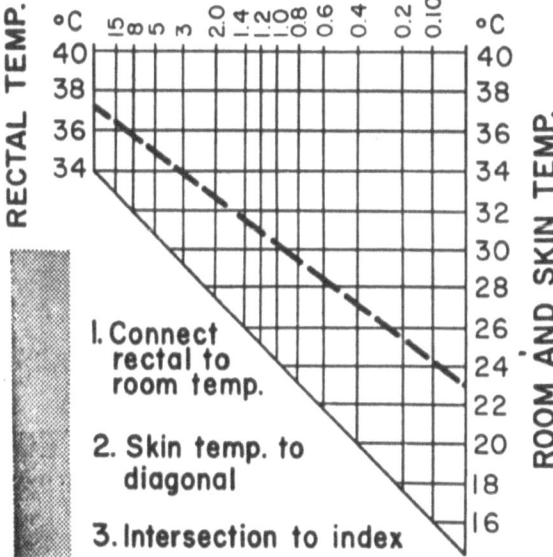

Fig. 2. Nomogram of Burton relating core temperature to room temperature and skin temperature to circulation. The circulatory index is at the top of the graph.

dashed diagonal line is superimposed on this graph for practical use. It should be pointed out that increased skin temperatures, which vary little with time, may be due to increased local metabolic processes such as inflammation or cancers, while cool but constant temperatures may represent areas of low metabolic heat or insulation by subcutaneous fat. Rapid changes in skin temperature when the environment is constant usually represents changes in the blood flow.

There are three parts of the body which can be considered as radiators. First are the hands and feet where there is a small tissue volume and large blood content and large surface area. In these areas there are wide skin temperature variations which occur under the control of the sympathetic nervous system. The second set of radiators consists of the arms and legs, and here the relationship between heat, tissue and blood content and skin surface is less favorable for the regulation of heat loss. Here the circulation is also under the control of the parasympathetic nerves and bradykinin which can produce active vasodilatation. The third set of radiators is formed by the head and trunk. Here the large tissue volume and small variations in skin circulation create a skin temperature which is quite constant (12, 13).

Infrared energy in the form of 'invisible light' is emitted by the human body and by all objects whose temperatures are above absolute zero. This invisible energy may be gathered and displayed optically in the form of the thermogram. The human body is constantly broadcasting electromagnetic signals which are related to the metabolic state of the body and the temperature and emissivity of the skin. It is known that the human skin is partically transparent and partially reflective to visible light, and also to the near infrared. Its optical properties in the region of the longer wavelengths are different. From about 3 μm to about 15 μm human skin is essentially unreflective and nontransparent. In fact, it is an almost perfect absorber or 'black body', therefore the body is an almost perfect emitter of infrared energy. A black body has a heat emissivity of 1.0. This indicates that it absorbs and radiates far infrared but does not reflect far infrared. The human skin at ordinary skin temperatures has an emissivity of approximately 1.0. The maximum emissivity of energy is in the 8–9 μm range (Fig. 3).

4.   INSTRUMENTS

There are various instruments available for thermography. Most instruments consist of an optical system, an infrared detector and its processing electronics and a display system. All systems receive infrared radiation from the subject. The radiation is focused on the detector and voltage

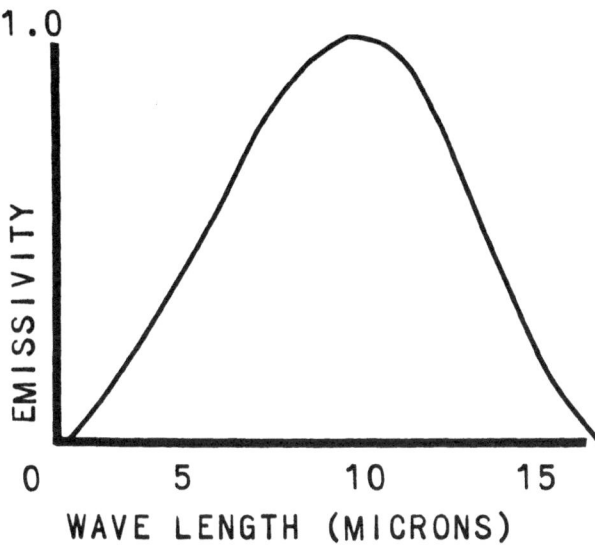

Fig. 3. The emissivity of human skin in the far infrared range is similar to that of a black body at a comfortable room temperature.

variations result which produce the display on a cathode ray tube or other format. The optical system scans the body in a series of lines comprising from 100 to 600 lines per frame, which produce the picture. In the original Barnes thermograph the scanning optic is a mechanically moveable mirror that receives heat rays from different points of the body as the mirror is moved in two directions, from side to side and up and down. In other instruments, such as the AGA, spinning mirrors have been employed to receive the heat being emitted from the body. The optical system focuses the heat on the detector and voltage variations are recorded on Polaroid or other film.

The detectors are devices which convert infrared energy into voltage changes in proportion to the amount of infrared falling on the detector. The thermistor bolometer records maximum energy emission from the body at a maximum of 9.5 μm wavelength. The indium antimonide detector has a peak energy detection of about 4.5 μm wavelength. The mercury cadmium telluride detector has a maximum detection of about 12 μm wavelength.

The voltage variations are amplified and converted into a suitable form for display. In the Barnes instrument, a white light moves mechanically and in synchrony with the moving mirror. The light is focused onto black and white or colour Polaroid or X-ray film. The display system may also be a cathode ray oscilloscope with an appropriate camera for photographing from the face of the tube. Black and white Polaroid film type 084 or 667, 70 mm film or sheet X-ray film may be used for making permanent records.

Some commonly used terms relating to thermographic instruments are defined as follows:

Resolving power is the ability of the system to detect clearly and with detail small heat temperature differences. The resolving power is often related to the number of horizontal scan lines and the number of points measured per line as well as the size of the minimal detector spot for measurement.

Thermal sensitivity is the ability of the device to display two different shades of gray. Sensitivity of 0.1 °C is considered adequate for thermographic purposes.

Field of view is the field which is displayed on a cathode ray oscilloscope. In most instances the closer the camera is to the subject the smaller the field of view. The field of view for the Spectrotherm, for example, is 16 in. × 16 in. at a distance of 2 f.

Focal range is the distance over which the camera will produce a sharp image. With the Texas Instrument unit this is from zero to infinity and in the AGA from 3.1 f. to infinity.

Detector is the type of thermistor or other device which converts infrared energy into a voltage change. Some detectors require liquid nitrogen for reference while other use an electric internal heat reference source.

Spectral range is the energy range to which the instrument responds most efficiently.

Display is the manner of revealing the thermographic record which may be on a TV monitor or cathode ray oscilloscope tube or photographic film. The display is often on Polaroid or other film. It is important that the film used has high resolution and is capable of recording many shades of gray.

Format is the size of the display which may vary depending upon the system employed. Often 4 in. × 5 in. Polaroid film is used.

Frame time is the length of time it takes to record a picture, i.e., 2 sec in the Spectrotherm and 1/16 sec in the AGA.

Angle of view is the angle at the camera within which the picture is recorded.

Angular resolution is the resolution which is obtained at different angular settings.

Scan time is the length of time it takes to scan the subject when recording a thermogram.

Thermal resolution is the limit of temperature differentiation between two shades of gray.

Temperature range is the extremes of temperature which the equipment is able to detect, generally from zero to 50 °C. Commerical instruments record a wider range.

Optical system consists of the pick-up system and optics which are employed to collect infrared radiation. The system may be a mechanical moving mirror or spinning mirrors.

Chopper is a spinning wheel or device which allows a thermistor to receive energy from a reference source such as a black body and alternately receive infrared from the subject.

Isotherm is a display pattern of many temperature points, all of which have the same temperature. Often isothermic measurements are made in 1 °C intervals.

Infrared is a portion of the spectrum at the red end of the thermal radiation scale and are wavelengths longer than those of visible light.

Comparison of the Spectrotherm, Texas Instruments and AGA shows that the Spectrotherm has more lines per field than the AGA and hence greater thermal resolving power (Table 1).

5. TECHNIQUE

COMMENTARY

A skillfully recorded thermogram is a basic requirement for a good thermographic interpretation. Good technique involves the proper room and environment, good patient preparation, proper positioning of the patient, accurate focusing of the instrument, careful setting of the contrast and brightness of the instrument and proper selection and processing of the recording film.

When an elastic bandage has been over the area of examination it is advisable to expose the area to room temperature for longer than 30 min. The effect of the elastic bandage lasts longer than we expect.

Thermographic room: The walls, ceilings, floor and objects in the room

Table 1. Comparative competitive characteristics of three different thermographic instruments.

Characteristics	Spectrotherm 1000	Texas Instruments	AGA
Resolution; elements/frame	525 lines; 600 elements/line	525 lines horizontal 525 elements/line	140 lines
Thermal sensitivity	<0.2 °C	0.07 °C	<0.2 °C
Field of view	30° × 30° (16 in. × 16 in. at 2 ft.)	33° × 33° (19 in. × 19 in. at 2 ft.)	25° × 25°
Focal range	4 in. to 20 in. ft.	0 to infinity	3.1 ft. to infinity
Detector	Mercury/cadmium telluride	Mercury/cadmium telluride	Indium antimonide
Detector cooling	N (>4 h)	N (4 h)	N (4 h)
Spectral range	to beyond 13 μm	6–14 μm	2–5.6 μm
Display	TV monitor	CRT	TV monitor
Format	3 in. × 3 in.	3 in. × 3 in.	3.5 in. × 3.5 in.
Power requirements	100/200 W 110, 50 or 60 Hz	200 W, 115 V, 60 Hz	200 W, 115 or 23, 50 or 60 Hz
Size			
Scanner	23¼ in. × 21¾ in. × 12 in.	18 in. wide × 14.25 in. high × 18.75 in. long	7.9 in. × 9.4 in. × 20.8 in.
Display		20 in. × 15.75 in. × 22 in.	17.7 in. × 7.9 in. × 20.8 in.
Weight			
Scanner	85 lb	35 lb	30 lb
Display		45 lb	52 lb
Frame time	2 sec	4.5 sec	16 sec

70 °F is equal to 21 °C. It feels rather cold to most patients, particularly when undressed. However, the coldness of the room would have a provocative effect in reproducing the clinical signs such as dysthesia and discoloration of the fingers in cases of Raynaud's disease and related disorders.

should be as close to the same temperature as possible, preferably within 1 °C of each other. This is to prevent interchange of heat back and forth between the patient and objects within the room. A constant temperature of 70 °F is optimum for most instruments and patients. At this temperature most instruments work well and the patient's skin is constricted but he is not shivering. The air flow should be constant as drafts will cause cooling and artifacts. A constant down draft of 15 ft./min through a perforated diffusing ceiling provides an adequate system; however this technique for producing constant air flow is not mandatory.

Preparation for the test: Normally the patient should cool in the room environment where the test will be performed for at least 15 min with appropriate clothing removed. One should avoid contact with other parts of the body such as touching the skin, rubbing or scratching. The skin should be observed by the technician and notes made concerning local skin blemishes, scars or unusual contour of the skin such as a deep depression along the spine. The skin should be observed for sweating, but no perspiration should occur after cooling and a rest period.

Position of the subject: The subject may be supine in which case a front silvered mirror is used to collect the infrared radiation, or the subject may be standing or sitting for direct photography without use of a mirror. The scan lines should pass from one side of the body to the other, for example from right to left or left to right so that accurate comparisons of comparable areas on each side of the patient can be made.

Focus of the thermograph: The part of maximum interest should serve as the site for focusing, i.e., the forehead. Since the depth of field is often narrow, particularly at close range, accurate focus is mandatory for accurate thermographic representation.

The *brightness* setting of the machine is adjusted in accordance with the temperature of the parts of the body being studied. This setting brings various parts of the body of different temperature into the visible range of the camera and film, thus allowing warm and cool parts to appear visible on the film. A complete black or complete white represents a loss of information. It is only the ranges of gray between black and white that make useful displays in the thermogram.

The *sensitivity* setting refers to the range of temperatures which will be displayed. The camera may be operated in a white-hot or dark-hot mode. All thermograms should have within the picture a heat standard or thermal gray scale with temperatures of known increments. The gray scale usually consists of a scale with increments of temperatures ranging from 29 to 38 °C. The Spectrotherm 2000 displays an analogue graph of the temperature going across the part of the body of interest. The scale for the temperature graph is displayed as a single digit number at the right of the graph. For example, a setting of 6 means that the distance from the bottom horizontal line to the top horizontal line represents a change of 6 °C.

When photographing onto Polaroid film, the Polaroid type 084 and type 667 black and white films for diagnostic recordings have sufficient contrast, gray scale, resolution and exposure range to accurately reproduce data from the CRT imaging displays. This is the same film that is commonly used with ultrasound scanners and computerized axial tomographic instruments. If X-ray film is used a separate film processor is often desirable for best results.

Special thermographic techniques: Special techniques for peripheral vascular disease are used. These include body heating to indirectly warm the patient's limbs or acra, dynamic thermography which shows temperature changes with the legs in different positions, i.e., elevated, flat or down for venous disorders; sympathetic blocks to promote vasodilatation; cooling such as the application of alcohol sprays to the head for cerebral vascular disease; clamps for occluding the carotid arteries to facilitate visualization of internal carotid arteries; mirror devices for showing more than one view of a part in one film, and exercize testing used for demonstrating peripheral arterial insufficiency.

6. HEAD AND CEREBRAL VASCULAR DISEASE

Thermography has been useful for evaluating the cerebral vascular circulation, namely the internal carotid, common carotid and innominate artery in patients with signs or symptoms suggesting a vascular disorder. Studies may be made before and after carotid artery surgery. A survey of the literature indicates that thermography can reveal 90% of patients with complete occlusion of one internal carotid artery. With internal carotid artery stenosis of 70% or greater, about 70% of the thermograms are diagnostic. With common carotid artery occlusion about 95% are positive and with common carotid artery stenosis of greater than 70% the yield is about 95%. With bilateral or common carotid artery occlusion about 90% of thermograms are positive (14). The following conditions seldom give abnormal thermograms: occlusions of the cerebral arteries, generalized cerebral atherosclerosis, subarachnoid hemorrhage, arteriovenous malformations, brain tumors, external carotid occlusion, and carotid cavernous fistula. One can anticipate an improved pattern on the thermogram after successful carotid artery surgery.

Although we have only limited experience on arteriovenous malformations or carotid cavernous fistulas, there is evidence to suggest that thermography may be helpful to rule out arteriovenous malformations when it is positive. In one of our cases of chronic headache, thermography revealed 2.25 °C increased temperature over the branches of the left superficial temporal and facial arteries. The patient was found to have an A-V malformation of the occipital lobe.

6.1. *Technique*

A high resolution camera should be employed at a room temperature between 68 and 72 °F, humidity of approximately 30–50% and a rest period of 15 min. A temperature variation from dark gray to light gray of

2 or 3 °C is desirable. Heat reference standards should be in the picture. Two pictures are usually made, one light and one dark. Pictures may be made with or without temporal artery head clamp. The clamp increases the sensitivity of the test (15, 16). The rate of rewarming after cooling the forehead with alcohol or with tepid water in a plastic bag has been less successful than the use of a head clamp.

6.2.   *Normal*

The normal facial thermogram shows a reproducible thermal pattern. Normally the nose has a variable temperature and may be cool or warm (Fig. 4 and 5). The cheeks and ears are usually cool. The anterior portion of the forehead is warm with a narrow range of temperature variation over the surface (Fig. 5). Frontal artery and supraorbital artery heat is often detectable. Heat is normally trapped by skin folds along the edge of the cheek, around the mouth, at the internal canthi and along the free margins of the eyelids. The eyeballs of the open eye are slightly warm and like the bridge of the nose. Facial heat patterns are symmetrical.

The arterial circulation of the face through the external carotid artery and the internal carotid artery must be understood to appreciate heat patterns that occur with disease (Figs. 6, 7 and 8). The external carotid artery courses over the angle of the jaw along the nasolabial fold to the side and tip of the nose, continuing to the inner canthus of the eye where it meets branches of the internal carotid (Figs. 6 and 7). The external carotid artery is one of the collateral pathways to the internal carotid. With internal carotid artery obstruction blood carried by the external carotid artery could account for a warm spot at the tip of the nose (Figs. 6 and 7). The external carotid artery from the neck then courses along the side of the face just anterior to the tragus of the ear. At this point the external carotid gives off a superficial branch, the lateral orbital division, that goes to the lateral aspect of the orbit and supplies the skin in this area (Fig. 7). The temporal division of the external carotid then courses up over the forehead to connect with the frontal and supraorbital branches of the internal carotid artery (Fig. 7). The temporal artery becomes a large collateral pathway when internal carotid artery obstruction occurs. Branches of the internal carotid artery emerge from the inner canthus of the eye and supply blood to the bridge of the nose and the forehead. Also, branches emerge from the frontal and supraorbital arteries and supply heat to the forehead (Fig. 8). With internal carotid artery obstruction one can see cool areas at the inner canthus of the eye, above the nose, and above the eyebrow. There are anastomotic connections between the external and internal carotid arteries through the temporal nasal and supraorbital branches. With internal carotid artery obstruction, blood flows in an abnormal direction

There is always an exception. When collateral circulation has developed through the external carotid artery over the face in the case of complete obstruction of the carotid artery, thermography may show elevation of the from the temporal into the nasal arteries instead of in the reverse direction which is the normal direction of flow. Blood will always flow from the level of higher pressure to one of lower pressure; thus lowering the pressure in the internal circuit causes a reversal of flow.

Wood (14) has shown that a significant difference in the temperature on the two sides of the head is not invoked until the blood vessel is 60% closed. This was shown by use of the progressive closure of a clamp on the internal or common carotid artery. Generally, it is felt that about a 75% narrowing of the blood vessel is required before a stroke occurs. With these findings it would appear that thermography can provide a means for detecting approaching stroke prior to a neurologic deficit (15, 16).

temperature ipsilateral to the obstruction. This finding may cause some difficulty in determining the side of the carotid artery occlusion. However, with awareness of this possibility one may correctly determine the site of the occlusion, since the increased temperature due to superficial collateral circulation is usually a diffuse and unusually elevated temperature pattern relative to the normal physiological one. Similar phenomenon can occur in cases of arterial obstruction of limbs.

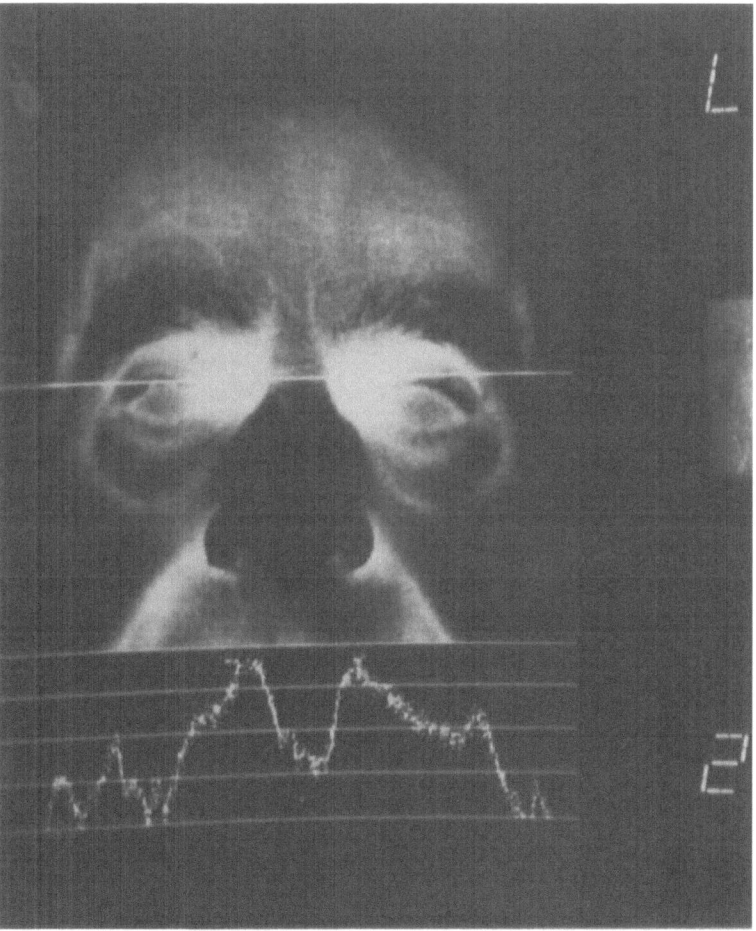

Fig. 4. Normal thermogram of the head with analogue scale at the bottom. The heat pattern is symmetrical. The nose is cold.

6.3. *Abnormal*

The heat abnormalities indicating unilateral internal carotid artery disease are a loss of inner canthus heat by approximately 0.7 °C, a decrease in eyeball temperature by approximately 0.7 °C, a decrease in unilateral forehead temperature by about 0.7 °C and a hot tip of the nose. Evidence of unilateral common carotid stenosis produces additionally ipsilateral cooling of the cheek, lateral aspect of the orbit, and temporal artery area. The pattern of the positive thermogram is the same regardless of whether there is stenosis or occlusion of the artery; however, stenosis is not as evident as is a total occlusion.

The changes described generally pertain, if the lesion is in the internal

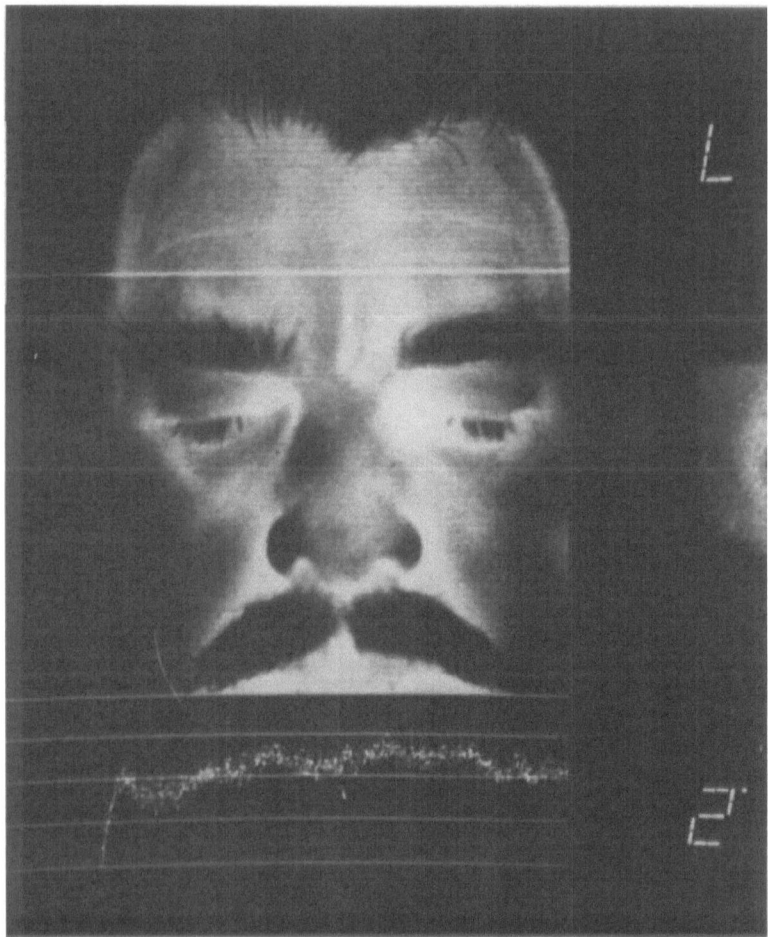

Fig. 5. Normal heat pattern. Eyebrows, eyelashes and moustache are cool, having low metabolic activity. The heat patterns are symmetrical from side to side. The nose is warm.

carotid artery, just adjacent to the bifurcation near the origin of the common carotid artery or in the distal cervical intrapetrosal or cavernous portion of the internal carotid artery and proximal to the origin of the ophthalmic branch.

Bilateral compromise of the internal system is a more complex pattern since a complete occlusion promotes a large collateral flow. Thus, occlusion of an internal carotid artery on one side with contralateral internal carotid stenosis produces an apparent paradox in that the stenotic side is cooler than the occluded side since total occlusion, if long standing, may promote a large ipsilateral collateral circulation. Collateral flow is often observed through branches of the superficial temporal artery anastomosing with the supraorbital artery. Extensive collateral flow across the midline may occur through deep or superficial paramedian vessels.

Case 1, Mr. E.N., 58-year-old male, had transient ischemic attacks in 1967. The thermogram at that time showed a 1 °C cooling of the left forehead compared with the right. Also there was an area of decrease in inner canthus heat on the left compared with the right. The tip of the nose was warm (Fig. 9). Ten years later the patient had an isotherm thermogram which showed, on the left, decreased supraorbital heat and decreased inner canthus heat (Fig. 10). There was a temperature increase at the tip of

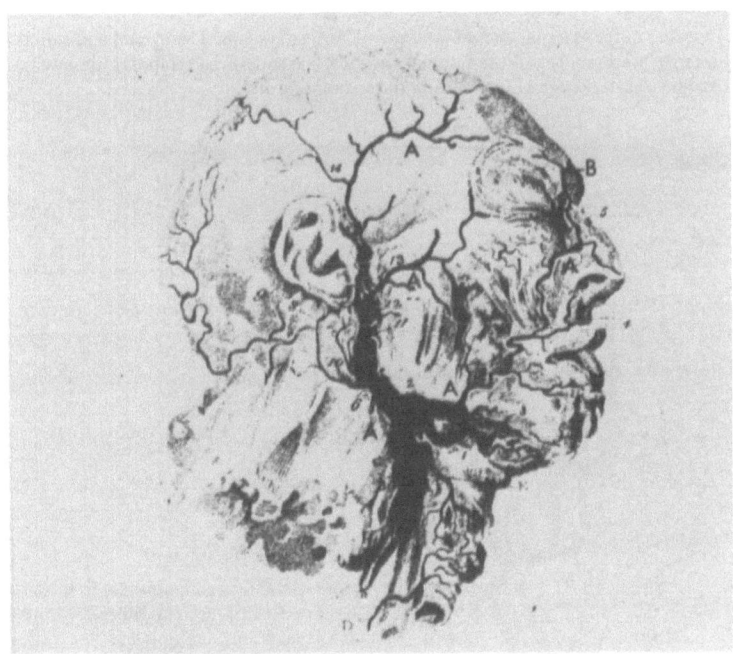

Fig. 6. External carotid artery at A, and supraorbital or nasal branches from the internal carotid artery at B.

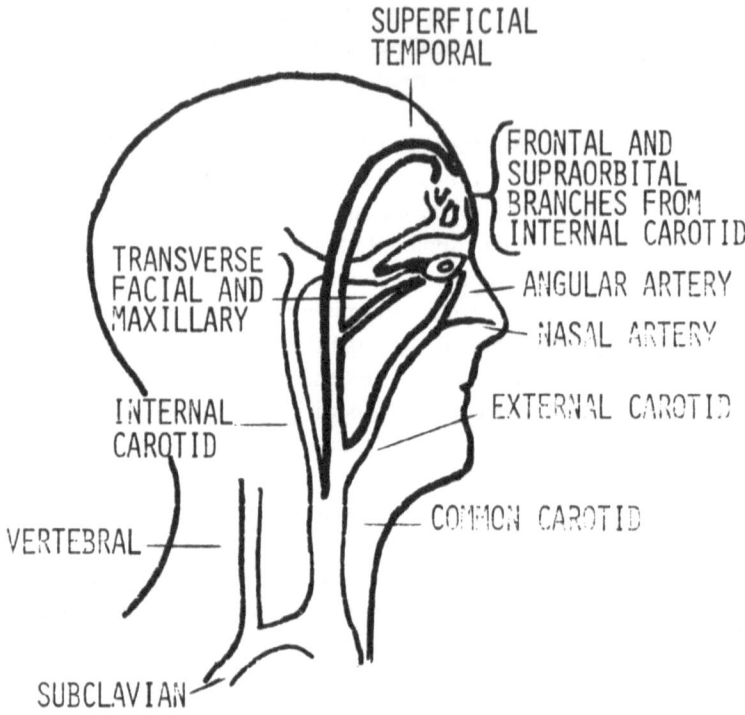

Fig. 7. Drawing of the external and internal carotid artery systems. The frontal and supra-orbital arteries are branches of the internal carotid. The superficial temporal, transverse frontal and nasal arteries are branches from the external carotid.

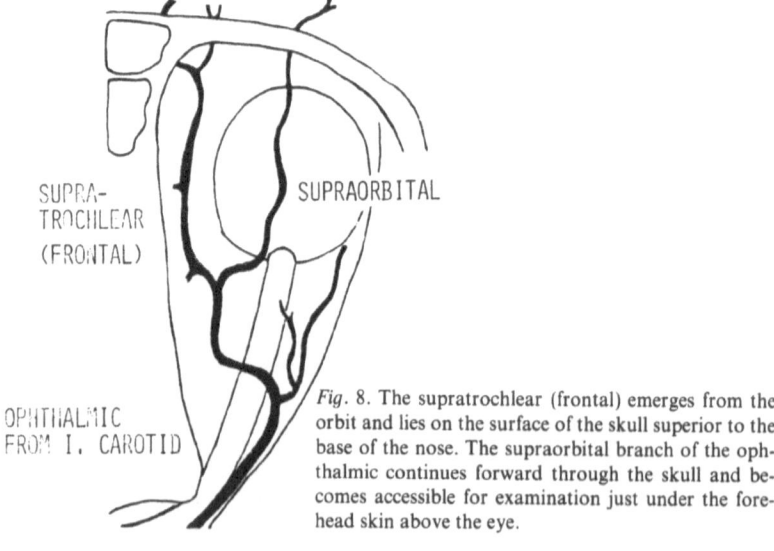

Fig. 8. The supratrochlear (frontal) emerges from the orbit and lies on the surface of the skull superior to the base of the nose. The supraorbital branch of the ophthalmic continues forward through the skull and becomes accessible for examination just under the forehead skin above the eye.

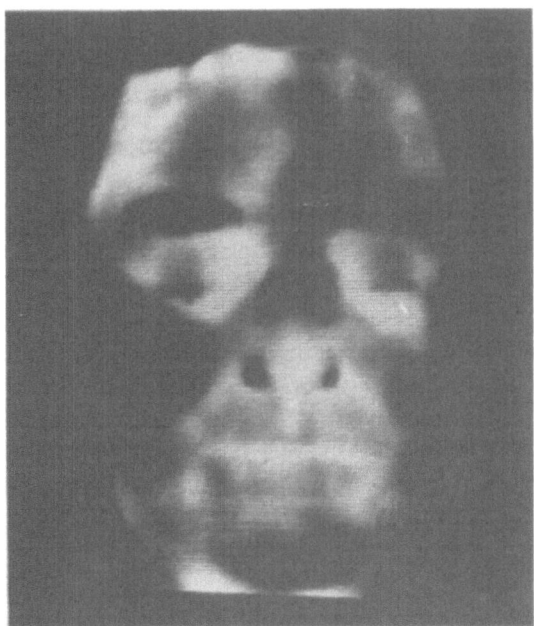

Fig. 9. Patient E.N. shows cooling above the left eyebrow with decreased left inner canthus heat. The tip of the nose is warm.

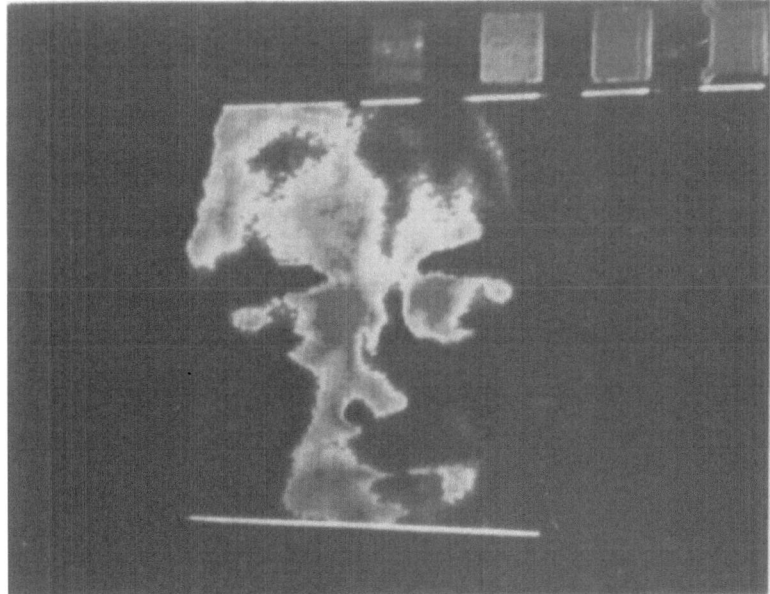

Fig. 10. Patient E.N. 10 years later. The color isotherm showed, on the left, decreased left frontal artery heat and decreased left canthus heat with decreased heat along the course of the external carotid artery along the side of the face and in the temporal artery area.

the nose. There was cooling of the left forehead and left nasolabial fold. This picture suggested left common carotid artery occlusion (Fig. 10). Pulse propagation time measurements made from the ECG to the time of arrival of pulsations of the supraorbital arteries showed a 20 msec delay of the time of arrival of the pulse on the left forehead. Doppler studies over the left eye showed decreased frequency in the signal over the left nasal artery (Fig. 11). This patient had not had a stroke. He had diabetes, angina pectoris, hypertension and peripheral arterial disease. Clinically the arterial pulse at the neck was low on the left compared with the right. There was no bruit on the left. Angiogram showed complete occlusion of the left common carotid artery at the bifurcation which extended into the internal and external carotid arteries. Surgery was not performed. This case is important in that the decreased forehead heat, canthus cooling and increased nose heat are all displayed. It is significant that this patient went for 10 years with very few symptoms and only occasional transient ischemic attacks with complete obstruction of the left common carotid artery.

Case 2, Mr. H.Q., is a 65-year-old male with transient ischemic attacks. The thermogram was taken with a ΔT of $2\,^{\circ}$C. Thus each horizontal line at the bottom of the film represents $0.5\,^{\circ}$C change. The analogue temperature trace at the bottom of the film is a record of temperature change at the

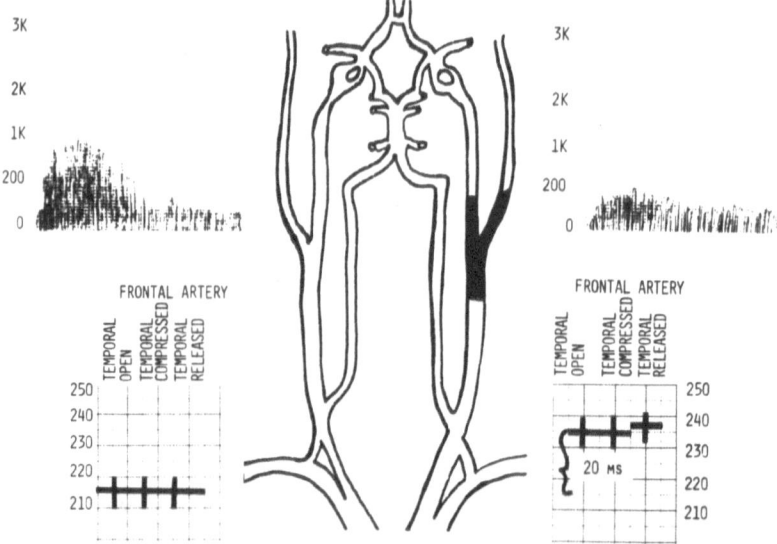

Fig. 11. Drawing of angiogram showing complete obstruction of the internal and external carotid artery on the left. The Doppler flow signals as analyzed with the Kay Sonagraph show low frequencies on the left. The timing from the beginning of the QRS complex to the arrival of the foot of the pulse wave over the nasal arteries was delayed to 20 msec on the left. Temporal artery compression did not add any additional information.

fiducial line over the forehead. The left forehead was 0.5 °C less than the right. Inner canthus heat on the left was definitely less than the right. Left eyeball heat was cooler than the right. There was an increased temperature of the tip of the nose, increased heat in the region of the left nasolabial fold and, also, slight increase of heat over the left temporal artery. The cool forehead, canthus and eyeball represent decreased internal carotid circulation. The increased temperature at the tip of the nose, at the left nasolabial fold and at the left forehead represents collateral circulation (Fig. 12). A color thermogram three years later showed a cool left forehead and canthus. The left external maxillary area was warm with a warm nose which indicates well-developed collateral circulation (Fig. 13). The external carotid artery was patent. The angiogram showed complete occlusion of the left internal carotid artery. Pulse propagation time from the ECG to frontal arteries showed a 20 msec delay on the left compared with the right. Compression of the left temporal artery caused an additional

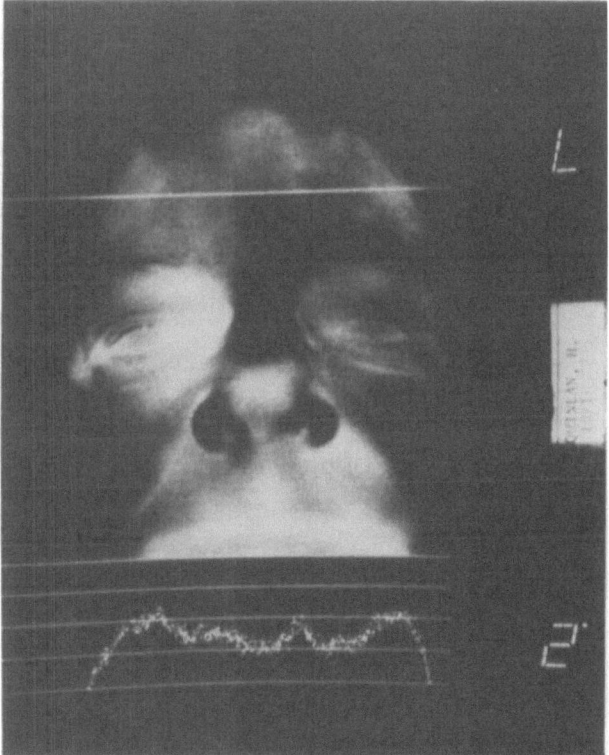

Fig. 12. Patient H.Q. showed, on the left, coolness of the forehead, decreased left inner canthus heat and a temperature increase at the tip of the nose. The left nasolabial heat was increased suggesting a collateral pathway through the external maxillary artery.

delay on the left. Pneumatic plethysmographic studies over the frontal arteries showed pulse loss on the left with left temporal compression.

This patient clearly shows the effect of occlusion of just the internal carotid artery on the left with the thermograms, pulse timing and head pneumoplethysmograms all indicating abnormal circulation on the left. This case is in contrast to case 1 in which the common carotid was obstructed and showed minimal collateral circulation through the external carotid artery, whereas case 2 showed the external carotid serving as a major collateral pathway to the circle of Willis.

The patient had previously had a small stroke involving the right arm with almost no residual. He had had slight aphasia but there was none at the time of the examination. He has arteriosclerosis of the arteries of both legs.

6.4. *Comment*

The accuracy of thermography for the detection of carotid arterial insufficiency is probably greater than any other of its clinical, noninvasive

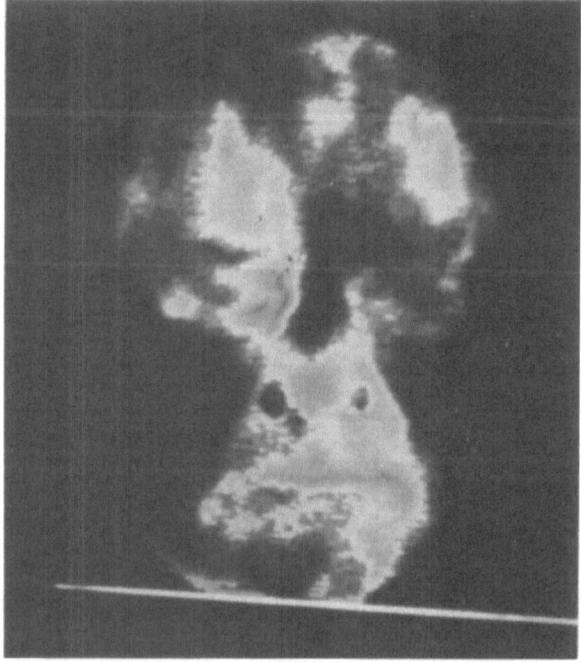

Fig. 13. Patient H.Q. 3 years later demonstrated in a color isotherm coolness over the left eye, coolness of the left eye, coolness of the left inner canthus with increased collateral circulation along the left nasolabial fold and in the region of the left temporal artery.

counterparts. Experience shows that patients with 60% occlusive or stenotic lesions in the common or internal carotid artery have abnormal patterns to the extent of 88%. The cases of failure may be because of poor photographic technique on the part of the thermographer. Other modalities, such as ophthalmodynamometry, arm to retina dye appearance times, isotope studies, carotid compression tests and analysis of carotid bruits are procedures of established value. To these, thermography must be considered complimentary and should not be neglected by the careful diagnostician. Some of the procedures above are of limited value. Hollenhorst found that about 30% of patients with occlusive disease readings are equal on the two sides. The prolonged arm to retina dye appearance time appears to be dependent on high grade obstruction with fluorescein taking a more devious route on the obstructed side (17). There was no direct relationship between the appearance time and retinal artery pressure as demonstrated by Heyman (18). Thermography and ophthalmodynamometry are often complimentary in bilateral carotid artery insufficiency. With internal carotid occlusion on one side and stenosis on the other, thermographic cooling is usually found on the stenotic side while the retinal artery pressure is lower on the occluded side. This discrepancy may help reveal the true status of the vascular insufficiency (14).

It is probably as well to record thermograms with the patient in the sitting or standing position. Hollenhorst noted that retinal artery pressure differences, significant of disease, were greater when patients were upright (17). Wood described one patient in whom the thermogram was normal supine and abnormal in the sitting position (14).

Articats. Positive thermograms have been shown in patients with boils or pimples on the face, sunburn, scratching of the skin and inadequate cooling. Infections of the tear ducts and conjunctivitis may also produce misleading results. Trauma to the face, carotid cavernous fistula. angiomas of the brain and a few anteriorly situated meningiomas may alter the skin temperature.

7. DISORDERS OF THE ARTERIAL SYSTEM

In examining the hands and feet thermographically, attention to detail is necessary to prevent the occurrence of artifacts produced by rubbing or scratching the skin, clenching the fists, pulling, pushing, smoking or drafts. It is often necessary to have an observer present in the room during the equilibration period so that artifacts will not occur.

Arteriosclerosis obliterans with or without diabetes is by far the most common arterial abnormality of the extremities. Arterial emboli, laceration of arteries, contusion, collagen diseases, for example scleroderma, vascular tumors, AV fistulas, and Buerger's disease are less common (19, 20).

7.1.   *Normal arms and hands*

Normally the arms and hands are symmetrical in temperature from side to side. The temperature over the bones such as elbows and the wrists is slightly lower than the forearms. The temperatures of the fingers with respect to the hand vary a great deal depending upon vasoconstriction or vasodilatation. With vasoconstriction the fingers are cooler than the palms and backs of the hands, whereas with vasodilatation the reverse is true. Normally the hand vein distribution is prominent and this occurs when the fingers are warm and there is a high rate of blood flow through the hands. Fig. 14A shows normal heat distribution of a hand before, and Fig. 14B after, one ounce of whiskey with a resultant increase in finger temperature and the appearance of a venous pattern. Here the Love (10) formula can be applied and the blood flow determined.

7.2.   *Arterial disease of the arms and hands*

An early sign of vascular disease is the 'bite deficit' (Fig. 15). This figure shows a typical cool spot at the tip of the middle finger which was due to digital arterial vascular disease. This patient had peripheral arteriosclerosis related to diabetes (2).

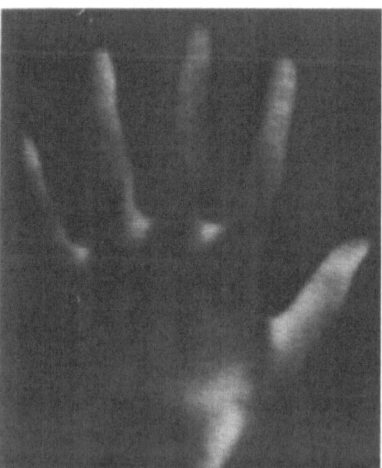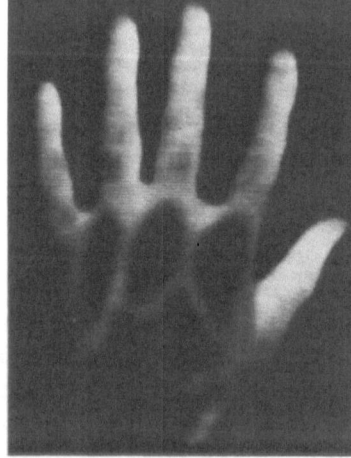

Fig. 14. In A, to the left, the vein pattern on the back of the hand is not readily visualized. In B, to the right, after one ounce of whiskey orally the fingers became warmer and the vein pattern became prominent indicating an increased rate of blood flow.

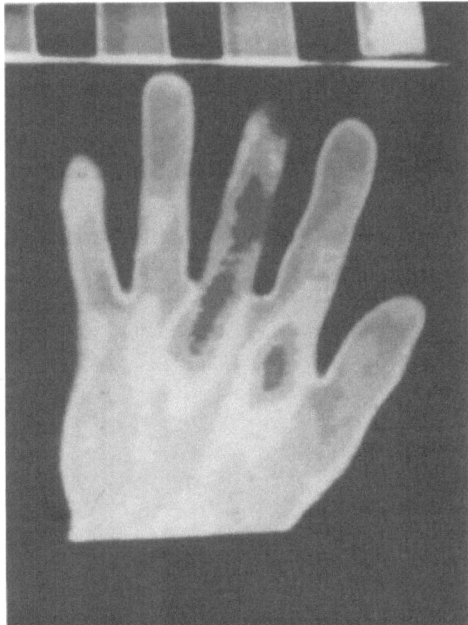

Fig. 15. A 'bite defect' showing an early avascular lesion at the tip of the finger.

Bilateral or unilateral arterial abnormalities of the hands occurs in certain vascular disorders. Bilateral disease is often systemic in origin while unilateral disease is often due to trauma. Fig. 16 shows a cool index finger on one hand and a cool middle finger on the other hand. Bilateral hand disease is common in generalized disease states such as arteriosclerotic disease, with or without diabetes. This patient was a 38-year-old male with diabetes mellitus.

Buerger's disease produces a 'motheaten display' of the thermogram of the hands (Fig. 17). There is scattered disease of islands of small blood vessels which results in a heat pattern showing a variability of temperature zones of the hands. The figure shows a thermogram of a 35-year-old male with Buerger's disease who had painful fourth fingers on each hand. These fingers did not show in the thermogram because they were so cold that they exceeded the sensitivity setting of the thermograph. The compression test at the wrist demonstrated ulnar artery occlusion on the right hand and radial artery occlusion on the left hand.

Smoking has a profound effect on the skin circulation of the hands in some subjects. The hands of a nonsmoker before and during smoking one standard brand cigarette are shown in Fig. 18. There is a large decrease in the temperature of the hands from light gray (warm) to dark gray (cool). This represents $4\,^{\circ}C$ temperature change (from 33 to $29\,^{\circ}C$) or a calculated

change in blood flow of the digits from 14 cu.mm/4 ml/sec to 4 cu.mm/
4 ml/sec.

7.3.   *Normal legs and feet*

The normal leg has thigh and calf temperatures which are warmer than the
kneecap area which is cool. The ankle is cooler than the calf. The toe
temperatures may be cooler or warmer than the dorsum of the foot.

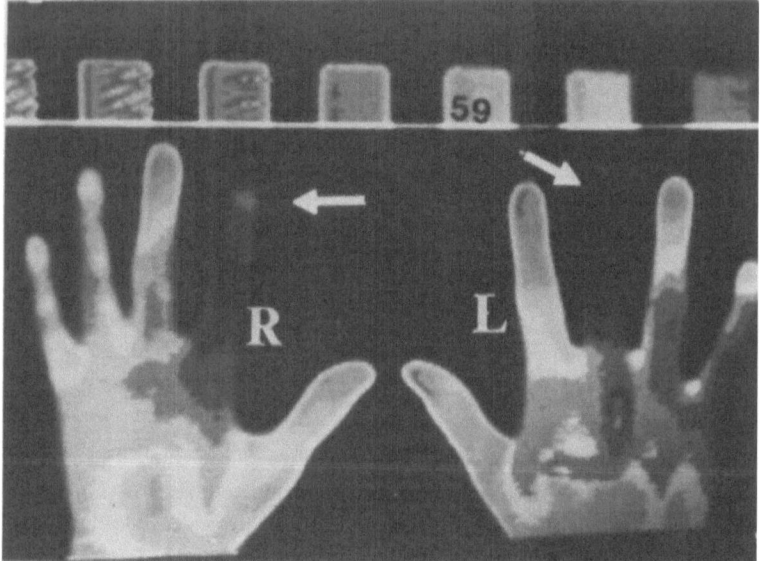

Fig. 16. Ischemic fingers are present on both hands indicating a systemic disorder, often
diabetes mellitus.

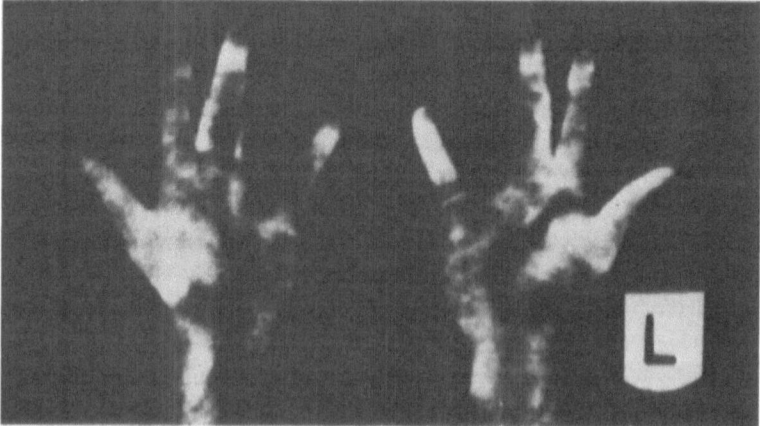

Fig. 17. 'Motheaten' appearance of fingers indicates diffuse vascular disease typical of
thromboangiitis obliterans (Buerger's disease).

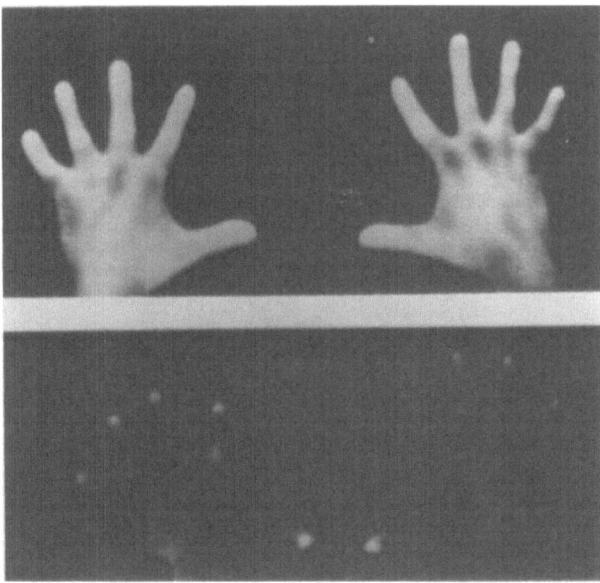

Fig. 18. Smoking: above, hands of normal temperature are shown. Below, after smoking one cigarette, marked vasoconstriction occurred. Only the tips of the fingers remain warm.

7.4. *Arterial disease of the legs and feet*

With an acute arterial occlusion the limb will be cool above and below the embolus because the collateral circulation may not have developed early. With chronic arterial occlusion a rich collateral circulation develops around the occluded area and the limb will be warm above and cool below the occlusion. An acute right superficial femoral artery occlusion is shown in Fig. 19. Here there is very little collateral circulation. A chronic left superficial femoral artery obstruction extending to the popliteal space is shown in Fig. 20. The left leg shows a temperature line just below the knee. The left thigh is warm but the left calf is cool.

Ischemic ulcers are shown in Fig 21A and B. The thermograms (A) show bilateral ischemic limbs with a nonhealing arterial ischemic ulcer on the outer aspect of one leg. There is no inflammatory reaction around the ulcer since the tissues are ischemic. Fig. 21B shows an ulcer in nonischemic limbs in which inflammation with warm blood occurs, draining the cephalad.

Thermography of the feet and toes is rewarding as it is difficult to determine the toe circulation with other techniques (21-23). Fig. 22 shows a case in which the temperatures of the right toes and foot to be generally lower than the left. All the toes have a similar circulation and this finding is consistent with disease higher up in the leg. The patient's right leg is cool

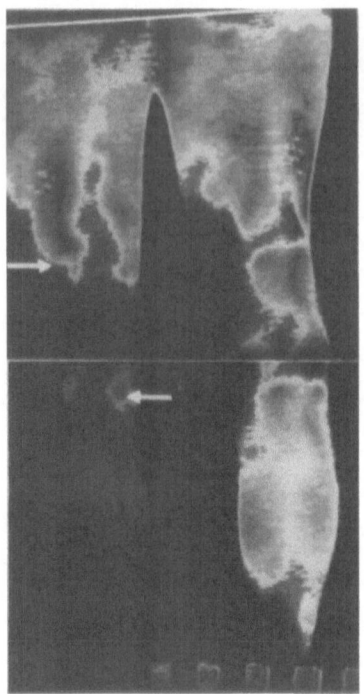

Fig. 19. Acute right superficial femoral artery occlusion with no significant collateral circulation (labeled R).

from the point of obstruction distally. There is a good run-off of blood. A superficial femoral artery obstruction was present in this case. Digital artery disease is shown in Fig. 23. The second and third toes on one side are cool, indicating small vessel disease and a poor run-off.

Dramatic changes are seen in the circulation before and after sympathetic block or sympathectomy. In Fig. 24 the feet before the block showed a rainbow appearance which is significant of high grade vasoconstriction. A lumbar sympathetic block was performed on one side and there was a marked increase in the temperature of the ipsilateral foot, the temperature increasing approximately 10 °C.

Various dynamic tests can be performed to determine the characteristics of the arterial circulation. Cooling of the part with bags of cool water at 10°C for 5 min and determining the rate of rewarming may reveal the presence of disease. The relatively avascular tissue will rewarm more slowly than normal tissue. Raynaud's disease may be studied by placing the hands in gloves and the gloved hand in water at 10 °C for 5 min after which measurements can be made. The effect of body heating often indirectly promotes rapid increases in heat in the vascular area but slow or no increase in an avascular area. Here the body is warmed and measurements can be made on the hands or feet which are at room temperature.

8. VENOUS THROMBOSIS AND INSUFFICIENCY

Venous thrombosis may be either superficial or deep. The thermograph is an ideal instrument for the detection of superficial or deep vein thrombophlebitis. There is a good correlation between thermographic and venographic techniques (24).

8.1. *Method*

Patients are examined in a proper room environment (vide supra). The ankles are elevated 10 in. off the bed to promote venous drainage. Equilibration time is 15 min. One may use an ethanol spray to cool the legs and watch the rate of rewarming. The phlebitis side rewarms faster than the

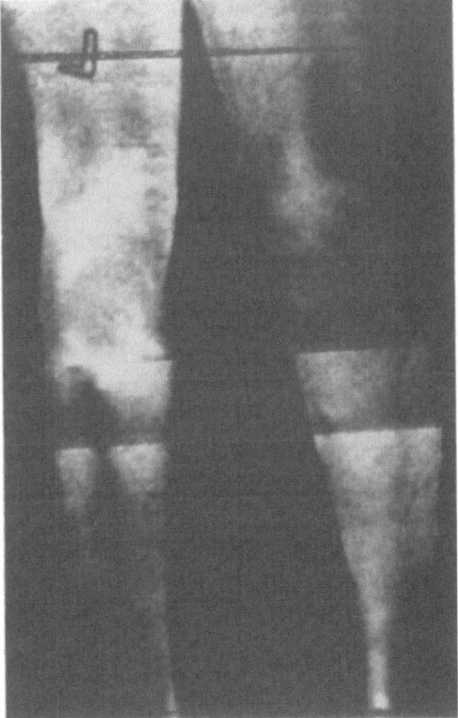

Fig. 20. Chronic superficial femoral artery obstruction shows, on the left, a warm collateral circulation above the knee extending to below the knee with cool calf and ankle in the ischemic zone.

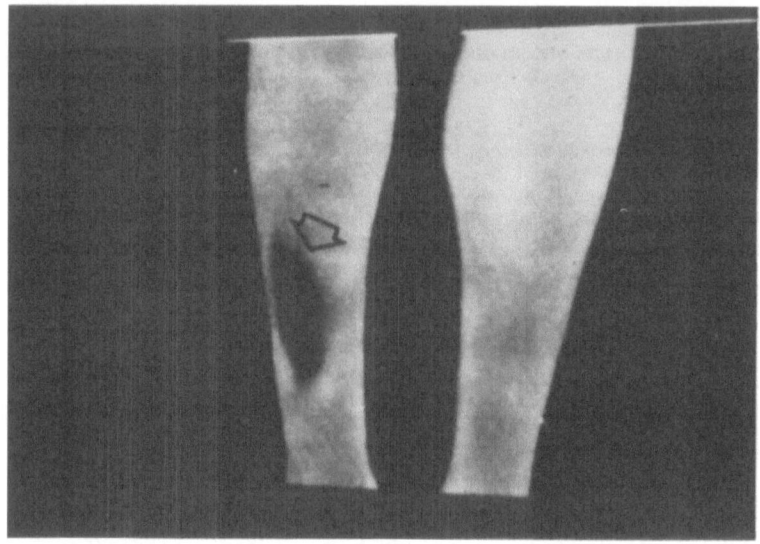

A

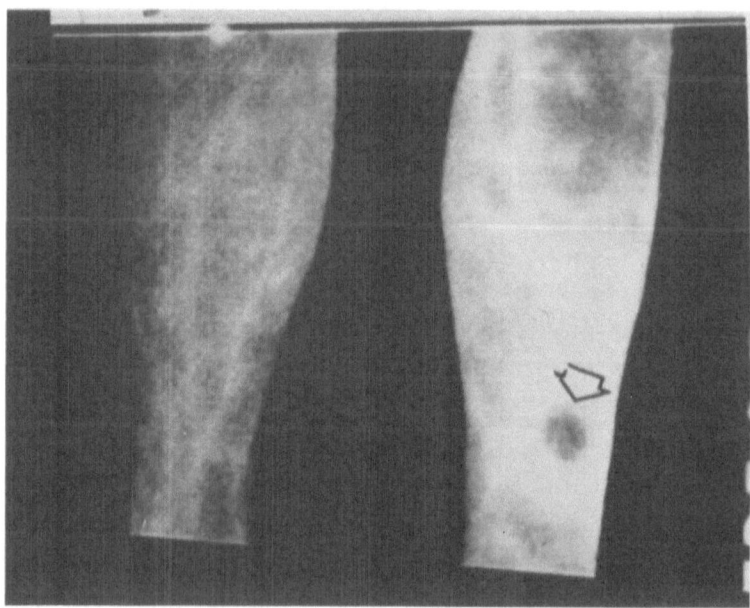

B

Fig. 21. 'A' shows ulceration in an ischemic leg which produces no inflammatory reaction. B shows ulceration in a nonischemic leg which produces a warm inflammatory reaction around the ulcer.

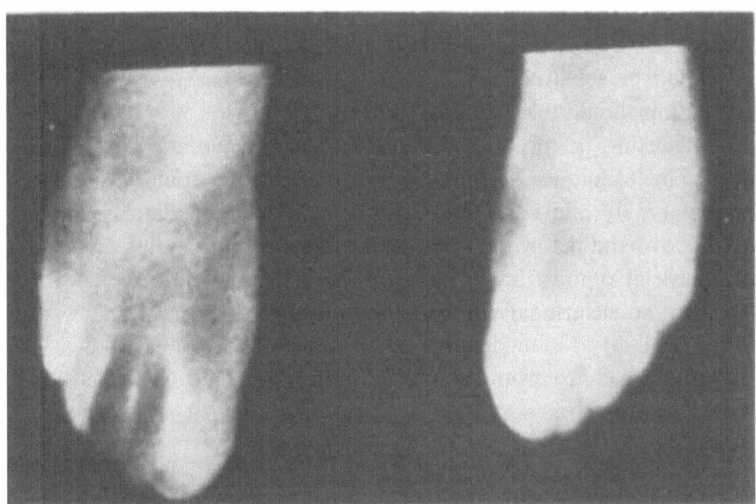

Fig. 22. A high, obstructive lesion in a medium sized artery produces coolness in the foot and all ipsilateral toes.

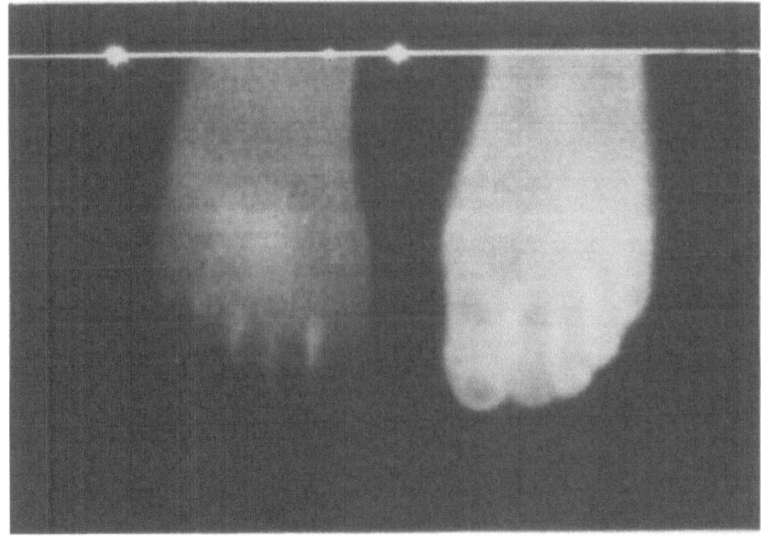

Fig. 23. Digital artery disease produces coolness of only the digits involved, characteristic of small vessel disease.

normal side. It is desirable to have the position of the camera such that it receives rays from the patient through a mirror, causing the radiation to strike the lens of the camera at right angles. This prevents distortion. The legs should be separated by 6 in. to prevent crossheating. The whole examination should take about 20 min.

For detecting perforator veins the following technique may be employed. The technique of Patel (25) places the patient supine with the legs elevated at a 30° angle and the heels resting on a stool. Tourniquets are placed above and below the site of suspected perforator veins to exclude the superficial venous flow. The leg is then cooled with ice or cool wet towels and an electric fan for 5 min and the feet are exercized. Thermograms are obtained immediately and 20, 40 and 60 sec after exercize and cooling. The exercize produces heat and warming of the deep vein blood.

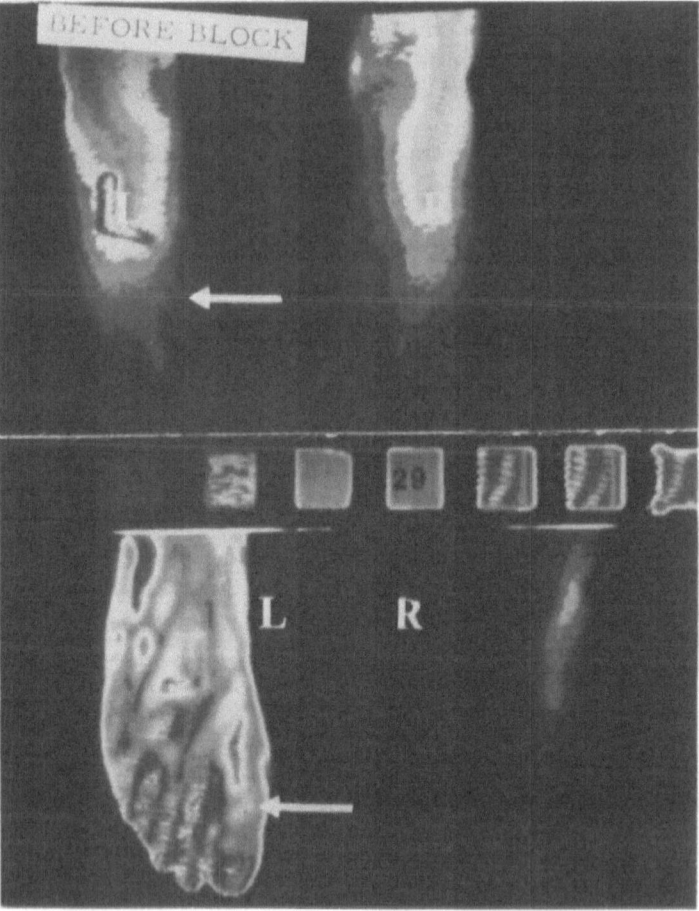

Fig. 24. A posterior tibial nerve block produces a large increase in skin circulation in patients who have functional vasoconstriction.

The presence of deep perforator veins makes a sharp contrast between the site of the perforator vein and the cool skin.

8.2. *Normal*

Normal leg thermograms are cool at the knees. Symmetrical temperatures are present throughout both legs (24). The calves and thighs may display a smooth set of temperature grays or may be mottled. A mottled normal pattern is usually found in obese individuals.

8.3. *Superficial vein phlebitis*

Superficial vein thrombophlebitis is shown in Fig. 25. The thermogram shows on one leg an area of increased heat which in the original picture was red (now white-hot). Thermographically there was a difference of 2 °C between the thrombosed area and the surrounding normal skin. Clinically the patient had a palpable, cord-like lesion identifiable as a thrombosed vein.

8.4. *Deep venous thrombosis*

Deep venous thrombosis is of considerable significance because of pul-

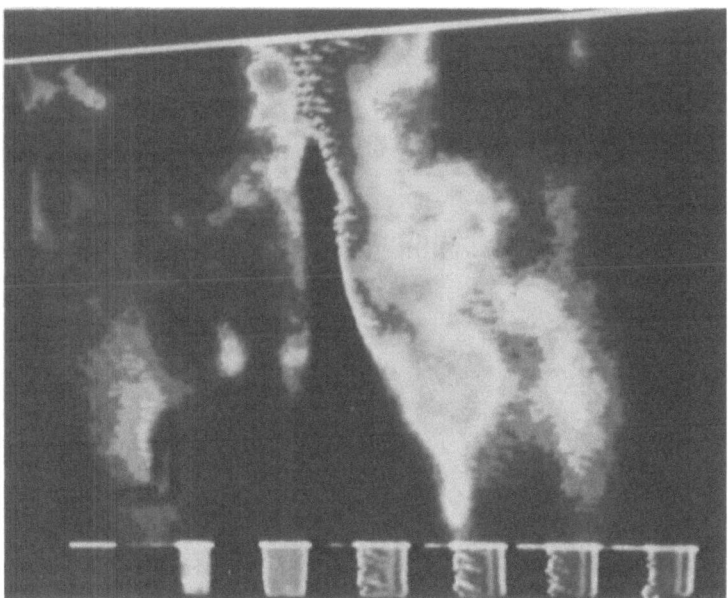

Fig. 25. Superficial vein thrombophlebitis shows as a white circuitous pattern involving the upper portion of the thigh (superficial femoral vein, white is hot).

monary emboli and because of the high incidence of deep venous thrombosis with such situations as pelvic surgery where the incidence of thrombosis is about 50%. Iliofemoral venous thrombosis is shown in Fig. 26–28. In Fig. 26 there is a small area of iliofemoral thrombosis which appears as a small hot area. In Fig. 27 there is a lesion in a similar place, however there is high grade collateral circulation over the lower abdomen. Pelvic phlebitis may be present. In Fig. 28 the femoral vein as well as the iliofemoral was occluded giving a white (warm) area which includes the thigh and groin.

Deep venous thrombosis of the calves warms the whole calf below the knee as shown in Fig. 29. In this picutre the right leg is warmer than the left by 1.5 °C. In another patient (Fig. 30) the deep venous thrombosis shows increased heat in one leg, the heat encroaching on the normal cool kneecap.

The reason for the increased heat with thrombophlebitis is not clearly known. Inflammation of the part, bradykinin, platelets, serotonin, prostaglandins (E2 and E2 alpha) may be involved.

8.5. *Venous insufficiency*

The detection of perforator veins and venous insufficiency has been highly successful (25). Special techniques are often employed. The Patel technique of cooling and exercize is shown in Fig. 31. The picture was supplied

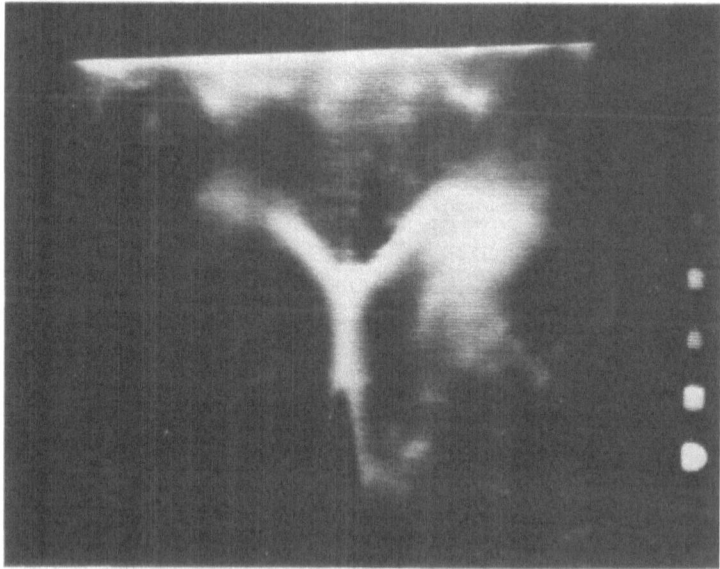

Fig. 26. There is a white-hot area of thrombophlebitis under the left inguinal ligament.

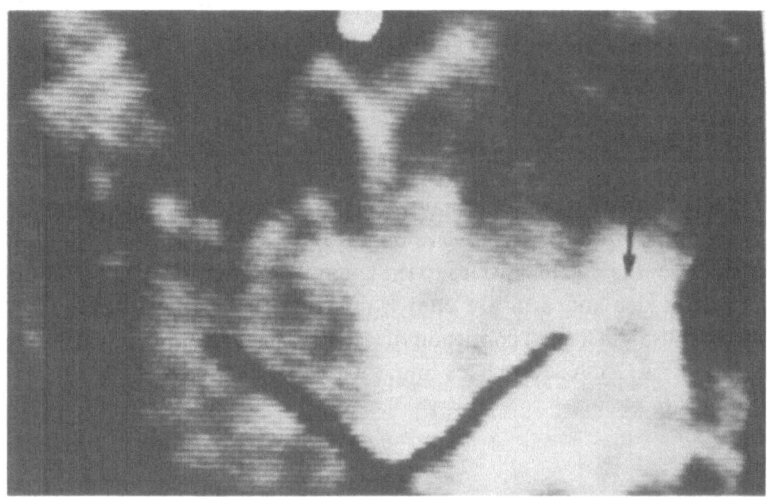

Fig. 27. There is a left iliofemoral thrombophlebitis with considerable collateral circulation over the abdomen.

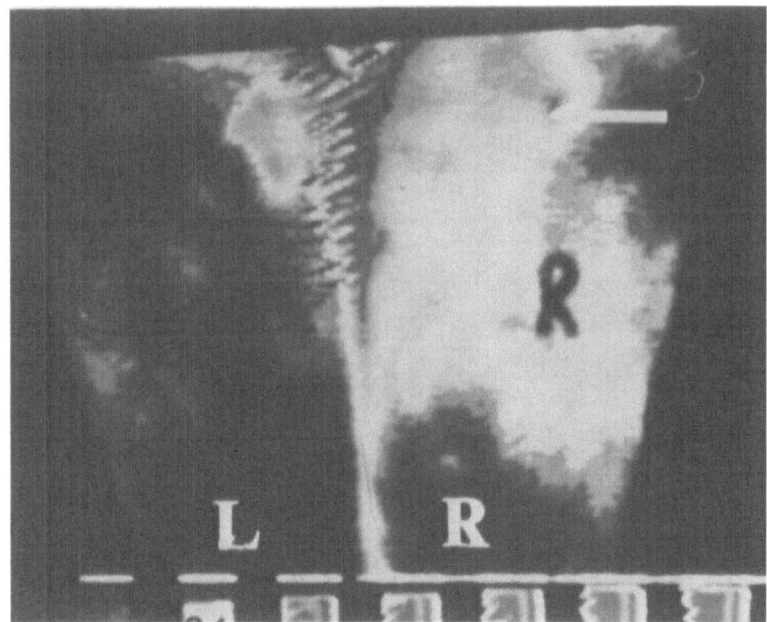

Fig. 28. Large iliofemoral thrombophlebitis in the patient's right leg. This thermogram was taken through a mirror and therefore reverses right and left.

One of the significant contributions of thermography in recent years is differential diagnostic value in chronic pain due to obscure causes. Diagnosis of reflex sympathetic dystrophy, Sudeck's atrophy, or causalgia-like syndrom is often unduly delayed until development of irreversible typical signs, such as atrophy of soft tissue and arthropathy. Earlier diagnosis and proper management of these processes promote optimal results. Thermography fulfills this need by earlier detection of the temperature change, as this author clearly demonstrates in Fig. 32, 33 and 34.

It is important to note that the temperature change occurs without any damage and without clinical signs of somatosensory or motor nerve impairment. The patient may present with intractable pain with psychoneurotic state, yet with normal neurological findings. It is frequently difficult to detect convincingly abnormal temperature changes in such patients by routine clinical examination. I strongly believe that it is our obligation to have these patients undergo thermography before labeling their problems as 'psychogenic' or 'malingering'. The significant temperature change of the involved limb in cases which have been treated as psychogenic or functional or even malingering is often surprising. Recognition of the temperature change in the painful limb on the photograph, which can be reviewed not only by the treating physician, but also by the patient, has, itself, therapeutic value to these patients, who have been distrusted and ignored by physicians, family members and friends. If the temperature change is reproducible on different days and at different times, and the pain is relieved by sympathetic block, these cases can be properly treated by a vasodilator or denervation of sympathetic nerves.

by Elizabeth Bell of the United Kingdom. Perforator veins are evident often with the patient supine at rest without cooling.

9.   LESIONS OF NERVES

One must differentiate abnormal heat patterns from vasoconstriction or vasodilatation produced by nerve damage or destruction of nerves (28). An injury of the brachial plexus to the left arm is shown in Fig. 32. The left neck, shoulder and arm are cool from functional vasoconstriction. A typical causalgia from a contusion of the wrist with cooling of the hand is shown in Fig. 33. A severe back injury with sciatica produced the cold leg seen in Fig. 34.

10.   SUMMARY

Thermography is an important noninvasive technique for revealing the effect of arterial stenoses, especially of the small vessels of the fingers and toes and in revealing the presence of deep venous thrombosis and cerebral vascular disease. One must understand the effect of neurogenic heat abnormalities to avoid misinterpretation.

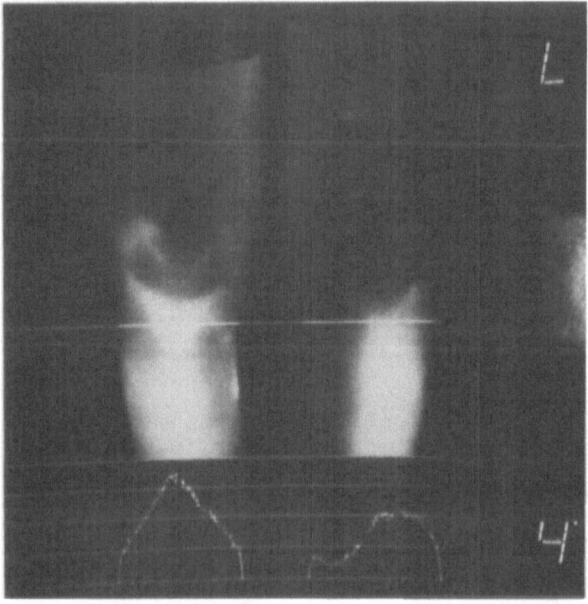

Fig. 29. There is thrombophlebitis of the right calf area. The right calf is warm.

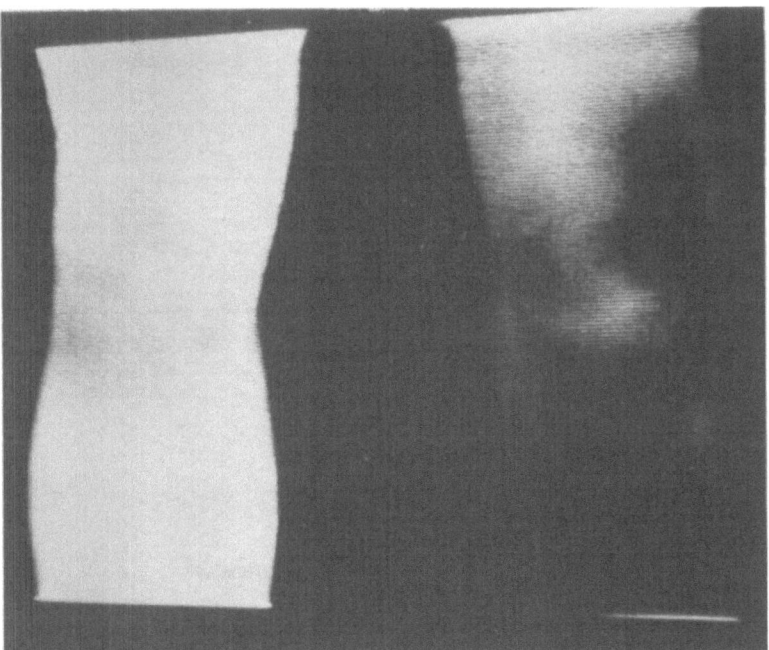

Fig. 30. There is extensive deep calf popliteal and superficial femoral vein thrombosis on the right which increases the heat throughout the entire calf and thigh and obliterates the normal cool knee pattern.

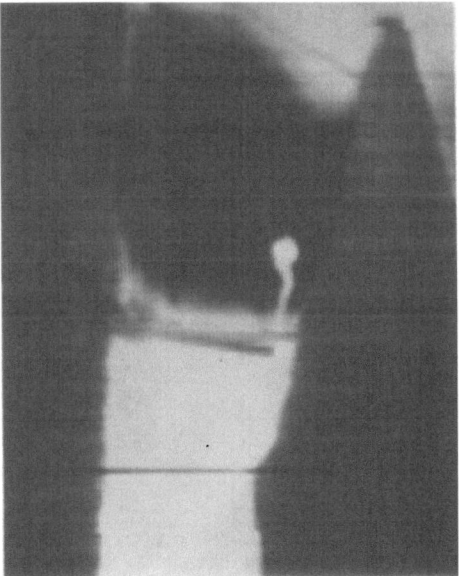

Fig. 31. Perforator vein obtained with the Patel technique. Picture supplied by Elizabeth Bell of the United Kingdom.

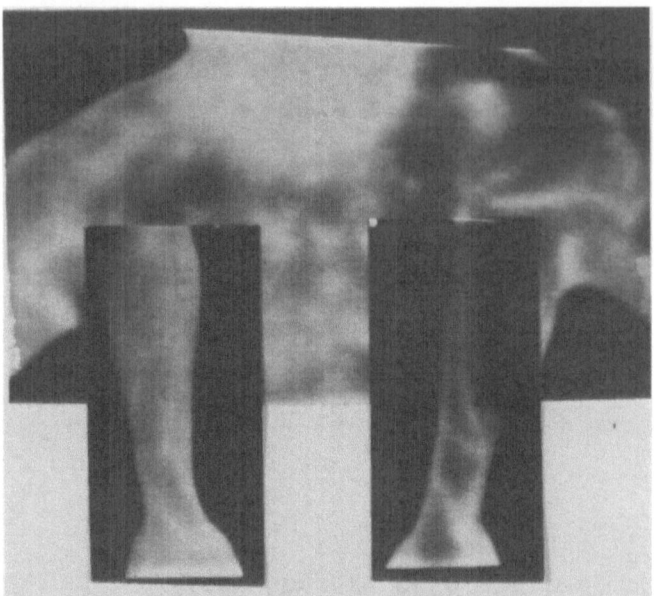

Fig. 32. Brachial plexus injury showing cool left shoulder with cool arm ipsilaterally.

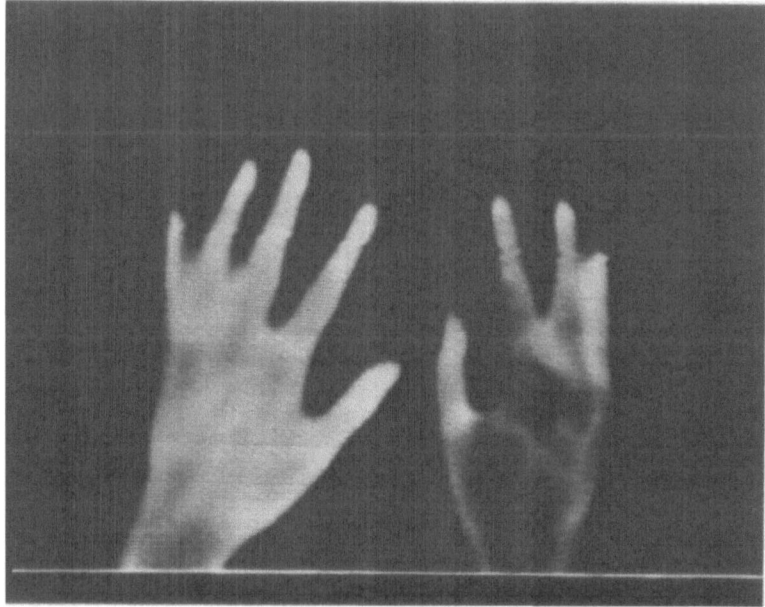

Fig. 33. Nerve injury at the wrist producing coolness of the hand due to nerve irritation.

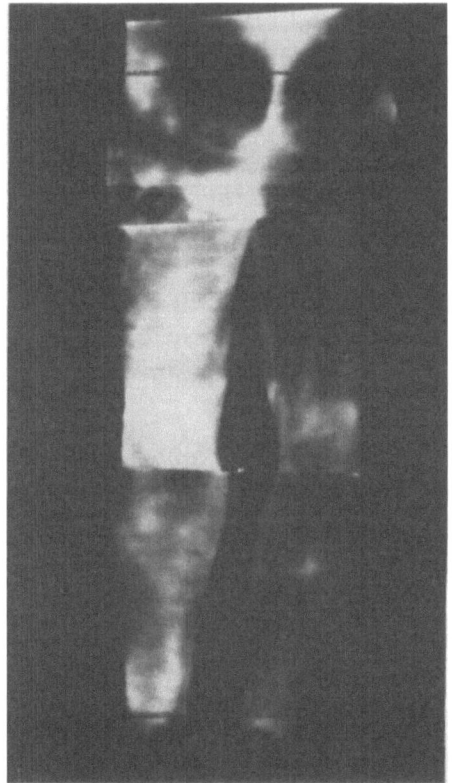

Fig. 34. Coolness (dark) of the right leg due to back and sciatic nerve injury.

REFERENCES TO MAIN TEXT

1. Uetmatsu S, (Editor): Medical Thermography. Theory and Clinical Applications, Los Angeles, CA, Brentwood Publ.
2. Barnes RB, Gershon-Cohen J: Clinical thermography. Amer. med. Assoc. 185: 949–952, 1963.
3. Ryan J: Thermography. Aust. Radiol. 13, 23–36, 1969.
4. Herschel W: Investigations of the powers of prismatic colours to heat and illuminate objects. Phil. Trans. Roy. Soc. 90: 255-92, 1800.
5. Herschel JFW: On the distribution of the colorific rays in the solar system. Phil. Trans. Roy. Soc. 131: 51–2, 1840.
6. Hardy DL: The radiation of heat from the human body. III. The human skin as a black-body radiator. J. Clin. Invest. 13: 615, 1934.
7. Astheimer RW, Wormser EM: High speed infrared radiometers. J. Opt. Soc. Amer. 49: 179–181, 1959.
8. Lawson RN: Thermography – A new tool in the investigation of breast cancer. Can. Serv. Med. J. 13: 517–518, 1957.
9. Lloyd-Williams K, Lloyd-Williams FJ, Handley RS: Infrared radiation thermometry in clinical practice. Lancet 2: 958–959, 1960.

10. Love TJ, Lindsted RD: ASME Publication 75-WA/Bio-6 Proceedings of Annual Meeting, Nov/Dec 1975.
11. Burton AC: Application of theory of heat flow. J. Nutrit. 7: 497–533, 1934.
12. Mali JWH: In: Medical Thermography, Von Voss H, Leiden PI (eds), Basel, Switzerland, Karger, 1969.
13. Haberman JD, Reed DA, Love TJ: Thermographic technique. Appl. Radiol. Sept/Oct., p 55, 1975.
14. Wood, Ernest H: Thermography in the diagnosis of cerebrovascular disease. Radiology 85: 270–283, 1965.
15. Capistrant TD, Gummit RJ: Detecting carotid occlusive disease by thermography. Stroke 5: 57–64, 1973.
16. Capistrant TD, Gummit RJ: Thermogram and cerebrovascular disease. Arch. Neurol. (Chic.) 22: 499–504, 1970.
17. Hollenhorst RW: Neuro-Ophthalmologic Aspects in Cerebral Vascular Diseases. Siekert RC, Wishnant JP (eds), New York, Grune and Stratton, 1961, p 8–12.
18. Heyman A: Discussion of ophthalmodynamometry as a diagnostic procedure. Neurology (Minneap.) II: 104–106, 1961.
19. McLoughlin BA, Rawsthorne GB: Thermography in the diagnosis of occlusive vascular disease of the lower limbs. Brit. J. Surg. 60: 655–656, 1973.
20. Winsor T, Bendezu J: Thermography and the peripheral circulation. N.Y. Acad. Sci. 121: 135–156, 1964.
21. Winsor T, Winsor D: Disorders of the cardiovascular system: The thermographic technique. Acta Thermographica 1: 142–150, 1976.
22. Winsor T, Winsor D: Thermography in cardiovascular disease. App. Radiol.: 117–148, Nov/Dec, 1975.
23. Winsor T, Winsor D: Thermography in cardiovascular disease. In: Medical Thermography, Theory and Application. Uematsu S (ed) Los Angeles, Ca, Brentwood Publ. p 121–142.
24. Cooke ED, Pilcher MF: Deep vein thrombosis: preclinical diagnosis by thermography. Brit. J. Surg. 61: 971–978, 1974.
25. Patel KO, Williams JR, Lloyd-Williams K: Thermographic localization of incompetent perforating veins in the leg. Brit. med. J. 24: 195–197, 1970.
26. Lloyd-Williams K: Thermography in the diagnosis of varicose veins and venous insufficiency. In: Medical Thermography. Proceedings of a Boerhaave Course for Postgraduate Medical Education, Leiden 1968. Bibl. Radiol. 5, Basel/New York, Karger, p 127–129, 1969.
27. Elem B, Shorey BA, Lloyd-Williams K: Comparison between thermography and fluorescein test in the detection of incompetent perforating veins. Brit. Med. J. 4: 651–652, 1971.
28. Marinacci AA: Thermography in the detection of non-neurological imitators of peripheral nerve complexes. Bull. LA Neurol. Soc. 30: 1–11, 1965.

6. Noninvasive pressure measurements in arterial disease

R. VERHAEGHE

Commentary by J. Gundersen

1. INTRODUCTION

Numerous methods have been developed for assessment of the arterial system in the limbs but none of them provides a complete picture of the peripheral circulation. Undoubtly, indirect pressure measurements with noninvasive techniques have gained a widespread popularity during the last decade because of their simplicity and reliability. The basic principle of sphygmomanometric blood pressure measurement is well-known: a distensible cuff is applied around the limb and inflated above systolic pressure; reappearance of flow or a related phenomenon during deflation is detected by a sensor and indicates the systolic pressure value. In the present chapter, the application of this principle to the extremities of patients with arterial disease will be reviewed.

2. THE CUFF

From the early days of the sphygmomanometric blood pressure measurements, it has been recognized that the size of the cuff was of critical importance. Ideally, the dimensions of the inflatable bag should be such that the values of the indirect pressure readings are identical to the intra-arterial pressure determinations. To comply with this principle, the American Heart Association (1) and the World Health Organization (2) have ruled that the inflatable bag be 20% wider than the diameter of the limb on which it is to be used. A bag 12–14 cm wide fulfills this criterion for the arm of the average adult. A considerably higher pressure would have to be applied before the brachial artery is occluded by a smaller bag, leading to an overestimation of the systolic blood pressure. The length of the compression bag is equally important. The WHO recommends it to be at least 22 cm for the upper limb. The AHA admits that a bag is long enough when it covers half the limb circumference if care is taken to apply it directly over the compressible artery, but advises to use bags which completely encircle the limb to obviate any risk of misapplication. In practice, 35 cm bags are sufficiently long to go around a normal arm. To date, no similar official recommendations have been issued on the size of cuffs for the legs and digits. In general, the problems of measuring indirect blood pressure in lower limbs are essentially the same as in the upper, although even more variation in anatomy may be encountered. For instance, the thigh has usually a more conical shape in females compared to males and the relative mass of subcutaneous fat and muscle may vary individually. On the other hand the exact relation between the intra-arterial blood pressure in the brachial artery and the deep arteries of the calf or the digital arteries is largely unknown: therefore it is almost impossible to determine which compression bag ought to give the most reliable pressure values. Furthermore, whereas the use of the 20% rule may still be valid for the thigh and perhaps for the calf, it is questionable for the ankle where bony structures and tendon mass may hamper the compression of the arteries.

In practice, essentially two attitudes have been adopted to cope with the problems of the cuff size. Gundersen (3, 4) proposed that a cuff be used which wherever applied gives approximately the same pressure readings as those recorded in the arm. He therefore introduced a single cuff of 18 cm × 60 cm for thigh, calf and ankle and a 2.4 cm × 9 cm cuff for thumb and toe. His proposal gained wide acceptance in the Scandinavian countries. The more pragmatic view is to care less about the actual size of the cuff but to determine the range of 'normal' pressures obtained in healthy subjects with a particular cuff. For instance, several authors use the conventional arm cuff for the ankle (which is still well above the 20% rule) and a larger cuff (e.g., 15 cm × 40 cm) for calf and thigh. Obviously, the 'normal' pressure range may then be considerably higher than the arm pressure. Others even take deliberately narrow cuffs for the thigh (e.g., 8 cm width) in order to be able to measure at a proximal and a distal level (5). The AHA recommends a deflation rate of 2–3 mm Hg/sec for measurements of blood pressure in the arm with the auscultation technique (1). For digital pressure measurements, Gundersen (3) found the smallest error rate in the range between 4 and 6 mm Hg/sec.

3. THE SENSOR

Whereas the classic auscultatory and palpatory techniques for indirect measurement of blood pressure may still be applicable to the lower limb of healthy subjects, they are certainly no longer adequate for patients with arterial occlusive disease. However, several sensitive devices are available which enable to pick-up blood flow distal to an arterial obstruction and thus can be used as a sensor for pressure measurement. The most commonly used in clinical practice are the Doppler flow velocimeter and, to a lesser extent, the strain-gauge plethysmograph.

The principle of flow detection with ultrasound is outlined elsewhere in this book. Determination of the ankle blood pressure is probably the most widespread application of the ultrasound flow velocimeter. The Doppler probe is placed over one of the tibial arteries with a cuff around the ankle which is inflated to a suprasystolic level (Fig. 1). Reappearance of the flow signal during deflation indicates the systolic pressure at the site of the cuff. There is a good agreement between systolic pressures obtained at the ankles by listening over the different vessels (6). Pressure measurements can be made in the same way at the level of the calf or the thigh by only moving the cuff. The great advantage of this technique is its extreme simplicity; with the currently available pocket-size Doppler flow velocimeters it can be applied as a routine bedside screening method for peripheral arterial disease. It should be remembered though that only sys-

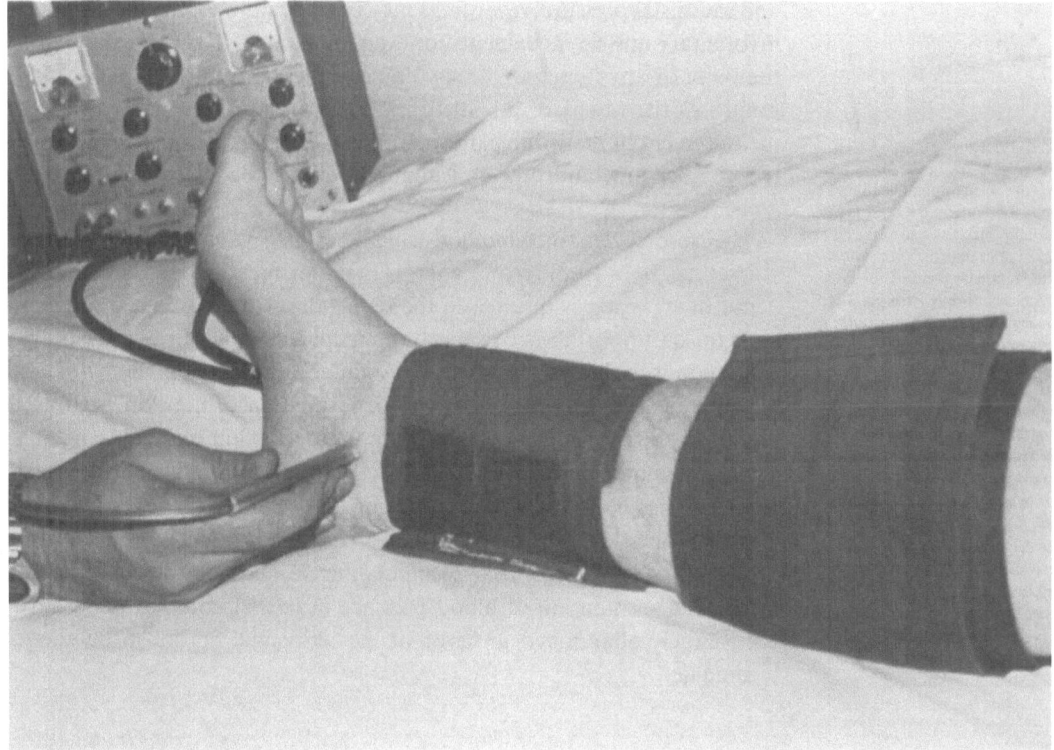

Fig. 1. Indirect systolic pressure measurement with ultrasound. A cuff is wrapped around the calf and above the ankle; the probe of a Doppler velocimeter is held over the posterior tibial artery.

tolic pressure is measured; ultrasonic instruments which sense arterial wall motion corresponding to systole and diastole instead of red blood cell motion have been developed but are only useful in patients with patent peripheral arteries (7–10) As the ultrasonic beam is narrow, the probe has to be directed exactly and at a fixed angle over the blood vessel. The method is difficult to apply to digital arteries and is unreliable in toes of patients with advanced arterial insufficiency (3).

The mercury-in-silastic strain-gauge plethysmograph (see Chapter 2), mainly used for measurement of blood flow, can be adapted for recording blood pressure as well. Therefore, the strain-gauge is placed around the first toe distally to one or more occluding cuffs (Fig. 2). The systolic pressure is indicated by the change in volume of the toe or the reappearance of pulses which occurs when the inflated cuff is slowly deflated. The cuff pressure is recorded simultaneously with a suitable transducer; in this way any subjective element in pressure reading is eliminated. Gundersen (3) designed special cuffs which can be applied around the proximal phalanx of the toe or thumb for digital pressure recording. It should be noted, however, that in some patients with advanced ischemia and low distal pressure, recordings may be difficult to evaluate, because of involuntary muscle movements, or even impossible due to the absence of toe pulse or any increase in toe volume. Other conventional plethysmographs as the water- or air-filled have been used as sensor for pressure measurement but failed to gain wide clinical acceptance, the former being too cumbersome and time-consuming, the later too susceptible to artefacts.

The isotope clearance method which was originally designed for flow studies has been employed in a few centers for pressure measurement. A depot of ^{133}xenon is injected in the tissue distal to an arterial occlusion cuff; the cuff pressure necessary to interrupt the wash-out of the isotope corresponds to the systolic pressure. An interesting development with this technique is that it can be adapted for estimation of the skin perfusion blood pressure by injecting the isotope into the skin and subsequently applying counter-pressure over the injection site (11). Similar skin pressure recording has been attempted by placing an occluding cuff over a photo-electric probe (12).

Several other devices and techniques have been described for non-invasive determination of blood pressure (Table 1); most of them have been largely abandoned in favor of the ultrasonic or the strain-gauge technique.

COMMENTARY

It is of course impossible to measure blood pressure if there are no pulsations in the digital arteries at all. Even in patients with severe arterial disease there is, however, practically always some pulsation in the digital arteries. Of course a reservation should be taken for acute arterial emboli.

If there is a problem to detect the toe pulses when the patient is in the recumbent position it is a good idea to have the patient sitting and measure blood pressure in that position. Of course the height from the heart to the level of the great toe or to the ankle should be subtracted in these cases. Using this refinement it is sometimes possible to get a more detailed information of the distal blood pressure.

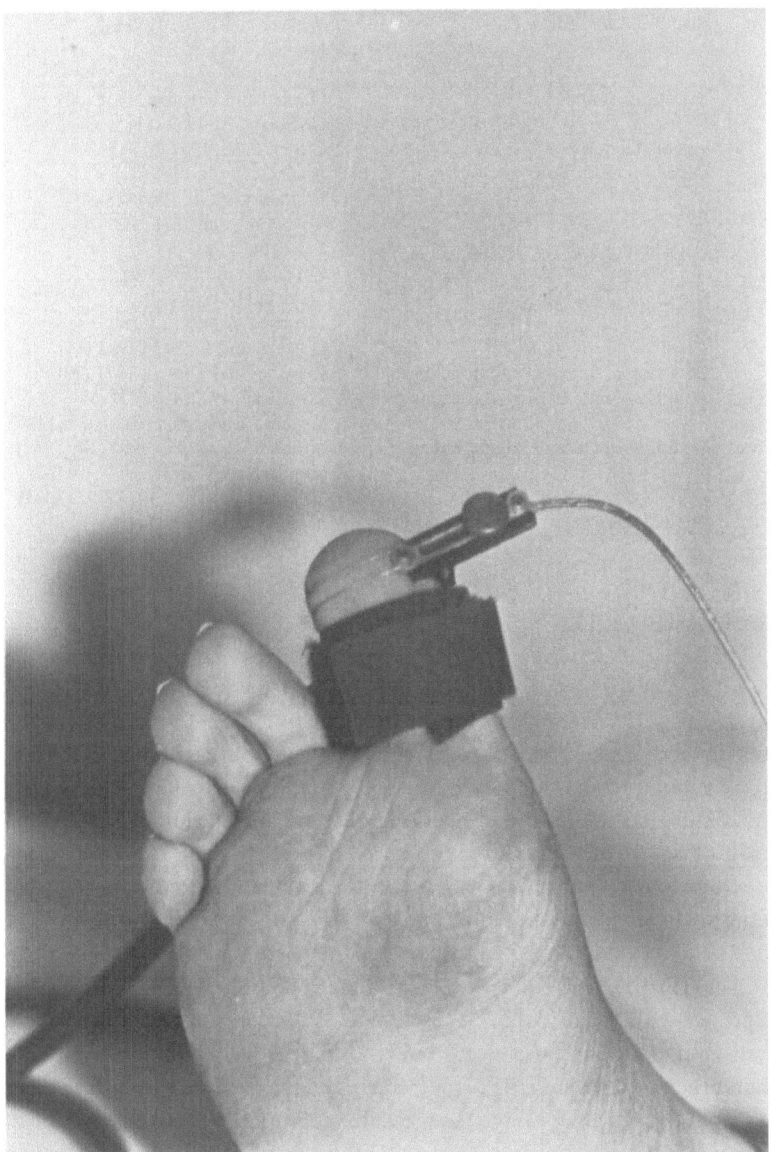

Fig. 2. Pressure measurement in the first toe with the mercury strain-gauge.

Table 1. Devices and techniques used as a sensor in indirect blood pressure measurement.

Sensor	Principle	Selected references
'Flush', spectroscopic method	Reappearance of flow	Weaver and Bohr, 1950 (48) Gaskell, 1965 (49) Carter, 1968 (24)
Auscultation (cup, microphone)	Korotkoff-sounds	Gaskell and Krisman, 1958 (50) Geddes et al., 1959 (51)
Capacitance pulse pick-up	Pulse detection	Carter, 1968, 1969 (6, 24)
Ultrasound	Detection of (in)flow	Rushmer et al., 1966 (52) Strandness et al., 1966 (53) Yao et al., 1969 (27)
	Detection of wall movement	Felix et al., 1973 (9) Poppers et al., 1973 (10)
Isotope clearance	Detection of (out)flow	Dahn et al., 1967 (54) Lassen et al., 1972 (25) Holstein and Larssen, 1973 (11)
Plethysmograph: water-filled	Detection of pulse or volume changes	Celander and Thoren, 1971 (20)
air-filled	Detection of pulse or volume changes	Lorentsen, 1972, 1973 (21, 55) Siggaard-Andersen et al., 1972 (39)
strain-gauge	Detection of pulse or volume changes	Strandness and Bell, 1965 (38) Gundersen, 1972 (3) Nielsen et al., 1972, 1973 (12, 13, 23)
photo-electric	Flow of pulse detection	Nielsen et al., 1973 (12)

4. NORMAL VALUES

Pressure measurements can be made either at rest or after a period of muscle exercise. To account for the moment-to-moment variation in systemic blood pressure, it is customary to relate pressure readings in the leg to the simultaneously measured brachial pressure. This can be achieved by calculating either the gradient between the arm and the lower limb or the ratio of leg to arm pressure; the latter figure is usually referred to as pressure index. Normal values for both parameters at rest have been reported in several studies in recent years (Table 2). The following factors may help to explain the apparent discrepancy between data from different studies: (1) differences in cuff size: as already discussed, lower values are expected with larger cuffs; (2) age of the subjects: indirectly measured systolic pressure in lower limbs tends to increase more rapidly with age than brachial pressure (13, 14); (3) the individual scatter within the same study is considerable; (4) the toe pressure measured in the supine position has to be corrected for the difference in height between the arm and the toe. As a general guideline it appears fair to accept as the lower limit of normal ankle pressure the value of the brachial pressure when 10–12 cm cuffs are used; with 18 cm cuffs, however, only an ankle pressure 20 cm lower than the arm pressure is significant. Many clinicians use distal pressure measurements after exercise to evaluate the functional reserve of the peripheral

Table 2. Systolic pressure at rest in lower limbs of healthy subjects measured by indirect methods.

	Reference	Number	Cuff width (cm)	Sensor	Normal value Δ arm–leg (mm Hg)	Index leg/arm	Other
Thigh	Carter, 1968 (24)	85 limbs	15	capacitance pulse pick-ups		1.07–1.27	
	Gundersen, 1972 (3)	14 subjects	18	strain-gauge plethysmograph	−3.6 ± 10.2		
	Siggaard-Andersen 1972 (39)	10 limbs	12	air-plethysmograph			arm 138 ± 12 mm Hg thigh 126 ± 17 mm Hg
	Bell et al., 1973 (14)	30 subjects	18	strain-gauge plethysmograph	−2.8 ± 12.8		
Calf	Thulesius and Gjöres, 1971 (29)	40 limbs	18	ultrasound	−2 ± 9	1.0 ± 0.08	
	Gundersen, 1972 (3)	14 subjects	18 12	strain-gauge plethysmograph	2.1 ± 7.6 −5.5 ± 10.2		
	Bell et al., 1973 (14)	30 subjects	18	strain-gauge plethysmograph	−5.2 ± 12.2		Δ thigh–calf: −2.4 ± 8.7
	Lorentsen, 1973 (21)	12 subjects	12	air-plethysmograph	0.9 ± 2.3		
Ankle	Carter, 1968 (24)	44 limbs	12.5	capacitance pulse pick-ups		0.97–1.24	
	Yao et al., 1969 (27)	25 subjects	?	ultrasound		>1.0	
	Bollinger et al., 1970 (28)	13 subjects	8.5	ultrasound	−15.4 ± 13.7		
	Gundersen, 1972 (3)	14 subjects	18	strain-gauge plethysmograph	1.4 ± 11.7 −4.7 ± 10.6		
	Nielsen et al., 1972 (13)	10 subjects <31 years 14 subjects >43 years	12	strain-gauge plethysmograph	−23.6 ± 9.5		
	Siggaard-Andersen, 1972 (39)	10 limbs	12	air-plethysmograph			arm 138 ± 12 mm Hg ankle 113 ± 19 mm IIg
	Lorentsen, 1973 (21)	13 subjects	10	air-plethysmograph	−11.6 ± 2.4		
	Yao, 1973 (31)	50 subjects	?	ultrasound		>1.0	
Toe	Gundersen, 1972 (3)	27 subjects	2.4	strain-gauge plethysmograph	22.2 ± 11.8		Δ ankle–toe:
	Nielsen et al., 1972 (13)	10 subjects < 31 years 14 subjects > 43 years		strain-gauge plethysmograph	4.8 ± 6.6 9.8 ± 10.7		24.3 ± 7.3 33.3 ± 12.1
	Bell et al., 1973 (14)	30 subjects	2.4	strain-gauge plethysmograph	5.1 ± 14.7*		Δ calf–toe: 10.4 ± 12.8*
	Lezack and Carter, 1973 (35)	45 limbs	1.9	flush technique or strain-gauge plethysmograph	>70	0.64–1.10	

* Corrected for difference in height between arm and toe.

circulation. For this purpose, the patient is asked to perform a standardized exercise test on a treadmill or using a footpedal ergometer and pressure is recorded before and at regular intervals after exercize. In normal subjects, the ankle pressure is reduced during the vasodilatation which accompanies exercise (15, 16). When sequential measurements are made, flow velocity and ankle pressure show an inverse relationship, both returning to control levels at the same time. With noninvasive techniques the pressure gradient between arm and ankle becomes unmeasurable within 30–40 sec after stopping the exercise (17). Thus, when the first postexercise recording is made 1 min after exercise, it is probably correct to consider any decrease in pressure relative to the pre-exercise value and to the expected rise in systemic pressure as indicative of arterial obstructive disease. Comparable results may be obtained when the exercise is replaced by a period of arterial occlusion and measurements are made during the reactive hyperemia which follows the release of the arterial compression (17, 18).

5.   VALIDITY AND REPRODUCIBILITY

The validity of indirect blood pressure measurements with the ultrasonic velocimeter or the plethysmograph has been tested in several studies. Kazamias et al. (19) measured pressure with a Doppler transducer applied over the radial artery of one arm and through an indwelling needle in the brachial artery of the opposite arm: in 65 measurements in 12 subjects in whom arterial pressure was lowered artificially the correlation coefficient was 0.99 and the maximum error 10 mm Hg. Stegall et al. (7) reported an excellent correlation between intra-arterial and indirect pressure measured with an ultrasonic device in the same and the opposite arm in 10 normotensive patients; the largest difference between the two methods being 5 mm Hg. The maximum difference between forearm pressure values obtained by Celander and Thoren (20) with the water-filled plethysmograph and simultaneous intra-arterial measurements in 6 young subjects was 4 mm Hg. Gundersen (3) compared the systolic thumb pressure obtained with a strain-gauge in 8 subjects (187 measurements) with simultaneously recorded intra-arterial blood pressure in the radial artery and reported a correlation of 0.93. The same correlation was maintained during induced hypotension (2 cases). Fewer data are available on leg pressure measurements. A comparison between plethysmographically and intra-arterially measured calf blood pressure was reported by Lorentsen (21) in two patients: the indirect pressure obtained with a cuff of 12 cm was slightly lower in both: 18 and 9 mm Hg, respectively. Grüntzig and Schlumpf (22) obtained a correlation of 0.95 in 15 patients with femoral occlusion but patent crural arteries, in whom they compared ankle blood pressure with the ultrasonic technique (12 cm cuff) and direct pressure with a catheter in the distal popliteal artery.

Errors originating in the technical procedure as well as the biological variation of blood pressure may influence the reproducibility of indirect pressure measurements. Grüntzig and Schlumpf (22) measured on three consecutive days the ankle pressure in 10 patients with segmental femoral occlusion and found a similar variability for the pressure in the leg as for the auscultatory arm pressure. Nielsen et al. (13, 23) reported an acceptable reproducibility of duplicate measurements at the finger, ankle and toe in 24 normal subjects and at the ankle and toe in 20 patients, the standard deviation being 5 mm Hg or less. Gundersen (3) found that the measuring technique did not influence the pressure during 3 consecutive readings on each of two different days in a series of normal subjects and patients with arterial disease.

Several sensors used for indirect pressure recording have been compared with each other: the capacitance pulse pick-up with the visual 'flush' technique, the spectroscopic method and the ultrasonic flow detector (6, 16, 24), the strain-gauge versus the xenon clearance (25), the air-filled plethysmograph (26) and the Doppler flow velocimeter (3, 27). In general a good to excellent agreement is found between these different sensors although the differences in individual persons are not always negligible and in some studies a systematic difference between two sensors (Fig. 3) was discovered (26).

6.   CORRELATION BETWEEN FLOW AND PRESSURE MEASUREMENTS

No clear correlation can be demonstrated between resting calf flow measured by venous occlusion plethysmography and calf or ankle pressure in patients with arterial insufficiency, resting flow remaining nearly constant in spite of circulatory impairment. By contrast, a significant relationship exists (Fig. 4) between pressure measurements at rest and calf flow during reactive hyperemia elicited by temporary arterial occlusion (3, 28, 29).

As in normal subjects (17) a strong inverse relationship has been reported between ankle systolic pressure and calf blood flow after exercise in patients with arterial obstruction (30, 31) but the reduction in pressure and the postexercise hyperemia last longer in the latter group. The slope of the regression line is even different according to the site and extent of the occluding process due to the complex pressure-flow relationship in the presence of obstruction of the main artery which involves both a variable collateral resistance and the muscular arteriolar resistance.

When systolic calf or ankle pressures of patients with arterial obstructive disease are plotted against their claudication distance or the work they can perform on a treadmill, a much weaker or no correlation at all is found (32–34). This is not surprising because other than hemodynamic factors may contribute to the working capacity of ischemic muscle.

7.   LIMITATIONS

Indirect pressure measurements are easily accepted by patients and normally well tolerated; therefore they can be frequently repeated. Only patients with severe ischaemic disease in the extremities may occasionally experience some discomfort when the cuffs are inflated. Whereas local systolic pressure recordings allow a sensitive evaluation of obstructive disease along the main arterial pathway of the limb proximally to the occluding cuff, they provide no information on the presence of isolated

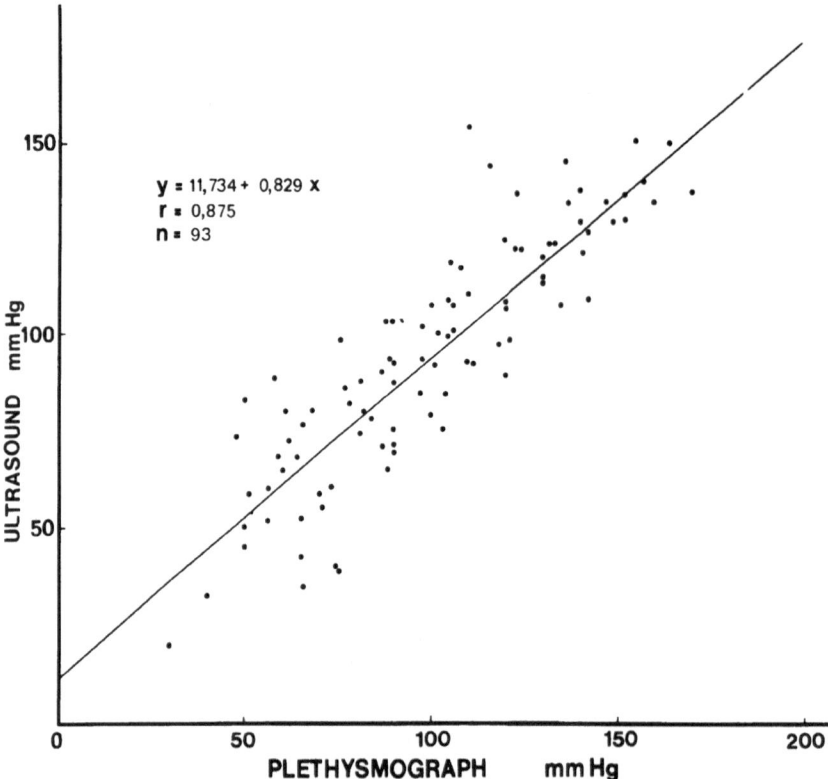

$$y = 11,734 + 0,829 \ x$$
$$r = 0,875$$
$$n = 93$$

Fig. 3. Correlation between systolic pressure measured with a Doppler probe over the tibial artery and with a strain-gauge around the first toe in legs with arterial obstructive disease (Verhaeghe and Beyens, unpublished).

lesions in side branches of the main vessels as in the internal iliac or deep femoral artery. Fortunately, isolated occlusive disease in these branches is rare. Combined disease of both the main vessel and the side branch may well influence the distal pressure; for instance when the superficial femoral artery is occluded, the deep femoral becomes the main source of collateral blood supply and therefore any lesion on this vessel will cause an additional reduction of the ankle pressure. In limbs with heavy calcification of the arterial media as observed in diabetes, indirect pressure measurements may become impossible because of the incompressibility of the calcified vessel wall. The distal flow signal over these arteries does not disappear, even at cuff pressures which exceed largely the brachial pressure. Finally, digital occlusions distally to the occluding cuff can not be diagnosed, but this is not frequently observed.

8. Clinical application

Measurement of the systolic blood pressure along the arterial tree of a limb can be applied both for diagnostic and prognostic purposes in the evaluation of peripheral arterial insufficiency. Physicians traditionally rely on a

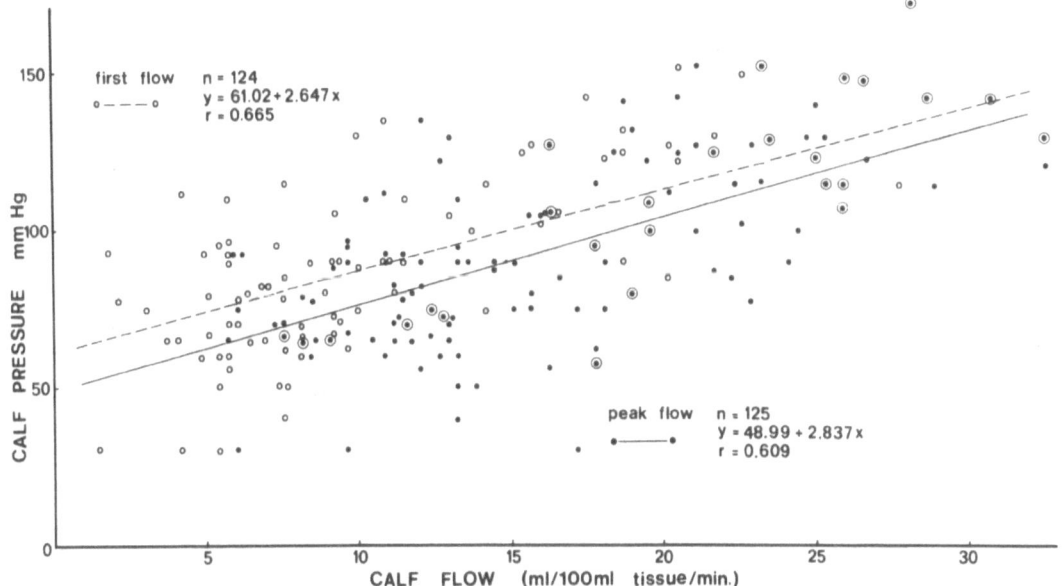

Fig. 4. Correlation between calf pressure at rest (measurement by ultrasound) and flow parameters (recorded with strain-gauge plethysmograph) during reactive hyperemia after arterial compression for 5 min. First flow = flow recorded during first period of venous occlusion after release of arterial compression. Peak flow = highest flow during reactive hyperemia (Verhaeghe and Beyens, unpublished).

detailed history and a meticulous physical examination in making the diagnosis of arterial obstructive disease. Claudication pain in conjunction with absent distal pulses, color changes, a cooler temperature and a poor nutrition of the skin are valuable guides to an impaired circulation. However these observations are fairly subjective and difficult to record with precision. In addition, the characteristics of intermittent claudication are not readily apparent from the complaints in some patients or the pedal pulses may remain palpable. Here, a practical method for objective assessment of the peripheral circulation such as noninvasive systolic pressure measurements is extremely valuable. As a general rule, muscle ischemia is not the cause of calf pain if the systolic pressure at the ankle is identical to the brachial pressure. In our experience, measurements at rest are sufficient to distinguish vascular pain for other causes of exertional discomfort in most patients and recordings after leg exercise are rarely required. However the problem may be quite different in preventive medicine or in epidemiological studies where arterial pathology has to be detected before symptoms arise: in the latter case, a pressure drop after exercise is a more sensitive indicator.

Evaluation of the functional importance of atherosclerotic lesions in peripheral arteries is often difficult and presents a real challenge to the clinician. Particularly an patients with atherosclerotic disease in consecutive arterial segments, it may be important to predict the functional significance of the disease in the individual segments. For instance, in patients with irregularities in the aorto-iliac arteries combined with marked stenosis of the superficial femoral artery, the decision where to operate first will be influenced by the functional importance of the disease in the proximal segment. The severity of the lesions cannot adequately be estimated from the encroachment of the diameter of the arterial lumen in a single plane angiogram; by contrast, assessment of the pressure gradient over an arterial segment is a reliable measure of the hemodynamic significance of an angiographically demonstrated stenosis. A mild degree of arterial narrowing has no functional significance if a hemodynamic abnormality is absent. A similar degree of functional impairment may be caused by a severe stenosis and a complete occlusion of the superficial femoral artery as indicated by a comparable pressure gradient between arm and calf in the two cases (Fig. 5). Patients with obstruction of both the iliac and femoral arteries have a more profound pressure drop between arm and calf or ankle than these with a single anatomical occlusion (ref. 31, see also Fig. 5). Thus it appears that the more extensive the occlusive process the larger the pressure gradient. That pressure measurements are a convenient method for objective assessment of the severity of ischemic symptoms is further demonstrated by the finding that patients with ischemic rest pain and/or gangrene have a significantly lower ankle pressure than those with only exertional pain (3, 31, 35, 36). Patients with ankle systolic pressure of less than 50 mm Hg usually have ischemic rest pain in the foot: they are incapable of nourishing their distal tissues at rest.

Angiography undoubtly remains the method of choice to obtain a precise anatomical picture of atherosclerotic lesions on the main arteries. Usually, palpation of the peripheral pulses gives a first indication on the location of the most proximal occlusion. Segmental pressure measurements substantiate this clinical impression and provide additional information: a drop in systolic pressure reflects an increased resistance proximal to the inflated cuff. For instance, when three cuffs are applied around the leg, occlusive lesions can be located either above the level of

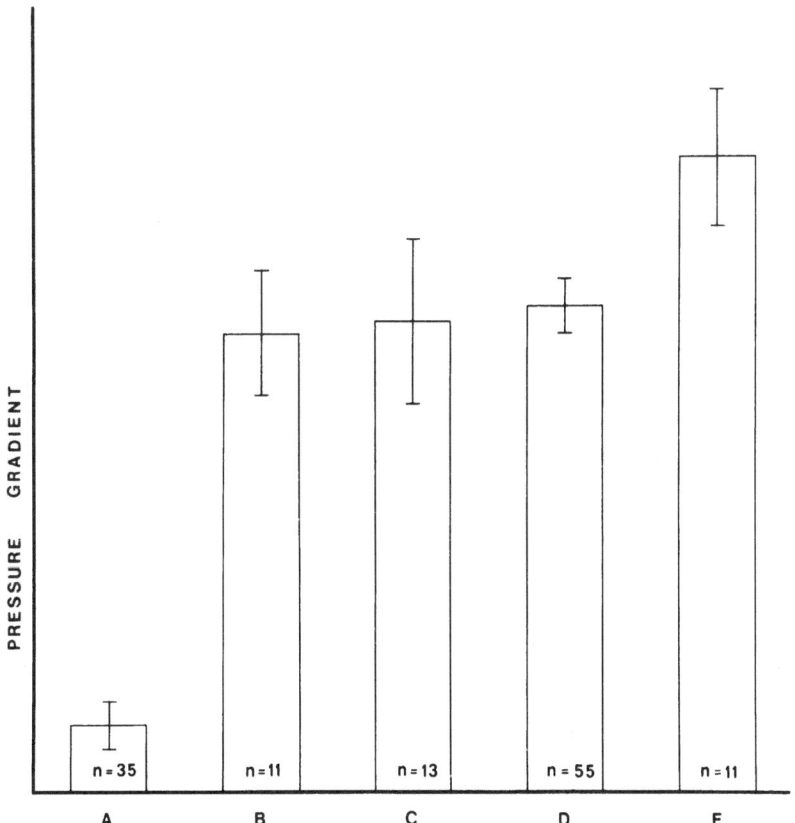

Fig. 5. Arm–calf pressure gradient in legs with arterial obstructive diease. A = nonstenotic lesions on angiography; B = occlusion of external iliac artery; C = severe stenosis of superficial femoral artery; D = occlusion of superficial artery; E = occlusion of iliac and superficial femoral artery. The gradient is similar in disease of iliac and femoral artery but is larger when both segments are occluded (Verhaeghe and Beyens, unpublished).

the midthigh (aorto-iliac, common femoral and upper part of the super-ficial femoral artery), between midthigh and calf (lower part of the super-ficial femoral and popliteal artery), between calf and ankle (crural arte-ries), or in more than one of the above segments. Recently, Barnes' group has advised again to use two narrow cuffs around the thigh, one around the proximal part and the second one above the knee, as originally proposed by Winsor (37) and later by Strandness and Bell (38). Even admitting that the narrow cuff technique records artifically elevated arterial pressures, they found that the use of a fourth cuff permits a better anatomical distinction of regional occlusive disease especially between the aorto-iliac, femoral and popliteal segments (5).

Patency of the blood vessels distal to an arterial obstruction is a factor of paramount importance when vascular reconstruction is considered. Angiography may appear inadequate to evaluate the distal run-off because the arteries in the lower leg fill only slowly and often incompletely with contrast medium in the presence of an iliac or femoral occlusion due to the considerable resistance in collateral vessels. Segmental blood pressure recordings can help to overcome this obstacle: the presence of a significant pressure gradient between calf and ankle or toe indicates in this case hemodynamically important lesions in the tibial or pedal arterial bed. Siggaard-Andersen et al. (39) reported a gradient of 19 mm Hg between distal thigh and ankle in 42 extremities with functioning distal run-off (at least one crural patent) against 53 mm Hg in 18 legs with poor run-off (all crural arteries occluded). Such information on the function of the distal vascular bed is useful in deciding whether or not surgery should be done in an individual patient and as a consequence may help to avoid unnecessary angiography in a number of patients with poor surgical prognosis.

Reappearance of palpable distal arterial pulses is rarely observed during follow-up of medically treated patients with atherosclerotic obstructive disease. General measures such as a weight-reducing diet, refraining from tobacco and exercise training can improve the claudication symptoms but whether this is accompanied by an improvement in flow or distal pressure remains debatable. In a recent study, we followed 45 patients with mild intermittent claudication over a 13-month period: their performance on the treadmill improved from 285 ± 21 m to 400 ± 29 m ($p < 0.01$) but their ankle pressure index at rest remained remarkably stable (0.61 ± 0.02 versus 0.64 ± 0.02, $p > 0.05$), suggesting that mechanisms other than an augmented blood supply are responsible for the symptomatic improve-ment (Fig. 6). By contrast, successful vascular reconstruction results in an almost immediate augmentation of the distal pressure, even when distal palpable pulses do not reappear. Consequently, repeated pressure re-cording in the leg is an easily obtained and convenient parameter to

It is true, as stated, that measure-ment of the difference between arm and for instance great toe pressure is a rather constant value even when measured on three consecutive days. An interesting observation was, however, made when comparing these three measurements. The blood pressure in the arm (the central blood pressure) was, namely, highest on the first day, lower on the second day and lowest on the third day of measurement. Evidently the patients were a little nervous when the first measurement was to be performed but the excitement was less on the second day and the patients completely calm on the third day. As the toe blood pressure, however, reacts in parallel with the arm blood pressure the difference is unchanged. Therefore, the peripheral blood pressure should always be related to the central blood pressure.

I do agree that the run-off blood in the lower leg sometimes is diffi-cult to evaluate. This technique may however be refined by in-jecting large amounts of contrast in reactive hyperaemia and also by waiting a fair time (20–30 sec) before the exposure is made. Robert Tyson in Philadelphia and his coworkers have since many years performed very delicate work with distal bypass proce-dures to the small arteries of the lower leg. The background for the very good results in this group is the outstanding angiographic work by the X-ray department of the Temple University in Philadelphia.

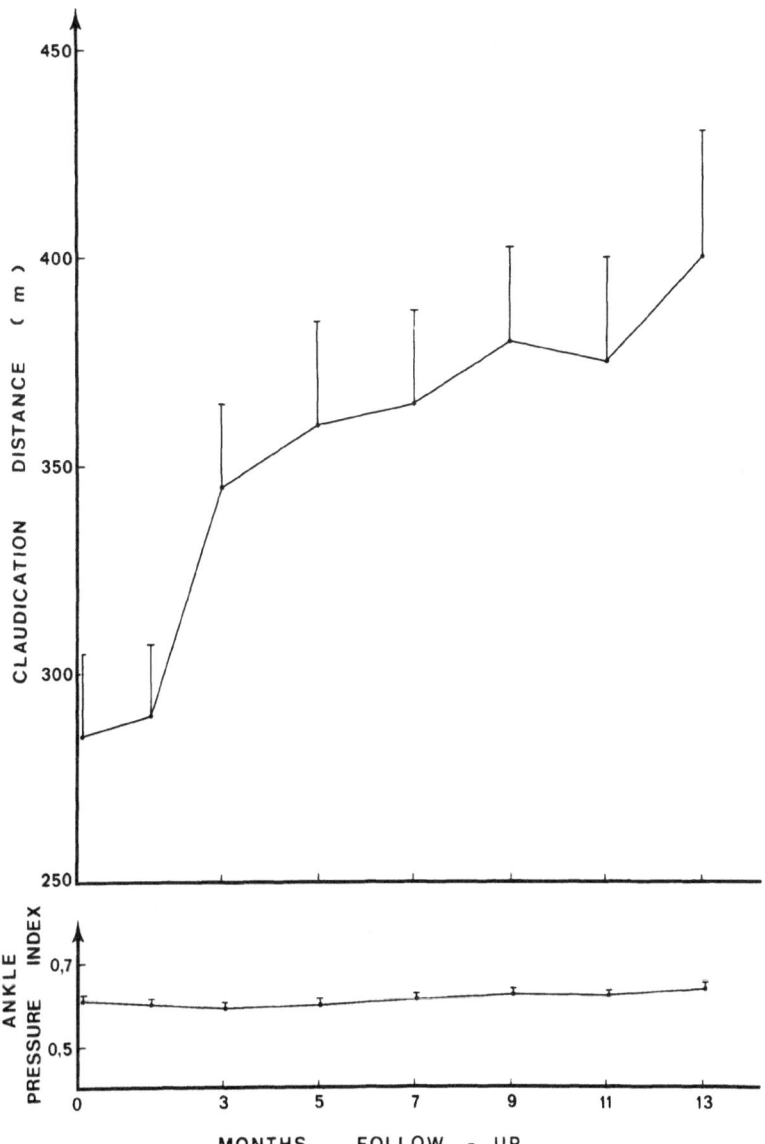

Fig. 6. Evolution of claudication distance measured on a treadmill (upper) and ankle pressure index (lower) measured with ultrasound in 45 patients with mild intermittent claudication followed over a 13-month period. Whereas claudication distance increased progressively, ankle pressure remained constant (Verhaeghe and Beyens, unpublished).

As a conclusion it could be stated that pressure measurements are easy and fast to perform. They are nonintrusive and without discomfort for the patient. The pressure difference from the arm to the distal level of the lower limb gives a reliable picture of the arterial disease. The only situation where the pressure values sometimes may give a false positive high value is in cases of a short stenosis in the aorta-iliac region.

In patients with normal distal pressures and a history of claudication a supplementary investigation should be made making blood pressure measurements immediately after intensive work with the leg muscles.

Additional literature: refs. 1–5.

monitor graft patency in the early postoperative period and a reliable indicator of re-occlusion during long term follow-up.

The prognostic value of leg blood pressure measurements has been stressed in various circumstances. Bone et al. (40) analyzed the value of the pre-operative proximal thigh pressure index, the pre-operative pressure gradient between adjacent leg segments and the early postoperative increase in ankle pressure index in predicting the result of aortofemoral reconstruction. A low pressure index in the proximal thigh which reflects severe aorto-iliac disease was uniformly predictive of a beneficial reconstruction; extremities with an increasing number of abnormal pressure gradients between adjacent segments were less and less likely to benefit from the aorto-femoral bypass and a clear increase in ankle pressure index immediately after the surgical procedure was an excellent predictor of subsequent symptomatic improvement. Nielsen et al. (41) found that the decreased systolic toe blood pressure in patients with occlusive arterial disease drops further after sympathetic blockade while the skin temperature rose, indicating that this procedure reduces the peripheral resistance more than the collateral resistance. Hence, they concluded that abolition of the sympathetic vasomotor tone is potentially harmful in patients with severe distal hypotension. A similar conclusion was reached by Yao and Bergan (42) who correlated ankle pressure with response to sympathectomy; in their study a pressure index above 0.35 was needed for a favorable clinical result of sympathectomy. In an effort to predict whether limited amputation has a real chance of success in cases of digital gangrene, several authors have correlated pressure measurements with healing or non-healing of the amputation wound. The minimal pressure associated with a successful minor amputation varied from 40 (43) to 60 mm Hg (44) the reason for this discrepancy being unclear. Barnes et al. (45) also reported that a below-knee amputation fails if no Doppler signal and thus no pressure is detectable below the knee; by contrast healing occurs in 75% of the extremities with a below-knee pressure less than 70 mm Hg and in all extremities with a pressure greater than 70 mm Hg. Closely related to the latter problem is the question of whether amputation is avoidable in the presence of incipient gangrene when vascular reconstruction appears impractical. Carter (46) observed that foot and toe ulcerations would not heal if the ankle pressure was less than 55 mm Hg whereas healing occurred at higher pressures. In our own series of 47 patients with rest pain of gangrene, 26 underwent a major amputation within the next 6 months; their ankle pressure (34 ± 3.4 mm Hg) was significantly different ($p < 0.05$) from that in 21 patients who did not require amputation (50.0 ± 5.2 mm Hg) within the same time period. From all these data it would appear that distal pressure is certainly related to the prognosis of a severely ischemic leg but prospective data from larger studies are needed to indicate more precisely the critical value of ankle pressure with regard to foot viability.

Whereas a large number of studies have concentrated on various aspects of the clinical application of distal pressure measurements in arterial obstructive disease, relatively few information is available on its use in other vascular disorders. By measuring digital blood pressure after step-wise local cooling, Nielsen and Lassen (47) were able to demonstrate an abrupt increase in arterial tone leading to complete closure of the digital arteries in patients with Raynaud's phenomenon; in normal subjects, a gradual increase in arterial tone was observed without closure of the arteries.

REFERENCES TO MAIN TEXT

1. Kirkendall WM, Burton AC, Epstein FH, Freis ED: Recommendations for human blood pressure determination by sphygmomanometers. Circulation 36: 980, 1967.
2. Rose GA, Blackburn H: Cardiovascular survey methods. WHO, Geneva, 1968, p 91.
3. Gundersen J: Segmental measurements of systolic blood pressure in the extremities including the thumb and the great toe. Acta chir. scand. Suppl. 426: 1, 1972.
4. Gundersen J: Standardized multisegmental measurements of blood pressure for quanti-tative evaluation of the circulation in the limbs. Scand. J. clin. Lab. Invest. Suppl. 128, 31: 111, 1973.
5. Heintz SE, Bone GE, Slaymaker EE, Hayes AC, Barnes RW: Value of arterial pressure measurements in the proximal and distal part of the thigh in arterial occlusive disease. Surg. Gynecol. Obstetr. 146: 337, 1978.
6. Carter SA: Clinical measurement of systolic pressures in limbs with arterial occlusive disease. J. Amer. med. Assoc. 207: 1869, 1969.
7. Stegall HF, Kardon MB, Kemmerer WT: Indirect measurement of arterial blood pres-sure by Doppler ultrasonic sphygmomanometry. J. appl. Physiol 25: 793, 1968.
8. Hernandez A, Goldring D, Hartmann AF, Crawford C, Reed GN: Measurement of blood pressure in infants and children by the Doppler ultrasonic technique. Pediatrics 48: 788, 1971.
9 Felix WR, Hochberg HM, George MED, Schmalzbach EL, Vaserberg R: Ultrasound measurement of arm and leg blood pressures: J. Amer. med. Assoc. 226: 1096, 1973.
10. Poppers PJ, Hochberg HM, Schmalzbach EL: A method for ultrasonic measurement of blood pressure in the adult leg. Anesthesiology 38: 490, 1973.
11. Holstein P, Lassen NA: Radioisotope clearance technique for measurement of distal blood pressure in skin and muscles. Scand. J. clin. Lab. Invest. Suppl. 128, 31: 143, 1973.
12. Nielsen PE, Lonsmann Poulsen H, Gyntelberg F: Skin blood pressure measured by a photoelectric probe and external counterpressure. Scand. J. clin. Lab. Invest. Suppl. 128, 31: 137, 1973.
13. Nielsen PE, Bell G, Lassen NA: The measurement of digital systolic blood pressure by strain gauge technique. Scand. J. clin. Lab. Invest. 29: 371, 1972.
14. Bell G, Nielsen PE, Lassen NA, Wolfson B: Indirect measurement of systolic blood pressure in the lower limb using a mercury in rubber strain gauge. Cardiovasc. Res. 7: 282, 1973.
15. King LT, Strandness DE, Bell JW: The hemodynamic response of the lower extremities to exercise. J. Surg. Res. 5: 167, 1965.
16. Carter SA: Response of ankle systolic pressure to leg exercise in mild or questionable arterial disease. N. Engl. J. Med. 287: 578, 1972.
17. Mahler F, Koen L, Johansen KH, Bernstein EF, Fronek A: Postocclusion and post-exercise flow velocity and ankle pressures in normals and marathon runners. Angiology 29: 721, 1978.

18. Johnson WC: Doppler ankle pressure and reactive hyperemia in the diagnosis of arterial insufficiency. J. Surg. Res 18: 177, 1975.
19. Kazamias TM, Gander MP, Franklin DL, Ross J, Jr: Blood pressure measurement with Doppler ultrasonic flowmeter. J. appl. Physiol. 30: 585, 1971.
20. Celander O, Thoren O: Validation of a plethysmographic method for measuring the systolic and diastolic blood pressure in man. Scand. J. clin. Lab. Invest. 27: 129, 1971.
21. Lorentsen E: Calf blood pressure measurements. Scand. J. clin. Lab. Invest. 31: 69, 1973.
22. Grüntzig A, Schlumpf M: The validity and reliability of post-stenotic blood pressure measurement by Doppler ultrasonic sphygmomanometry. VASA 3: 65, 1974.
23. Nielsen PE, Bell G, Lassen NA: Strain gauge studies of distal blood pressure in normal subjects and in patients with peripheral arterial disease. Analysis of normal variation and reproducibility and comparison to intra-arterial measurements. Scand. J. clin. Lab. Invest. Suppl. 128, 31: 103, 1973.
24. Carter SA: Indirect systolic pressures and pulse waves in arterial occlusive disease of the lower extremities. Circulation 37: 624, 1968.
25. Lassen NA, Tuedegaard E, Jeppesen FJ, Nielsen PE, Bell G, Gundersen J: Distal blood pressure measurement in occlusive arterial disease, strain-gauge compared to Xenon[133]. Angiology 23: 211, 1972.
26. Bell G, Nielsen PE, Wolfson B, Ulrich J, Engell HC, Lassen NA: Measurement of systolic pressure in the limbs of patients with arterial occlusive disease. Surg. Gyn. Obstetr. 136: 177, 1973.
27. Yao ST, Hobbs JT, Irvine WT: Ankle systolic pressure measurements in arterial disease affecting the lower extremities. Brit. J. Surg. 56: 676, 1969.
28. Bollinger A, Mahler F, Zehender O: Kombinierte Druck- und Durchflussmessungen in der Beurteilung arterieller Durchblutungsstörungen. Dtsch. med. Wsch. 95: 1039, 1970.
29. Thulesius O, Gjöres JE: Use of Doppler shift detection for determining peripheral arterial blood pressure. Angiology 22: 594, 1971.
30. Sumner DS, Strandness DE: The relationship between calf blood flow and ankle blood pressure in patients with intermittent claudication. Surgery 65: 763, 1969.
31. Yao JST: New techniques in objective arterial evaluation. Arch. Surg. 106: 600, 1973.
32. Yao ST, Needham TN, Gourmoos C, Irvine WT: New techniques in objective arterial evaluation. Surgery 71: 4, 1972.
33. Bollinger A, Schlumph M, Butti P, Grüntzig A: Measurement of systolic ankle blood pressure with Doppler ulstrasound at rest and after exercise in patients with leg artery occlusions. Scand. J. clin. Lab. Invest. Suppl. 128, 31: 123, 1973.
34. Quin RO, Evans DH, Fyfe T, Bell PRF: Evaluation of indirect blood pressure measurement as a method of assessment of peripheral vascular disease. J. Cardiovasc. Surg. 18: 109, 1977.
35. Lezack JD, Carter SA: The relationship of distal systolic pressures to the clinical and angiographic findings in limbs with arterial occlusive disease. Scand. J. clin. Lab. Invest. Suppl. 128, 31: 97, 1973.
36. Lennihan R, Mackereth M: Ankle blood pressure in vascular insufficiency involving the legs. J. clin. Ultrasound 1: 120, 1973.
37. Winsor T: Influence of arterial disease on the systolic blood pressure gradients of the extremity. Amer. J. med. Sci., 220: 117, 1950.
38. Strandness DE, Jr, Bell JW: Peripheral vascular disease; diagnosis and objective evaluation using a mercury strain gauge. Ann. Surg. Suppl. 1, 161: 3, 1965.
39. Siggaard-Andersen J, Ulrich J, Engell HC, Bonde-Petersen F: Blood pressure measurements of the lower limb. Angiology, 23, 350, 1972.
40. Bone GE, Hayes AC, Slaymaker EE, Barnes RW: Value of segmental limb blood pressures in predicting results of aortofemoral bypass. Amer. J. Surg. 132: 733, 1976.
41. Nielsen PE, Bell G, Augustenborg G, Lassen NA: Reduction in distal blood pressure by sympathetic nerve block in patients with occlusive arterial disease. Scand. J. clin. Lab. Invest. Suppl. 128, 31: 59, 1973.
42. Yao JST, Bergan JJ: Predictability of vascular reactivity relative to sympathetic ablation. Arch. Surg. 107: 676, 1973.

43. Verta MJ, Gross WS, Van Bellen B, Yao JST, Bergan JJ: Forefoot perfusion pressure and minor amputation for gangrene. Surgery 80: 729, 1976.
44. Baker WH, Barnes RW: Minor forefoot amputation in patients with low ankle pressure. Amer. J. Surg. 133: 331, 1977.
45. Barnes RW, Shanik GD, Slaymaker EE: An index of healing in below knee amputation: leg blood pressure by Doppler ultrasound. Surgery 79: 13, 1976.
46. Carter SA: The relationship of distal systolic pressures to healing of skin lesions in limbs with arterial occlusive disease, with special reference to diabetes mellitus. Scand. J. clin. Lab. Invest. Suppl. 128, 31: 239, 1973.
47. Nielsen SL, Lassen NA: Measurement of digital blood pressure after local cooling. J. appl. Physiol. 43: 907, 1977.
48. Weaver JC, Bohr DF: The digital blood pressure. I. Values in normal subjects. Amer. Heart J. 39: 413, 1950.
49. Gaskell P: Measurement of blood pressure, the critical opening pressure and the critical closing pressure of digital vessels under various circumstances. Canad. J. Physiol. Pharmacol. 43: 979, 1965.
50. Gaskell P, Krisman AM: The brachial to digital blood pressure gradient in normal subjects and in patients with high blood pressure. Canad. J. Biochem. Physiol. 36: 889, 1958.
51. Geddes LA, Spencer WA, Hoff HE: Graphic recording of the Korotkoff sounds. Amer. Heart J. 57: 361, 1959.
52. Rushmer RF, Baker DW, Stegall HF: Transcutaneous Doppler flow detection as a non-destructive technique. J. appl. Physiol. 21: 554, 1966.
53. Strandness DE, McCutcheon EP, Rushmer RF: Application of a transcutaneous Doppler flowmeter in evaluation of occlusive arterial disease. Surg. Gynec. Obstr. 112: 1039, 1966.
54. Dahn I, Lassen NA, Westling H: Blood flow in human muscles during external pressure or venous stasis. Clin. Sci. 32: 467, 1967.
55. Lorentsen E, Hoel BL, Hol R: Evaluation of the functional importance of atherosclerotic obliterations in the aorto-iliac artery by pressure/flow measurements. Acta med. scand. 191: 399, 1972.

REFERENCES TO COMMENTARY

1. Gundersen J: Measurement of systolic blood pressure in all the toes. VASA 1: 281–284, 1972.
2. Gundersen J: Temperature induced disparities between the systolic blood pressure in the arm and in the thumb and the great toe. VASA 1: 247–258, 1973.
3. Gundersen J: Measurement of systolic blood pressure in all the fingers. Danish med. Bull. 20: 129–131, 1973.
4. Gundersen J, Dahlin K: Measurement of systolic blood pressure in fingers of newborn infants. Acta pediatr. scand. 64: 741–744, 1975.
5. Gundersen J: The peripheral blood pressure in legs with venous ulcers. Acta chir. scand. 141: 514–516, 1976.

7. Intra-arterial pressure

K.L. GOULD

Commentary by H.L. Falsetti

COMMENTARY

Pressure is a force per unit area. When using units of mercury, it always refers to a force per unit area.

1. BASIC CONCEPTS

The force of cardiac contraction is transmitted to the arterial system as pressure which maintains patency of blood vessels and perfusion of capillaries. The term pressure is derived from the Latin verb, premere, meaning to act on with steady force or weight. It is defined as the static force per unit area exerted by a column of fluid according to the equation: $P = h \times d \times a$, where h and d are the height and density of the column of fluid and a is the acceleration of gravity. In physics or engineering, the units of pressure are expressed in absolute units of the cgs (centimeter-gram-second) system as $cm \times g/cm^3 \times cm/sec^2$. This expression reduces to g/sec^2-cm or $g\text{-}cm/sec^2\text{-}cm^2$ or $dynes/cm^2$, where the dyne is the unit of force. However, for biological systems, these units are simplified to the height in millimeters of a standard reference fluid, mercury by convention, with the density of mercury, d, and the acceleration of gravity, a, omitted since they are constants. In physiology, the units of pressure are then expressed as mm Hg. Mercury is used as a standard fluid because of its high density, thereby permitting measurement of arterial pressure with a relatively short tube. The relation between mm Hg and cgs units can be calculated as follows: 1 mm Hg = $(0.1\ cm)$ $(13.6\ g/cm^3)$ $(980\ cm/sec^2)$ where 0.1 cm is 1 mm height of the column, 13.6 g/cm^3 is the density of mercury, and 980 cm/sec^2 is the acceleration due to gravity. One mm Hg, therefore, equals 1333 $dynes/cm^2$ or 0.019 lb/in^2; 52 mm Hg equals 1 lb/sq. in.

As an alternative, the unit centimeter of saline is also used for low pressures such as venous pressure. In absolute units, 1 cm saline would be equal to $(1.0\ cm)$ $(1.04\ g/cm^3)$ $(980\ cm/sec^2)$, where 1.04 g/cm^3 is the density of saline. Therefore, 1 cm saline equals 1019 $dynes/cm^2$ of pressure. Similarly, the units of pressure could be expressed as centimeters of blood (density 1.055 g/cm^3) and 1 mm Hg calculated to equal to 1.29 cm of blood,

1 mm mercury equals 1.31 cm of water or 1.29 cm of blood.

an important point in establishing a zero pressure reference.

Arterial pressures are measured relative to a reference point outside the body arbitrarily defined as zero and chosen as the level of the mid-right atrium. Actual or absolute pressure at this level outside the body is, in fact, not zero but atmospheric pressure or approximately 760 mm Hg. There-fore, an arterial pressure of 95 mm Hg means that the pressure is 95 mm Hg above atmospheric pressure. The reference zero point of a catheter-external pressure manometer system is determined by the position of the manometer relative to the atria. If the external manometer is 12.9 cm below the level of the atria, the manometer will record that pressure at the tip of the catheter plus the pressure produced by a column of blood 12.9 cm high equivalent to 10 mm Hg. It is important to understand the relation of body position to the zero reference point when measuring arterial pressure. Different pressures will be recorded with the external manometer located at the level of the atria as compared to having the transducer at the level of the head or feet, as illustrated in Fig. 1. In the

Pressures are always measured relative to a reference point. The importance of the reference point or transducer reference is emphasized.

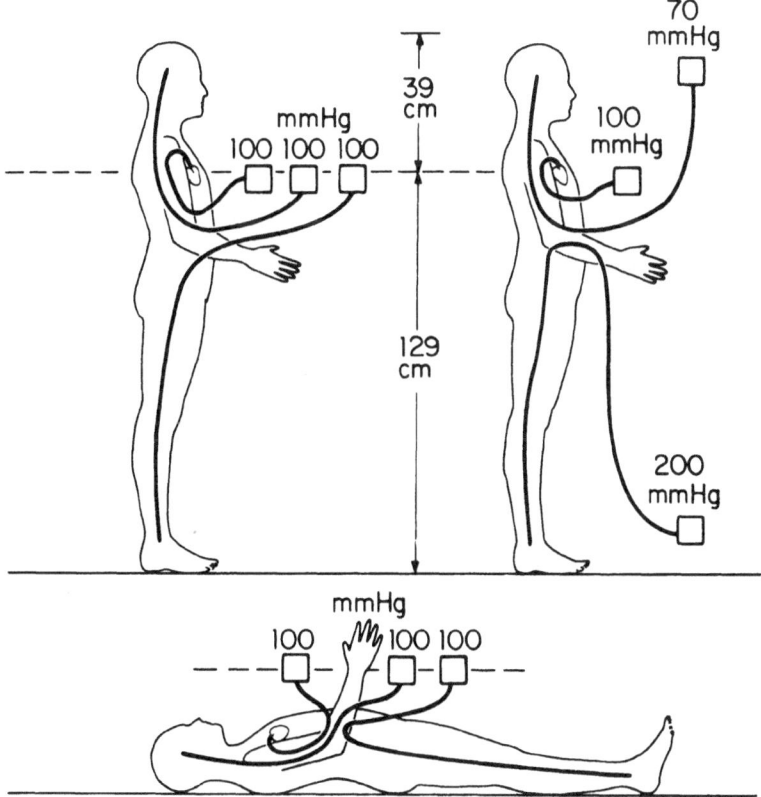

Fig. 1.

supine position, arterial pressures measured at the head, feet and aortic root relative to the zero reference at the atria are all equal. In the standing position, arterial pressure at the level of the head, feet and aortic root relative to the zero reference at the atrial level are also equal. However, the arterial pressure at the level of the feet relative to a zero reference also at the level of the feet is increased by that amount of pressure produced by the column of blood between the atria and the feet. This pressure is termed the transmural pressure and is the pressure 'seen' or sustained by the arterial wall. It is equal to the standard intra-arterial pressure (referenced to the atria) plus the pressure produced by the column of blood above the feet. At the level of the head, the transmural pressure relative to a zero reference also at the level of the head is equal to the standard arterial pressure relative to an atrial zero reference minus the pressure due to the column of blood between the head and atria. The force or pressure generated by the heart is described by the standard arterial blood pressure with zero reference at the atria. The transmural force or pressure on the arterial wall is described by the arterial pressure plus (for anatomic sites below the heart) or minus (for the anatomic sites above the heart) the pressure due to the column of blood between the atria and the anatomic site at which the transmural pressure is being determined. Blood pressure measurements by sphygmomanometer measure transmural pressure and are therefore affected by the position of the limb on which the blood pressure cuff is placed. A cuff blood pressure on an arm raised overhead in a standing patient will be lower than in a standing patient with the arm at the level of the atria even though actual arterial pressure is contant.

Pressure per se is a force per unit area and is by definition static, involving no motion, fluid displacement, distance, or time increment. However, in cardiovascular systems, pressure fluctuates periodically with cardiac contraction. A pressure recording apparatus must, therefore, have not only static accuracy but also dynamic accuracy for recording pressure at each instant in time during rapid fluctuations of pressure. The dynamic responses of fluid-filled catheter-manometer systems have been previously described in mathematical and experimental detail (1–6). A brief review of wave form analysis is appropriate here in order to understand how to measure and optimize dynamic accuracy and how to recognize 'bad' or 'good' pressure recordings during clinical studies.

This paragraph contains an analysis of the pressure wave. It contains basic theoretical information.

Cardiac contraction generates a transient pulse of force which passes along the aorta and arteries as a pressure wave. This pressure wave may be described and analyzed mathematically as the sum of a series of theoretical sine wave pressures which, when added together, reconstitute or equal the original wave form. Each of these theoretical sine waves is called a harmonic and is characterized by harmonic number, amplitude, and phase shift. The process of determining the number and characteristics of the harmonics necessary to reproduce the original wave form when added together is called harmonic or Fourier analysis. Fig. 2 illustrates an example. At the top is a recording of a left ventricular pressure wave. For purposes of analysis, the zero pressure baseline has been moved up so that the pressure wave can be described in terms of pressures above and below zero, e.g., a wave −40 to +50 mm Hg rather than in conventional terms of 0 to 90 mm Hg. The pressure wave can then be defined by a series of sine wave pressures shown below the left ventricular pressure trace. The harmonic number is the number of complete sine waves falling within the time period of the original cycle, in this case 1.1 sec. The first harmonic has one complete sine wave within this period. The second harmonic has two complete sine waves within this period, etc. The amplitude of the harmonic

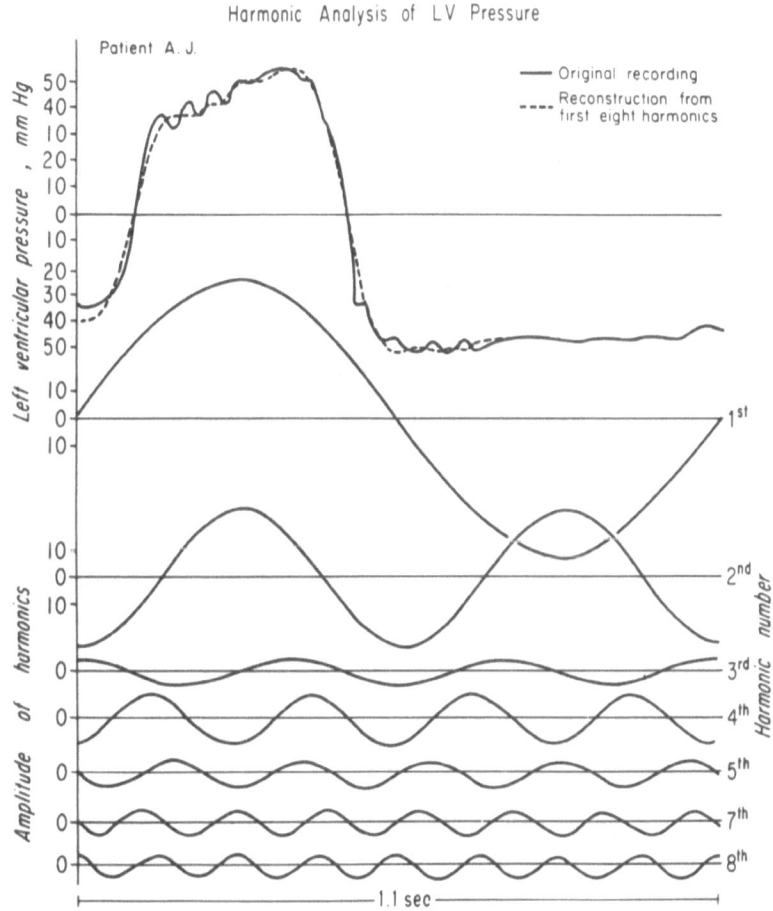

Fig. 2. Harmonic analysis of LV pressure.

is the maximum displacement of the sine wave above or below the midline zero reference. The phase shift defines the beginning of a harmonic sine wave in time relative to the basic cycle or first harmonic. When the harmonics are added up, the various deflections above or below zero reference accumulate to produce the positive wave during systole and cancel each other during diastole.

Poor dynamic accuracy or distortion of pressure waves by fluid-filled catheter-manometer systems may be understood in terms of the failure to faithfully record the amplitude and phase shifts of all essential harmonics of the pressure wave. Exaggeration of some harmonics by pressure resonance or oscillation in the fluid-filled catheter, failure to record some harmonics due to damping, or changes in the phase of some harmonics but not others will distort the recorded pressure wave form. There are mathematical equations corresponding to the sine waves of the harmonic analysis conceptually illustrated in Fig. 2 (1–3). However, in practice, it is not necessary to utilize sine wave equations in the analysis of dynamic accuracy of a given catheter-manometer system, and details will not be given here.

In general, at least 20 harmonics are required to exactly reconstitute a left ventricular pressure wave, particularly the rate of rise or upstroke, dp/dt, of the pressure trace (7–12). The exact number of harmonics changes with the heart rate as discussed subsequently (10, 11). Only 8–10 harmonics are required to reconstitute an approximation of the left ventricular pressure with the correct peak systolic pressure. Other details such as the rate of pressure rise and abrupt fluctuations in pressure cannot be reconstituted with the first 8 harmonics, illustrated in Fig. 2 and Fig. 3. If only 4 harmonics are used, the reconstituted pressure wave is grossly distorted, as shown in Fig. 3a. A catheter-manometer recording system which fails to record higher harmonics, therefore, produces a distorted pressure wave as shown; this type of distortion is called overdamping since the higher harmonics are damped out. However, most fluid-filled catheter-manometer systems are underdamped. In this case, the column of fluid in the catheter oscillates or resonates at one or several of the higher harmonics. The harmonic at which resonance occurs, therefore, becomes accentuated and its amplitude becomes artifactually large. The reconstituted pressure is therefore distorted, as shown in Fig. 4D, with parts of the recorded pressure wave being greater than the actual or real undistorted pressure wave.

These concepts of harmonic analysis may be related functionally to a catheter-manometer system by testing its dynamic accuracy with a device which generates sine wave pressures at any selectable frequency. A number of different types of sine wave pressure generators have been described and are also commercially available. The device consists of a

Although 20 harmonics will accurately reproduce the pressure wave, in practice only 8–10 harmonics are required for a reliable left ventricular pressure. If rates of pressure changes are used, as dp/dt, higher frequency response is required. The effect of heart rate on frequency is noted. The higher the heart rate, the greater the frequency response required.

fluid-filled chamber into which the tip of a catheter is inserted and sealed. The pressure in the chamber fluctuates in a sine wave pattern with waves of 20–30 mm Hg amplitude at variably controlled frequencies. This pressure is recorded by a reference pressure transducer attached directly to the chamber. Thus, two pressures are recorded: the standard or reference pressure and the pressure through the catheter attached to a second or test transducer. Fig. 5 shows an example of testing a catheter-manometer system with a sine wave pressure generator. At the top is the electrical driving signal. At the bottom is the reference sine wave pressure in the test chamber having an amplitude of 20 mm Hg. In the middle is the pressure recorded through the catheter-manometer system being tested. The numbers at the bottom of each panel indicate the frequency of the pressure waves or cycles per second, also termed Hertz, where 1 Hz equals 1 cycle/sec. For frequency of pressure waves up to 20 Hz, the catheter-manometer system recorded the pressure waves fairly accurately. How-

A method to test the fidelity of catheter systems is presented. The frequency characteristics of a catheter are best described by the natural frequency and degree of damping. These may be calculated as noted by the formulas included in these paragraphs or more simply by noting the peak amplitude response, for example, in Fig. 6. The peak amplitude response corresponds to the natural frequency. The degree of damping can be approximated by dividing the amplitude response by two. For example in Fig. 7 the Gensini catheter with one stopcock would have a natural frequency of approximately 50 Hz and a damping ratio of $1/2 \times 0.5 = 0.25$.

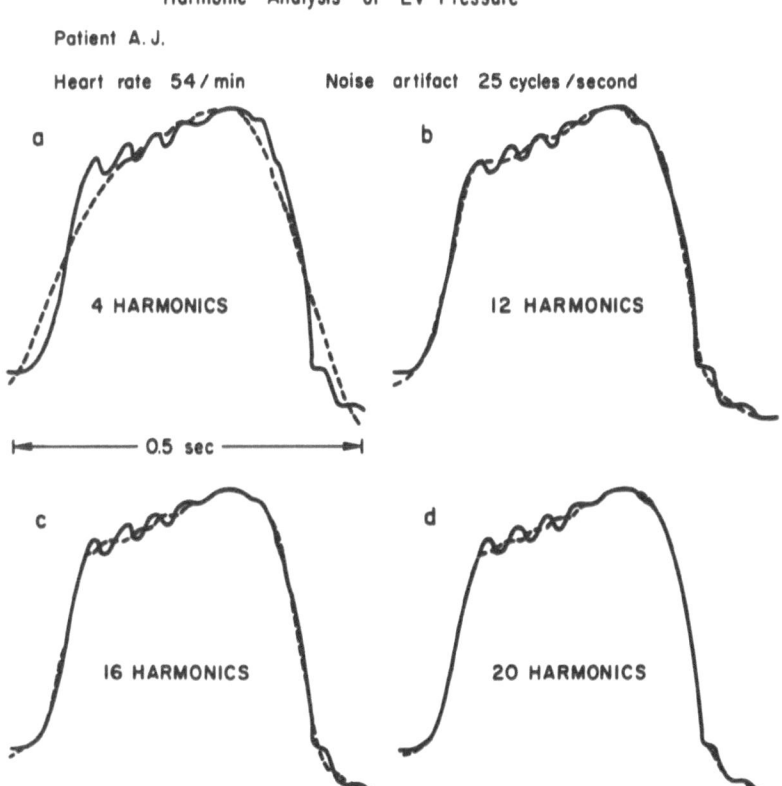

Harmonic Analysis of LV Pressure

Patient A. J.

Heart rate 54 / min   Noise artifact 25 cycles / second

a   4 HARMONICS

b   12 HARMONICS

|— 0.5 sec —|

c   16 HARMONICS

d   20 HARMONICS

Fig. 3. Harmonic analysis of LV pressure.

ever, at 50 Hz, the catheter pressure is distorted, i.e., is amplified to approximately 45 mm Hg even though the pressure waves in the chamber remain at 20 mm Hg amplitude. At 103 Hz, the pressure waves recorded through the catheter were 150 mm Hg in amplitude compared to 20 mm Hg in the reference chamber. Thus, the catheter-manometer system distorted or amplified the actual pressure waves to 7.5 times the actual amplitude of the pressure waves in the test chamber. Such distortion is

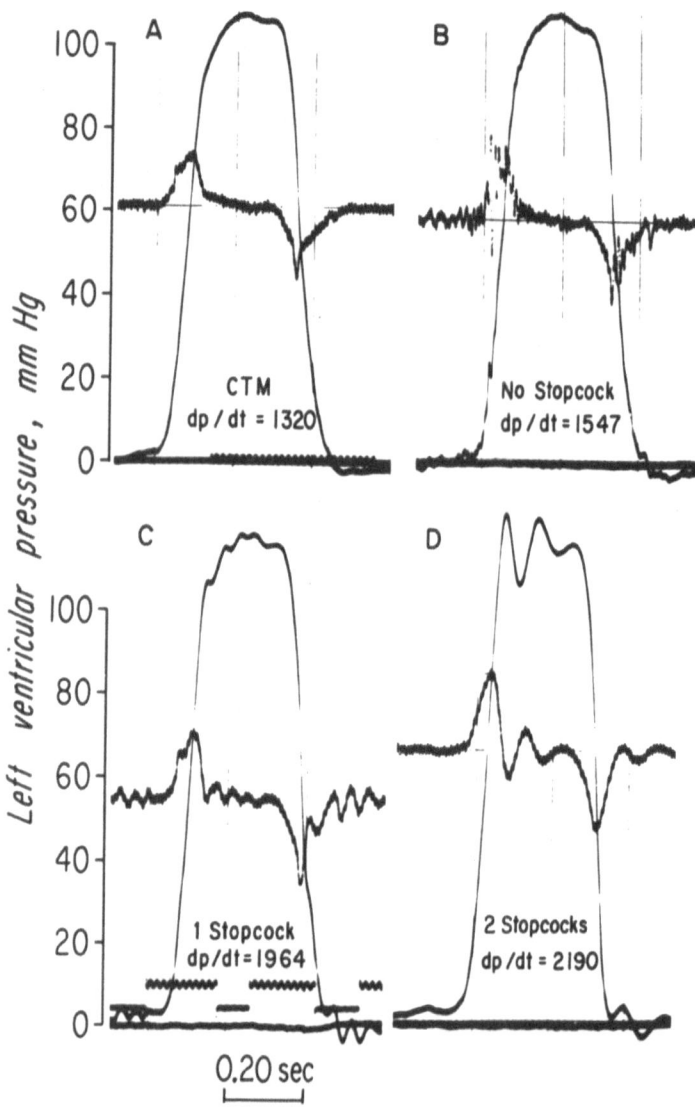

Fig. 4.

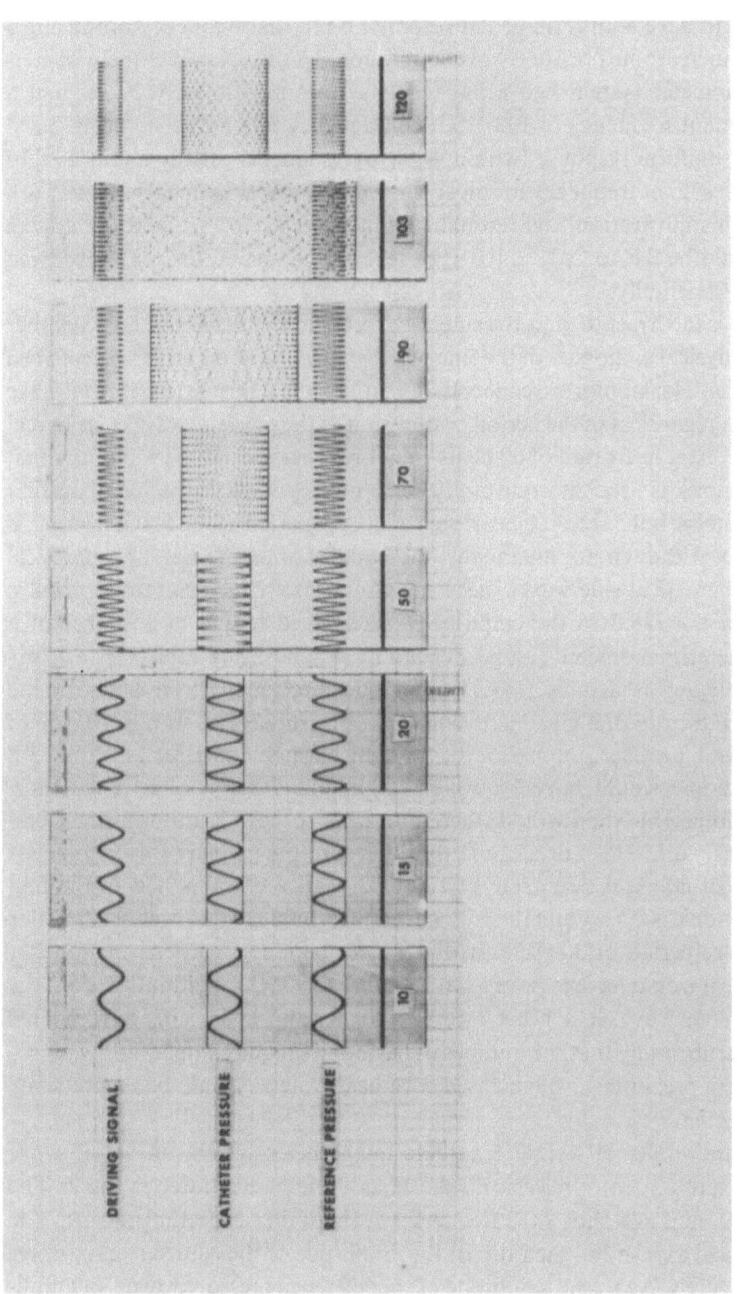

Fig. 5.

due to underdamping. That frequency at which maximum amplification occurs is called the resonant frequency. A catheter-manometer system is said to have a uniform or flat response up to that frequency producing a 5% increase in pressure wave amplitude. In this example, the catheter-manometer system had a flat response to approximately 20 Hz and a resonant frequency of 103 Hz. The frequency to which the system has a flat, uniform response (within $+5\%$ overshoot) is usually about 20% of the resonant frequency for most clinical, i.e., underdamped, catheters (4). In this illustration, the resonant frequency was 103 Hz and the system should be flat to 20% $\times$ 103 Hz or 21 Hz compared to 20 Hz observed experimentally.

It is incorrect to view the sine wave pressures in the above test chamber as physical analogues of the sine waves in the harmonic analysis described earlier. Harmonics are conceptual, mathematical forms describing a wave form regardless of the period or duration of the pressure wave cycle in real time. At a heart rate of 60 beats/min, or 1 beat/sec, the period of the first harmonic is 1 sec. At a rate of 120 beats/min, or 2/sec, the period of the first harmonic is 0.5 sec. At a heart rate of 30, the period of the first harmonic is 2 sec. Although not analogous, the number of harmonics, or theoretical mathematical sine waves, necessary to faithfully reconstitute a pressure wave is related to the empirically determined frequency response of a catheter-manometer system depending on the heart rate (11). For example, let us assume that 15 harmonics are required for approximate reproduction of a given left ventricular pressure wave. At a heart rate of 60 or 1 beat/sec, the period of the first harmonic is 1 sec and the 15th harmonic would have 15 cycles within this 1 sec period. A catheter-manometer system would, therefore, have to have a uniform or flat response to 15 Hz in order to faithfully record the pressure wave at a heart rate of 60. At a heart rate of 120 or 2 beats/sec, the period of the first harmonic is 0.5 sec and the 15th harmonic would have 15 cycles within this 0.5 sec period or 30 cycles within a 1 sec period. A catheter-manometer system would have to have a flat response to 30 Hz to faithfully record the pressure wave at a heart rate of 120. Knopp et al. (10) have shown experimentally that the number of harmonics required to faithfully reproduce a pressure wave increased with heart rate as would be theoretically expected.

The results of testing a catheter-manometer system on a sine wave pressure generator may be displayed as a graph, illustrated in Fig. 6. The horizontal axis shows the frequency in Hz of the generator pressure. The vertical axis shows the ratio of the amplitude of the catheter-manometer pressure wave to the amplitude of the reference pressure wave. An amplitude ratio of 1.0 indicates no error or overshoot. An amplitude ratio of 2.0 indicates that the catheter-manometer pressure wave has an amplitude two times as large as the actual amplitude of the reference pressure wave. An amplitude ratio of 1.05 indicates an overshoot of $+5\%$ and is conventionally defined as the limit of acceptable error for a catheter system. A 'fast' system has a frequency response curve to the right side of the graph, such as the transseptal catheter. It faithfully records pressure waves up to 25 Hz. A 'slow' system falls to the left side of the graph, such as a 7F Gensini with one stopcock; it faithfully records pressure waves up to only 10 Hz. In addition, this slower system is more damped than the others, as indicated by a lower peak amplitude ratio of 6.0 compared to 13.0 for the faster systems. All the catheters in Fig. 6 are underdamped. A critically damped system (not shown) would have no peak amplitude ratio; it would be flat to some input frequency, and thereafter its response would fall off to less than 1.0. Standard 8 French Gensini and 8.5 French transseptal catheters without intervening stopcocks have natural frequencies of 115–120 Hz and are flat to 20–25 Hz. One stopcock decreases uniform amplitude response to 12–15 Hz. In these relatively large catheters, blood or hypaque increased damping slightly, i.e., lowered height of the resonance peak, but did not change the frequency at which peak resonance occurred.

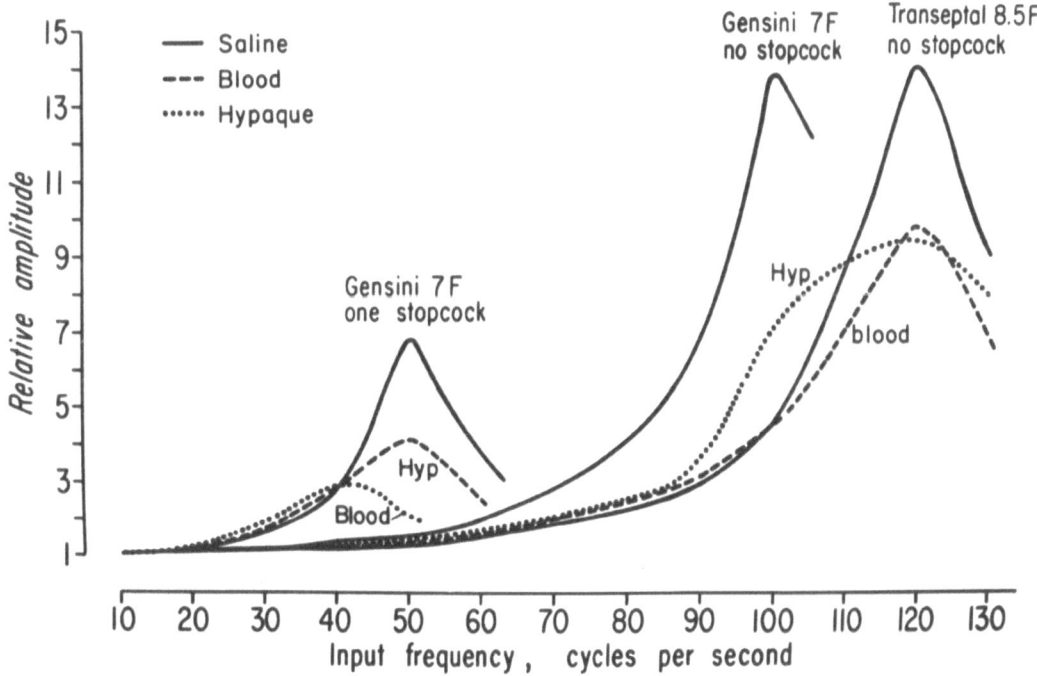

Fig. 6.

Another approach may also be used to test the dynamic accuracy of a catheter-manometer system called transient analysis. In this technique, the saline-filled catheter system is shock excited by a square wave pressure change, and the resulting oscillations recorded. A number of different methods for producing a sudden square step in pressure have been described. The simplist is a partially fluid-filled chamber into which the catheter is inserted through a sealed side hole and the chamber covered with a rubber diaphragm balloon or finger of a rubber surgical glove. A positive pressure is applied through a separate side tube so as to tense the rubber diaphragm outward. With the recorder running, the diaphragm is burst with a flame. The sudden release of pressure creates a square wave drop in pressure recorded by the catheter. If undamped, the catheter-manometer system oscillates producing a series of fluctuating pressure waves which die out with time, as shown in Fig. 7. By measuring the amplitude and period of these pressure oscillations, the characteristics of the catheter manometer system can be calculated with the following three relationships published by Fry (2):

Degree of damping is expressed as the damping ratio, h, which is the ratio of actual damping to critical damping and is calculated as:

$$h = \sqrt{\frac{ln^2\,(b/a)}{\pi^2 + ln^2\,(b/a)}}$$

where b/a is the ratio of amplitudes shown in Fig. 7 and $(100) \times (b/a) = \%$ overshoot. π is 3.1416. ln is the natural logarithm to base e, and ln^2 is this value squared.

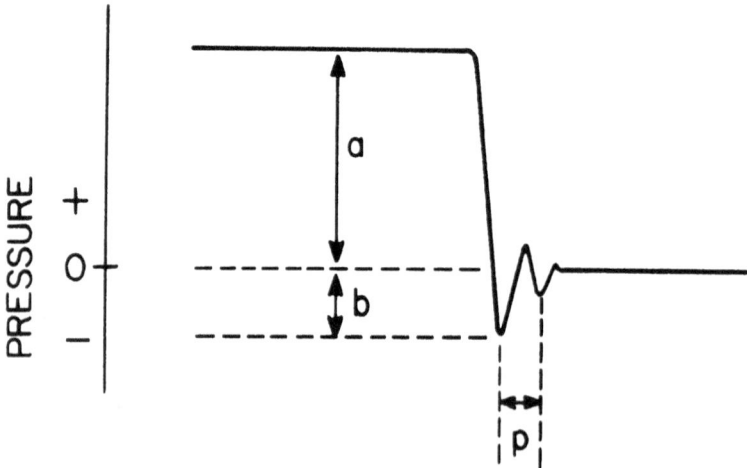

Fig. 7.

The undamped natural frequency, F_u, is calculated as follows:

$$F_u = F_d / \sqrt{1-h^2}$$

Where F_d is the observed frequency of the recorded oscillations, termed the damped natural frequency, and is equal to $1/p$ where p is the period of damped oscillation, i.e., the time between successive wave peaks shown in Fig. 7. On a clinical left ventricular pressure, the number of pressure oscillations at the leading edge of peak systolic pressure (See Fig. 4D) can be used in a similar manner to estimate approximately the damped natural frequency of the catheter system in vivo.

Amplitude response, R, is calculated as:

$$R = 1/\sqrt{(1-\beta^2)^2 + (2h\beta)^2}$$

where β = ratio of the system undamped natural frequency, F_u, to any arbitrarily selected driving frequency from 1 Hz up to 100 Hz.

Phase lag in degrees, θ, is calculated as:

$$\theta = tan^{-1} \frac{2h\beta}{1-\beta^2}$$

Phase lag or phase shift are terms used to describe the delay in each harmonic of a pressure wave. A shift of a whole sine wave cycle of a given harmonic is a 360° phase shift, a shift of one-half cycle is 180°, a shift of one-quarter cycle is 90°. A half-cycle or 180° phase shift of a low frequency, e.g., the first harmonic, is a much longer delay in real time in seconds than a half-cycle phase shift of a high frequency, e.g., the 20th harmonic. Thus, if all harmonics of a pressure wave were delayed 90°, each harmonic would have a different delay in real time in seconds and the recorded wave would be grossly distorted. For undistorted pressure recordings, the phase shift in degrees must be directly proportional to frequency of the harmonics and the shift in real time in seconds must be the same for all harmonics. For catheter systems which have damping ratios of 0.125–1.0, phase lag is approximately linearly related to frequency over a range of frequencies up to 30–40% of resonant frequency (2). Thus, for a catheter system with a resonant frequency of at least 80 Hz or flat to 20–25 Hz, there is little distortion due to phase lag.

As an example of the use of these equations, let the ratio of b/a in Fig. 7 equal 0.5 and the period $p = 0.02$ sec. Per cent overshoot would be 50%. The damping ratio, h, would be calculated as: $b/a = 0.5$, $\ln b/a = 0.693$, $\ln^2 b/a = 0.480$, and, therefore, h can be calculated to be 0.22, which indicates considerable underdamping. Critical damping occurs at $h = 0.707$ in which case there is only 4–5% overshoot. The damped natural frequency, Fd, would be $= \frac{1}{p}$ or $F_d = 1/0.02$ sec $= 50$ Hz and the undamped natural frequency would be $F_u = (50)/\sqrt{1-(0.22)^2} = 51$ Hz or cycles/sec. Thus, there is so little damping in this system that the undamped natural frequency is approximately the same as the damped natural frequency.

The phase lag which would occur at a given driving frequency, for example 10 Hz, would be calculated as: $\beta = 10/51 = 0.20$ and $h = 0.22$ from above. Therefore, $\theta = tan^{-1}(2)(0.22)(0.2)/0.96$ and $\theta = 5.2°$ phase shift. For a heart rate of 1 beat/sec, the real time delay, t, at 10 Hz would be $t = (1\ sec)(\frac{1}{10})\left(\frac{5.2°}{360°}\right) = 1.5 \times 10^{-3}$ sec or 1.5 msec. At another driving frequency, for example, 20 Hz, $\beta = 20/51 = 0.39$ and $\theta = tan^{-1}(2)$ $(0.22)(0.39)/0.85$ and $\theta = 11.5°$. For the same heart rate of 1 beat/sec, the delay, t, at 20 Hz would be $t = (1\ sec)(\frac{1}{20})\left(\frac{11.5°}{360°}\right) = 1.6 \times 10^{-3}$ sec or 1.6 msec. Thus, for a doubling of the frequency, the phase lag doubles and the delay in seconds is comparable for all frequencies. Therefore, there would be no distortion due to phase shift for the example above which is typical of most clinical catheters if well flushed with only one stopcock in the system.

The terms damped natural frequency, undamped natural frequency, and resonant frequency are not interchangeable in general. The damped natural frequency is the observed frequency of oscillation of a catheter-manometer system after a sudden square wave pressure change. The undamped natural frequency is the theoretical calculated frequency of oscillations of a system after a square wave pressure change if there were no damping. These two terms apply only to the transient analysis technique. Resonant frequency applies only to the technique of testing a catheter system with a sine wave pressure generator. The resonant frequency, F_r, is related to the undamped natural frequency, F_u, according to the equation:

$$F_r = F_u\sqrt{1-2h^2}$$

The resonant frequency is related to the damped natural frequency according to the equation:

$$F_r = F_d\sqrt{\frac{1-2h^2}{1-h^2}}$$

both relations being derived from Fry (2). At low damping ratios of $h \leq 0.31$, F_r, F_u, and F_d are within 10% of each other which applies to most, if not virtually all, standard, single lumen, saline-filled, clinical catheters of 5 French or greater size. At higher damping ratios 0.31–0.707, resonant frequency is always less than the undamped natural frequency and greater than the damped natural frequency. At critical damping with *h* approaching 0.707, there is no resonance, and these terms have no physical meaning.

2.   ANALYSIS AND USE OF CLINICAL CATHETER-MANOMETER SYSTEMS

Several reports have analyzed catheter-manometer systems; most of them have used a sine wave pressure generator and most have shown similar results (4, 6, 12–21).

Table 2 illustrates typical data, in this case obtained from studies by the author in the cardiac catheterization laboratory of the Seattle Veterans Administration Hospital, Seattle, Washington. Resonant frequencies and the frequency to which the system had a flat response (within $+5\%$ overshoot) are shown for a variety of catheters used clinically. Also shown are the effects of microdisplacement (Honeywell Kulite) compared to plastic dome, fluid-filled transducers (Statham), the effects of stopcocks in the system, and the effects of filling the catheter with saline, blood, or viscous contrast media.The data can be summarized as follows. Short, stiff, large bore catheters, e.g., the 8.5 F transseptal catheter, have the best response characteristics with resonant frequencies of 155 Hz and flat responses to 23–25 Hz. Long, soft, small bore catheters, e.g., 7F Cournard, have poor response characteristics with resonant frequencies under 50 Hz and flat to 13 Hz or less. Stopcocks, even wide bore types, between the catheter and transducer markedly deteriorate frequency response, probably due to the entrapment of tiny air bubbles in the stopcock interstices. Two or more stopcocks have cumulative worse effects than one. The type of fluid filling the system affected the degree of overshoot. For example, viscous Hypaque 60% increased damping and altered the shape of the frequency response curve as shown in Fig. 6; it might also lower the resonant frequency. However, the more viscous fluid did not change the frequency to which the catheter-manometer remained flat and therefore did not alter the adequacy of the system for recording pressure waves. In small catheters, 4 French or less, contrast media caused sufficient damping to prevent recording pressure waves adequately. The microdisplacement Kulite and Statham P23Gb pressure transducers with the catheters shown had similar frequency responses in our study. There is another report that the Statham P23 Db with clinical catheters had a lower resonant frequency than a microdisplacement pressure transducer (15). The Statham P23Gb pressure transducer had a stiffer membrane than the P23 Db and would be expected to have a higher resonant frequency when used with clinical catheters (4, 5) and, therefore, more comparable to a microdiscplacement catheter. Our data support this expectation. Other results in Table 2 are similar to previous reports (4, 6, 13–21).

Table 1. Physical characteristics of standard cardiac catheters.

Catheter	OD size French scale	Length (cm)	Inside diameter		Outside diameter		Material	Manufacturer and number
			mm	inches	mm	inches		
Gensini	8	100	1.73	0.068	2.67	0.104	teflon	USCI* 7435
Gensini	7	100	1.47	0.058	2.33	0.091	teflon	USCI* 7435
Transseptal	8.5	70	1.52	0.060	2.83	0.111	teflon	USCI 7730
Cournand	7	125	1.17	0.046	2.33	0.091	dacron	USCI 5500
Cournand	6	125	0.91	0.036	2.00	0.078	dacron	USCI 5500
Lehman	7	125	1.47	0.058	2.33	0.091	dacron	USCI 5400
Lehman	6	125	1.17	0.046	2.00	0.078	dacron	USCI 5400
Lehman	4	118	0.58	0.023	1.33	0.052	teflon	USCI 7450
Miscellaneous	8.5	70	2.16	0.085	2.80	0.110	polyethylene	B-D**
(thin wall)	3.7	132	0.79	0.031	1.20	0.047	polyethylene	B-D

* United States Catheter and Instrument Company.
** Becton, Dickinson and Company.

Virtually everyone who has studied frequency responses of catheters have found that consistent reproducible clinical recordings or frequency response testing requires repeated careful flushing of the catheter-manometer system with boiled or deaerated sterile saline (2, 4–6, 12, 14–17, 20, 23). For example, Futamura (17) has quantified the progressive improvement in frequency response with successive flushing up to 5 flushes in sequence. Thereafter, frequency responses remained stable. Similarly, elimination of stopcocks and connector tubing is important for obtaining good frequency responses (2, 12, 14–16).

In laboratory practice, there are three types of pressure wave distortions, all visually recognizable. Clinical catheter-manometer systems are either underdamped and slow, underdamped and fast, or overdamped. Examples are illustrated in Fig. 4. The pressure recording 4A is an ideal reference left ventricular pressure trace recorded by catheter tip micromanometer and therefore unaffected by catheter-induced distortion. Pressure 4B is a recording through an underdamped, fast catheter-manometer system. There is considerable high frequency resonance or hash due to underdamping, but the system has a flat dynamic response to 20–25 Hz and a resonant frequency of greater than 100 Hz. Therefore, the recording contains accurate pressure information, and the basic wave form is correct. The high frequency 'hash' is visually unattractive but does not deform the pressure wave. It can be removed by filtering the signal through an electronic analog filter, a frequency-limited galvanometer recorder or digital computer filtering as discussed subsequently. Pressure 4C is a recording through an underdamped, moderately slow catheter-manometer system flat to 10–13 Hz with a resonant frequency of 40–50 Hz in which the pressure wave is somewhat distorted but clinically useful for measuring peak systolic and end-diastolic pressure. Pressure 4D is a grossly distorted recording through an underdamped, very slow catheter-manometer system flat to 3–5 Hz with a resonant frequency of 13–17 Hz. It is so distorted that the pressure information and basic wave form have been lost. No type of processing can extract a correct pressure wave from this recording. The cause of such distortion is due to one or several of the following: improper flushing of the system, two or more stopcocks or multiple manifold connectors in the system, or long, soft extender tubings between the catheter and transducer.

Maximum dp/dt or rate of pressure rise is very sensitive to catheter-induced distortion of the pressure wave. Underdamping causes pressure overshoot at any given instant on the rising pressure trace and therefore results in an erroneously high dp/dt as shown in Fig. 4. Even the fast system in 4B has enough artifact to give a dp/dt that is artifactually 17% too high compared to the reference or true value determined by catheter tip manometer. The dp/dt in 4D is 66% higher than the true value.

The importance of careful flushing of the catheter system cannot be overemphasized.

Common types of pressure wave distortion are discussed. With practice, these can be easily recognized.

Table 2. Frequency responses of standard cardiac catheters.

Catheter	Size (French)	Honeywell K7lite PSL 126-6 Pressure Transducers						Statham P23Gb	
		Saline		Blood		Hypaque 60%		Saline	
		No sc	sc	No sc	sc	No sc	sc	No sc	sc
Gensini	8	115/20**	81/13	100/20	73/20	85/20	72/20	103/25	41/13
Gensini	7	103/20	51/12	104/20	52/12	95/23	45/12	101/27	60/13
Transseptal	8.5	155/33	51/16	102/22	45/17	120/20	44/12	155/45	52/13
Cournand	7	41/13	—	37/7	—	35/6	—	83/7	—
Cournand	6	75/13	—	74/21	53/12	—	—	—	—
Lehman	7	80/18	—	74/17	—	54/15	—	—	—
Lehman	6	91/12	—	80/18	—	75/21	—	—	—
Lehman	4	86/16	—	76/17	—	50/17	—	—	—
Miscell.	8.5	110/16	83/16	110/17	87/14	100/20	59/14	100/22.	67/21
Miscell.	3.7	58/13	44/11	65/14	30/12	50/17	over damped	—	27/11

* A single wide bore Ole Dich stopcock, Ole Dich Instrument Makers, Denmark.
** The numerator is resonant frequency. The denominator is the frequency to which the system has a flat amplitude response (+5% overshoot).

Fig. 8 illustrates overdamped pressures. The reference pressure recorded by catheter tip manometer is shown in 8A, an underdamped fast catheter manometer recording in 8B, a slightly overdamped catheter manometer recording in 8C, and a grossly overdamped recording in 8D. In the clinical laboratory, overdamped pressures are due to one or more of the following: small, long catheters less than 2–3 French, to damping needles intentionally placed between the catheter and transducer, to entrapment or abutment of an end hole catheter against the arterial or left ventricular wall, or to blood clotted in the catheter. Unclotted blood in standard catheters down to 3 French will not produce overdamped pressures as illustrated in 8C and 8D. Observation of such tracings that persist after ruling out causes other than clot and which cannot be corrected by aspirating the contents of the catheter usually requires removal of the catheter since forward flushing carries the risk of embolization. Contrast media in catheters down to 4 French will not produce overdamping shown in Fig. 8.

Pressure recordings obtained by catheter-manometer systems are technically good only if the system is fast, i.e., flat to 20–25 Hz and the pressure waves look like those shown in Fig. 4A, B, or Fig. 8B. Technically acceptable tracings for recording peak systolic, end-diastolic, and the approximate pressure wave can be obtained with a system flat to about 15 Hz and the pressure waves look like those in Fig. 4C or Fig. 8C. A slower system producing recordings like those of Fig. 4D or an overdamped system as in Fig. 8D are not technically acceptable for any quantitative measurements. Virtually all standard clinical catheters 125 cm long or shorter and 5 French or greater in diameter, if properly flushed with sterile deaerated saline and with no more than a single stopcock between the transducer and catheter, will produce adequate pressure recordings for qualitative evaluation of the wave form and quantitative measurement of systolic or diastolic pressure. The following procedure is recommended. Initially record pressure with only one three-way large bore stopcock in the system flushed as follows with sterile, deaerated saline (e.g., Abbott). Pour saline gently into a basin and draw gently into a syringe, preferably plastic, without creating bubbles. Attach the filled syringe to the side arm of the stopcock and flush back through the stopcock being careful to flush out all bubbles. Attach the transducer to the stopcock while flushing gently. If a transducer with a plastic dome is used, the entire dome should be flushed through. Then turn the stopcock so as to flush forward through the male end. Remove any other stopcocks from the catheter, let it bleed backward, and attach to the male end of the flushed stopcock with the syringe in place on the side arm. Aspirate blood into the syringe and then flush forward. While flushing, turn the stopcock through to record pressure. Remove the syringe, turn the stopcock to air to establish zero baseline, then turn the stopcock to pressure for recording. If optimized high fidelity recordings

This section is required reading. It gives the practical details for obtaining reliable left ventricular pressure tracings.

are desired, then record a second pressure after removing all stopcocks and attaching the bleeding catheter directly to the gauge. Zero reference is recorded while the gauge is being held waiting for the back bleeding to wash out all saline. After recording 3–4 heart beats, quickly reintroduce a stopcock, aspirate a syringe of blood, and flush the system with saline in order to avoid blood clotting in the catheter. Any other routine such as a continuous flush-through system is acceptable as long as the basic requirements are met, i.e., careful repeated flushing and no more than one stopcock in line between the catheter and transducer.

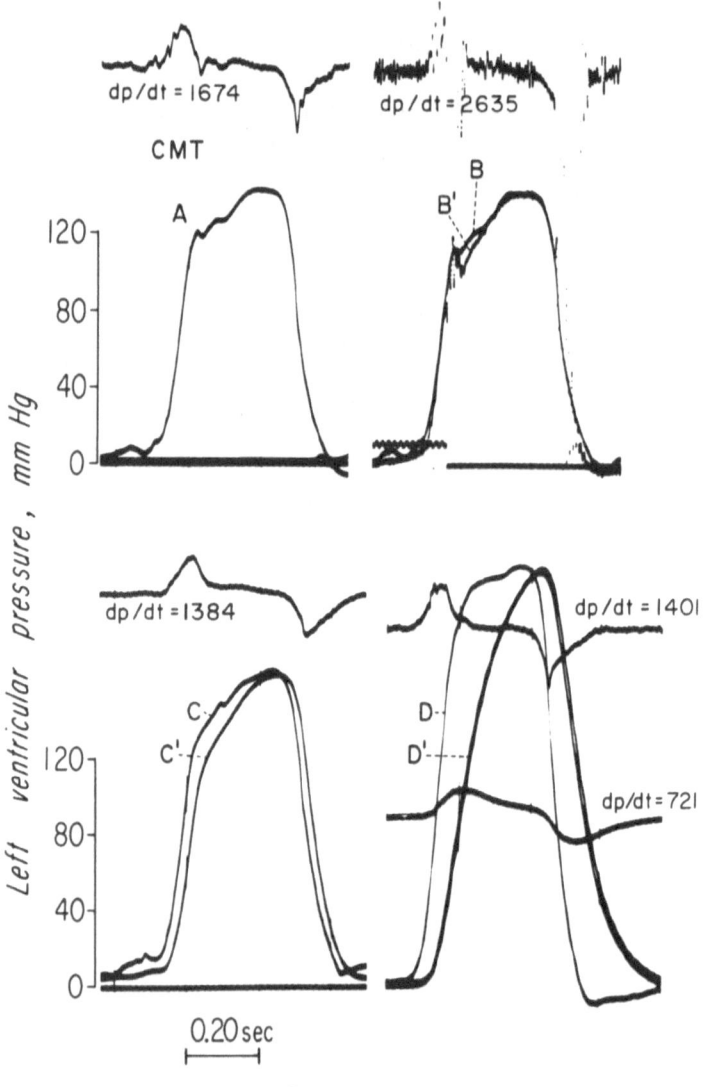

Fig. 8.

Peripheral artery (e.g., brachial, radial) systolic pressures are greater than central aortic systolic pressures because the peripheral artery itself acts like an underdamped catheter causing overshoot as the pressure wave is transmitted distally (19). Thus, some overshoot in peripheral arteries may not indicate a poor recording system but may be a physiologic in vivo phenomenon. However, even peripheral artery pressures do not have the undulations seen in the tracing Fig. 4D.

3. SPECIAL PROCESSING OF PRESSURE RECORDINGS

Unprocessed, standard catheter-manometer recordings are not adequate for quantitative analysis of the exact pressure wave form, e.g., measurement of dp/dt or rate of pressure rise. A catheter system may be fast enough to record the basic pressure wave form, i.e., flat to 25 Hz, but since such fast systems are invariably underdamped, there is high frequency resonance or hash which prevents the direct determination of dp/dt. A number of approaches have been developed to alter the catheter system itself or process the recording, thereby eliminating the high frequency components and extracting a smooth, accurate pressure wave which can be differentiated to obtain a reliable dp/dt. All correction techniques require fast catheter systems. The pressure wave is so distorted by a slow system that no correction method is adequate. The most extensively developed method of processing pressure recordings uses analog or electronic filters. Knopp et al. (10) processed pressure signals through a 15 Hz low pass analog filter before differentiation and compared the resulting value of dp/dt to a reference measurement with a direct manometer system. In their system peak dp/dt was underestimated by 12% at 2000 mm Hg/sec and by 20% at 3300 mm Hg/sec. Gould et al. (12) processed pressure signals through two, in series, variable low pass filters with very sharp roll off. By studying a range of cut-off frequencies, they determined that dp/dt could be measured within $\pm 12\%$ accuracy in comparison to the catheter tip manometer by passing the catheter-manometer pressure signal through a high quality 22 Hz low pass filter. Lower cut-off frequency caused peak dp/dt to be consistently underestimated. Falsetti et al. (16) and later Futamura (17) developed a more complex analog compensator consisting of cascaded variable low pass-band pass filters which were manually set according to the experimentally determined undamped natural frequency and damping ratio of each catheter used. Brower et al. (18) carried this approach further by developing an ingenious, fully automatic device which in effect automatically on line determined the natural undamped frequency and damping ratio of a pressure recording and thence automatically set a band pass filter to eliminate artifacts. How-

The special processing of pressure recordings is currently of little interest. The last paragraph summarizes this whole section.

ever, the system required a dedicated miniprocessor and hardware. All of these systems worked fairly well provided fast catheter-manometer systems with high resonant frequencies were used. Another related approach was described by Rowell et al. (19) utilizing a galvanometer recorder with a 24 Hz frequency limiting galvanometer. The effect of this system is the same as utilizing a 24 Hz low pass filter but avoided the phase shifts inherent in analog filters.

The other major approach for correcting the distortions of catheter-manometer systems utilized damping devices inserted between the catheter and the transducer. The purpose of these devices was to increase damping to a critical damping ratio, thereby eliminating overshoot or resonance. Krovetz et al. (20), subsequently Lapointe and Roberque (22), and recently Li et al. (21) utilized this approach but found it of limited value. Dear and Spear (23) utilized still another approach. They flushed the catheter system with CO_2 gas before flushing, thereby reducing the content of microscopic air bubles which cause resonance in the system. They reported accurate measurements of dp/dt with this approach, but it is somewhat awkward to use clinically.

Currently there appears to be little role for compensating or correction procedures for catheter-manometer recordings. Since peak dp/dt or related pressure measurements are now infrequently used clinically to assess myocardial performance, there is little practical use for them. If highly accurate pressure wave forms are required, as for measuring dp/dt for research purposes, modern catheter tip micromanometers mounted within angiographic catheters are relatively easy to use at acceptable costs. For routine clinical data, a well-flushed catheter-manometer system with a single stopcock permits accurate quantitative measurements of systolic and diastolic pressures, pressure gradients, and adequate qualitative assessment of the wave form.

REFERENCES TO MAIN TEXT

1. Hansen AT, Warburg E: The theory for elastic liquid containing membrane manometers. Acta physiol. scand. 19: 306–349, 1950.
2. Fry DL: Physiologic recording by modern instruments with particular reference to pressure recording. Physiol. Rev. 40: 753–788, 1960.
3. Attlinger EO, Anne A, McDonald DA: Use of Fourier series for the analysis of biological systems. Biophys. J. 291–304, 1966.
4. Yanof HM, Rosen AL, McDonald NM, McDonald DA: A critical study of the response of manometers to forced oscillations. Phys. med. Biol. 8: 407–422, 1963.
5. Yanof HM: Biomedical Electronics, Davis, 1965, p 265–284.
6. Fry DL, Noble FW, Mallos AJ: An evaluation of modern pressure recording systems. Circulat. Res. 5:40–46, 1957.
7. Gleason WL, Braunwald E: Studies on the first derivative of the ventricular pressure pulse in man. J. clin. Invest. 41: 80–91, 1962.

8. Wallace AG, Skinner NS, Mitchell HJ: Hemodynamic determinants of the maximal rate of rise of the left ventricular pressure. Amer. J. Physiol. 205: 30–36, 1963.

9. Patel DJ, Mason DT, Ross J, Braunwald E: Harmonic analysis of pressure pulses obtained from the heart and great vessels of man. Amer. Heart J. 69: 785–794, 1965.

10. Knopp TJ, Rahimtoola SH, Swan HJC: The first derivative of ventricular pressure recorded by means of conventional cardiac catheter. Cardiovasc. Res. 4: 398–404, 1970.

11. Gersh BJ, Hahn CEW, Prys-Roberts C: Physical criteria for measurement of left ventricular pressure and its first derivative. Cardiovasc. Res. 5: 32–40, 1971.

12. Gould KL, Trenholme S, Kennedy JW: In vivo comparison of catheter manometer systems with the catheter tip micromanometer. J. appl. Physiol. 34: 263–267, 1973.

13. Cronvich JA, Burch GE, Frequency characteristics of some pressure transducer systems. Amer. Heart J. 77: 792–797, 1969.

14. Shapiro GG, Krovetz LJ: Damped and undamped frequency responses of underdamped catheter manometer systems. Amer. Heart J. 80: 226–236, 1970.

15. Scruggs V, Pietras RJ, Rosen KM: Frequency response of fluid filled catheter micromanometer systems used for measurement of left ventricular pressure. Amer. Heart J. 89: 619–624, 1975.

16. Falsetti HL, Mates RE, Carroll RJ, Gupta RL, Bell AC: Analysis and correction of pressure wave distortion in fluid filled catheter systems. Circulation 44: 165–172. 1974.

17. Futamura Y: Correction of distortions of pressure waves obtained with catheter-manometer systems. Jap. Heart J. 18: 664–678, 1977.

18. Brower RW, Spaans W, Rewiersma PAM, Meester GT: A fully automatic device for compensating for artifacts in conventional catheter-manometer pressure recordings. Biomed. Eng. 10: 305–310, 1975.

19. Rowell LB, Brengelmann GL, Blackmon JR, Bruce RA, Murray JA: Disparities between arotic and peripheral pulse pressures induced by upright exercise and vasomotor changes in man. Circulation 32: 954–964, 1968.

20. Krovetz LJ, Jennings RB, Golgbloom SD: Limitation of correction of frequency dependent artefact in pressure recordings using harmonic analysis. Circulation 50: 992–997, 1974.

21. Li JKJ, van Brummelen AGW, Noordergraaf A: Fluid filled pressure measurement systems. J. appl. Physiol. 40: 839–843, 1976.

22. Lapointe AC, Roberge FA: Mechanical damping of the manometric system used in the pressure gradient technique. IEEE Trans. Biomed. Eng. 21: 76–78, 1974.

23. Dear HD, Spear AF: Accurate method for measuring dp/dt with cardiac catheters and external transducers. J. appl. Physiol. 30: 897–899, 1971.

8. Blood viscosity and red cell deformability

JOHN A. DORMANDY

Commentary by S. Chien

1. INTRODUCTION

Blood flow is determined by the pressure gradient, the calibre of the vessels and the viscosity of the blood. For too long a disproportionate emphasis has been placed by clinicians interested in circulatory diseases on the pathology of the vessels. The physical flow properties of the blood have only recently been investigated systematically and this chapter will attempt to summarise the available techniques of measurement and outline the clinical significance of the results obtained. These have defined the physiological and pathological importance of such measurements and reports are beginning to appear of therapeutic manoeuvres, aimed at lowering whole blood viscosity, improving patients with various circulatory diseases. These will be briefly reviewed.

Whilst a reasonably coherent picture is emerging regarding the viscosity of bulk blood, clinicians have only recently begun to investigate the flow properties or deformability of individual red cells; and these will be discussed briefly in the last section of this chapter.

1.1. Some basic definitions

1.1.1. *Viscosity, shear rate and shear stress.* The viscosity of a fluid is due to the internal friction between adjacent layers of the fluid. Most of this discussion will be concerned with streamlined flow, where adjacent layers of a fluid move parallel to each other, usually at different velocities. The velocity difference between adjacent layers is a measure of the shearing within the flowing fluid and this velocity gradient is termed the shear rate. The velocity of flow in the fluid and the shearing within the fluid is produced by a force which is called the shear stress.

The viscosity of the fluid is then defined as the ratio of the shear stress to the shear rate it produces. The greater the viscosity of a fluid, the more shear stress or force will be required to produce a certain shear rate or velocity. Alternatively, an increase in the viscosity will decrease the shear rate produced by a constant shear stress.

Fig. 1 illustrates these definitions: Let A be two layers of fluid flowing in relation to each other at velocities v_1 and v_2' pushed by a force F. The shear rate is the velocity gradient, $\dfrac{dv}{dx}$, where v is the difference between v_1 and v_2 and x is the distance between the layers of fluid being considered. The units of shear rate will be distance per time divided by distance, which equals the reciprocal of time, usually expressed as inverse seconds (sec^{-1}). The shear stress is expressed as force per unit area, F divided by A, and will be in units of dyne/cm^2 (1 dyne $= 10^{-5}$ Newtons). The viscosity of the fluid, being the shear stress over the shear rate it produces, will be expressed in units of dynes, sec/cm^2, which equals one poise or a hundred centipoises (cP). (In SI. units, the shear stress is expressed in pascals, which are equivalent to 10 dynes/cm^2. The shear rate remains in sec^{-1} and the unit of viscosity is the Pascal second. One pascal second is equivalent to 10 Poise and therefore rather conveniently a millipascal second equals one centipoise.)

For practical purposes, as a rough approximation, the shear stress can be thought of as the force pushing the blood along the vessels and the shear rate as the velocity of flow. The relationship between these two will be determined by the viscosity of the fluid. Although the shear stress will be constant across the tube, the velocity gradient will vary, from a high value near the wall to zero in the axis of the tube.

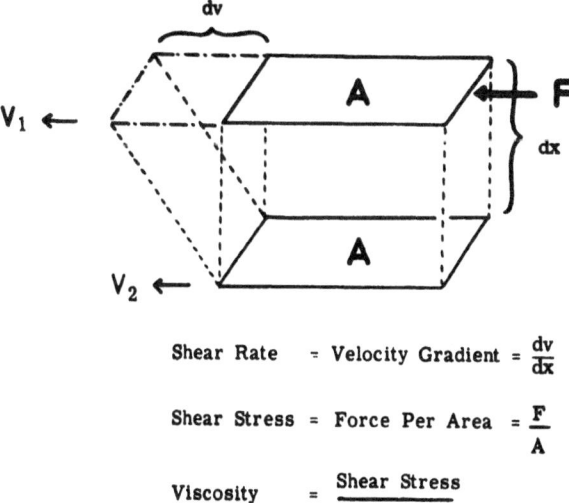

$$\text{Shear Rate} = \text{Velocity Gradient} = \frac{dv}{dx}$$

$$\text{Shear Stress} = \text{Force Per Area} = \frac{F}{A}$$

$$\text{Viscosity} = \frac{\text{Shear Stress}}{\text{Shear Rate}}$$

Fig. 1. Definition of viscosity.

COMMENTARY

Author's figure 1 illustrates the flow of a Newtonian fluid (a fluid whose viscosity does not change with shearing condition, see page 216) between two parallel plates. Under such conditions the shear rate, or the velocity gradient, is the same everywhere in the fluid. In flow through a cylindrical tube, however, the velocity of flow approaches zero near the wall and is at the maximum in the center. Thus, the velocity distribution of a Newtonian fluid flowing in a cylindrical tube is parabolic in nature, and the velocity gradient also varies accordingly (Fig. 1 p. 265). The shear rate is given by the change in velocity per unit distance along the radial direction of the tube; it is zero in the center of the tube, where the velocity profile is essentially flat and has maximum values near the wall, where the change in velocity with radial distance is the steepest. If the fluid is non-Newtonian (viscosity varies with shear rate), then the velocity profile in a tube is more blunted in the middle and steeper near the wall as compared with the Newtonian fluid.

Shear stress should be thought of as the shearing force *per unit area* of fluid being sheared. In the case of flow through a tube, the shear stress is *not constant* across the tube, but rather varies across the tube in the same manner as the shear rate for a Newtonian fluid. Due to this radial variation of shear stress, one usually uses the shear stress – shear rate relationship at the tube wall to determine blood viscosity in tube flow. The wall shear stress can be calculated from the pressure gradient (i.e., the change in pressure, ΔP, over a tube length (L) and the tube radius (R): shear stress $= R\,(\Delta P/2L)$.

Wall shear rate is a function of the mean linear velocity of flow (v, in cm/sec, is the mean of velocity values across the tube) and the tube radius (R, in cm): wall shear rate for a Newtonian fluid $= 4\,v/R$. It can also be expressed as $4Q/\Pi R^3$, where Q is the volumetric flow rate (in cm^3/sec), since $Q = \Pi R^2 v$.

The term 'relative viscosity' has more than academic usefulness. It serves to focus on the behaviour of the red cells (e.g., changes in their deformability or aggregation, especially when determined at a fixed cell concentration), after normalizing for variations in plasma viscosity.

Sometimes the term 'relative viscosity' is used, to mean the viscosity of the whole blood divided by that of its plasma. Its usefulness is more academic than practical.

1.1.2. Non-Newtonian behaviour of blood. Newton first described the concept of viscosity and believed that all fluids have a single constant viscosity. In other words, for a given fluid the ratio of shear stress to shear rate will be constant and a certain change in the shear stress applied to the fluid will produce an exactly proportional change in the resulting shear rate. This situation is shown diagrammatically by the continuous line in Fig. 2. The slope of the straight line in Fig. 2a will represent the viscosity of the fluid.

It was only in 1915 that it was realised that blood does not behave in a Newtonian manner in that it has a variable viscosity (1). As the shear stress decreases, the resulting shear rate decreases out of proportion as shown by the interrupted line in Fig. 2. The ratio of shear stress to shear rate, that is, the viscosity, thus increases at lower shear rates.

The word 'relatively' is used to indicate 'proportionately'. That is, in a given tube, when the flow velocity is reduced to 1% of the initial value, the shear stress required is greater than 1% of the initial value. The absolute value of shear stress needed is still less than that of the initial value.

This non-Newtonian behaviour means that it requires a *relatively* larger force to move blood slowly than to move it fast. As can be seen from Fig. 2b, at higher shear rates blood does become Newtonian and normal blood reaches a constant viscosity value at shear rates above 100 sec^{-1}. The implications of this in the measurement of blood viscosity are clearly vital and are described in Section 1.2.1. while the probable reason for this non-Newtonian behaviour is briefly discussed in Section 3.3.1. (It should be noted that plasma alone is Newtonian.)

Normal blood approaches a constant viscosity value at shear rates above 100 sec^{-1}, but probably 200–400 sec^{-1} or even higher are needed to attain a constant viscosity.

There are other reasons than non-Newtonian behaviour which make the application of concepts of fluid viscosity to the living circulation difficult. For instance, blood flow is not streamlined in the microcirculation or even in large vessels under pathological conditions. (The relationship between

The text seems to imply that turbulence is more likely to occur in the microcirculation than in large vessels. Actually, it is extremely unlikely for turbulence to occur in the small vessels where the radii are small and the linear velocity is slow; it is in large vessels, especially in regions with complicated geometry (e.g., branching or curvature) where turbulence is more likely to occur.

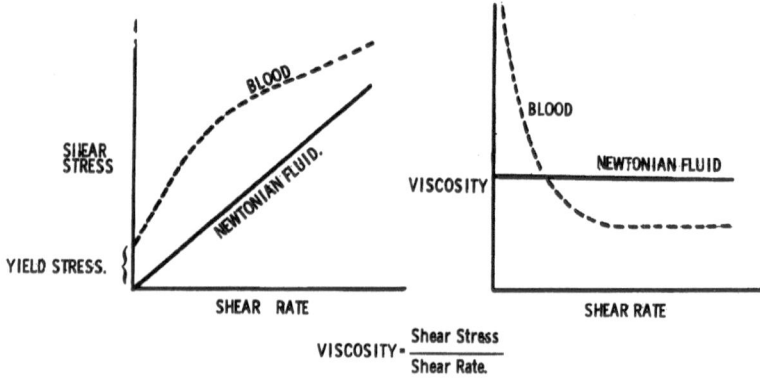

$$VISCOSITY = \frac{Shear\ Stress}{Shear\ Rate.}$$

Fig. 2. Relationship between shear stress, shear rate and viscosity in a Newtonian fluid and blood.

viscosity and turbulence is briefly discussed in Section 1.2.1.) Finally, measurements of blood flow in isolated animal circulations suggest that the non-Newtonian behaviour of blood is less marked 'in vivo' than 'in vitro' (Section 1.3.1.).

1.1.3. *Yield stress.* Another feature of the non-Newtonian behaviour of blood is that it possesses a yield stress. This is the minimum shear stress necessary to produce a minimum shear rate or flow. The yield stress has to be exceeded to begin flow in stationary blood and similarly flow will cease if the shear stress falls below the yield stress. This is also illustrated diagrammatically in Fig. 2. (It is the yield stress, as well as surface tension, which prevents some fluids from dripping if the yield stress exceeds the force of gravity.)

Thixotropy is sometimes mentioned in relation to blood viscosity. It is applied to the time dependence of viscosity; that is, a spontaneous alteration in viscosity as a consequence of the fluid being exposed to a shearing force. It has never been properly characterised for human blood largely because of methodological problems.

The concept of yield stress in blood is still debatable. The values reported in the literature are generally obtained by extrapolating the shear stress – shear rate relationship to zero shear rate. Because of the strong aggregation tendency of red cells as near zero shear rate is approached, it is extremely difficult to obtain reliable data needed to obtain such an extrapolated yield stress value. As a result, widely scattered 'yield stress' values have been reported in the literature for normal blood, depending on the method of measurement. In general, the 'yield stress' value obtained is extremely small; it amounts to approximately a pressure drop of 0.0001 mm Hg per mm vessel length in a 100 μm vessel. This is not sufficient to prevent fluid dripping by gravity. It appears that the rheological properties of the blood can be described without using the term 'yield stress'.

1.2. *Some physiological considerations*

1.2.1. *Physiological shear rates.* Since the viscosity of blood changes with the shear rate, it is necessary to consider what shear rates blood is exposed to in the living circulation since it is at these shear rates that ex-vivum measurements should be carried out. In larger vessels with streamlined flow, the shear rate will vary, at any one time, from zero in the axis to a high value (probably from 100 to 1000 sec^{-1}) near the vessel wall.

If the blood flow is pulsatile, there will be a superimposed fluctuation which in some arteries, for instance the femoral artery in normal subjects, may actually result in opposite flow near the wall and the axis of the vessel. There will then be an additional annulus of zero shear rate in the vessel.

The mathematical complexity of this problem can be simplified by calculating an average shear rate for different parts of the circulation, based on the dimensions of the vessels and the average velocity of flow in them (2–5). The results of some of these calculations are shown in Table 1.

Table 1. Calculation of mean shear rates in the circulation.

Source and reference	Arteries and arterioles	Capillaries	Venules and veins
Chien (2)	500–1000	2000	80–100
Whitmore (3)	100–500	500	50–150
Wells (4)	—	0–20	—
Replogle et al. (5)	Over 200	0–200	Over 200

Leaving the microcirculation aside, there is general agreement that the lowest shear rates are in the smaller veins and the highest in the large arteries. Under normal circumstances, distinctions between shear rates above approximately 100 sec^{-1} are irrelevant because the blood is Newtonian at this range and its viscosity is therefore independent of the shear rate.

This relatively simple concept of blood flow in larger vessels does assume that flow is streamlined. Blood flow however becomes turbulent if its Reynolds number exceeds approximately 700. This probably never occurs in the normal circulation, but almost certainly does exist in pathological arteries and will be favoured by low blood viscosities as Reynolds number is inversely related to the viscosity of the fluid. Turbulent flow is inefficient in terms of energy use and may be harmful.

Turbulence occurs near the root of the aorta in the normal circulation.

1.2.2. The microcirulation.

The relevance of bulk blood viscosity to flow in the microcirculation, where the dimensions of the vessels are comparable to that of individual red cells, is doubtful. Most calculations based on mean flow velocity and vessel size will produce very high figures for the average shear rate (Table 1).

Studies by Cokelet (1) indicate that blood viscosity in narrow tubes with size approaching that of individual red cells agrees with the bulk viscosity measurement made in the viscometer, if the proper tube haematocrit values are used. Studies on pressure-flow relations in individual microvessels in the cat mesentery (2) indicate that the in vivo apparent blood viscosity determined in single microvessels also agrees well with bulk viscosity data obtained in vitro at high shear rates.

On the other hand, we know that some capillaries are often completely collapsed and that in others blood flow is intermittent. In such a stop-start situation, one may well argue that the yield stress, that is, the force necessary to begin movement in blood, is the most significant. Determination of yield stress is discussed in Section 2.6.5.

Finally, one may well argue that measurements carried out on bulk blood (as occurs in all viscometers) do not reflect the situation in the microcirculation at whatever shear rate they are carried out. And this is where considerations of the flow properties of individual red cells is really relevant.

Some capillaries do not have blood flowing through them at times, but they usually do not collapse. The cessation of flow is usually due to the constriction of terminal arterioles or precapillary sphincters upstream.

1.2.3. Red cell deformability.

As soon as Leeuwenhoek looked down the first microscope and saw a living circulation, he observed that red cells are flexible. Every time this experience is repeated, one is astonished at the extreme deformations undergone by individual red cells as they negotiate the capillary passages. The visco-elastic properties of the red cells is probably of paramount importance in determining flow in the microcirculation. Red cell deformability is also thought to be important at the other end of the circulatory spectrum, in large arteries. Because of the high shear stresses in these vessels, red cells are exposed to great forces tending to deform them in such a way as to offer least resistance to forward flow. It has been shown that making the red cells rigid would considerably increase the viscosity of bulk blood at high shear rates. It is indeed the deformability of the red cells which probably contributes to the non-Newtonian behaviour of blood. Normal blood remains fluid at cell concentrations of over 90%, while rigid particles the shape of red cells would assume the consistency of a brick at a concentration of 60%.

1.3.   *Are measurements of blood viscosity relevant to flow in the circulation?*

Before describing the techniques for assessing blood viscosity in the laboratory, it is necessary to examine the evidence that such measurements do relate to a function of blood influencing its flow in the circulation. Apart from the purely in vitro experiments showing that viscosity is related to flow of blood in an artificial system, three types of evidence are available from observations on the living circulation.

1.3.1. *'In vivo' viscometry.*   A number of studies have been carried out using isolated animal circulations, for instance in the ear or the leg, where viscosity of blood could be related to the known viscosity of an artificial fluid or of plasma by measuring the flow rate at fixed perfusion pressures. These values for 'in vivo' viscosity could be related to simultaneous measurements of the viscosity of the same samples in viscometers. In most of these experiments a very accurate correlation was formed. In many cases, however, the increase in viscosity at low flow rates measured 'in vivo' was less than would be predicted from 'in vitro' measurements (6–9). In other words, the non-Newtonian behaviour of blood is less apparent in the living circulation than in viscometric measurements.

1.3.2. *Relating viscosity to actual in vivo blood flow.*   These experiments form the crux of the evidence justifying in vitro viscometry. In most of these studies changes in measured blood viscosity have been related to changes in blood flow, using noninvasive techniques of measurement. In dog experiments, changes in viscosity have been related to changes in total cardiac output (10). Changes in cardiac output were largely due to alterations in stroke volume rather than heart rate. The mean arterial blood pressure did not alter significantly and the responses were unaltered by blocking the baroreceptor reflex (11). In humans, changes in blood viscosity have been related to changes in particular circulations such as the leg (12) or the brain (13). Fig. 3 illustrates the close correlation between the percentage change in blood viscosity and resulting change in calf blood flow measured by plethysmography in a number of normal human legs (12).

Although the correlation between flow and viscosity is excellent in all these studies (with coefficients of correlation from 0.80 to 0.95) the size of the effect on flows depends on the shear rates at which the viscosities are

In measurements on blood viscosity in vivo, except for the study carried out directly on individual microvessels (see comments for Section 1.2.2.), one has to compare the pressure–flow relationships between the whole blood and the suspending medium (plasma or other equivalent fluid) and to obtain only a relative apparent viscosity. When the cell-free suspending fluid is used, due to its low viscosity and hence low Reynolds number, there may be a significant degree of inertial pressure dissipation (3). Therefore, the calculated relative apparent viscosity may be in error.

In the studies of Messmer (4), the haematocrit of the dog was altered by isovolemic exchange transfusion. The changes in viscosity *resulting from such haematocrit variations* have been found to correlate inversely with the cardiac output.

The correlation of changes in blood viscosity determined in vitro with blood flows measured in vivo is an important finding.

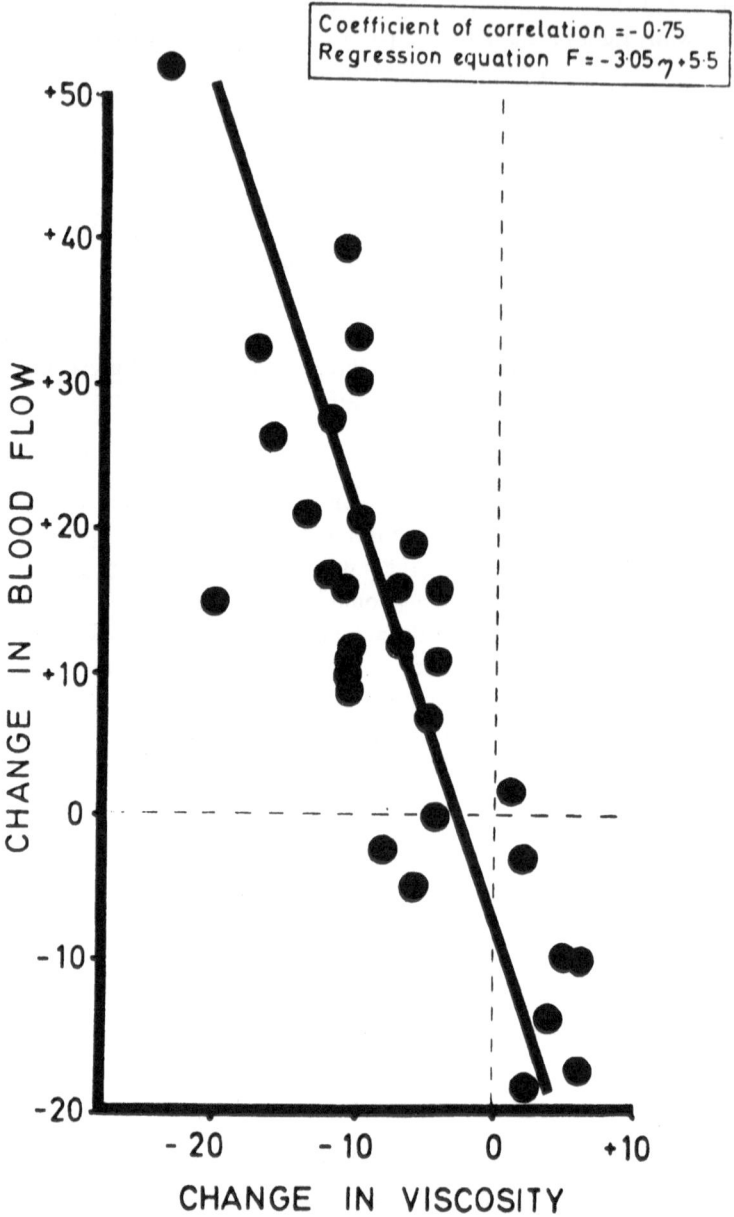

Fig. 3. Results of a series of observations in humans. The percentage change in viscosity during intravenous infusion is related to the percentage change in calf blood flow.

measured. For instance, in general a 20% change in flow results from a 10% change in viscosity measured at a high shear rate (230 sec^{-1}) while it requires only a 5% change in viscosity at lower shear rates. One may use this kind of evidence to argue the case for and against particular physiological shear rates.

1.3.3. *Clinical evidence.* Finally, there is now a mass of evidence, outlined in Section 4, that a high measured blood viscosity is accompanied by clinical states of circulatory insufficiency. Also, therapeutic measures shown to lower blood viscosity have been seen to improve patients with diseases of blood flow and have been supported by objective measurements of flow.

In summary, there is now little room for doubting the physiological validity of current techniques of viscometry. The results obtained are not an artefact of the techniques employed but relate closely to a genuine flow property of the blood in the living circulation.

> The material presented by the author does not seem to justify such a strong conclusion. The comments given above by this reviewer may help to strengthen somewhat these concluding remarks.

2. VISCOMETERS

2.1. *Capillary viscometers*

Most of the viscometers until the early 1960s were of the capillary tube type. They were all based on the principle of measuring the rate of flow through a narrow glass tube of specified dimensions. The contemporary example of this type of viscometer available commercially is the Harkness viscometer (14).* The sample is isolated by two columns of mercury and pushed through a tube measuring 20 cm in length and 0.38 cm in diameter at a constant pressure of mercury. In the latest model there is an automatic timing device which allows the viscosity to be read off directly.

These viscometers are the cheapest, most robust, easiest and probably the quickest to use. They all have the basic disadvantage that because the sample travels along a tube at changing pressure heads it is exposed to a whole range of shear rates and it is therefore impossible to define a single shear rate at which measurements are made. Since whole blood is non-Newtonian, with changing viscosities at different shear rates, capillary viscometers are unsuitable for absolute measurements on whole blood viscosity. (In practice, the range of shear rates tend to be very high, that is mostly in the Newtonian range of normal blood.) On the other hand capillary viscometers are ideally suitable for the measurement of plasma viscosity, which behaves as a Newtonian fluid.

---

* Available in England from Coulter Electronics Ltd, Cold Harbour Lane, Harpenden, Herts, AL5 4 UN.

2.2.   Wells-Brookfield viscometer

2.2.1. Principle of rotational viscometers.

The exact assessment of whole blood viscosity depends on being able to carry out measurements at a range of single specified shear rates. This became possible with the development of rotational viscometers, the first to become widely available being the Wells-Brookfield.*

In all rotational viscometers the sample is sheared between two surfaces, of varying complexity, moving in relation to each other. Usually one surface is static and the other can be rotated at varying speeds equivalent to different single shear rates. With the correct geometry, the whole sample can be exposed to this single shear rate. The stress exerted on one or the other surface by the sheared blood is then recorded.

A more elaborate and more accurate rotational viscometer also widely used is that made by Contraves and will also be considered in detail. Finally a number of other rotational viscometers, less often used and frequently purpose made will be discussed briefly. Table 2 compares some of the features of the commercially available viscometers mentioned in the text. Many practical details of viscometry, such as sampling and anticoagulation, are common to all viscometers and will be considered together in a final section (2.6).

2.2.2. Construction of the Wells-Brookfield viscometer.

This machine was first described in 1961 (15) and is of a cone-on-plate or cone-in-cup construction. Fig. 4 is a photograph of the machine and Fig. 5 is a diagram illustrating the principle on which it works. A 1 ml blood sample is placed in a detachable sample cup which is surrounded by a water jacket to control the temperature. When replaced in the viscometer a shallow cone comes into contact with the surface of the sample. The cone is rotated on the surface of the sample by a variable speed motor to which it is connected by a beryllium copper spring suspension. The torque in this spring gives a

* Available in England from Baird and Tatlock (London) Ltd, Freshwater Road, Chardwell Heath, Essex.

Table 2. Comparison of commercially available viscometers.

	Harkness	Wells-Brookfield	Contraves	Weissenberg	Deer	Haake
Range of shear rate	Very high	High	Full range	Full range	Full range	Full range
Reliability	Very good	Average	Average	?	?	?
Ease of operation	Very easy	Very easy	Average	Difficult	Easy	Easy
Sample volume (ml)	0.5	1.0	1.0	10.0	1.0	0.5
Oscillatory function	No	No	No	Yes	No	No
Approx. cost in pounds	850	800	6000–8000	10,000–15,000	5000–6000	9000–10,000

measure of the drag applied to the cone by the blood and is recorded on a rotating scale at the top of the viscometer. Different speeds of rotation will expose the sample to different shear rates and the shear stress can be calculated directly from the torque on the spring suspension, provided its physical properties are known. Alternatively, the machine can be calibrated using fluids of known viscosity.

The cone-on-plate construction ensures that the whole sample is exposed to the same shear rate. The velocity difference between the two surfaces will increase towards the periphery, but so will the distance between them, thereby ensuring that the velocity gradient remains constant.

2.2.3. Operation of Wells-Brookfield viscometer. The clearance between the sample cup and the rotating cone has to be carefully adjusted before measurements can be made. This can be achieved by means of a collar on a screw thread which adjusts this clearance (Fig. 4b). The aim is to have the apex of the cone just clear of the sample cup. Removing the sample cup, a 1 ml sample of blood is pipetted into it and the cup replaced. A choice of 8 speeds can be selected by a gear, ranging from 60 to 0.3 re./min, equivalent to shear rates of 230–1.15 sec^{-1}. As soon as the cone is rotated, its spring suspension will twist as a result of the drag applied to the cone by the

The tip of the cone is slightly truncated. The adjustment is made such that the imaginary apex of the cone would just 'touch' the surface of the sample cup.

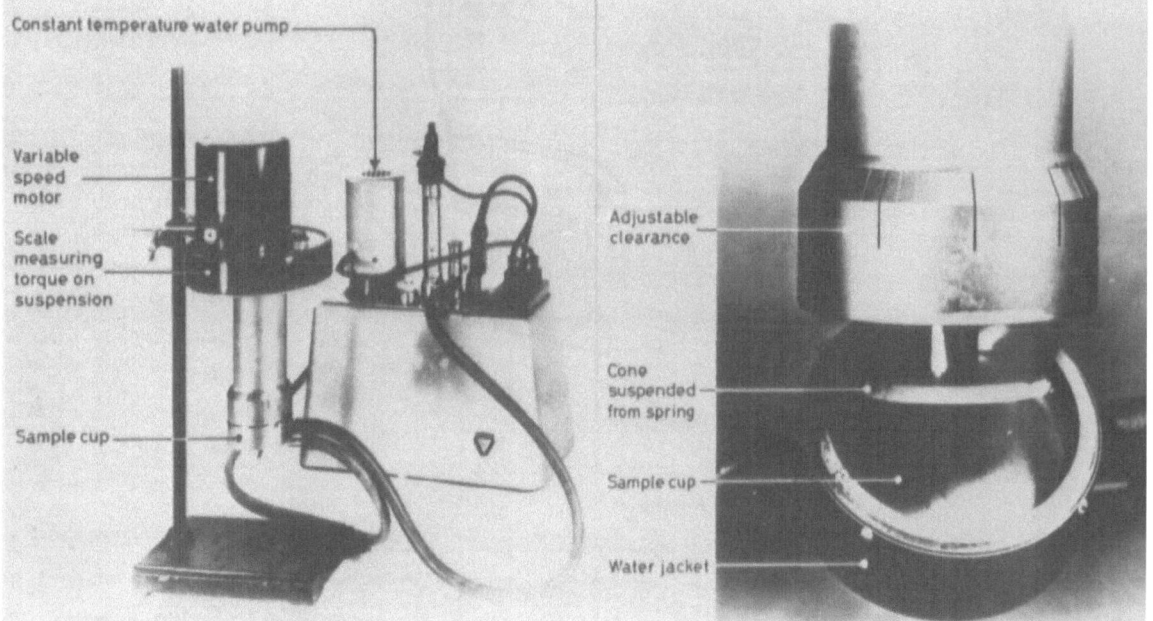

Fig. 4. Photograph of the complete Wells-Brookfield microviscometer and of the sample cup removed for insertion of a sample

blood. The torque can be read off from a pointer on a rotating scale and usually gives a stable reading within 2–3 min. For measurements at a new shear rate, it is probably best to change the sample after carefully cleaning the sample cup and the cone.

The formation of protein film at the air–blood or air–plasma interface will cause a falsely high viscosity reading, particularly at low shear rates (see Section 2.3.2). This artifact can be reduced by floating a drop of oil (e.g., mineral oil) on the surface of blood or plasma sample.

2.2.4. *Performance of the Wells-Brookfield viscometer.* The principal limiting factor to the accuracy of all viscometers is the sensitivity of the stress measuring system. In the case of the Wells-Brookfield viscometer, the shear stress is measured by the twisting of the cone's spring suspension. This also acts as the link driving the rotating cone and therefore has to be reasonably robust. The result is that measurements are most accurate at maximum torques, that is, at high shear rates. The coefficient of variation of individual readings on different aliquots of the same sample varies from 2% at high shear rates ($230 \sec^{-1}$) to over 15% at the lower shear rates. The minimum shear rate at which reliable readings can be obtained is probably $23 \sec^{-1}$, where the coefficient of variation is around 8%.

The instrument is stable and day to day variations in the calibration factor usually stay under 2% over several months. Breakdowns are infrequent, the commonest accident being a broken spring suspension, which can be quite easily replaced by the user.

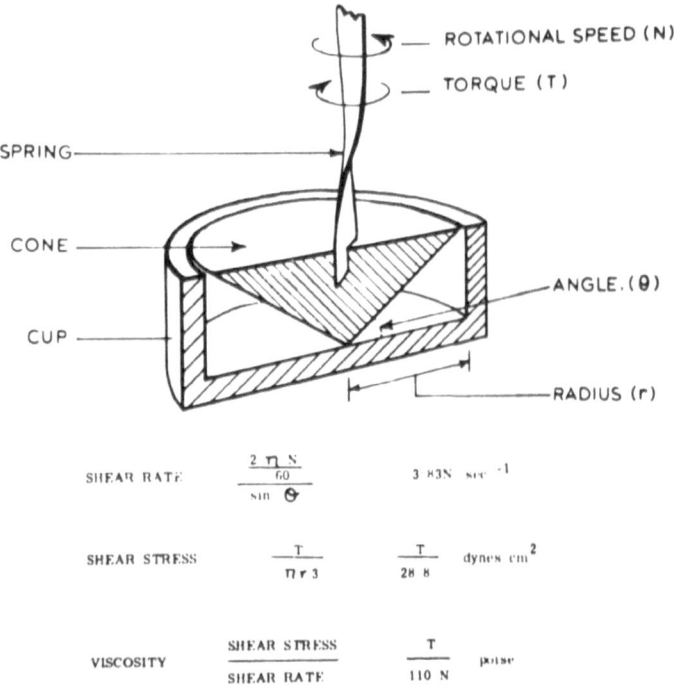

Fig. 5. Diagram showing the principle of the Wells-Brookfield instrument.

2.3.   *Contraves viscometer**

2.3.1. Construction of the Contraves viscometer.   This is a more sensitive instrument than the Wells-Brookfield because one component of the sample chamber is used to apply the shear rate, while the stress is measured by the other component. (Compared with the Wells-Brookfield where the cone suspended on the spring is used to apply the shear and to measure the stress, the cup being totally passive.) Fig. 6 is a photograph of the viscometer and Fig. 7 illustrates its mechanism of operation (16, 17). The sample is introduced into a stainless steel cup, surrounded by a water jacket which controls the temperature. A small cylindrical stainless steel bob, held by a suspension wire, is lowered into the sample cup. The bob and cup are designed so that the distance between them containing the sample is small compared with the cross-sectional radii of the bob and cup. Under these circumstances, the shear rate is nearly constant within the sample between the cup and the bob. The cup is rotated at a known speed by a motor, while the bob remains stationary. The output of the motor unit can be adjusted so that rotational speeds corresponding to shear rates of 90 sec^{-1} down to approximately 0.01 sec^{-1} can be obtained. The torque applied to the bob through the sample fluid produces a turning effect on the bob, which is prevented from twisting by an equal and opposing torque, applied by an electromagnet. An automatic feedback mechanism from a mirror attached to the suspension wire regulates the strength of the electromagnetic field. The shear stress in the test fluid is directly related to the measured torque 'M' as follows:

$$\text{(Shear stress)}\ T = ML/2R^2\ \text{(dynes/cm}^2\text{)}$$

where L = effective height of bob, and R = radius of inner cylinder.

A time dependent record of the electrical output, that is, the current necessary to prevent the bob from turning, has to be recorded at low shear rates as the output is time dependent. The viscometer itself has a galvanometer registering the current which can be used without a recorder for measurements at high shear rates and for non-Newtonian calibration fluids. The meter has three sensitivity ranges and is arbitrarily divided into divisions from 0 to 100% deflection. Tables are supplied giving shear stress values for known percentage deflection at each sensitivity range. Therefore, by knowing the shear rate it is possible to construct viscosity/percentage deflection curves for each sensitivity range. In practice, the accuracy of this calculation would be checked by using a calibration fluid.

* Available in England from Contraves Industrial Products Ltd, Times House, Station Approach, Ruislip, Middlesex HA4 8LH.

2.3.2. *Operation of the Contraves viscometer.* The bob has to be centred carefully in the middle of the cup. It is then lifted out of the cup into which a 0.7 ml sample of blood is introduced with a pipette. After lowering the bob into the sample, the meniscus of the blood around the bob and cup is evened to help centralise the bob. For measurements at low shear rates a guard ring has to be used to break the surface of the sample and prevent the

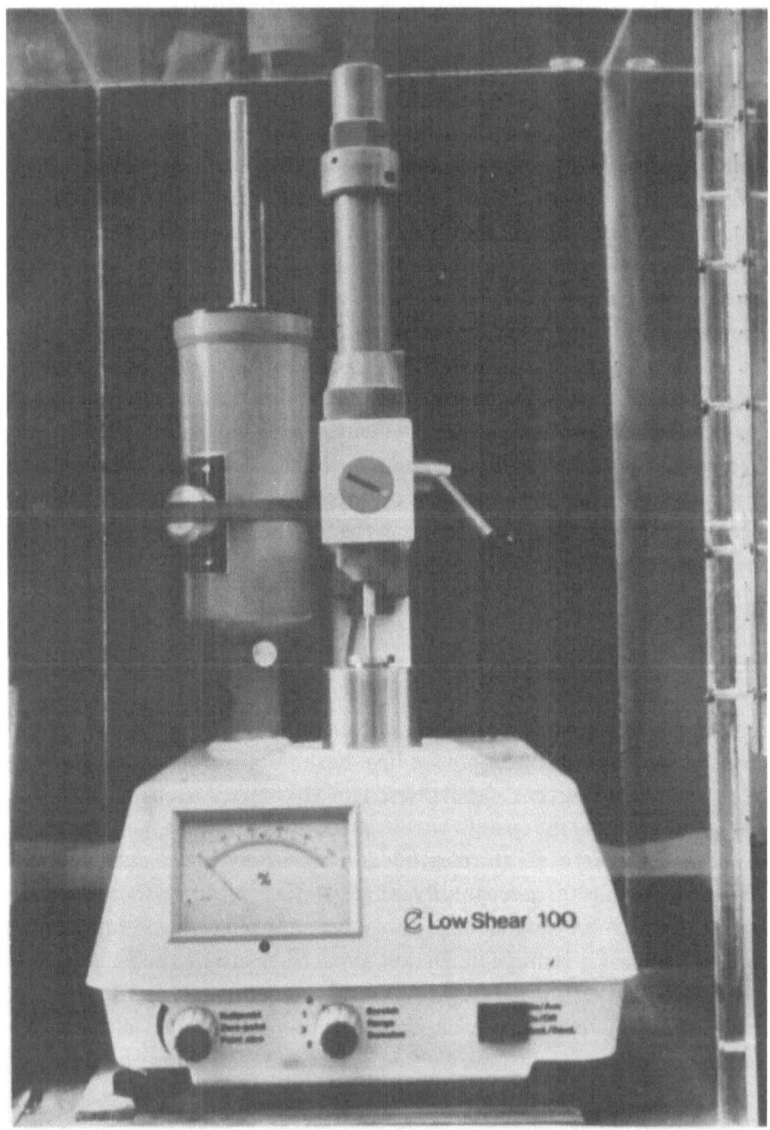

Fig. 6. Photograph of the Contraves microviscometer.

organised protein layer at the air–blood interface from applying an extra torque to the bob. The time the bob is lowered into the sample has to be marked on the recorder. The motor is switched on and a record obtained for approximately the first 3 min. At low shear rates a tracing is obtained with an initial overshoot, followed by a decline in torque and a later increase. These later changes are probably due to plasma skimming and then sedimentation of the red cells as illustrated in Fig. 8. To calculate the torque at zero time, the initial linear decline is extrapolated back as shown in practice in Fig. 9. There are considerable problems in interpreting tracings obtained at very low shear rates (17–19).

A comparison of Fig. 8 and Fig. 9 (the tracings for shear rate = 2.62 sec^{-1}) indicates that the extrapolation technique is not consistent. A major problem in extrapolation is that the decay is usually not a simple linear or exponential function of time.

2.3.3. Performance of the Contraves viscometer.

With the earlier models, problems were experienced by most users of this machine; usually due to imperfect electronic circuits. These have taken variable lengths of time to sort out. Thereafter the viscometer is remarkably stable, with less than 0.5% variations in its performance during the course of a day, and less than 5% over a year. (These variations are recognised and corrected by a calibration procedure.)

It is not clear from the wording whether the problems have already been solved by the manufacturer or still need to be sorted out by the users.

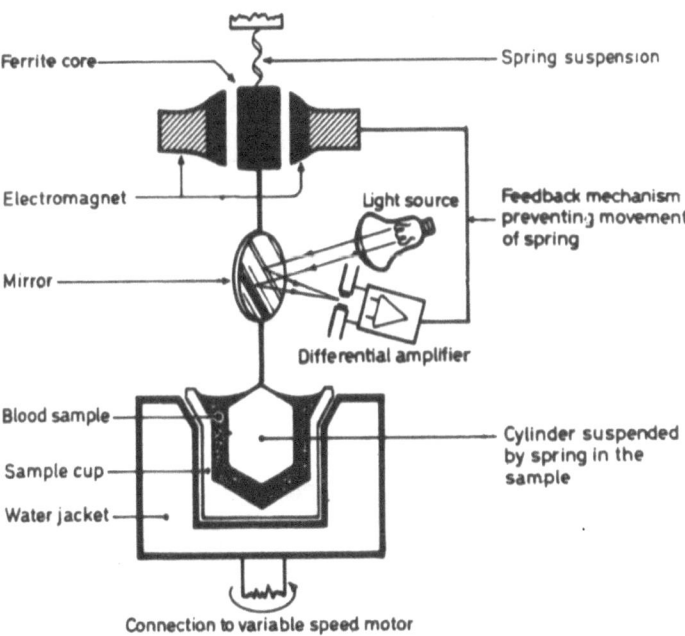

2.4.   *Other viscometers*

2.4.1.   *Weissenberg rheogoniometer.** This is the most sophisticated apparatus available and has long been used for measuring the viscosity of materials other than blood, such as various pastes, suspensions, emulsions and creams. Various platens can be fitted and either cone-on-plate or concentric cylindrical configurations are available for use with blood. It is very versatile, for instance it can apply an oscillatory or sinusoidal movement to the sample. It can thus be adpated to assess the visco-elastic properties of red cells (20) as well as measuring whole blood viscosity. The shear rate is applied by movement of the lower platen and the shear stress is transmitted through the sample to the upper platen where it is very accurately detected by a sophisticated measuring device based on a torsion bar.

The Weissenberg rheogoniometer is the most accurate of the commercially available viscometers, but it is correspondingly delicate and requires more technical skill to use reliably. It has the added disadvantage of requiring larger sample volumes than most other viscometers. Most machines are used in industrial research; only a very few in medical research and none for anything approaching routine medical investigation. It is undoubtedly a tool for the totally committed reseacher who has considerable technical resources.

* Available in England from Sangamo Weston Controls Ltd, North Bersted, Bognor Regis, Sussex, PO22 9BS.

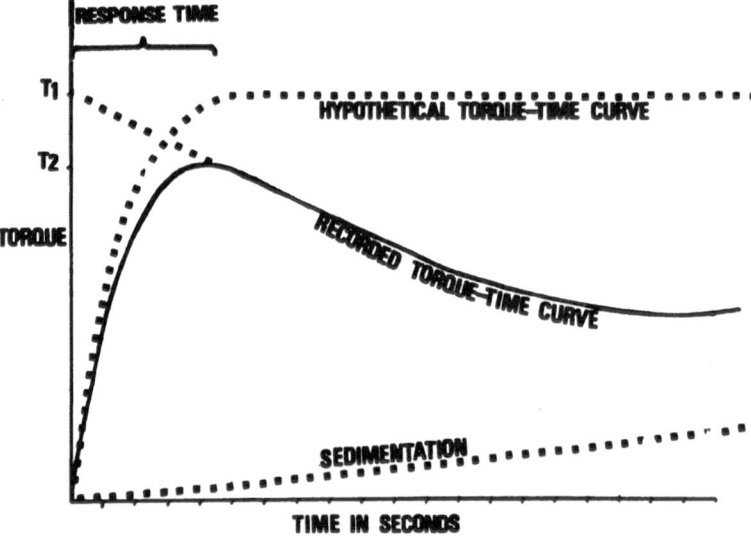

Fig. 8. Theoretical interpretation of time dependent tracing obtained at low shear rates. T_2 is the actual peak deflection, while T_1 is the torque derived by extrapolating back to zero time the initial linear decay in the tracing obtained. It is this value, T_2, which is used to calculate the viscosity.

2.4.2. *Deer rheometer.** The Deer rheometer is a recent viscometer on the market and is fundamentally different from those previously described. It neither rotates one component of the sample container while measuring the torque in the other, as in the Contraves of the Weissenberg machines, nor does it measure the torque in the transmission of the rotating element as in the Wells-Brookfield. Instead it applies a constant torque to a cylinder suspended in the sample and measures the resultant rate of rotation of the cylinder. While all the other rotational viscometers measure the shear stress at a fixed predetermined shear rate, the Deer viscometer measures the shear rate produced by a fixed shear stress. This effect is achieved by a special electric motor which can be driven at a predetermined stress.

With the use of the Deer rheometer, Kiessewetter et al. (5) were not able to detect a yield stress for normal blood.

This system has the theoretical advantage of being more relevent to the circulation, where one is usually interested in the flow that will result when a certain force is applied to the blood, rather than the force necessary to

* Available in England from Deer Rheometers, 2 Chessington Close, West Ewell, Surrey.

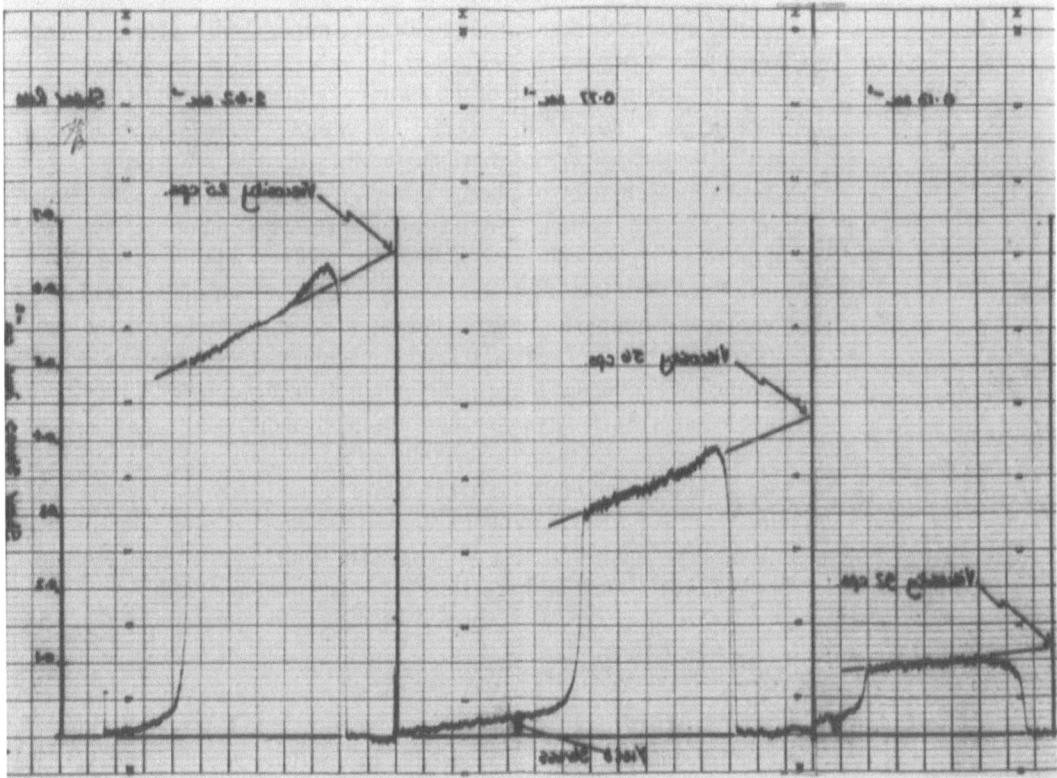

Fig. 9. Actual tracings obtained with the Contraves viscometer at three low shear rates on three separate samples of the same blood. The shear stress is recorded at the shear rates of 0.13, 0.77 and 2.62 sec⁻¹.

produce a certain flow. In practical terms, it means that yield stress and visco-elastic properties of blood can be measured more directly. Because it is relatively new, there have so far been very few published results using this viscometer[21].

2.4.3. *Haake Biovisco.*

2.4.3. *Haake Biovisco.** Although the company have had considerable experience with industrial viscometers, this is their first model specially designed for blood. It is basically of the same design as the Contraves, with some theoretical advantages, but at the moment there is no published work with this machine. It could prove to be the ideal machine for sensitive routine measurements.

2.5. Comparison of viscometers

There have been few published comparisons of the results obtained with different types of viscometers (22, 23) but the results using plasma are usually similar while it seems that the whole blood viscosity is often 10–20% higher in a concentric cylindrical compared with a cone-on-plate rotational viscometer (22).

Table 2 compares some of the features of the commercially available viscometers mentioned in the text. The choice is really determined primarily by the purposes for which the measurements are needed. For routine measurement of plasma viscosity, the Harkness capillary tube viscometer is the best buy. For measurement of whole blood viscosity, one of the rotational machines is required. The Wells-Brookfield is about one-tenth the cost of the others, but is only reliable at high shear rates and is therefore unsuitable for research purposes. The other four are in the same price bracket. The Deer and Haake machines are relatively new and insufficient experience makes a definite judgment impossible; they both have features which may make them ultimately more useful than the either of the other two. Of these two established viscometers, the Weissenberg is more suited for fundamental research into the basic physical properties of blood, but is far less suitable for clinical use either in a research or in a routine investigation context. For clinical use the Contraves is undoubtedly the most practical of the established widely used machines.

2.6. General techniques in viscometry

2.6.1. *Sampling and anticoagulants.* Venous blood is used routinely, avoiding stasis. (If it is only possible to insert the needle if the vein is artificially distended, then the occlusion should be released for 1 min

* Available in England from MSE Scientific Instruments, Menor Royal, Crawley, Sussex, RH10 2QQ.

before a sample is withdrawn.) It is important to avoid excessive trauma to
the blood during withdrawal and therefore a wide bore needle (such as a
21-gauge needle) and minimum suction on the syringe should be used. The
specimen is then placed in an anticoagulant container and gently mixed. If
allowance is made for slight differences in haematocrit, none of the commonly used anticoagulants other tham citrate or oxalate have a significant
effect on the blood viscosity (23–25). (Citrate and oxalate may cause
shrinkage of the red cell.) This has been confirmed by measurements
carried out immediately without anticoagulation (26). The commonly
used anticoagulants in the viscosity literature are solid lithium heparin and
ethylene-diamino tetra acetic acid (E.D.T.A.).

The packed cell volume must be measured on the same sample of blood
as is used for measuring viscosity. A duplicate microhaematocrit technique
is perfectly adequate.

2.6.2. *Storage and delay before measurement.*

One of the biggest logistic
problems in viscometry is the very marked effect of storage on the physical
properties of whole blood. This is probably at least in part due to the well
documented metabolic changes which take place in blood outside the
circulation. The results of measurements of whole blood viscosity begin to
change in an unpredictable fashion within a few hours of withdrawal of the
blood (27). If the sample has been kept at room temperature all measurements should be carried out within 4–8 h (28, 29). At 4 °C the sample may
maintain its essential physical characteristics for approximately 12 h (30).
These changes will be greater if measurements are made at low rather than
high shear rates.

2.6.3. *Temperature of viscometer.*

Measurements of viscosity are usually
carried out at 37 °C and all viscometers are equipped with systems for
thermostatically maintaining the sample at a particular temperature.
Where readings have to be taken rapidly after delivery of the sample into
the machine, as in the Contraves viscometer, equilibration of the sample to
37 °C may be a problem. In this case, the blood, pipettes and the sample
holder, if this is removable, should be preheated to 37 °C in an incubator.

The viscosity of normal plasma increses 2–3% for every degree fall in
temperature from 37 to 15 °C (31). The parallel increase in whole blood
viscosity is of the same order so that in normal subjects the relative
viscosity of blood is unaltered between 15 and 37 °C (32–34). It may be
clinically relevant to carry out measurements of blood viscosity at temperatures below 37 °C, for instance in investigating patients with Raynaud's phenomenon (Fig. 10) or the effect of hypothermic surgery (Section
4.4.6.). In some patients grossly abnormal patterns of viscosity have been
described at temperatures below 37 °C (34).

2.6.4. *Calibration of viscometer.* All viscometers should be recalibrated every day, preferably at the beginning and end of each series of measurements to ensure that there has been no drift. Although theoretically the resuls of measurements can be calculated in absolute units in some viscometers, such as the Wells-Brookfield, without calibration, in practice it is wiser to calculate all readings on the basis of a daily calibration control.

There are a number of calibration fluids available, usually available through the manufacturers of the viscometers. These are usually oils and all have the inevitable drawback of being Newtonian liquids. This is unavoidable if the manufacturers are to quote a single constant and stable viscosity value for a particular fluid. Accurately standardised non-Newtonian fluid with blood-like behaviour does not exist. Calibration should be carried out at the same shear rates as will be used for the measurements of blood; on the other hand, the absolute values obtained can only be in the haematological range at a few of the shear rates. This problem, which is probably of theoretical importance only, can be partly overcome by using several calibration fluids of different viscosities for calibration at different shear rates.

As commented before, the usefulness of 'yield stress' is questionable. The difficulty in using the residual torque to measure the yield stress is apparent when one examines the middle panel of Fig. 9 (shear rate $= 0.77 \, \text{sec}^{-1}$). Although a vertical marking of 'yield stress' is made on the tracing, it seems arbitrary, and the tracing actually returns to the baseline without a demonstrable yield stress. Casson plots of the square root of the shear stress versus the square root of the shear rate often do not lead to the linear relationship shown in Fig. 11, especially when viscometric data on shear rates lower than 10 sec^{-1} are included.

2.6.5. *Determination of yield stress.* The yield stress of normal blood is very low and direct measurementts in viscometers are of doubtful validity

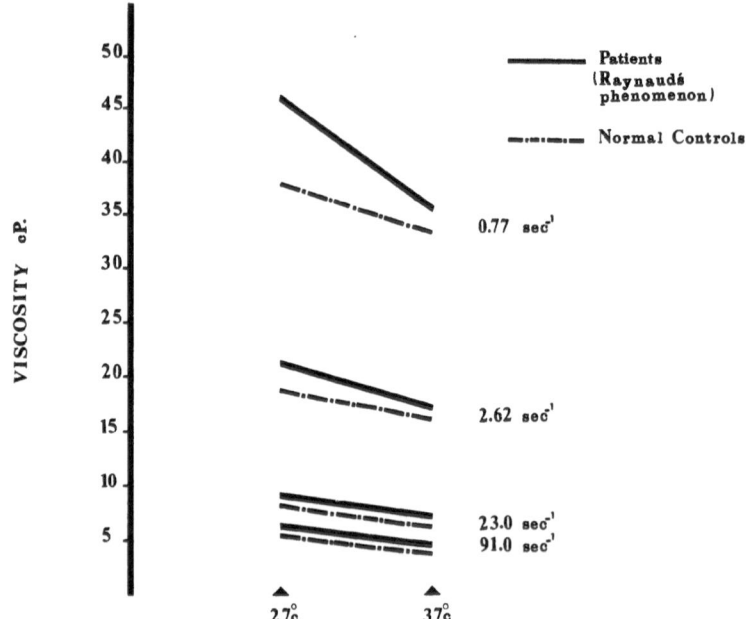

Fig. 10. The whole blood viscosity at four shear rates measured at 37 °C and 25 °C in a group of normal subjects and patients with Raynaud's phenomenon.

because of the many inevitable artefacts at low shear rates. The variable shear stress Deer viscometer should be able to measure yield stress directly. In theory, the residual torque, after stopping movement of the sample, should in a conventional rotational viscometer also be a direct measure of the yield stress (35). Finally, other special apparatus has been devised for its direct measurement (36). In practice the simplist and probably the most accurate determination of yield stress is by extrapolations from viscosity measurements at high shear rates assuming a linear relation between the square root of the shear stress and the square root of the shear rate as originally suggested by Casson (37–39). Fig. 11 illustrates this principle. The intercept of the linear regression line on the zero shear rate axis gives the square root of the yield stress.

3. INTERPRETATION OF RESULTS

3.1. Haematocrit correction

3.1.1. Importance. The haematocrit, or packed cell volume, is by far the most critical determinant of whole blood viscosity in vitro. Some method for attempting to eliminate this effect has been used by most workers for three reasons. Firstly, because the haematocrit in different parts of the circulation can vary at any one time as well as from hour to hour depending on the subject's activity. To eliminate unnecessary random fluctuations in the measured viscosity some form of haematocrit correction has to be applied. Secondly, the effect of the haematocrit on the measured viscosity can be so overwhelming, that the influence of other determinants cannot be analysed until the haematocrit effect has been removed. Lastly, and possibly most importantly, there is mounting evidence that although haematocrit is an important determinant of viscosity in larger vessels and as measured in viscometers, the in vivo viscosity of blood in the majority of the circulation is independent of haematocrit (18, 40, 41). In order to compare the effective viscosity in the microcirculation of two examples of blood, it is therefore necessary to eliminate differences due to haematocrit, which only exist in bulk blood.

The statement that the in vivo viscosity of blood in the majority of the circulation is independent of haematocrit is debatable.

Whatever system of correction is used, the haematocrit is adjusted to either an arbitrary value (usually 45%) or to the mean haematocrit of the group observed.

3.1.2. Character of the haematocrit–viscosity relationship. It seems proper to discuss the nature of the effect of haematocrit on whole blood viscosity before considering the techniques used for applying a haematocrit correction to the measured blood viscosity.

The most unifying concept of blood viscosity and its dependence on shear rate and haematocrit is the concept of the effective cell volume put forward by Chien (42). This suggests that a low shear rates the effective cell volume and therefore the viscosity is increased because red cell aggregates 'immobilise' a larger volume of surrounding plasma than individual red cells. For similar reasons the effect of haematocrit will be greater at low than high shear rates. (The effect of red cell deformability on blood viscosity can also partly be explained on this basis, as the effective cell volume of a deformable red cell will be less than that of a rigid particle of the same true volume.)

'For similar reasons the effect of cell aggregation on effective cell volume will be greater at low than high shear rates'.

A number of different mathematical relations between haematocrit and viscosity have been postulated, ranging from a double arithmetic linear to a double logarithmic linear relationship. It now seems likely that the simplest relationship true within the physiological range is most closely described by the following formula:

$$log\ \eta = log\ \eta o + kC$$

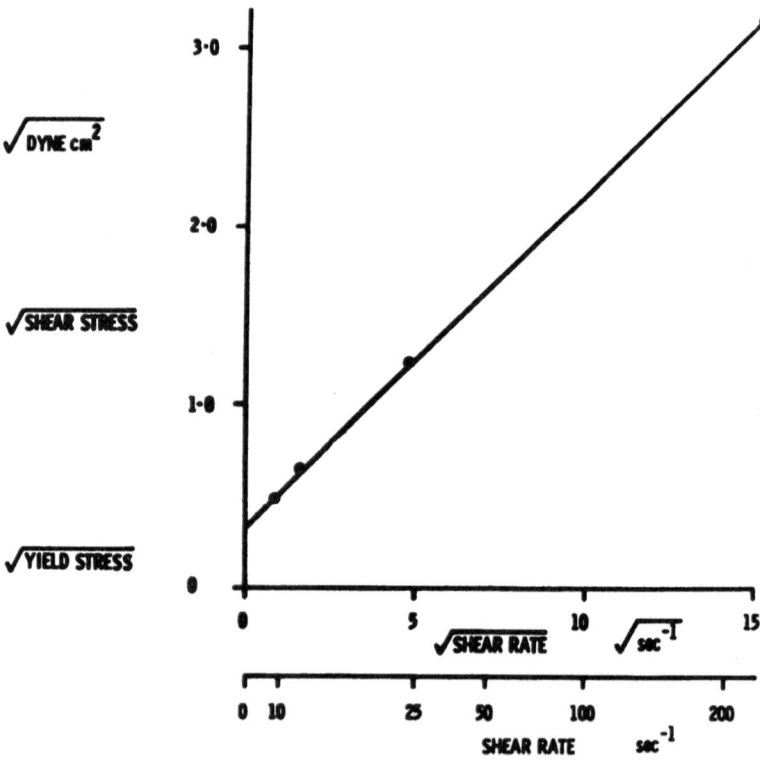

Fig. 11. Diagram to show how the yield stress can be derived from viscosity measurements at two or more shear rates using the linear Casson relationship between the square root of the shear stress and square root of the shear rate.

where C is the packed cell volume expressed as a percentage, η is the viscosity of that packed cell volume, $log\ \eta\ o$ is the intercept when $C = 0$ and the slope of the line is k. The value of k increases as the shear rate gets less, in other words the effect of haematocrit becomes more critical at lower shear rates. This relationship is approximately true within the physiological range of haematocrit and it has been verified experimentally by several workers, with coefficients of correlation between 0.85 and 0.98 (43–46). Fig. 12 gives some idea of the magnitude of the haemotocrit effect on viscosity. Using a semilogarithmic plot the best fitting linear regression has been calculated for a group of normal control bloods. It can be seen that when measurements are carried out on bulk blood in vitro, the effect of haematocrit is greater when measurements of viscosity are made at lower shear rates. This effect may be less marked in the living microcirculation. There are two principal techniques used for applying a haematocrit correction.

3.1.3. *Correction by reconstruction of the sample.*   The most obvious way to determine what the viscosity of a sample would have been at a standard haematocrit, is to artificially reconstitute the sample at that haematocrit. This involves centrifuging the sample and then removing some of the plasma or red cells to reproduce the chosen standard haematocrit (47).

There are two drawbacks to this technique. Firstly, it requires double the volume of blood so as to allow measurements at both the original (or native) haematocrit and at the reconstituted standard haematocrit. Secondly, inaccuracies may be introduced by the process of reconstitution, partly due to the inevitable error in achieving exactly the correct new haematocrit and partly because the concentration of both formed elements, such as platelets and white cells, as well as the plasma constituents may be slightly altered during reconstitution.

3.1.4. *Mathematical correction.*   Having defined or accepted a particular haematocrit–viscosity relationship, this may be used to convert mathematically the viscosity at the measured haematocrit to what it would be at the chosen standard haematocrit. This is clearly an indirect method and depends on the accuracy of the haematocrit–viscosity relationship employed for the calculation. On the other hand, it does not have either of the disadvantages of the first method described.

The simplest way to apply a mathematically derived coorection is to accept a log-linear relationship between viscosity and haematocrit in the physiological range and use a simple calculator to derive a regression line. The slope of this line can then be used to 'slide' the measured viscosity value up or down the scale to read off the corrected viscosity value at a chosen standard haematocrit. This technique is illustrated in Fig. 11.

3.2. *Normal values*

3.2.1. *Normal plasma viscosity.*   Plasma is a Newtonian liquid and therefore has the same viscosity at all shear rates. The normal range at 25 °C is from 1.50 to 1.72 cP and is uninfluenced by age or sex (48). It remains very constant, within this range, for any given individual.

The fact that plasma is more viscous than water is almost totally due to its protein content. Even the massive changes in the non-protein contents of plasma found in conditions like uraemia and diabetes do not have a significant effect on plasma alone (31). (This no longer applies if red cells are added.) There is general agreement among the many studies of the relative influence of different proteins; fibrinogen is by far the most important, followed by globulin and then albumin (31, 49, 50).

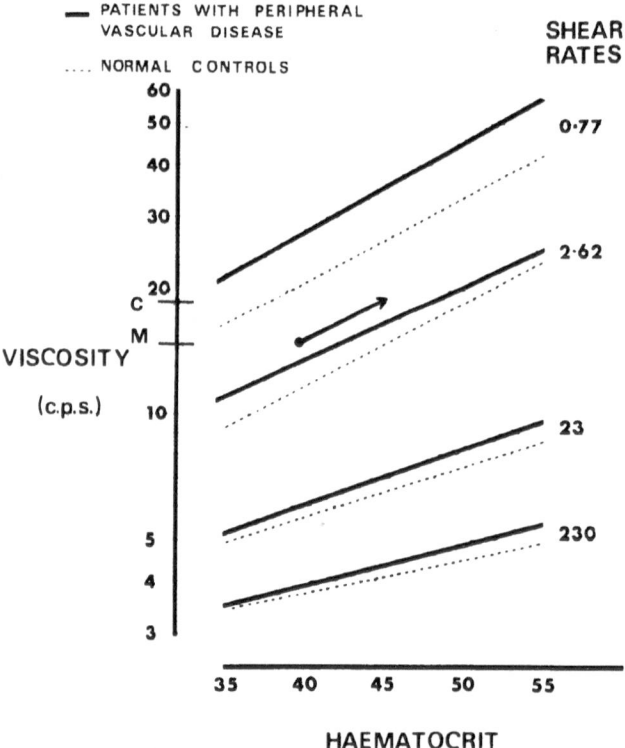

Fig. 12. Linear regression lines between the logarithm of the viscosity and haematocrit in a group of patients with ischaemia of the leg and a matched group of controls. Viscosity was measured at four shear rates. M indicates the measured viscosity at 2.62 sec^{-1} of a sample of blood with a haematocrit of 39%. This is converted to a 'corrected' viscosity, C, at a haematocrit of 45% by moving the result along a line parallel to the appropriate regression line derived from the whole group.

3.2.2. *Normal whole blood viscosity.*   The normal range of whole blood viscosity will vary slightly according to the details of measurement such as the viscometer employed, the range of haematocrit of the samples and of course the shear rate at which measurements are carried out. If the measurements are corrected to a standard haematocrit of 45%, then the range (average $\pm$ 2 standard deviations) of a normal population will be of the order of 3.70–4.85 (at 230 sec^{-1}), 5.3–7.8 (at 23 sec^{-1}), 12.0–19.0 (at 2.62 sec^{-1}) and 24–40 (at 0.77 sec^{-1}) expressed in centipoises. From the practical clinical standpoint, it is undoubtedly best to determine the normal range at frequent intervals and compare patient's values of the current normal values. If a correction is applied for differences in the plasma fibrinogen content, the ranges will be decreased, particularly at the lower shear rates.

At a haematocrit of 40%, the normal yield stress is in the range of 0.01–0.06 dynes/cm^2, depending mostly on the fibrinogen (39).

3.2.3. *Effect of age and sex on blood viscosity.*   Neither age, after the first few weeks of life, nor sex have an effect on blood viscosity if differences in plasma fibrinogen and haematocrit are eliminated (51). (There may be a slight haematocrit independent variation with menstruation (52).) The differences between the sexes is probably wholly due to a difference in haematocrit, while the slight increase in blood viscosity with age is probably due to the increasing plasma fibrinogen with ageing. This may be the result of the inevitable inclusion of older subjects with occult chronic disease, most of these conditions being associated with a raised fibrinogen.

3.2.4. *Daily and seasonal fluctuations in blood viscosity.*   Eating does not seem to influence blood viscosity (28, 53). Exercise and posture probably only have an effect by virtue of changes in plasma volume and the haematocrit. Diurnal changes in blood viscosity have been described, but are again due to changes in haematocrit (54); similarly with seasonal changes, where variation in fibrinogen may also play a part (55).

3.3.   *Determinants of blood viscosity*

3.3.1. *Causes of the non-Newtonian behaviour of blood.*   It is now generally believed that the increase in the viscosity of whole blood with decreasing shear rate is principally due to the aggregation of red cells at low shear rates and the deformation of red cells at high shear rates. Fig. 13 taken from Chien's work[2] illustrates diagrammatically the experimental evidence for this. The aggregation of red cells is promoted principally by the fibrinogen in plasma tending to bind the cells together and this is opposed by the shearing effect of flow tending to separate the cells. Red cells will therefore aggregate increasingly as the shear rate decreases, thus raising the viscosity of the blood.

The concept of effective cell volume, already mentioned, postulates that red cell aggregates trap more plasma than the red cells individually and therefore have a higher effective cell volume and thus a higher viscosity.

At the other end of the scale, at high shear rates, red cells flow individually and are distorted by the higher mechanical forces. This results, not only in the alignment of the long axis of the cell in the direction of flow, but also the deformation of the cells so that they offer less resistance to flow and therefore a lower blood viscosity.

The curve composed of round dots in Fig. 13 is obtained for suspensions of normal cells in an albumin solution (i.e., fibrinogen- and *globulin*-free plasma).

Fig. 13 shows that removal of the fibrinogen from the blood largely abolishes the increased viscosity at low shear rates, while making the red cells artificially rigid increases the viscosity at high shear rates. After the haematocrit, which has already been considered, probably the two most important determinants of blood viscosity are plasma fibrinogen and red cell deformability. (The latter will be considered in more detail in the last section of this chapter.)

3.3.2. *Role of plasma fibrinogen.* Fibrinogen's effect on plasma viscosity has already been mentioned; quantitatively much more significant is its

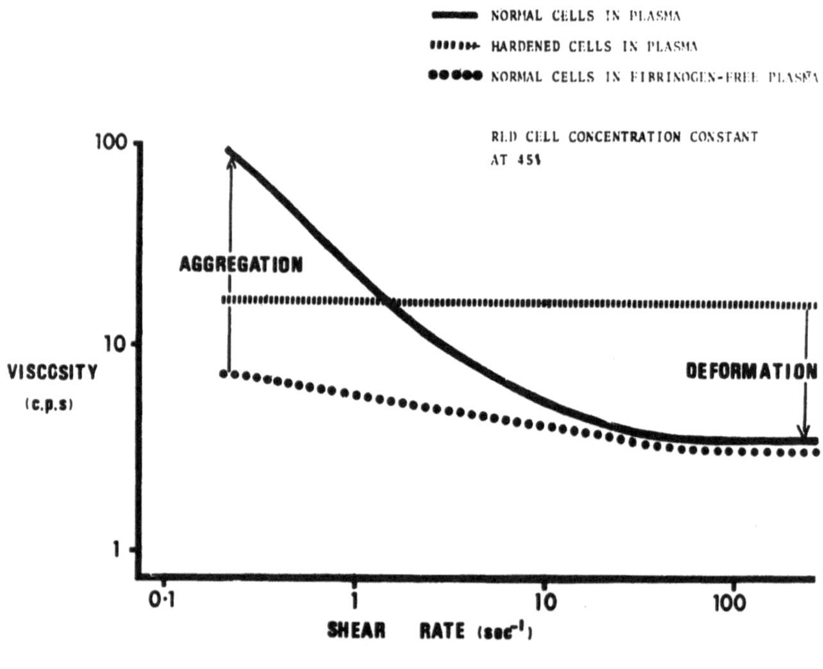

Fig. 13. Mechanism of shear rate dependence of blood viscosity, adapted from Chien.

effect on whole blood viscosity at low shear rates where a difference of 0.1 G% of fibrinogen may double the whole blood viscosity by increasing red cell aggregation. After eliminating the effect of haematocrit in populations of patients, blood viscosity is very closely correlated to plasma fibrinogen, particularly at low shear rates (35, 56, 57). For instance, at a shear rate of 1 sec^{-1} the correlation has been found to be as high as 0.95 (44). Fig. 14 illustrates the usual increase in plasma fibrinogen observed after any major operation, together with the changes in whole blood viscosity measured at two shear rates; the parallelism between the changes in fibrinogen and viscosity at low shear rates can be seen.

Some globulin fractions in plasma (e.g., a-2 and β-1) also play a significant role, similar to that of fibrinogen, in affecting blood viscosity. This role is exaggerated in macroglobulinaemia.

There has been a suggestion that the effect of fibrinogen may be more complex than originally thought. Some workers have described a phenomenon, termed 'fibrinogen sensitivity' (58), which is illustrated in Fig. 15. This shows the extremely close correlation between haematocrit corrected blood viscosity and plasma fibrinogen in three patients with circulatory disease. The slope of the regression lines is however very different; changes in fibrinogen seem to have a much greater effect in one patient than another. Much more work needs to be done in this area; for instance, the

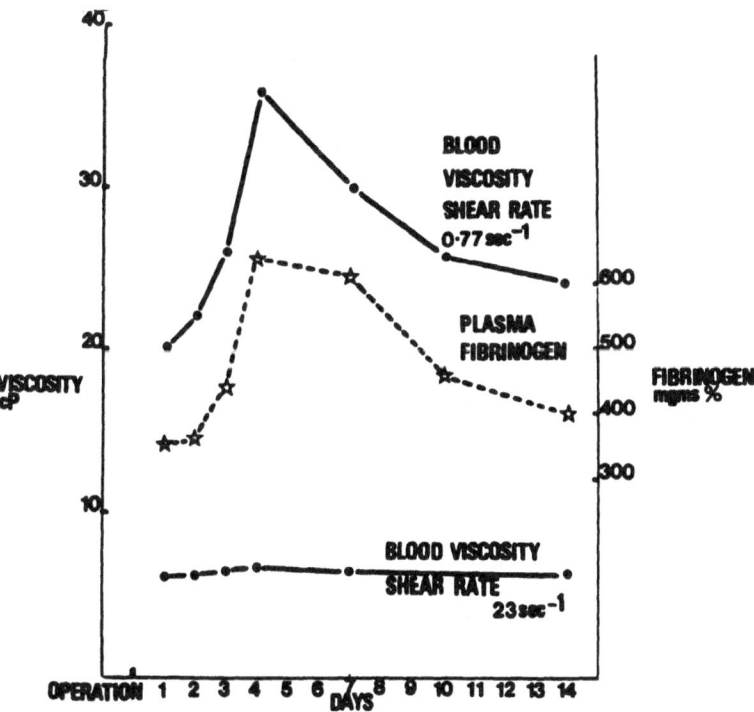

Fig. 14. Comparison of plasma fibrinogen and blood viscosity, measured at high and low shear rates, in the postoperative period.

importance of the various fibrinogen and fibrin degradation products is quite unclear. There is also evidence that at a constant haematocrit the yield stress is dependent on the fibrinogen concentration (39).

3.3.3. *Effect of other plasma factors.*   Because of their smaller and more symmetrical shape, other proteins have much lesser effect than fibrinogen on blood viscosity (59). However, if they are present in abnormal quantities, as in macroglobulinaemia, their effect may be significant (49).

Lipids (23) and glucose (60) have been shown to have no effect on blood viscosity. The pH and osmolarity of the blood however can play a significant role, although this is probably indirectly through their effect on the red cell deformability, by influencing the volume and shape of the red cells. Both a fall in pH and an increase in osmolarity raise whole blood viscosity, but the effect of hypotonicity is less clear (56, 61–63). The necessary changes in osmolarity may not occur even in pathological circumstances; the effect of pH however may well be significant in ischaemia.

The effects of changes in osmolarity on blood viscosity depend on whether comparisons are made at the same haematocrit or at the same red cell count (6).

3.3.4. *Summary: Determinants of whole blood viscosity.*   The factors affecting whole blood viscosity may be divided into three groups: plasma

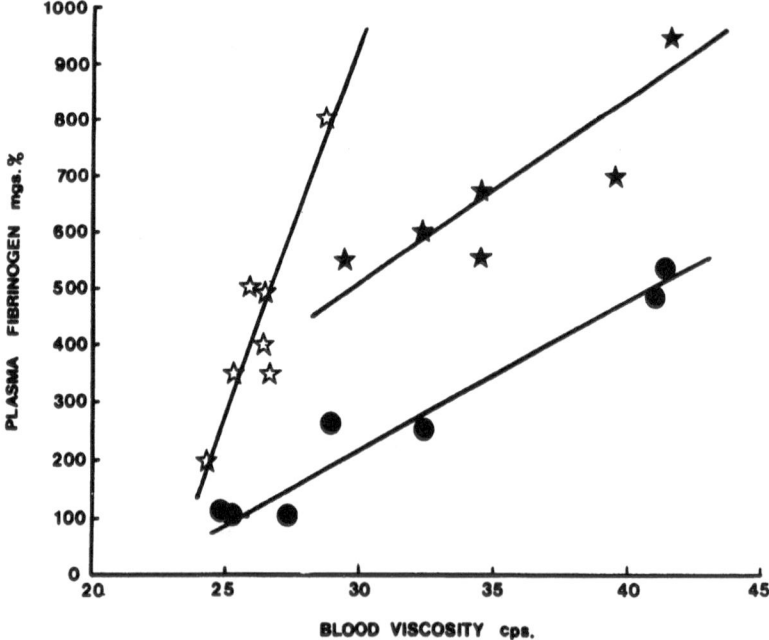

Fig. 15. Plasma fibrinogen and blood viscosity at a shear rate of 0.77 sec^{-1} measured on different occasions in three patients. There is a very close correlation between viscosity and fibrinogen in any one patient, but the slope of the regression lines can be very different.

factors, factors affecting the red cell directly and most importantly the concentration of red cells in the plasma. In fact all these influence interact; for instance the plasma fibrinogen largely exerts its effect by influencing the aggregation of red cells. Although their mechanisms of action may be complex, the various determinants of whole blood viscosity may be considered as originating in a property of the red cell or plasma. Platelets and white cells in normal concentrations do not seem to influence the viscosity of whole blood (35, 64).) This does not take into account the shear rate to which the blood is exposed or at which its viscosity is measured. For practical purposes, the effective viscosity of blood in a particular part of the living circulation will be most influenced by the shear rates and haematocrit in that part of the circulation as well as the plasma fibrinogen concentration. This approach can be applied usefully to a classification of hyperviscosity states. The clinical relevance of blood viscosity including a consideration of the hyperviscosity states will be discussed in the next section.

4.   CLINICAL APPLICATIONS OF BLOOD VISCOSITY MEASUREMENT

Polycythaemia has long been recognised as a hyperviscosity disease. Virtually all its clinical manifestations are the result of poor blood flow in the presence of normal vessels and a normal heart. The poor flow must be due to the considerable increase in blood viscosity associated with the high haematocrit. Despite the increased oxygen carrying capacity of the blood, the decreased flow apparently results in an overall decrease in oxygen delivery to the tissues.

Despite this example of polycythaemia, the concept of hyperviscosity being responsible for circulatory insufficiency in other conditions did not gain widespread consideration till the last 10–20 years, when the modern techniques of viscometry began to be applied clinically.

Plasma viscosity will be considered briefly only, as in the circulation the viscosity of whole blood, albeit at low haematocrits, in some areas is clearly more relevant. Hyperviscosity diseases will be considered in two groups: those conditions where an abnormally high blood viscosity is invariably present and is a constant important feature of the clinical picture, as in polycythaemia for instance, and those diseases where hyperviscosity is found in only some circumstances and is only one of many important aetiological factors.

Table 3 shows an aetiological classification of hyperviscosity states. Diseases in groups A, B and C are invariably associated with high blood viscosity and can be considered as the pure hyperviscosity states. These conditions are however all quite rare. More interesting perhaps are the

Table 3. Hyperviscosity states.

'Pure' hyperviscosity states			
A. Plasma abnormality	B. High haematocrit	C. Cellular abnormality	D. Conditions partly, or occasionally, associated with hyperviscosity
Congenital hyperfibrinogenaemia	Primary polycythaemia	Spherocytosis	Venous thrombosis
Macroglobulinaemia	Secondary polycythaemia	Sickle cell disease	Intermittent claudication
Myeloma	'Stress' polycythaemia	Other haemoglobinopathics	Malignancy
Some collagen diseases	Neonates	Leukaemia	Raynaud's phenomenon
Cryoglobulinaemia			Some paediatric conditions
			Diabetes
			Myocardial ischaemia
			Dehydration
			Hypovolaemic shock

much more common diseases in group D where a proportion of patients have a high blood viscosity and where this is of clinical importance only under certain circumstances. The causes of the hyperviscosity in this last group is more obscure than in the 'pure' hyperviscosity diseases. The distinction between these groups is of course artificial and somewhat blurred.

4.1.   *Plasma viscosity in clinical medicine*

It is implied here that plasma viscosity and erythrocyte sedimentation rate are alternative measurements for the same purpose. It is true that both tests reflect alterations in plasma protein concentrations. It should be noted, however, that sedimentation rate also depends on the concentration and properties of the erythrocytes and that excessively high plasma viscosity may retard erythrocyte sedimentation.

There is one important area where the measurement of plasma viscosity alone has become accepted as being of definite clinical value. In many laboratories it is a preferred alternative to the measurement of erythrocyte sedimentation rate. This has almost wholly been the result of a lifetime's dedicated work by Harkness (31). The plasma viscosity is probably a more useful measurement, particularly in hyperproteinaemic states, for instance in the assessment of treatment in myeloma and macroglobulinaemia. Measurements of plasma viscosity have also been shown to be related more closely than the sedimentation rate in the clinical status of patients with a variety of other chronic diseases such as rheumatoid arthritis (65). Its measurement also has some technical advantages over measurement of the sedimentation rate in that it uses a smaller sample, gives a result within a minute and the samples can be stored before testing if necessary.

4.2.   *Pure hyperviscosity diseases*

As shown in the aetiological classification of hyperviscosity states (Table 3), in some diseases, hyperviscosity is always or usually found as the result of a single identifiable primary abnormality of the plasma, red cells or the concentration of red cells in plasma.

4.2.1. *A. Due to a plasma abnormality.* These are all relatively rare diseases where either a normal protein is present in abnormally high concentrations, for instance in congenital hyperfibrinogenaemia, or where an abnormal protein is found. The largest group of diseases exemplifying hyperviscosity due to the presence of abnormal proteins are the plasma cell dyskresias (66), characterised by excess production of various immunoglobulins. The increase in viscosity is most noticeable at low shear rates and depends on the level of immunoglobulins and their tendency to polymerise. Clinically apparent consequences of the hyperviscosity are found in about half the cases of Waldenström's macroglobulinaemia, but in only about 10% of multiple myeloma cases, because of the lower molecular weight of the immunoglobulins concerned. Plasmapheresis is extremely successful in the treatment of these conditions (67). Hyperviscosity due to plasma abnormalities has also been described in rheumatoid arthritis (68) and some other collagen diseases (69, 70).

But by far the commonnest plasma cause of hyperviscosity are the many conditions associated with a non-specific increase in plasma fibrinogen, some of which are considered in group D of hyperviscosity diseases (Section 4.3.).

4.2.2. *B. Due to a high haematocrit: Polycythaemia.* As far as the blood viscosity, and therefore blood flow, is concerned it is the high haematocrit and not the red cell mass which matters. This is not quite equivalent to polycythaemia, which is a haematological disease usually defined in terms of the red cell mass. Polycythaemias are commonly subdivided into pure polycythaemia rubra vera where there may be also an increase in other formed elements in the blood and secondary polycythaemia, where haemoconcentration of red cells only occurs as a reaction to hypoxia or erythropoetin producing tumours. The fascinating question arises: at what level does the polycythaemia secondary to hypoxia cease to be beneficial in terms of oxygen delivery because of the decreased flow due to the accompanying hyperviscosity? This is the inverse of the question posed by the treatment of circulatory failure by haemodilution (Section 4.5.1). It has recently been advocated that the management of these patients should be aimed at keeping their whole blood viscosity below a certain limit, rather than to control treatment by measurements of haematocrit or by the, less relevant and more complicated, measurement of red cell mass. In addition, a group of patients, with a relatively high haematocrit but a red cell mass within the normal range, have been variously described as having stress polycythaemia or Gainsbock's disease. There has been an increasing realisation that blood flow and symptoms of ischaemia in various circulations (13, 71) as well as mortality (72) is significantly related to haematocrit levels even within the so-called normal range.

The high incidence of arterial and venous thromboses (73), cerebral symptoms, myocardial ischaemia and intermittent claudication (74) in patients with a high haematocrit is most likely to be due to the decreased blood flow secondary to the high viscosity.

4.2.3. C. Due to abnormality in the cellular components.

Accurate and quantitative assessment of red cell deformability is a very·new measurement, which will be considered in the next section (Section 5). Haematologists have however long recognised a group of diseases where the red cells are assumed to be abnormally rigid or undeformable and where this is thought to give rise to associated haematological and circulatory problems. This group of diseases has sometimes been described as sclerocytotic (75) and include spherocytosis, malaria and sickle cell disease.

These and other conditions altering red cell deformability are discussed in more detail later in Section 5.4. They are mentioned here because the red cell abnormality may often be sufficient to alter the whole blood viscosity as well.

Mention must also be made of the white blood cell, which is recognized to be more rigid than red cells (76) and some of the clinical features of leukaemia have been shown to be due to a hyperviscosity state (77, 78).

4.3. D. Other clinical conditions where hyperviscosity may play an important role

This is a group of very varied and common conditions, associated with a circulatory impairment where abnormally high blood viscosity is sometimes found. It is probably only one of several aetiological factors, but it may be important in that it is often of prognostic significance and its correction may be of therapeutic use.

4.3.1. Venous thrombosis.

Changes in blood viscosity will directly affect velocity of blood flow, which is one of Virchow's triad of causes of venous thrombosis. There is much circumstantial evidence linking hyperviscosity to venous thrombosis. For instance, most of the clinical conditions recognised as predisposing to venous thrombosis, such as dehydration, polycythaemia, myocardial infarction and surgery are known to be frequently associated with a high blood viscosity.

A more direct relation has been demonstrated in prospective studies where whole blood viscosity or yield stress immediately before operation has been correlated with the development of postoperative deep venous thrombosis (79, 80). A relationship between viscosity and retinal vein thrombosis has also been described (81). The level of the hyperfibrinogenaemia after myocardial infarction has also been shown to be related to the development of venous thromosis (82).

In one interesting but small study it was shown that for unknown reasons a few women develop a sudden and considerable increase in blood viscosity when taking oral contraceptives and it was also these same women who suffered thrombotic complications (83).

4.3.2. *Myocardial ischaemia.* There have been repeated reports that patients with myocardial ischaemia have a higher haematocrit, fibrinogen and blood viscosity than normal controls (82, 84, 85). An increased incidence of myocardial ischaemia has also been shown in patients in the Framingham study who had a high haematocrit (86).

There is no doubt that the blood viscosity is markedly increased immediately after a myocardial infarction, partly due to haemoconcentration and partly hyperfibrinogenaemia (87–89). The crucial question remains to be answered as to whether a transient hyperviscosity, for whatever reason, may not have precipitated the infarction?

In any event, the postinfarction hyperviscosity must contribute to the circulatory impairment following acute myocardial ischaemia. This has been demonstrated in a study of blood viscosity in patients immediately on admission to hospital with a myocardial infarction (90). Patients with a higher viscosity were more liable to develop circulatory shock and the patients who subsequently died had the highest blood viscosity on admission.

4.3.3. *Intermittent claudication.* Ischaemia of the legs is an excellent example of a very common condition, where arterial stenosis had always been assumed to be the only cause, but in fact an abnormally high blood viscosity has been demonstrated in about a quarter of all patients (91, 92) (Fig. 16). In these cases, there is often remarkably little arterial narrowing, the principal defect being the hyperviscosity. If there is co-existent disease of the arteries as well as of the flow properties of blood within them, the prognosis has been shown to be particularly bleak (93).

The mechanism of the hyperviscosity is not always certain; but in the majority it is due to a hyperfibrinogenaemia, often aggravated by a relatively high haematocrit. The concept of a dual pathology in peripheral circulatory disease, that is arterial disease combined with a raised blood viscosity, throws a new light on the significance of biochemical changes in the blood which may exert an aetiological influence on either or both these pathological processes.

4.3.4. *Diabetes.* Early measurements of whole blood viscosity in diabetics yielded conflicting results. The most recent, largest and most detailed study has shown a significantly higher whole blood viscosity at low shear rates in diabetics compared with matched non-diabetic controls (94). Abnormally high values were particularly common in diabetics with circulatory abnormalities. This may have been due to a raised plasma fibrinogen, which has also been described by others (95) and has been shown to be correlated with an increase in mortality (96).

Especially high levels of blood viscosity have been described during ketoacidosis and may be related to the frequent thromboembolic complications. Abnormal red cell rigidity has also been described in poorly controlled diabetics (97) and those with widespread microangiopathy (94).

In hypertensive patients, blood viscosity has been found to be correlated with the plasma renin levels (normalised for urinary sodium excretion). The elevated blood viscosity, especially in high renin patients, has been shown to be due to a combination of several factors, including slight elevations of haematocrit, plasma fibrinogen and globulin concentrations, and red cell aggregation (7).

4.3.5. *Essential hypertension.* The hypothesis that the basic defect in essential hypertension is an increase in whole blood viscosity has many attractive features. An otherwise normal cardiovascular system could only maintain a normal circulation of hyperviscous blood by increasing the perfusion pressure. This hypothesis has received little attention so far although in one study the blood viscosity of young patients with essential hypertension was shown to be higher than that of age matched normo-

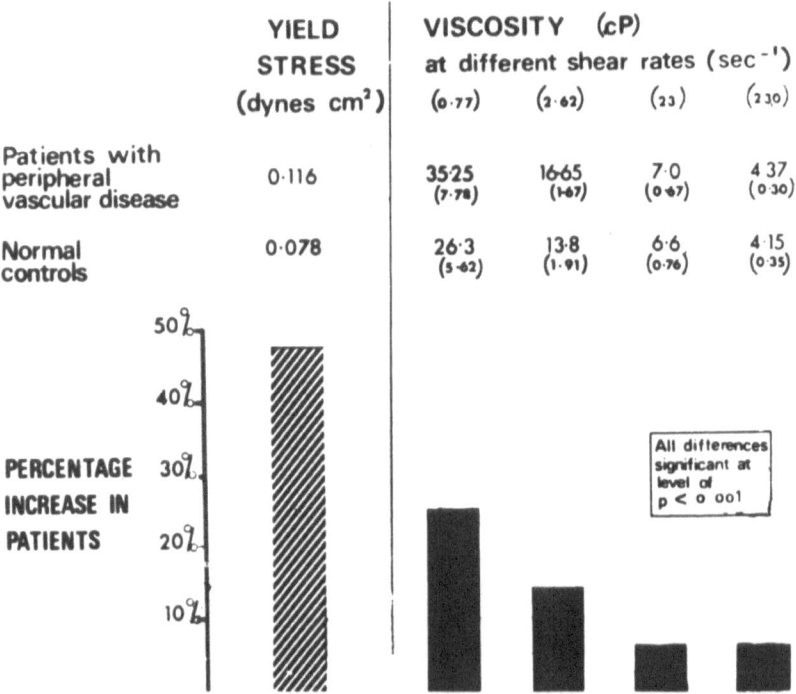

Fig. 16. The mean values and standard deviation of blood viscosity at four shear rates and yield stress in a group of patients with intermittent claudication and a matched control group. (Derived from the same data as Fig. 12.) The histogram indicates the increased values in the patients as a percentage of the controls.

tensive controls (98). The concept of viscoreceptors in the body has not so far received widespread acceptance, but a malfunction of such viscosity receptors has been postulated as the primary disorder in essential hypertension (99).

4.3.6. *Raynaud's phenomenon.* One of the most puzzling features of Raynaud's phenomenon is that although a wide variety of quite different underlying pathological conditions appear to be associated with the phenomenon, the clinical manifestations of the attacks are so very similar in all cases, the precipitation of attacks by cold. It has already been mentioned that the viscosity of blood increases at lower temperature (Section 2.6.3). Routine viscosity measurements are carried out usually at 37 °C, but in patients with Raynaud's phenomenon it would seem reasonable to make measurements at lower temperatures as well, since the temperature of the blood in the digits at the beginning of an attack may be very low. One such study has been carried out and an abnormal response of the blood viscosity to a fall in temperature demonstrated in patients suffering from Raynaud's phenomenon(34). This may well be the effect of cryoglobulins (100).

4.3.7. *Paediatric conditions.* Blood viscosity is normally increased for the first few weeks of life, partly due to the higher haematocrit (78) and partly the increased rigidity of foetal erythrocytes (101). Extreme elevations of haematocrit with a correspondingly high blood viscosity have been recorded in infants with neurological, cardiologic and respiratory diseases (102).

4.3.8. *Role of hyperviscosity in circulatory shock.* Whatever the aetiology of shock the major common pathway is tissue hypoxia, which is usually due to microcirculatory failure. Hyperviscosity may well play a leading role in many of the vicious circles which tend to perpetuate microcirculatory failure. For instance slowing of the circulation with decreasing shear rate automatically increases the viscosity of the non-Newtonian blood. Abnormalities of the yield stress will tend to favour stasis. Hypoxia renders red cells increasingly rigid, raising blood viscosity and further aggravating the hypoxia and the acidosis of hypoxic tissue will have a similar effect.

4.3.9. *Blood viscosity and surgery.* Anaesthetic agents by themselves, whether given intravenously or by inhalation, have no or only very little effect on blood viscosity (103). Other aspects of surgery may have very profound effects, which have been quite extensively studied, particularly in the postoperative period. Virtually all the factors known to affect blood viscosity and red cell deformability are radically altered by surgery. The considerable fluid exchanges are probably the most important, not only by altering the haematocrit, but by the effect of the fluid replacements which may be used. Stored blood is acidotic and has extremely rigid red cells, although this is probably partly corrected when they reach the living circulation. Nevertheless, abnormalities in the circulating red cells have been found after large blood transfusions (104). The protein fractions of blood are also affected; after an initial fall, the plasma fibrinogen increases to a peak around the fifth day. This not only affects the whole blood viscosity (105, 106), but also the red cell deformability (57, 104), although this latter effect is complicated by the changes in fibrinogen degradation products and is still very incompletely understood. Fig. 17 shows typical changes in some of these rheological values after major general surgical procedures. The situation is further complicated in open heart surgery, where denaturation of proteins and trauma to the red cells in the extra-corporeal circuit have profound rheological effects (23, 107). In a large study of several hundred operations a very close correlation was found between the preoperative haemoglobin and the failure of reconstructive vascular procedures; the higher the haemoglobin the greater the incidence of operative failure (108).

4.4. *Diagnosis of hyperviscosity states*

A hyperviscosity state may be suspected on clinical grounds if the circulatory impairment seems out of proportion to the vessel or cardiac disease. It is particularly important to remember that a normal peripheral arterial pulse does not necessarily guarantee good blood flow, it merely indicates the absence of a major mechanical block between the heart and the point where the pulse is felt. In pure hyperviscosity states the peripheral pulse will be normal although blood flow will be decreased. (Similarly in small vessel desease distal to the pulse, the pulsations may well be even exaggerated.)

A frequent practical clinical problem is how to exclude a hyperviscosity component to the circulatory impairment. A normal full blood count including sedimentation rate will exclude many of the pure hyperviscosity states. The sedimentation rate can be usefully replaced by screening plasma viscosity estimation using a capillary viscometer. This would save time and improve accuracy. A plasma fibrinogen estimation is by far the most relevant biochemical test and can be both simple and reasonably accurate. If there is a suspicion of a hyperviscosity state, in the first instance the blood viscosity need only be measured at two shear rates, one within the Newtonian range and another at as low a shear as is practical. For routine clinical purposes the Contraves is the most suitable of the established commercially available viscometers (see Section 2.5 for a discussion of the relative merits of different machines. It is relevant to point out that in virtually all clinical conditions where hyperviscosity has been described the abnormalities are most easily detected when measurements are made at low shear rates. Finally, the red cell deformability is most easily and quickly assessed by one of the filtration techniques. These initial tests of plasma and blood viscosity and red cell deformability take at most half an hour of an experienced technician's time per patient. (If several specimens are screened simultaneously, it would of course take less time

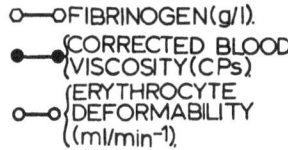

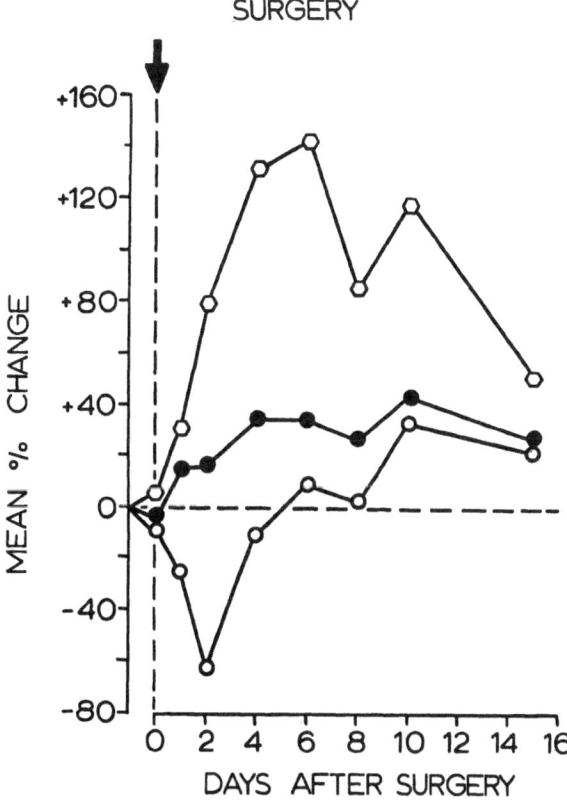

Fig. 17. Changes in red cell deformability following major surgery in relation to changes in plasma fibrinogen and whole blood viscosity.

per specimen.) If an abnormality is found in any of these basic tests a fuller characterisation of the rheological abnormality can be undertaken.

As with all diagnoses, the best safeguard that an underlying hyper-viscosity situation is not missed is the clinician's constant awareness of the possibility followed by a request for the appropriate screening tests just described.

4.5.   Treatment of circulatory disorders by lowering the blood viscosity

4.5.1. *Haemodilution.*   Haemodilution is the simplest and most effective technique for lowering blood viscosity, but of course it has the disadvan-tage of lowering the oxygen carrying capacity of the blood as well. There is however some evidence that there is an overall improvement in terms of oxygen delivery, which may explain some of the clinical success with blood-letting reported in the old medical literature. Phlebotomy has again been revived as a useful therapeutic manoeuvre in the treatment of angina (109) and even more recently in the treatment of cerebral ischaemia (13).

Normovolaemic haemodilution has also recently gained much popu-larity particularly in Germany as a preoperative measure following the pioneering work of Messmer (10). Normovolaemic haemodilution down to a haematocrit of approximately 30%, with replacement of the blood by a colloid solution, has been shown to increase oxygen availability to tissues (110) with a preferential increase in the coronary blood flow (111). As a preoperative measure it has the additional merit of relieving the demand for donor banked blood and making available for re-infusion the patient's own fresh blood should it prove necessary in the postoperative period.

Haemodilution using low molecular weight dextran (L.M.W.D.) infu-sion has been advocated on the grounds that additional benefits, in terms of red cell disaggregation, are produced by the L.M.W.D. But despite the widespread clinical use of L.M.W.D. for 30 years, its precise rheological effects are still disputed (12, 112).

4.5.2. *Plasmapharesis.*   Recently, it has been suggested that removal of immune complexes by plasmapharesis will lower blood viscosity and bene-fit patients (67, 77, 113). Most recently, this technique has been shown to be effective in lowering the blood viscosity and significantly improving patients with Raynaud's disease (114).

4.5.3. *Lowering fibrinogen to normal.*   There are widely used drugs which will lower fibrinogen levels to normal in patients where it is abnormally high. (A raised plasma fibrinogen is a common cause of hyperviscosity.) Normalising the fibrinogen in these cases has been accompanied by a parallel reduction in whole blood viscosity and there is beginning to be some evidence that this is of benefit to the patient, for instance in intermittent claudicants selected on the basis of a high viscosity due to a high fibrinogen (58, 115) (Fig. 18).

4.5.4. *Controlled defibrination.*   Lowering blood viscosity below normal would theoretically be of benefit to patients with circulatory disease due to arterial narrowing or possibly even cardiac disease. In the former case it would compensate for the arterial disease by increasing the flow down the unchanged narrow arteries. As far as we know an abnormally low viscosity has no harmful effects. Whilst haemodilution can lower blood viscosity below normal, it does so at the cost of lowering the oxygen carrying capacity of the blood as well. Controlled defibrination however would also lower blood viscosity below normal, but without reducing its oxygen carrying capacity. Since we know that less than 10% of the normal fibrinogen content of blood is sufficient for normal haemostasis, controlled defibrination down to this sort of level should be quite safe. As yet there is no accepted safe long term therapeutic technique for controlled defibrination; but the hypothesis can be tested by using such defibrinating agents such as Arvin for short periods. There have now been several clinical

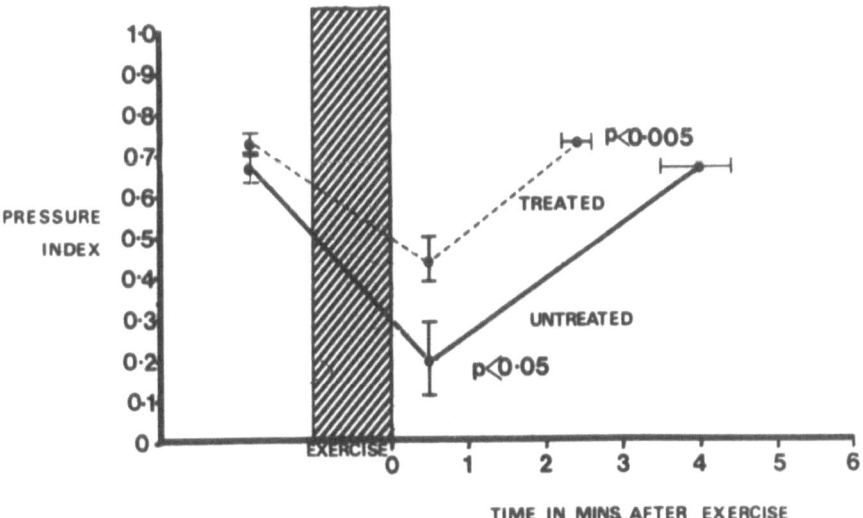

MEAN   PRESSURE   INDEX   RESULTS   IN   PATIENTS   WITH   HIGH   PLASMA FIBRINOGEN   CONCENTRATION

9 TREATED AND 13 UNTREATED PATIENTS WITH INITIAL PLASMA FIBRINOGEN CONCENTRATION ABOVE 400mgs%

TIME IN MINS. AFTER EXERCISE

Fig. 18. Ankle to arm systolic pressure ratio (pressure index) in patients with intermittent claudication. The untreated group had a high plasma fibrinogen, while in the treated group the fibrinogen had been lowered to normal with Clofibrate.

studies showing that such defibrination is indeed beneficial in circulatory conditions as assessed by objective measurements (Fig. 19) (116–118). It has also been shown to be a useful technique in improving vascular graft patency in animal models (119). Most importantly, these early studies, many of them in out-patients, have shown that controlled defibrination is safe.

4.5.5. *Conclusions: Clinical significance of blood viscosity measurements.* As a result of measurements of blood viscosity in a variety of diseases over the past two decades, there has been rapidly spreading realisation among clinicians that abnormalities of blood viscosity probably play a significant role in many circulatory conditions. More recently the first preliminary steps have been taken in attempting to develop therapeutic techniques for dealing with these hyperviscosity states. These represent a new and promising approach to the treatment of circulatory insufficiency.

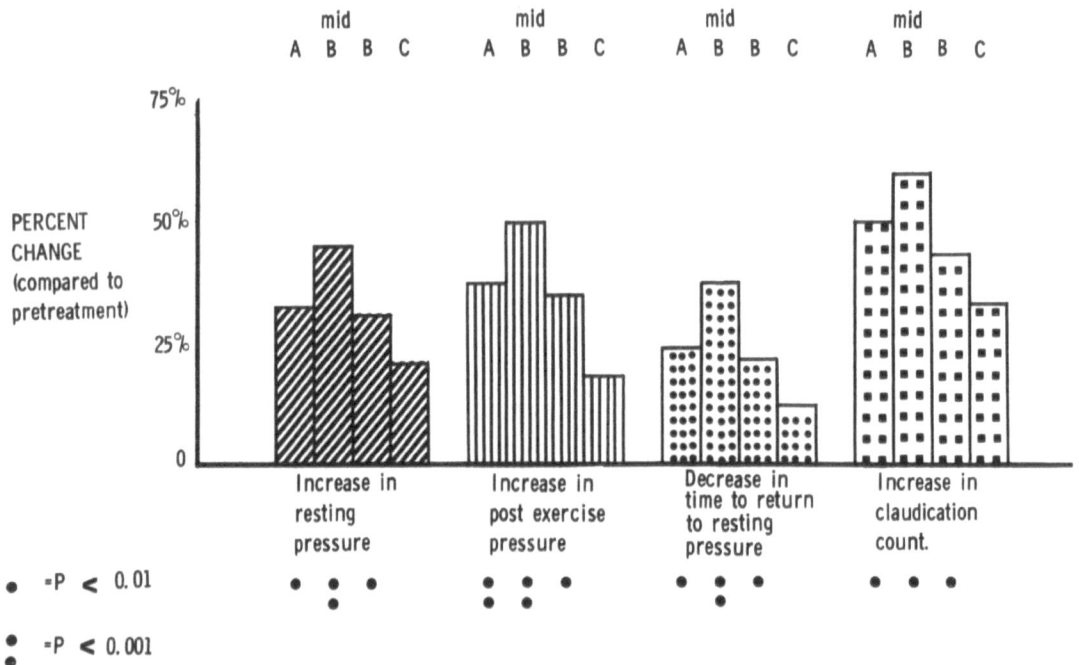

Fig. 19. Mean changes in the ankle to arm pressure index and the claudication count in 15 patients treated with subcutaneous Arvin. The changes are expressed as a percentage of the pretreatment value. A = end of induction period on the fourth day, mid B = two weeks later during the maintenance period, B = end of treatment at 4 weeks, and C = 2 weeks after stopping treatment.

5. RED CELL FLEXIBILITY

5.1. *Introduction*

This chapter has so far been mostly concerned with what could be termed macrorheology, that is the viscosity of bulk blood. This last section will consider the much newer and less understood area of microrheology or the flow properties of individual red cells.

The fact that red cells have to deform in order to negotiate the capillary passages was appreciated by Leeuwenhoek as long ago as 1672 (120), before we had any concept of blood viscosity. However it is only in the last very few years that any possible pathological or clinical significance has been attached to abnormalities in red cell deformability. This is undoubtedly due to the very considerable methodological problems which we are still in the very earliest stages of solving.

Some of the first techniques used for demonstrating red cell deformability, such as cinemicrophotography, were much too complicated to apply generally for medical investigation and will not be considered in detail. A number of fundamentally different techniques have been described recently, some of which are beginning to be applied clinically. Unfortunately, when these techniques have been compared they were often found to give totally incompatible results and consequently we do not even have any universally accepted units for expressing red cell deformability. Nevertheless, this is probably an area where rapid advances will be made in the near future towards a standardisation of methodologies. With a more accurate definition of the clinical role of abnormal deformability we may lood forward to the successful therapy of some circulatory abnormalities based on the pharmacological correction of some abnormalities in the physical properties of the red cells.

5.2. *Measurement of red cell deformability*

5.2.1. *Techniques based on the measurement of bulk viscosity.* The deformability of individual red cells is one of the components determining the viscosity of bulk blood. Its effect can be increased by resuspending the cells in fluids simpler than plasma, by altering red cell concentration and making measurements at selected shear rates. All these techniques have been advocated to try and devise a measure of red cell deformability from results obtained on relatively large samples in conventional viscometers. Such measurements have been carried out on blood of normal haematocrit at high shear rates (56), maximally packed red cells with a haematocrit of around 98% (121, 122) and on red cells resuspended in Ringer–albumin solution at very low shear rates (61, 123).

Determination of the negative pressure necessary to deform a small portion of red cell surface with a small micropipette yields information primarily on membrane properties, and it does not provide insight into the other aspects of cell deformability e.g., the geometric relation between cell volume surface area. This geometric factor (which is mentioned under Section 5.3.2) and the membrane composition (lipids, proteins and their interrelations) are important determinants of red cell deformability, and they should be included in Fig. 21.

All these techniques suffer from being even less physiological than other available techniques to be discussed. In the capillaries individual red cells have to deform in a plasma environment, not surrounded by either Ringer albumin or squeezed by other maximally packed red cells.

5.2.2.   *Micropipette technique.*   Using a micropipette with a diameter less than that of a red cell, the negative pressure necessary to deform the surface of a red cell is measured under a microscope (124–127). This is probably the most direct technique for assessing deformability and certainly most of our fundamental knowledge about the factors influencing red cell deformability has been gained using this technique. But the high degree of technical skill required and the logistics of the technique preclude its use in a truly clinical context.

Larger pipettes, comparable to the diameter of capillaries, have also been used at flow rates in the physiological range, with haematocrits as high as 80%.

5.2.3. *Measurement of red cell rate of packing.*   This technique was originally described and used most consistently by Sirs and his colleagues (128, 129). It is based on the principle that the more deformable the red cells the quicker they will pack when centrifuged. Speeds equivalent to $200–600 \times g$ are usually used although lower forces of $20–50 \times g$ have also been tried.

The advantages of this technique are its relative simplicity, no special equipment being necessary, its reproducability to within $\pm 2\%$ and the fact that fresh blood is used without any pretreatment or resuspension. Its principal disadvantage is the totally unphysiological forces applied to the red cells. The rate of packing of red cells, under pressures several hundred times those in the microcirculation, will depend on a number of factors possibly unrelated to red cell deformability in vivo.

5.2.4. *Filtration techniques.*   A number of systems have been devised based on the passage of red cells, either suspended in their own plasma or more often resuspended in various artificial solutions, through filters with narrow channels. These techniques all have the advantage of exposing a large population of red cells to a situation where each has to deform individually. A quantitative result may be obtained either by recording the pressure necessary to keep flow constant, the 'screen filtration pressure' (130), or by measuring the volume of cells filtered at a constant pressure. The latter is probably the more physiological.

Various types of filters have been used: paper-fibre filters have long branching channels which have an irregular bore but approximate that of the red cell (131). Millipore filters (124, 132) were probably the most widely used and also consist of irregular tortuous channels covering approximately 80% of an inert cellulose ester filter. The newer polycarbonate (Nucleopore) filters (133) have even more regular cylindrical channels but with a far lower and slightly variable pore density. Most of the filters used have a pore diameter of 5 μm, but pores with a 3 or 8 μm diameter have also been used (Fig. 20). For the screen filtration technique a metal grid with 20 μm gaps has been used.

In most of the filtration studies the red cells have been resuspended in artificial media, sometimes at very low concentrations. This will give more reproducible results and can be argued to be a purer reflection of the physical properties of red cells. On the other hand, measuring the deformability of red cells in their native plasma is probably more physiological and more relevant clinically. Possibly measurements of red cells both in plasma and washed in a buffer solution should be carried out.

5.2.5. *Other techniques.*   Recently an ingenious and new functional tech-

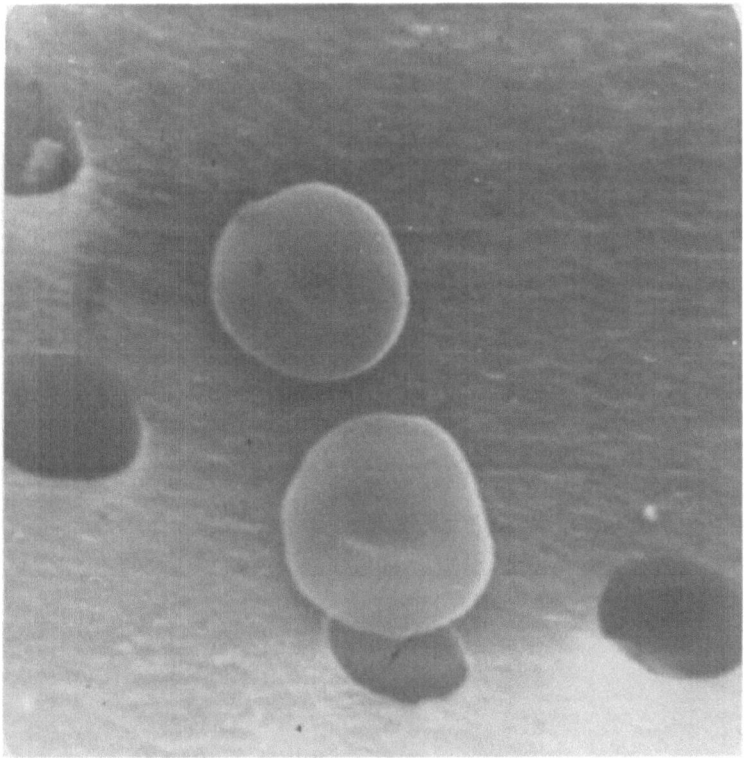

Fig. 20. Electron photomicrograph of the Nucleopore filter and red cells about to enter the pores.

nique has been developed based on the filming of the diffraction patterns produced by dilute suspensions of red cells exposed to various shear rates. The results are expressed in terms of the increase in the long axis of the red cells as a function of the applied shear stress (135).

   The counter-rotating rheoscope is a more direct technique allowing the filming of individual red cells exposed to various shear stresses so arranged that the red cell remains stationary in relation to the observer (136).

5.3.   Determinants of red cell deformability

5.3.1.   *Cell contents.*   Fig. 21 summarises the various groups of factors

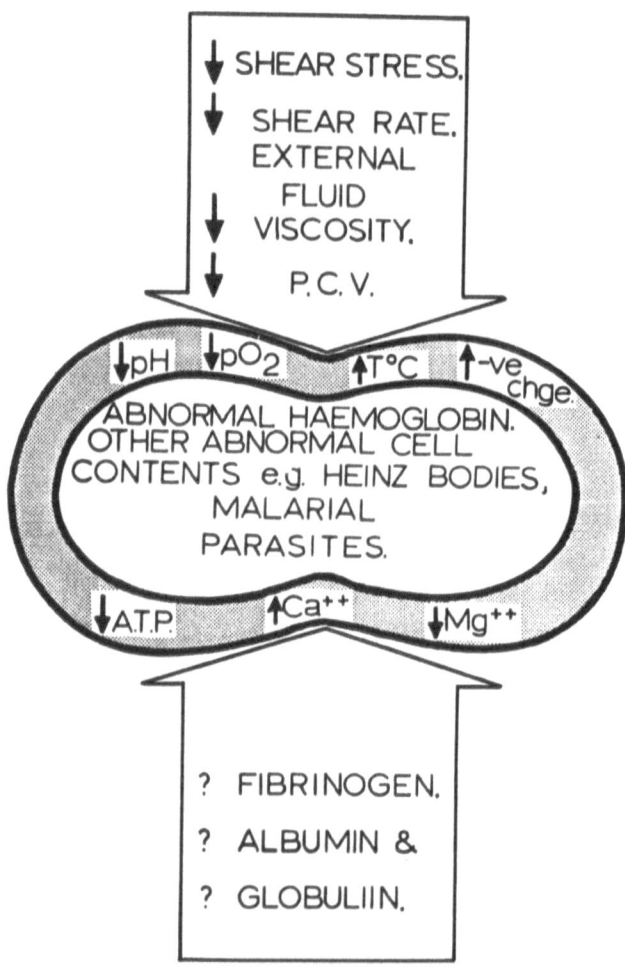

Fig. 21. Diagrammatic illustration of the various changes which may decrease red cell deformability.

which may determine the flow properties of individual red cells. The classification into influences acting from within the cell, on the cell membrane and from the outside is of course artificial as there is an infinity of interactions between individual factors. It does however serve a descriptive purpose.

The mean corpuscular haemoglobin concentration affects the internal fluid viscosity of normal red cells (137). The only other normal physiological factor observed to have an effect on the internal viscosity of red cells has been the presence of nuclei in immature red cells (138).

Under pathological conditions, decreased deformability has been observed in the presence of haemoglobin S, with the deposition of excess Heinz bodies (139) and in the infestation of red cells by mature malarial parasites (140).

Recent studies (8) raise questions on the role of A.T.P. on membrane flexibility. It is possible that A.T.P. depletion causes a reduction in red cell deformability primarily due to cell shape change, whereas the elastic properties of the membrane are little affected.

5.3.2. Properties of the membrane and red cell shape.

The relationship between A.T.P. and the membrane calcium/magnesium ratio is thought to be the most important determinant of membrane flexibility (124, 141, 142). The effect of temperature on the deformability of the membrane has been studied, but results are contradictory (143, 144). Similarly contradictory results have been obtained regarding changes in red cell deformability when the normal surface negative change is removed (145).

Both acidosis and hypoxia are believed to increase red cell rigidity, but to some extent both these effects may be exerted by making red cells more spherical. The shape of red cells is believed to be principally determined by membrane properties rather than factors within the cell and for the cell to be deformable it must have a large area to volume ratio. The maintenance of the normal discoid shape of red cels is also dependent on A.T.P. (146).

The trapping of older red cells in the spleen may be due to the increased sphericity of older cells and the increase in rigidity with acidosis and hypoxia (125, 134).

The effect of hypoxia on red cell rigidity is still controversial. Probably very low O_2 tension (less than 5 mm Hg) and a concurrent acidosis are needed to increase red cell rigidity.

5.3.3. External physical and biochemical factors.

The actual deformation undergone by the red cell will also depend on the external forces applied to it, that is the local shear stress at the cell plasma vessel wall interfaces. The forces acting on individual red cells will be greater if the concentration of red cells is increased (147) or if the viscosity of the suspending fluid is varied (148).

There have been very few studies of the effect of plasma constituents on the deformability of red cells, although this is clearly potentially of considerable clinical importance. Using the packing rate during centrifugation as an index of red cell deformability it would seem that plasma fibrinogen actually improves red cell flexibility (149); that is adding fibrinogen to normal blood increases deformability, while defibrination

In the studies quoted on the effect of fibrinogen on red cell sedimentation in refs 149, 150, the authors did not exclude the role of fibrinogen on red cell aggregation, which has an important influence on erythrocyte sedimentation rate. Therefore, their results should not be interpreted in terms of the effects of fibrinogen or defibrination on *red cell deformability*.

renders them more rigid (150). These rather surprising findings have not been confirmed in studies using a filtration technique to assess red cell deformability (29). Very little is known of the effect of albumin or globulin on red cell deformability.

5.4.   Clinical relevance of red cell deformability

5.4.1. *Haematological diseases where decreased red cell deformability is the principal defect.*   Gross abnormalities in red cell deformability in sickle cell disease with crosslinkage of haemoglobin S under hypoxic conditions can be easily demonstrated by any of the techniques described for assessing red cell deformability (151, 152). Much more subtle changes have also been described in sickle cell trait patients (125). It has also been shown that the presence of haemoglobin D or F can modify the rheological properties of the red cell (153). Patients with thalassaemia, even in the absence of Heinz bodies, show a reduced defomability. Gross abnormalities in deformability have also been widely documented in spherocytosis and in a patient with Hodgkins' disease (148).

5.4.2. *Abnormal red cell deformability in other circulatory diseases.*   The concept that decreased blood flow, particularly in the microcirculation, may be partly due to abnormally rigid red cells could have considerable clinical significance. A vicious cycle could be set up in the ischaemic tissues, where the hypoxia and acidaemia would increase red cell rigidity and further impair tissue perfusion. Whilst decreased red cell deformability has been reported by several workers in experimental haemorrhagic shock (154), it has not been studied in patients.

In the last few years there have been reports of an abnormally decreased red cell deformability in patients with impaired circulation to the legs (155) and angina (156). The majority of these patients also had atherosclerosis but a possible relationship between vessel wall disease and abnormal red cell deformability has not yet been studied. In one prospective investigation, intermittent claudicants with decreased red cell deformability had a higher incidence of amputation in subsequent years than patients with more normal red cell deformability (155) (Fig. 22). Red cell deformability has also recently been shown to be decreased in diabetics with circulatory complications (94).

5.4.3. *Therapeutic relevance.*   Whether a decrease in the deformability of the red cells is a primary cause or merely a secondary aggravating factor in tissue ischaemia, reversal of such an abnormality may be of therapeutic value. This has been quickly recognised by the pharmacological industry who have marketed a number of drugs claiming to improve red cell deformability. Unfortunately these claims are rarely, if ever, supported by experimental evidence or by good scientific evidence of clinical benefit in double-blind trials. A number of independent pilot studies, using a variety of techniques for measuring red cell deformability, have failed to confirm most of these claims. (These negative studies inevitably tend to remain unpublished.) Until the role of abnormal red cell deformability in circulatory disorders has been defined and until we know a little more about the causes of decreased red cell deformability, it would seem premature to attempt to develop therapeutic manoeuvres aimed at producing clinical improvement through a direct effect on the physical properties of red cells.

6.   CONCLUSIONS

It is now reasonably well established that the physical flow properties of bulk blood play an important part in determining blood flow. The viscosity of bulk blood can now be measured by a number of techniques, which have been validated in terms of in vivo blood flow. Abnormal blood viscosity plays a part in a number of circulatory disorders, some rare, some very common. Recently a number of therapeutic techniques based on the manipulation of blood viscosity have been shown to be clinically beneficial in some of these circulatory conditions.

The ability of individual red cells to deform must be an important factor in negotiating the microcirculation, as well as playing a probable role in the decreased whole blood viscosity at high flow rates. There is some

This is a valuable chapter on blood viscosity and red cell deformability, particularly in terms of their clinical applications. This referee has more comments on the sections discussing the basic principles and techniques of viscometry than on the section dealing with clinical application, which is excellent. It is hoped that these remarks and comments might help the reader to further his understanding and thinking as well as to provide different perspectives which the author cannot introduce readily in the flow of the text.

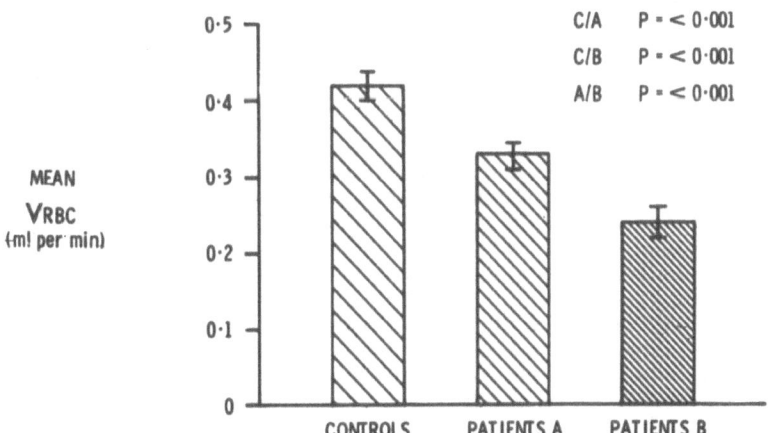

Fig. 22. Red cell deformability in a control group and two groups of patients with intermittent claudication. Groups A and B differed in that the latter subsequently required an amputation.

evidence that abnormalities in the deformability of red cells can be found in a range of circulatory diseases. But much work remains to be done in evaluating and standardising the different techniques used for assessing red cell deformability.

REFERENCES TO MAIN TEXT

1. Richardson DR, Intaglietta M, Zweifach BW: Simultaneous pressure amd flow measurements in the micro-circulation. Microvasc. Res. 3: 69, 1971.
2. Chien S: Present state of blood rheology. Haemodilution Int. Symp. Rottach-Egern, 1972, pl.
3. Whitmore RL: Flow behaviour of blood in the circulation. Nature (Lond.) 215: 123, 1967.
4. Wells RE: Blood flow in the microcirculation of man and the flow properties of blood. A correlative study. Bibl. anat. 9: 520, 1966.
5. Replogle RL, Meiselman HJ, Merrill EW: Clinival implications of blood rheology studies. Circulation 36: 148, 1967.
6. Skovborg F, Nielsen AV, Schlichtkrull J: Blood viscosity and vascular flow rate. Scand. J clin. Lab. Invest. 21: 83, 1968.
7. Rasmussen SN: Influence of plasma hypertonicity on blood viscosity in vitro and in an isolated vascular bed. Acta. physiol.scand. 84: 472, 1972.
8. Baeckström P, Folkow B, Kendrick E, Löfving B, Öberg B: Effects of vasoconstriction on blood viscosity in vivo. Acta physiol. scand. 81: 376, 1971.
9. Djojosugito AM, Folkow B, Öberg B, White S: A comparison of blood viscosity measured in vitro and in a vascular bed. Acta physiol. scand. 78: 70, 1970.
10. Messmer K: Acute preoperative haemodilution; an alternative to transfusion of donor blood. In: Acta Universitatis Upsaliensis. Symposium Dextran – 30 Years, Lewis D, Thoren L, (eds.), Uppsala, 1978, p 93–770.
11. Dormandy JA: Clinical significance of blood viscosity. Ann. roy. Coll. Surg.E 47: 211–228, 1970.
12. Dormandy JA: Influence of blood viscosity on blood flow and the effect of Low Molecular Weight Dextran. Brit. med. J. 2: 716–719, 1971.
13. Thomas DJ, Marshall J, Ross-Russell RW, Wetherleymein G, Duboulay GH, Pearson R, Symon L, Zilkha E: Effect of haematocrit on cerebral blood-flow in man. Lancet 5 Nov: 941, 1977.
14. Harkness J: A new instrument for the measurement of plasma viscosity. Lancet (2): 280, 1963.
15. Wells RE, Denton R, Merrill E: Measurement of viscosity of biologic fluids by cone plate viscometer. J Lab Clin Med 57: 646, 1961.
16. Spinelli FR, Meier ChD: Measurement of blood viscosity. Biorheology 11: 301, 1974.
17. Oiknine C, Mandret G, Goldman M: Détermination du comportement rhéologique du sang à l'aide d'un viscosimètre à cylindres coaxiaux. Biorheology 13: 127-132, 1976.
18. Schmid-Schönbein H: Microrheology of erythrocytes, blood viscosity and the distribution of blood flow: the microcirculation. Int. Rev. Physiol. 9: 1-62, 1976.
19. Copley AL: On biorheology – Joint Plenary Lect. Biorheology 10: 87, 1973.
20. Chien S, King RG, Skalak R, Usami S, Copley AL: Viscoelastic properties of human blood and red cell suspensions. Biorheology 12: 341–346, 1975.
21. Kiesewetter H, Kotitschke G, Schmid-Schönbein H: Yield stress measurements in red cell suspensions. Europ. J. Physiol. Suppl. 373: R23, 1978.
22. Charm SE, Kurland GS: A comparison of pipette, cone on plate and capillary tube viscometry for blood. Bibl. Anat. 10: 85, 1969.
23. Merrill EW: Rheology of blood. Physiol. Rev. 49: 863, 1969.
24. Galluzzi NJ, Delashmutt RK, Connolly VJ: Failure of anticoagulants to influence the viscosity of whole blood. J. Lab. Clin. Med. 64: 773, 1964.

25. Meiselman JJ, Frasher WG, Wayland H: Variable shear rate viscometry of native dog blood; effect of heparin injection. Biorheology 8: 91, 1971.

26. Meiselman JJ, Frasher WG, Wayland M: In vivo haemorheology employing outflow viscometric techniques. Biorheology 10: 361, 1973.

27. Barras JP: Blood rheology. General Review. Bibl. Haemat. 33: 277, 1969.

28. Zingg W, Sulev JC, Morgan CD: Study of possible sources of error in clinical blood viscosity determinations with the Wells-Brookfield viscometer. Biorheology 10: 585, 1973.

29. Reid H: Erythrocyte deformability: Its measurement in normal man and in patients with peripheral circulatory disease. Ph.D. Thesis, University of London, 1977.

30. Rosenblum WI, Warren EW: Elevation of blood viscosity produced by shearing in a rotational viscometer and its inhibition by refrigeration. Biorheology 10: 43, 1973.

31. Harkness J: The viscosity of human blood plasma; its measurement in health and disease. Biorheology 8: 171, 1971.

32. Barbee JH: The effect of temperature on the relative viscosity of human blood. Biorheology 10: 1, 1973.

33. Chien S, Usami S, Dellenback RJ, Bryant CA: Comparative haemorheology – Haematological implications of species differences in blood viscosity. Biorheology 8: 35, 1971.

34. Goyle KB, Dormandy JA: Abnormal blood viscosity in Raynaud's phenomenon. Lancet 1: 1317–1318, 1976.

35. Charm SE, Kurland GS (eds) Blood Flow and Microcirculation. New York, John Wiley, 1974.

36. Benis AM, Lacoste J: Study of erythrocyte aggregation by blood viscometry at low shear rates using a balance method. Circulat Res. 22: 29, 1968.

37. Scott-Blair GW: Equation of flow blood plasma and serum thru glass capillaries. Nature (Lond.) 183: 613, 1959.

38. Cokelet GR, Merrill EW, Gilliland ER, Shin H: The rheology of human blood measurement near and at zero shear rate. Trans. Soc. Rheology 7: 303, 1963.

39. Merrill EW, Cheng CS, Pelletier GA: Yield stress and endogenous fibrinogen. J. appl. Physiol. 26: 1, 1969.

40. Braasch D, Jenett W: Erythrocyte flexibility, hemoconcentration and blood flow resistance in glass capillaries with diameters between 6 and 50 microns. Bibl. Anat. 10: 109, 1969.

41. Skalak R, Chien PH, Chien S: Effect of hematocrit and rouleaux on apparent viscosity in capillaries. Biorheology 9: 67, 1972.

42. Chein S: Shear dependence of effective cell volume as a determinant of blood viscosity. Science 168: 977, 1970.

43. Begg TB, Hearns JB: Components in blood viscosity. Clin. Sci. 31: 89, 1966.

44. Weaver JPA, Evans A, Walder DN: The effect of increased fibrinogen content on the viscosity of blood. Clin. Sci. 36: 1, 1969.

45. Agarwal JB, Paltoo R, Palmer WM: Relative viscosity of blood at varying haematocrits in pulmonary circulation. J. appl. Physiol. 29:: 866, 1970.

46. Gregersen MI, Chien S, Peric B, Taylor H: Investigations of blood viscosity at low rates of shear. Bibl. Anat. 7: 383, 1965.

47. Yao ST, Shoemaker WC: Plasma and whole blood viscosity changes in shock after dextran infusion. Amer. J. Surg. 164: 973, 1966.

48. Phillips MJ, Harkness J: Plasma and whole blood viscosity. Brit. J. Haematol. 34(3): 347–52, 1976.

49. Somer T: The viscosity of blood, plasma and serum in Dysand paraproteinaemias. Acta med. scand. Suppl. 456: 180, 1966.

50. Eastham RD: The E.S.R. and plasma viscosity. J. clin. Path. 7: 164, 1954.

51. Ditzel J, Kampmann J: Whole blood viscosity, haematocrit and plasma protein in normal subjects at different ages. Acta. physiol. scand. 81: 264, 1971.

52. Dintenfass L, Yu JS: Changes in blood viscosity and the consistency of artificial thrombi in 17-year-old girls during the menstrual cycle. Med. J. Austr. 1: 181, 1968.

53. Merrill EW, Gilliland ER, Margetts WG, Hatch FT: Rheology of human blood and

hyperlipaemia. J. appl. Physiol. 19: 493, 1964.

54. Ehrly AM, Jung G: Circadian Rhythm of human blood viscosities. Biorheology 10: 577, 1973.

55. Tromp SW: Influence of weather and climate on the fibrin content of human blood. Int. J. Biometeor 18: 93, 1972.

56. Chien S: Biophysical behaviour of red cells in suspensions. The Red Blood Cell. Vol. II, New York, Academic Press, 1975.

57. Dupont PA, Sirs JA: The relationship of plasma fibrinogen, erythrocyte flexibility and blood viscosity. Thrombos. Haemostas 38: 660–667, 1977.

58. Postlethwaite JC: The importance of plasma fibrinogen in vascular surgery. Ann. roy. Coll. Surg. 58: 457, 1976.

59. Chien S, Usami S, Dellenback J, Gregersen MI: Shear-dependent interaction of plasma proteins with erythrocytes in blood rheology. Amer. J. Physiol. 219: 143, 1970.

60. Gordon W: The effect of ingested glucose, and intravenous injections of glucose, on the viscosity of whole blood in man. Clin. Sci. 36: 25, 1969.

61. Schmid-Schönbein H, Wells R, Goldstone J: Influence of deformability of human red cells upon blood viscosity. Circulat. Res. 25: 131, 1969.

62. Meiselman JG, Merrill EW, Gilliland ER, Pelletier GA, Salzman EW: Influence of plasma osmolarity on the rheology of human blood. J. appl. Physiol. 22: 772, 1967.

63. Ponder E: Red cell as osmometer. Cd Spr. Harbor Symp. quant. Biol. 8: 133, 1940.

64. Putnam TC, Kevy SV, Replogle RL: Factors affecting the viscosity of blood. Surg. Forum 16: 126, 1965.

65. Harkness J, Whittington RB: The viscosity of human blood plasma: its changes in disease and on the exhibition of changes. Rheol. Acta 10: 55–60, 1971.

66. Somer T: Hyperviscosity syndrome in plasma cell dyscrasias. Advanc. Microcirculation 6: 1, 1975.

67. Powles R, Smith C, Kohn J, Hamilton Fairly G: Method of removing abnormal protein rapidly from patients with malignant paraproteinaemias. Brit. med. J. 2: 664–667, 1971.

68. Jasin HE, Lospalluto J, Ziff M: Rheumatoid hyperviscosity syndrome. Amer. J. Med. 49: 484, 1970.

69. Editorial: Hyperviscosity syndrome. Brit. med. J. 2: 184, 1971.

70. Pruzanski W: Hyperviscosity and immunoglobulin complexes. Arch. int. Med. 80: 107, 1974.

71. Adar, R, Franklin A, Saltzman EW: Hemoconcentration in acute nonocclusive mesenteric ischaemia. J. Amer. med. Assoc. 228: 27, 1974.

72. Burge PS, Johnson WS, Prankerd TAJ: Morbidity and mortality in pseudopolycythaemia. Lancet 7 June: 1266, 1975.

73. Wasserman LR, Gilbert MS: Complications of polycythaemia vera. Sem. Hematol. 3: 199, 1966.

74. Edwards EA, Cooley MH: Peripheral vascular symptoms as the initial manifestation of polycythaemia vera. J. Amer. med. Assoc. 214: 1463–1467, 1970.

75. Wells R: Syndromes of hyperviscosity. New Engl. J. Med. 283: 183, 1970.

76. Steinberg MH, Charm SE: Effect of high concentrations of leukocytes on whole blood viscosity Blood 38: 299, 1971.

77. Preston FE, Sokol RJ, Lilleyman JS, Winfield DA, Blackburn EK: Cellular hyperviscosity as a cause of neurological symptoms in leukaemia. Brit. Med. J. (1): 476–478, 1978.

78. Wintrobe MM: Clinical Haematology, 7th Ed., Philadelphia, PA, Lea and Feburger, 1974.

79. Editorial: Haemorheology, blood-flow and venous thrombosis. Lancet 19 July: 113, 1975.

80. Dormandy JA, Edelman JB: High blood viscosity: an aetiological factor in venous thrombosis. Brit. J. Surg. 60: 187–190, 1973.

81. Ring CP, Pearson TC, Sanders MD, Wetherley-Mein G: Viscosity and retinal vein thrombosis. Brit. J. Opthalmol. 60: 397, 1976.

82. Fulton RM, Duckett K: Plasma-fibrinogen and thromboemboli after myorcardial

infarction. Lancet 27 Nov: 1161, 1976.

83. Aronson HB, Magora F, Schenker JG: Effect of oral contraceptives on blood viscosity. Amer. J. Obstet. Gynaecol. 110: 997, 1971.

84. Ditzel J, Dyeberg J, Grinstead P: Increased whole bloodviscosity at lower rates of shear and haematocrit levels in patients with previous myocardial infarction. In: 6th Europ. Conf. Microcirculation, Aalborg 1970, Basel, Karger, 1971, p 56.

85. Burch GE, Depasquale NP: Haematocrit, blood viscosity and myocardial infarction. Amer. J. Med. 32: 161, 1962.

86. Dawber TR, Kannel WB: Suspectibility to coronary heart disease. Mod. Concepts Cardiovasc. Dis. 30: 671, 1961.

87. Kellogg F, Goodman JR: Viscosity of blood in myocardial infarction. Circulat. Res. 8: 972, 1960.

88. Ditzel J, Bang HO, Thorsen N: Myocardial infarction and whole blood viscosity. Acta. med. scand. 183: 577, 1968.

89. Langsjoen PH, Inmon TW: Haemorrheologic observations in acute myocardial infarction. Angiology 19: 247, 1968.

90. Kung-Ming J, Chien S, Bigger JT: Observations on blood viscosity changes after acute myocardial infarction. Circulation 51: 1079, 1975.

91. McGrath MA: Tracy GD, Lord RSA, Penny R: Peripheral ischaemia caused by blood hyperviscosity. Austr. N.Z. Surg. 43: 109, 1973.

92. Dormandy JA, Hoare E, Colley J, Arrowsmith DE, Dormandy TL: Clinical, haemodynamical, rheological and biochemical findings in 126 patients with intermittent claudication. Brit. med. J. 4: 576–581, 1973.

93. Dormandy JA, Hoare E, Khattab A, Arrowsmith DE, Dormandy TL: Prognostic significance of rheological and biochemical findings in patients with intermittent claudication. Brit. med. J. 4: 581–583, 1973.

94. Barnes AJ, Locke P, Scudder PR, Dormandy TL, Dormandy JA, Slack J: Hyperviscosity: a treatable component of diabetic microcirculatory disease. Lancet (2): 789–791, 1977.

95. Wardle EN, Piercy DA, Anderson J: Some chemical indices of diabetic vascular disease. Postgrad. med. J. 49: 1–9, 1973.

96. Hart A, Cohen H, Thorp JM: Lipoprotein and fibrinogen studies in diabetes. Postgrad. med. J. (June) Suppl. 435, 1971.

97. Schmid-Schönbein MD, Volger E: Red cell aggregation and red cell deformability in diabetes. Diabetes 25 (Suppl. 2) 897: 902, 1976.

98. Tibblin G, Bergentz SE, Djure J, Wilhelmsen L: Haematocrit, plasma proteins, plasma volume and viscosity in early hypertension disease. Amer. Heart J. 72: 165, 1966.

99. Nihill MR et al: The effects of increased blood viscosity on pulmonary vascular resistance. Amer. Heart J. 92(I): 65–72, 1976.

100. Meltzer M, Franklin EC: Cryglobulinaemia – a study of 29 patients. Amer. J. Med. 40: 828, 1966.

101. Gross GP, Hathaway WE: Fetal erythrocyte deformability. Paediat. Res. 6: 593, 1972.

102. Baum RS: Hyperviscous blood and perinatal pathology Paediat. Res. 1: 288, 1967.

103. Aronson HB, Magora F, London M: The influence of Droperidol on blood viscosity in man. Brit. J. Anaesthes. 42: 1085, 1970.

104. Scholz PM, Karis JG, Gump FE, Kinney JM, Chein S: Correlation of blood rheology with vascular resistance in critically ill patients. J. appl. Physiol. 39: 1008, 1975.

105. Balas P, Bastounis E, Stamptopoulos CT, Lianov M: The influence of surgical trauma in blood viscosity. Angiology 25: 249, 1974.

106. Scholz PM, Kinney JM, Chein S: Effects of major abdominal operations on human blood rheology. Surgery 77: 351, 1975.

107. Aronson HB, Cotev S, Magora F, Borman JB: Blood viscosity and open heart surgery. Brit. J. Anaesthesia.

108. Bohmoutsos J, Morris T, Chavatzas D, Martin P: The influence of haemoglobin and platelet levels on the results of arterial surgery.

109. Burch GE, DePasquale NI: Haematocrit, viscosity and coronary blood flow. Dis. Chest. 48: 225, 1965.

110. Laks H, Pilon RN, Kloevekorn WP, Anderson W, MacCallum JR, O'Connor NE:: Acute hemodilution: its effect on hemodynamics and oxygen transport in anaesthetized man. Ann. Surg. 180: 103, 1974.

111. Kettler D, Hellberg K, Klaess G, Kontokollias JS, Loos W, de Vivie R: Haemodynamics, oxygen demand and oxygen uptake of the heart during isovolumic haemodilution. Anaesthetist, 25: 131, 1976.

112. Symposium. Dextran – 30 Years. Acta Universitatis Upsaliensis, Lewis D, Thoren L (eds), Uppsala, 1978.

113. Editorial: Plasmapheresis and immunosuppression. Lancet 22 May: 1113, 1976.

114. Talpos G, White JM, Horrocks M, Cotton LT: Plasmapheresis in Raynaud's disease. Lancet 1: 416–417, 1978.

115. Dormandy JA, Gutteridge JMC, Hoare E, Dormandy TL: Effect of clofibrate on blood viscosity in intermittent claudication. Brit med. J. 4: 259–262, 1974.

116. Wolf GK: Arvin in peripheral arterial circulatory disorders. Controlled multicentre trial. Europ. J. clin. Pharmacol. 9: 387, 1976.

117. Dormandy JA, Goyle KB, Reid HL: Treatment of severe intermittent claudication by controlled defibrination. Lancet 625–626, 1977.

118. Ehrly AH: Therapy of occlusive arterial diseases with ancrod. Artery 2: 98, 1976.

119. Postlethwaite JC, Goyle KB, Dormandy JA, Hynd JW: Improvement in experimental vascular graft patency by controlled defibrination. Brit. J. Surg. 64: 28–30, 1977.

120. Leeuwenhoek A: The Collected Letters of Antoni Van Leeuwenhoek. Vol. I, 1673–1676.

121. Dintenfass L: Viscosity of the packed white and red blood cells. Exp. molec. Pathol. 4: 597–605, 1965.

122. Dintenfass L: Internal viscosity of the red cell and a blood viscosity equation. Nature (Lond.) 219: 956, 1968.

123. Chien S, Usami J, Rowe AW: Rheological properties of red cells stored in liquid nitrogen. J. Lab. Clin. Med. 78: 175–180, 1970.

124. La Celle PL: Alteration of membrane deformability in haemolytic anaemias. Semin. Haematol. 7(4): 355–371, 1970.

125. La Celle PL, Weed RI: The contributions of normal and pathologic erythrocytes to blood. Progr. Haematol. 7: 1–37, 1971.

126. Rand, RP, Burton AC: Mechanical properties of the red cell membrane. 1. Membrane stiffness and intercellular pressure. Biophys. J. 4: 115–135, 1964.

127. Boyan CP, Underwood PS, William MD, Howland WS: The effects of operation, anaesthesia and plasma expanders on blood viscosity. Anaesthesiology 27: 279, 1966.

128. Sirs JA: The measurement of the haematocrit and flexibility of erythrocytes with a centrifuge. Biorheology 5: 1, 1968.

129. Rampling MW, Sirs JA: A survey of the variation of erythrocyte flexibility within a healthy population. Biorheology, 13: 101–105, 1976.

130. Swank RL, Davis E: Blood cell aggregation and screen filtration pressure. Circulation 33: 617, 1966.

131. Rosenmund MD, Binswanger MD, Straub PW: Oxidative injury to erythrocytes, cell rigidity and splenic hemolysis in hemodialyzed uremic patients. Ann. intern. Medicine 82: 460, 1975.

132. Protero J, Burton AC: The physics of blood flow in capillaries. The capillary resistance to flow. Biophys. J. 2: 199, 1962.

133. Gregersen MI, Bryant CA, Hammerle WE, Usami S, Chien S: Flow characteristics of human erythrocytes through polycarbonate sieves. Science 157: 825, 1967.

134. Schmid-Schönbein H, Volger E, Klose HJ, Weiss J: Blood microrheology and the development of 'stasis' in the microvasculature after injury. Advanc. Exp. Med. Biol. 33: 65, 1973.

135. Bessis M, Mohandas N: A diffractometric method for the measurement of cellular deformability. Blood Cells, 1: 307, 1975.

136. Schmid-Schönbein H, von Gosen J, Heinich L, Klose HJ, Volger E: A counter-rotating 'rheoscope chamber' for the study of the microrheology of blood cell aggregation by microscopic observation and microphotometry. Microvasc. Res. 6: 366, 1973.

137. Chien S, Usami S, Bertles JF: Abnormal rheology of oxygenated blood in sickle cell anaemia. J. clin. Invest. 49: 623, 1970.
138. LeBlond PF, La Celle PL, Weed RI: Cellular deformability: A possible determinant of the normal release of maturing erythrocytes from the bone marrow. Blood 37: 40, 1971.
139. Rifkind RZ, Danon D: Heinz body anaemia – an ultrastructural study. Blood 25(6): 885–896, 1965.
140. Miller LH, Usami S, Chien S: Alteration in the rheological properties of plasmodium knowlesi-infected red cells. A possible mechanism for capillary obstruction. J. clin. Invest. 50: 1451, 1971.
141. Wins P, Schonffeniels E: Studies on red cell ghost ATP-ase systems. Biochim. biophys. Acta (Amst.) 120: 341–350, 1966.

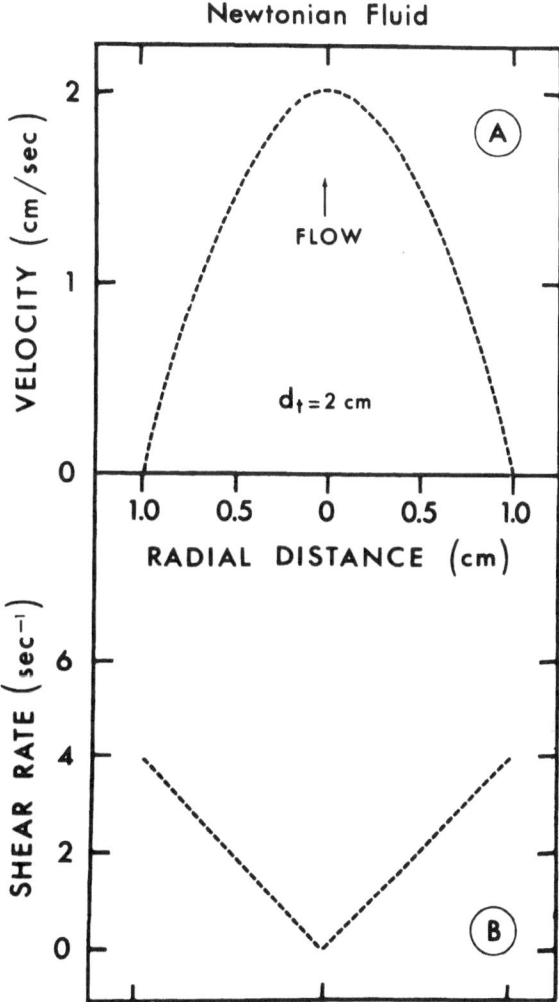

Fig. 1 to commentary. Flow of a Newtonian fluid between two parallel plates.

142. Weed RI, La Celle PL, Merrill EW: Metabolic dependence of red cell deformability. J. clin. Invest. 48: 795–809, 1969.

143. Schmid-Schönbein H, Weiss J, Ludwig H: A simple method for measuring red cell deformability in models of the microcirculation. Blut 26: 369-379, 1973.

144. Karle H, Handsen NE: Changes in the red cell membrane induced by a small rise in temperature. Scand. J. clin. Lab. Invest. 26: 169-174, 1970.

145. Weiss L: Studies on cell deformability. 1. Effect of surface change. J. Cell Biol. 26: 735, 1965.

146. Meiselman HJ: Flow behaviour of ATP-depleted human erythrocytes. Biorheology, 14: 111-126, 1977.

147. Goldsmith HL: Deformation of human red cells in tube flow. Biorrheology 7: 235, 1971.

148. Bessis M, Mohandas N: Deformability of normal, shape-altered and pathological red cells. Blood Cells 1: 315-321, 1975.

149. Rampling M, Sirs JA: The interactions of fibrinogen and dextrans with erythrocytes. J. Physiol. (Lond.) 223: 199, 1972.

150. Myers P, Rampling MW, Sirs JA: Interaction of Arvin with erythrocyte flexibility. J. Physiol. (Lond.) 230: 51P, 1972.

151. Schmid-Schönbein H, Wells R: Red cell aggregation and red cell deformation: Their influence on blood rheology in health and disease. Theoretical and Clinical Haemorheology. Mortent HH, Copley AL (eds) 1971.

152. Rampling MW: The flexibility and morphological reversibility of cells containing HbA or HbS after incubation. I.R.C.S. 2: 1637, 1974.

153. Charache S, Cowley CL: Rate of sickling of red cells during deoxygenation of blood from persons with various sickling disorders. Blood 24: 25, 1964.

154. Braasch D: Red cell deformability and capillary blood flow Physiol. Rev. 51: 679–701, 1971.

155. Reid HL, Dormandy JA, Barnes AJ, Lock PJ, Dormandy TL: Impaired red cell deformability in peripheral vascular disease. Lancet 666, 1977.

156. Nicolaides AN, Bowers R, Horbourne J, Kidner PH, Besterman EM: Blood viscosity, red-cell flexibility, haematocrit, and plasma fibrogen in patients with angina. Lancet, 5 Nov: 943, 1977.

REFERENCES TO COMMENTARY

1. Cokelet, In: Microcirculation, Grayson IJ, Zingg W (eds), New York, Plenum Press, 1976, Vol. 1, p 9–31.

2. Lipowsky HH, Usami S, Chien S: Microvasc. Res. 16: 153, 1978.

3. See ref. 10 in main text.

4. See ref. 21 in main text.

5. See ref. 56 in main text.

6. Chien S: Cardiovasc. Med. 2: 356, 1977.

7. Meiselman et al: Iaper presented at the IIIrd International Congress in Biorheology, La Tolla, CA, 1977.

9.   Diagnosis of deep vein thrombosis

VIJAY V. KAKKAR

Commentary by D.S. Sumner

1.   INTRODUCTION

Venous thromboembolism has become an increasingly important cause of disability and death during the past 50 years. There has also been a greater awareness of the ubiquity of the disease and of the possibility that we are experiencing an absolute as well as a relative increase in its occurrence.

One of the major difficulties in the management of deep vein thrombosis has been the lack of means for recognizing this condition. Several autopsy studies have shown that, in almost half the patients, there are no clinical signs or symptoms referable to the limbs and fatal embolism may be the first indication of thrombosis. The urgency of the physician's concern with venous thrombosis clearly lies in his inability to diagnose the condition accurately at an early stage, when treatment can be effective. During the past few years several diagnostic tools have become available, including the radioactive fibrinogen test, the ultrasonic technique, impedance plethysmography, radionuclide venography, and blood-coagulability assays. Improvements in the technique of venography have now reached a point where it can be relied upon as a reference standard for evaluating the accuracy of the new methods for detecting thrombi. It is now possible to determine the true incidence of this disease and to study its natural history with some precision. Attempts are being made to recognize individuals or groups of individuals at 'high risk' of developing deep vein thrombosis. It is now possible to evaluate the prophylactic efficacy of a number of choices either available or visible on the horizon, and the accepted methods of treatment are being challenged by several new drugs which are claimed to be significantly superior. There is real hope that the new knowledge arising from the use of improved diagnostic tools will help considerably in establishing a rational approach to the management of deep vein thrombosis. A brief outline of these new diagnostic techniques and how they may alter the management of this condition are presented in this article.

COMMENTARY

This introductory paragraph addresses the most critical issue in the field of venous thrombosis: the need for accurate, rapid and safe diagnostic techniques. Objective studies have uniformly demonstrated the fallibility of clinical diagnosis; which, because of its lack of sensitivity and specificity, cannot be relied upon to determine the necessity for treatment. Moreover, all reports in the literature that are based on clinical diagnosis alone must be viewed with skepticism. Vague histories, nonspecific symptoms, and physical signs that are often subtle, absent, or mimicked by other pathologic conditions account for the discrepancies. To support their position, the diminishing, but still vocal, ranks of those who defend clinical diagnosis usually cite the ease with which venous thrombosis is recognized in a diffusely swollen, cyanotic limb with tenderness over the femoral veins and with dilated superficial veins. Of course, most of these patients will have iliofemoral thrombosis, but not all! In fact, only 46–62% of those patients with clinical signs will actually have thrombi in their veins (1–3). When signs and symptoms are minimal, only 16% of suspected cases will have deep venous thrombosis (3). On the other hand, there may be no symptoms at all in 52–69% of limbs with venous thrombosis detected by the ^{125}I-fibrinogen uptake test (4, 5). Coon and Willis (6) found that a clinical diagnosis of venous thrombosis was made prior to death in only 19% of patients in whom the disease was demonstrated at autopsy.

2. FIBRINOGEN UPTAKE TEST (FUT)

The concept of using isotopes in the detection of venous thrombi was first introduced by Ambrus and others in 1957 (1), who produced radioactive thrombi in experimental animals by injecting ^{131}I-labeled fibrinogen followed by thrombin into artificially occluded vessel segments. Previously, McFarlane (2) had demonstrated that iodinated proteins are degraded at the same rate as the corresponding unlabeled protein. This led to the notion that fibrinogen, labeled with radioactive iodine, should behave in the same manner as endogenous fibrinogen, with normal conversion to fibrin under the action of thrombin. This hypothesis was first tested by Hobbs and Davies (3) in experimental animals, clearly demonstrating preferential uptake of ^{131}I-labeled fibrinogen by a forming thrombus and suggesting that such an approach might form the basis of a valuable clinical test for the detection of early venous thrombi. In 1964, Palko et al. (4) confirmed the earlier observations of Hobbs and Davies in experimental animals and in man. They were also able to show that ^{131}I-labeled fibrinogen was deposited in artificially induced thrombi in superficial veins; they then extended their experience of the technique to 75 patients (5). They did not, however, confirm their observations by venography.

In 1965, Atkins and Hawkins (6) introduced ^{125}I as an alternative to ^{131}I-labeled fibrinogen because of its many advantages. The isotope ^{125}I emits a soft gamma radiation; its longer half-life (60 days) leads to a greater differential between the thrombus and surrounding tissue, since catabolism of fibrinogen is unaffected by the isotope used; and lastly, the total body radiation with ^{125}I is less than that with ^{131}I. Although the thyroid gland receives a slightly higher dose, this is at a much slower rate. The only disadvantage is that tissue absorption with ^{125}I is greater than with ^{131}I; for example, at a depth of 3 cm, ^{131}I gives 50% of the surface count, whereas ^{125}I emits only 23%.

Flanc et al. (7) and, independently, Negus and his associates (8), in studies on postoperative patients and patients with a suspected deep venous thrombosis used venographic confirmation to establish the value of FUT for the detection of clinically silent thrombosis. However, the test at this stage was still very complicated; the equipment used for monitoring the radioactivity was heavy, cumbersome, and expensive. The test was simplified by Kakkar et al. (9), so that it could be adapted to screen a large number of patients and it could be performed at the patient's bedside.

2.1. *Preparation of fibrinogen*

Fibrinogen may be prepared by either Cohn fractionation or ammonium sulfate precipitation. The use of fibrinogen carries a small risk of transmitting serum hepatitis. This risk can be eliminated by using autologous fibrinogen, but this approach would limit widespread application of the test. Fibrinogen to be used, therefore, should be prepared from plasma obtained by repeated plasmapheresis of a small number of carefully screened donors. Such donors should meet the criteria established by strict biological standards. The recipients of fibrinogen prepared from such carefully selected donors must also be followed for at least 6 months to establish the fact that infusion of such material does not result in transmission of clinical or subclinical hepatitis, as demonstrated by acquisition of HAA, or induce an HAA antibody response in these recipients. We have now used FUT prepared in such manner in over 2500 patients and have not found evidence of clinical hepatitis after fibrinogen scanning.

2.2.   Labeling of fibrinogen

Fibrinogen can be radio-iodinated in several ways, including the iodine monochloride method (10), the chloramine-T method (11), the electrolytic method (12), and the enzymatic (lactoperioxidase) method (13). Physicochemical properties and kinetics of clearance from the circulation of canine fibrinogen labeled by these 4 methods have been investigated in detail (14), and it has been found that the iodine monochloride and enzymatic methods produce a more suitable labeled fibrinogen than either the chloramine-T or electrolytic method without significantly altering the molecule of fibrinogen. Furthermore, when the thrombus uptake of fibrinogen labeled by these 4 methods was compared in dogs, using a surgical model of venous thrombosis, the iodine monochloride preparations resulted in the greatest fibrinogen uptake and the highest thrombus-to-blood ratios (14).

2.3.   Dosimetry

The amount of radiation exposure has been calculated, following the injection of 100 μCi of ^{125}I-fibrinogen, to be approximately 200 mrem delivered to blood (15), 20 mrem to tissues (15), and 5 mrem to kidneys (16). This is less than the acceptable annual total body absorbed radiation dose (500 mrem/year) recommended for the general population by the British National Council on Radiation Protection.

Special studies have been preferred in antepartum (17) and postpartum patients (18) in order to determine the radiation risk to the fetus. Patients undergoing hysterotomy for termination of pregnancy and those with a known anencephalic fetus at term were given 100 μCi of ^{125}I-fibrinogen prior to delivery of the conceptus. After the death of the conceptus, samples of blood, amnionic fluid, placenta, and various fetal tissues were removed for determination of their radioactivity. The results showed no evidence that ^{125}I-fibrinogen crosses the placenta, but that free ^{125}I is present in small quantities. Table 1 shows the results obtained in one patient with a 15-week fetus, 3 days after the injection of 100 μCi of ^{125}I-fibrinogen to the mother. Although the amount of radioactivity to which the fetus is subjected is small, any extra activity to a developing fetus is undesirable.

Table 1. Concentration of radioactivity in the fetal tissues after administration of 100 μCi of ^{125}I-labeled fibrinogen to the mother.

Activity in μCi/g or ml (as appropriate)	
Fetal whole blood	0.00027
Fetal liver	0.00028
Fetal thyroid	0.017
Rest of fetus	0.003
Placenta	0.0074
Liquor amnii	0.00054
Maternal serum	0.0026
Maternal plasma	0.041

2.4.   Measurement of radioactivity

Immediately after intravenous injection of ^{125}I-labeled fibrinogen, a relatively higher radioactivity is present in the intravascular space. It is due to uneven distribution between intra- and extravascular spaces, as equilibrium is not complete.

Once the equilibrium is reached, 30% of labeled fibrinogen is confined to extravascular and 70% in the intravascular space. Under normal conditions the catabolic rate of ^{125}I-fibrinogen per 24 h is 15–20% for the extravascular and 25–30% for the intravascular space (19).

The radioactivity measured at leg surface is created by ^{125}I, free or bound to fibrinogen, fibrin, or fibrinogen degradation products and to that from the surrounding tissues, over an area which is free of thrombus; this activity, usually referred to as background activity, is built up by the intravascular and extravascular space, including the contribution of the lymphatic system. However, in an area overlying a developing thrombus, the surface radioacitivity is created by the intravascular and extravascular spaces, the thrombus and the phlebitic and periphlebitic reaction in the vein wall (Fig. 1). The rise in surface activity caused by a thrombus depends upon (1) the size of the thrombus, (2) the depth at which it is situated, and (3) the background activity. Adequate assessment of background activity is thus an essential basis for scan evaluation, which means

that preoperative measurements are mandatory in studies of post-operative thrombosis.

2.4.1. *Instrumentation used.*   The equipment used for measuring radioactivity consists of a detector system and a processing and display unit.
The detector system is composed of a sodium iodide crystal (thallium
activated) optically coupled to a photomultiplier. For measuring radioactivity, either a scaler or ratemeter can be used. The advantage of using a
scaler instrument is that measurement of radioactivity can proceed to a
predetermined number of counts, giving a predetermined measurement
error.

With a scaler, counts of a standard source of ^{125}I and of background
radioactivity are first taken; these are essential for the calculation of daily
machine variations. The radioactivity at the marked positions (Fig. 2) on
the thighs and calves is then recorded, as well as at the positions marked

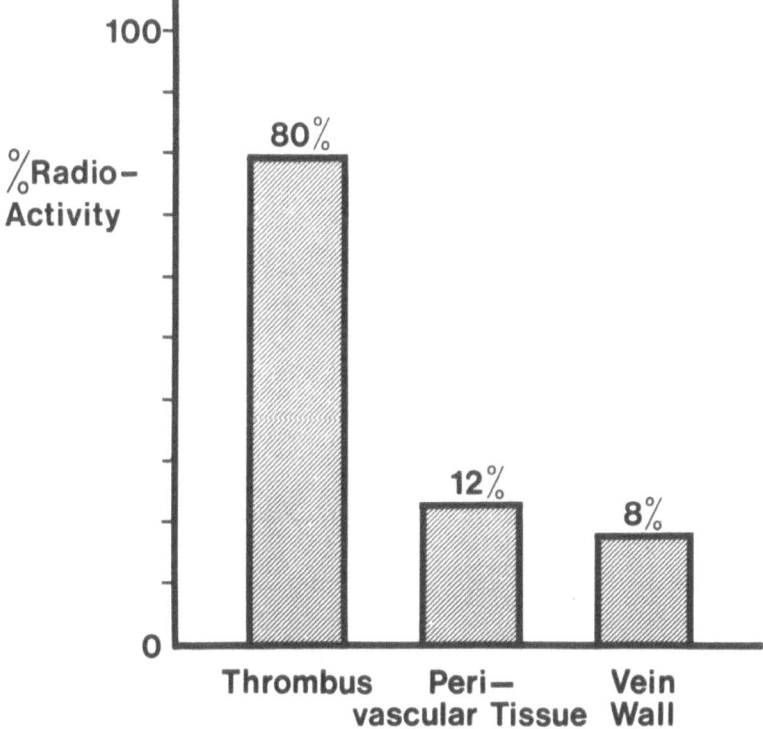

Fig. 1. ^{125}I-fibrinogen/fibrin radioactivity contained in a thrombus and contributed leg vein
wall and perivascular tissue. The figures represent the means of 8 thrombi which were
removed at autopsy. Radioactivity is expressed as a percentage of equal weight of blood
radioactivity.

over the heart. Three 10-sec counts are always obtained. Finally, the standard source and background are counted again. The results can be expressed as either absolute counts or as a percentage of heart counts in the manner described by Negus and his co-workers (8).

The ratemeter is switched on and the current provided by the two batteries is tested; the ^{125}I channel is then selected on the channel switch, and the CPS/per cent switch set to the position marked 'per cent'. The scintillation probe is adjusted to maximum or minimum depth, depending on the count rate; the probe is then placed over the heart (fourth left intercostal space just lateral to the sternal edge), and the range control adjusted until near full scale readings are obtained on the scale. The 'set per cent' control is adjusted so that the reading is exactly on the 100% mark.

With the machine adjusted to record the heart radioactivity as 100%, the probe is placed over each of the marked positions; as the collimator is placed over the limb, the 'fast constant' switch is turned on. Once the scale needles have settled, the 'slow constant' switch is turned on, and this helps to stabilize the needle. The reading obtained from the linear scale of the instrument is automatically represented as a percentage of the heart

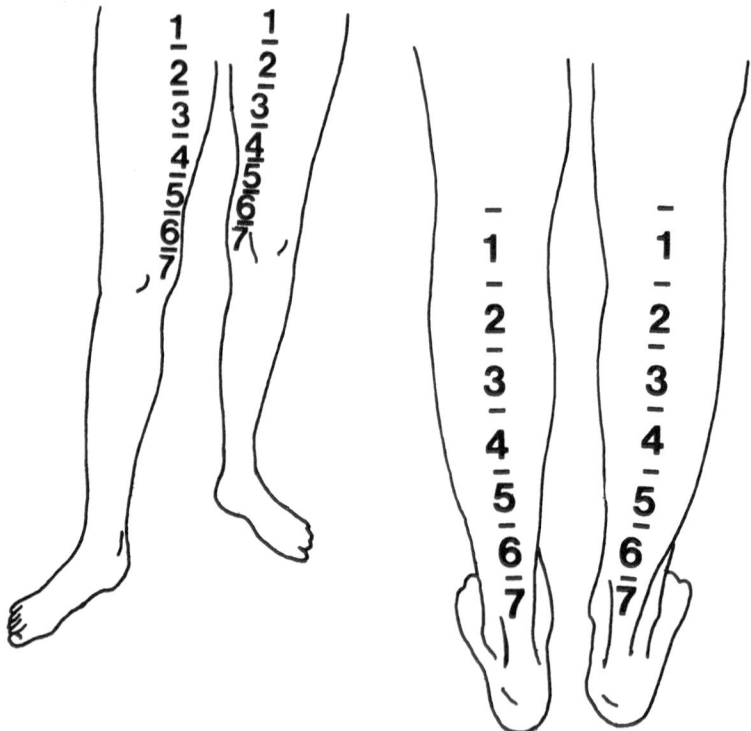

Fig. 2. Positions at which radioactivity is measured. These are marked at 2 in. intervals and counts are recorded over each position.

counts, and no calculation is necessary. Without moving the collimator away from the skin surface, it is gently slid to the next position and radioactivity recorded in the same manner. After counting one limb, the probe is again placed over the heart to check for any 'drift' in the machine.

2.4.2. *Test procedure.* The test can be used in every type of patient: surgical, orthopedic, obstetric, and medical. In surgical patients, the thyroid gland is blocked by sodium iodide (100 mg) given orally, in order to prevent excessive uptake of radioactive iodine. Twentyfour hours later, on the day before operation, 100 μCi of ^{125}I-fibrinogen is injected. Similarly, in medical patients, those with myocardial infarction for example, the thyroid gland can be blocked as soon as the patient is confined to bed. ^{125}Iodine-fibrinogen (100 μCi) is injected into an arm vein, and the radioactivity over the legs is measured 4 h later. Patients are scanned with their legs elevated 15–20° to minimize venous pooling in calf veins. Counting is carried out before operation, and this is taken as a baseline for comparison with subsequent counts. Radioactivity is again measured thereafter at daily intervals. In practice, it is probably sufficient to obtain counts preoperatively and on the first, third, and sixth postoperative days; if there are indications of a forming thrombus, then counting can be performed daily to see whether the thrombus is increasing in size or dissolving.

The statement that the FUT can be used in every type of patient is a bit broad. For example, patients with leg wounds or those who have undergone surgical procedures to the legs are not good candidates (8). Casts on the legs may decrease the counts. Moreover, in the United States, Abbott laboratories issues a warning that the drug should not be administered to children, pregnant patients, or to nursing mothers unless the expected benefits to be gained outweigh the potential risks. The medical letter (20: 63, 1978) states that iodides can cause both hypothyroidism and hyperthyroidism in elderly patients.

In Hume's (9) experience, the FUT first became positive after the sixth day in 48% of the patients. Most of the serious thrombi (72%) occurred during the second or third week in his series of patients undergoing hip reconstruction. Therefore, it would seem unwise to limit the test to the first 6 postoperative days.

2.5. *Criteria for diagnosis of deep vein thrombosis*

Several criteria have been advocated to diagnose deep vein thrombosis (DVT); these are based on comparison of the findings of venography. The primary aim is to determine whether a significant local increase in radioactivity and the different apparatus used require different diagnostic standards.

To assess a change in relative increase in radioactivity at a given point, it can be compared either to an adjacent point on the same leg, or to a corresponding point on the opposite leg, or to earlier measurements of the point iself. As discrepancies between the legs may be present, comparisons with points in the same limb are likely to produce more accurate results.

2.5.1. *Absolute counts in the limbs expressed as a percentage of the heart count.* Absolute counts of leg positions are expressed as a percentage of the heart counts and plotted against the thigh and calf positions. Only patients who had been examined by venography with unequivocal positive or negative results were included in this analysis. A total of 105 patients met these criteria for inclusion. The maximum count difference detected was used in compilation of these data. These values were then separated into two groups according to the positive or negative venographic results.

The count differences (corresponding sites) in the group with positive venography and in the group with negative venography are shown in Fig. 3. The point at which the two curves intersect (Δ 18%) represents the count difference at which incorrectly positive and incorrectly negative fibrinogen test results are minimal. The discrepancy between the fibrinogen test and venography could be explained by the fact that even with the recent modifications in the technique, it is doubtful if venography will ever show all small thrombi confined to the muscular veins of the calf, and these can be easily detected by fibrinogen test.

2.5.2. Radioactivity of the limbs expressed as percentage of heart counts. In order to determine the criteria that could be used for diagnosing DVT when a ratemeter is used, the results were compared in 40 patients (20 with and 20 without DVT) randomly selected from a group of patients who had

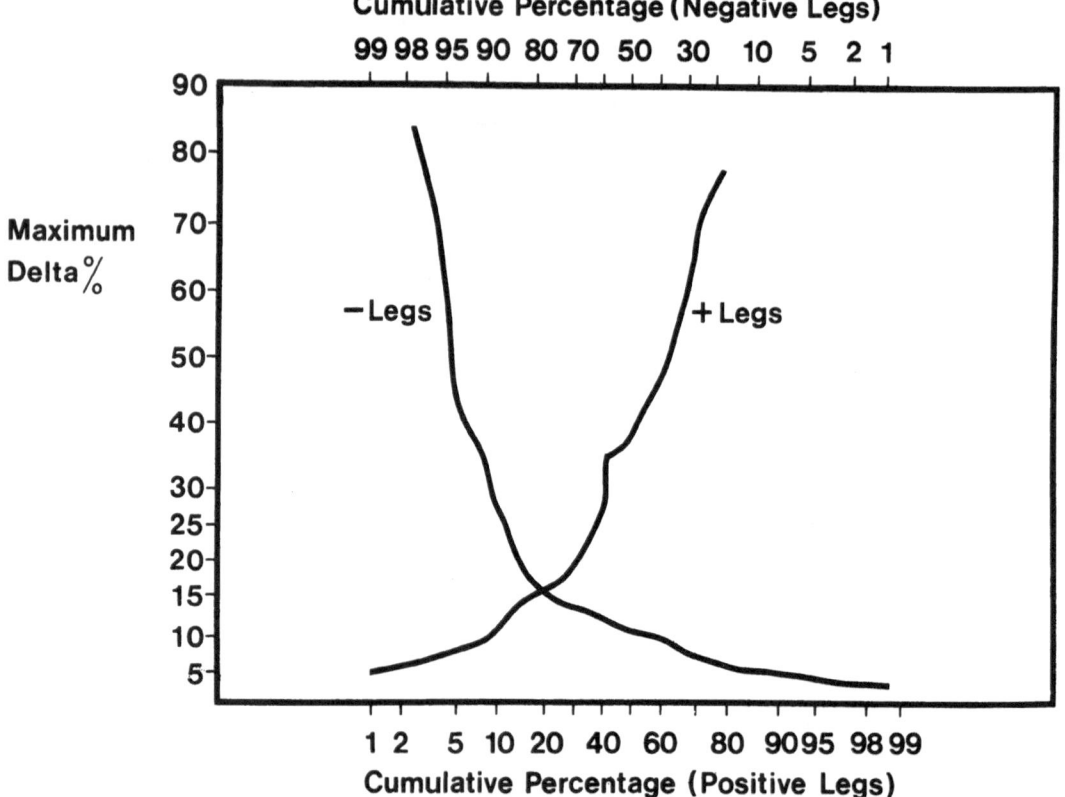

Fig. 3. The count differences in the group with positive and negative venographic results. The point at which the two curves intersect (18%) represents the count difference at which incorrectly positive and incorrectly negative fibrinogen test results are maximal.

been investigated with the scaler and the ratemeter, with the use of venography to confirm the presence or absence of thrombi. The data from these patients were expressed as a percentage of heart counts, and the percentage increase in radioactivity at the site of thrombosis on the day the diagnosis was noted. In patients who had no thrombosis the maximum rise in percentage at any position during the whole scanning period was also noted.

When the percentage increase in these readings was plotted against the number of patients, it was found that in all normal limbs the maximum percentage increase in radioactivity was never greater than 20. However, whenever a thrombosis was present, the increase was greater than 30% on the day of diagnosis, using the criteria of rises in the ratio of the ΔZ being greater than 0.05. Based on these observations, a criterion for diagnosing a thrombus was defined as an increase of 20 in the percentage reading on any day, compared with the reading at the same position on the previous day, provided this increase persisted for more than 24 h. However, Beeker (20), as well as Browse et al. (21), found radiologically identifiable thrombi at points where only a 5% increase in relative activity was demonstrated. Even if identical thrombi were formed at the same depth in different patients, the surface counts over these thrombi would differ between the patients, due to variations in the background activity. Therefore, although the fibrinogen test is an objective method of diagnosis, it requires a degree of objective assessment. Most patients considered to have a thrombus show an unequivocal scan, with a rise in relative activity of 40%–120% or more.

It is obvious from Fig. 3 that the selection of 20% change in radioactivity is the optimum point of division between positive and negative results. Although shifting the point to 15% would increase the sensitivity of the study, it would decrease its specificity. In the series reported by Morris and Mitchell (10), the sensitivity was 81% and the specificity was 100% when the 20% criterion was used; but when 15% was used, the sensitivity increased only slightly to 87% and the specificity fell to 87%.

2.6. Source of errors

Several factors may produce false-positive results, and these must be excluded by clinical examination of the limbs before analyzing the results of scans. Conditions that lead to accumulation of fibrinogen, fibrin, or degradation products (FDP), such as hematoma formation, gross edema, inflammatory reactions, incisions, arthritis, and ulcerations following bone fracture may give false-positive results. Although superficial thrombophlebitis may be associated with a phlebothrombosis in the deep veins, the results of scans in such patients should be interpreted with caution. Similar care should be taken in analyzing the results in the presence of varicose veins. Some areas showing especially high background activity, due to varicose veins, give a more variable relative activity from day to day, probably because of differing quantities of blood in the veins on different occasions, in spite of attempts to empty the veins prior to scanning.

After the injection of ^{125}I-fibrinogen, the period over which the level of

These deficits must not be passed over lightly. A high percentage of patients suspected of having or at risk of developing deep venous thrombosis will have one or more of the conditions listed.

Moreover, warfarin therapy may significantly reduce the accuracy of the test. Browse et al. (11) found 60% false negative studies in limbs after 6 days of warfarin treatment.

Fortunately, the distortions produced by ^{99m}Tc-albumin should be relatively brief, since this isotope has a short half-life. Usually, the FUT procedure can be re-instituted within 24–48 h.

radioactivity is sufficient to allow accurate counting depends to a large extent on the metabolic half-life of administered fibrinogen, which has been shown to be 3–4 days (22), and the 60-day physical half-life of ^{125}I. In practice, after the initial injection of 100 μCi of radioactive fibrinogen, counting is usually possible for 7–8 days. For a more prolonged period of scanning, additional injections of fibrinogen must be given. Low initial heart counts are due to the denatured fibrinogen molecule tagged to ^{125}I; when such radiolabeled fibrinogen is injected intravenously, large quantities of free ^{125}I released are excreted in the urine. Low initial precordial counts, therefore, require the administration of further labeled fibrinogen if scanning is to produce a valid conclusion. Unexpectedly high heart counts suggest that another isotope has been given to the patient. For example, labeled albumin for lung scanning in such a situation will produce erroneous results. ^{125}I-fibrinogen may also be accumulated in a myocardial infarct, thus giving a high precordial count.

Care should be taken to avoid the contamination of the collimator by radioactive urine; this can easily occur in patients who have some degree of urinary incontinence, or due to lack of care in handling the collimator probe.

These results are indeed impressive. From the data presented in Table 2, it is apparent that the sensitivity from both the limb (119 positive FUT's/121 positive phlebograms) and the patient series (96 positive FUT's/98 positive phlebograms) was 98%, implying that almost all developing thrombi were detected. However, the specificity was not quite so good, that of the limb series being only 74% (34 negative FUT's/46 negative phlebograms). Stated in another way, 26% of all radiologically negative limbs would be called positive by the FUT. As Browse et al. (11) point out, it is possible that clots were actually present in these limbs but were *too small or too remote* to be detected by X-ray; but this is an assumption that has not been proved. Kerrigan et al. (12) have demonstrated experimentally that thrombi incorporating ^{125}I-fibrinogen may lyse sufficiently to yield a negative phlebogram even though local radioactivity persists. Nevertheless, Harris et al. (13) used similar arguments to explain the opposite finding. In their study, three small fresh

2.7. Accuracy of the fibrinogen test

Although the precise establishment of the presence and extent of venous thrombosis requires detailed autopsy examination, improvements in venography technique have now reached a point where it can be relied upon as a reference standard for evaluating the accuracy of new methods for detecting thrombi.

The accuracy of the radioactive fibrinogen test in diagnosing deep vein thrombosis has now been confirmed by several workers (Table 2); it is apparent that there is a remarkably close agreement between the ^{125}I-fibrinogen technique and venography, with 92% agreement in the limb series and 94% in the patient series. False-positive ^{125}I-fibrinogen results were found in 9% of limbs and 7% of patients (Table 2). As already mentioned, it may be that these represent small calf vein thrombi which were not detected by venography. False-negative ^{125}I-fibrinogen results occurred in 6% of limbs and 4% of patients; these might be explained as static or resolving thrombi that have not incorporated ^{125}I-fibrinogen, but which are radiologically detectable. The summation of data from these studies leads to the inescapable conclusion that the fibrinogen test has a very high sensitivity and specificity and will detect the vast majority of venous thrombi.

Table 2. Correlation of venographic findings with the ^{125}I-fibrinogen test in reported series.

Reference	Leg scan positive		Leg scan negative	
	Positive phlebogram	Negative phlebogram	Positive phlebogram	Negative phlebogram
Flanc et al.	17	1	0	0
Negus et al.	24	2	0	3
Kakkar et al.	39*	1*	0	0
Lambie et al.	40	2	2	16
Pinto	20	2	0	3
Milne et al.	18	5	0	12
Bonnar and Walsh	15*	0*	0	0
Kakkar	32*	4*	2*	50*
Hume and Gurewich	10	2	0	0
Total limbs	19	12	2	34
Total patients	96*	7*	2	50*

* The numbers of patients rather than limbs.

2.8. Potential limitation of fibrinogen test

An important limitation of the fibrinogen test is its inability to detect thrombi in the pelvic veins and, to a lesser extent, in the upper third of thigh veins. Diagnosis by this method depends on a sufficient difference between the radioactivity in the thrombus and its surrounding background. In the pelvis, the proximity of the bladder containing radioactive urine or large arteries and other vascular structures gives an increased background count, which makes the test less reliable in these situations. The failure of the test to detect iliac vein thrombosis is clearly a disadvantage, but it is of little clinical significance because thrombi rarely start in this region. It is unusual for thrombosis to occur in the thigh or pelvis without concurrent thrombosis of the calf veins, except in patients undergoing total hip replacement. Secondly, the test cannot be used in patients in whom surgery is being performed over the limbs, but this does not include those having total hip replacement or surgery for fracture of the neck of femur. There are a number of situations where the use of ^{125}I-fibrinogen is contra-indicated. It should be avoided during pregnancy and lactation and, possibly, in younger patients below the age of 40.

2.9. Clinical significance of isotopic thrombi

The evidence that the fibrinogen uptake test is an accurate method for detecting thrombi in the deep veins of the lower limbs is irrefutable. However, it has been suggested that such thrombi are of little or no clinical significance. It is not known whether treatment of isotopic thrombi, de-

thrombi lying in the distal thigh were not detected by the FUT. They suggested that the thrombi were *too small* to produce the necessary accumulation of radioactivity. Can we have it both ways? Is it valid to explain false-positive and false-negative results by the same mechanism?

It is curious that the patient specificity in Table 2 (88%, 50 negative FUTs/57 negative phlebograms) was considerably better than the limb specificity, implying that some of the false-positive studies were in legs of the same patients in whom the other leg was positive by phlebography. Although this evidence could be construed as supporting the contention of Browse et al. (11), other explanations are, of course, possible.

Approximately two-thirds of all emboli originate from the iliac or femoral veins, and most fatal emboli have their origin in these segments (14). For this reason, it is important to examine carefully the statement that 'it is unusual for thrombosis to occur in the thigh or pelvis without concurrent thrombosis of the calf veins...'. While it is true that isolated iliac vein thrombi are rare, occurring in less than 1% of cases (15, 16), an appreciable number of ilio-femoral thromboses develop in the absence of radiologically demonstrable calf or popliteal vein thrombi (3.4%, Stamatakis et al. (17); 14%, Nicolaides and O'Connell (16); 38% Diener (15)). It is possible that phlebography, being a static assessment, fails to detect early calf thrombi that have lysed by the time that the iliofemoral thrombus develops. On the other hand, FUT, when used prospectively, may detect these transient calf vein thrombi and alert the clinician to the possible development of the more serious proximal disease. Nevertheless, attention to detail, careful followup, and supplementary means of diagnosis are necessary in order to avoid missing a significant number of thrombi in the iliofemoral segment when FUT is used for screening.

Mavor et al. (18) state: 'Its (FUT) routine use as some form of early warning system is not likely to be satisfactory. A positive finding is unlikely to be of clinical significance except in a few cases, and a negative finding will not necessarily exclude the probability of subsequent embolism or serious venous insufficiency from iliofemoral involvement.' They reviewed 72 cases where embolism was the initial sign of deep venous thrombosis. In only one of 6 cases showing a positive peripheral scan was the source considered to be the deep veins below the knee.

Of 11 deaths in the series reported by Gruber et al. (19) 8 had negative fibrinogen tests during the first postoperative week. This prompted them to state '... that one can die from fatal pulmonary embolus even though a fibrinogen test had been negative a couple of hours earlier.' Doouss (20) reviewed 176 limbs with positive scans. In 84% there was spontaneous lysis; in 7 propagation occurred to proximal segments; and only two had pulmonary emboli, both nonfatal. Cranley (21) considers minor intravascular clotting in the calf veins to be a part of life and points out that these clots are regularly dissolved by the fibrinolytic process. Unless thrombi reach a major vein, he feels that they have little clinical significance.

In contrast, Moreno-Cabral et al. (22) in a phlebographic study found that popliteal thrombi had an incidence of embolism of 66% and tibial thrombi had an incidence of 33%. Four of 9 tibial emboli involved greater than 20% of the total lung volume. Unfortunately, this study suffers from the fact that most of the patients had symptomatic deep venous thrombosis or were already known to have pulmonary emboli. Moreover, the

tected at an early stage in the development of the disease, also reduces the mortality due to pulmonary embolism. Therefore, the most direct way of assessing the clinical significance of such thrombi would be to determine whether treatment of the scan-detected thrombi would reduce the mortality due to pulmonary embolism.

The relationship between leg scanning and postoperative pulmonary embolism was investigated by Kakkar et al. (23), observing 132 consecutive surgical patients. They found no pulmonary emboli in 92 patients with negative leg scans and no emboli in 31 patients with scan evidence of calf vein thrombosis, but 4 pulmonary emboli were observed in 9 patients in whom proximal extension of the calf vein thrombosis occurred. Similarly, Scottish researchers (24) studied 386 surgical patients and found on pulmonary emboli among 292 patients with normal leg scans, but they detected pulmonary embolism in 8 of 94 scan-positive patients. The diagnosis of pulmonary embolism was confirmed by perfusion lung scanning in two patients, at necropsy in two others, but in 4 the diagnosis was based on clinical evidence alone. Similar results have been reported by several other workers (Table 3). Of 410 patients who had positive scans, 24 developed clinical evidence of pulmonary embolism, while 1 out of 1351 patients with negative scans developed this complication.

In other studies, objective methods have been used to diagnose the presence of pulmonary emboli. Browse et al. (25) used routine pre- and postoperative ventilation and perfusion lung scans and chest X-rays to diagnose postoperative pulmonary embolism in 40 surgical patients studied with ^{125}I-fibrinogen leg scanning. The diagnosis of pulmonary embolism was made without previous knowledge of the leg scan result. Pulmonary embolism was diagnosed in 6 of 11 patients with positive leg scans, but only in 1 of 29 patients with negative leg scans. However, different results have been reported by other workers (26).

Table 3. Reported incidence of pulmonary embolism in a group of patients who had a negative or positive leg scan following major elective surgery.

Reference	Positive leg scan	Pulmonary embolism	Negative leg scan	Pulmonary embolism
Murray et al.	13	4	37	0
Pinto	17	0	37	0
Williams	16	0	40	0
Rosengarten and Laird	8	1	17	0
Kakkar	248	9	687	0
Warlow et al.	18	4	12	0
Gordon-Smith et al.	32	1	118	1
Handley et al.	7	2	41	0
Bonnar and Walsh	16	1	246	0
Hills et al.	35	2	116	0
Total	410	24	1351	1

Further evidence regarding the clinical significance of isotopic thrombi is provided by a retrospective analysis of the incidence of fatal pulmonary embolism, as proved by autopsy, in two groups of surgical patients undergoing major elective operations. In one group, the FUT was used as a screening procedure to detect early thrombi and their extension, while, in the other group, no specific screening procedure was used, and treatment was based on the presence of clinical features suggestive of DVT. These patients formed th control group in a multicenter trial designed to assess the efficacy of low-dose heparin in preventing postoperative fatal pulmonary embolism; 2046 patients over the age of 40 years, undergoing only major elective surgical procedures, were included in this analysis. In 667 of these patients, the FUT was used to detect the development of DVT; these constituted the screened group, while, in the remaining 1409 patients, no specific screening procedure was employed, and these constituted the nonscreened group. The incidence of fatal pulmonary embolism as proved by autopsy was determined in both groups. In the nonscreened group, a clinical diagnosis of DVT was made in 72 patients (5.1%); while 164 patients (24.6%) in the screened group developed DVT; 9.5% of the screened patients and 4.1% of the nonscreened patients received heparin and/or anticoagulant drugs as treatment for DVT. One hundred patients died during the postoperative period, 29 (4.3%) in the screened group and 71 (5.0%) in the nonscreened group. Twenty-two of the patients who died were found at postmortem to have had pulmonary emboli: 19 in the nonscreened group and 3 in the screened group. Only one patient with the negative leg scan in the screened group died from pulmonary embolism (PE). There were two additional patients in the screened group with PE, one fatal and one nonfatal; both had positive leg scans several days before death, but did not receive treatment with anticoagulants. In contrast, 19 patients in the nonscreened group were found at autopsy to have PE: 14 fatal and 5 nonfatal. The difference in the incidences of fatal PE between the two groups is statistically significant (p < 0.05) and can be explained on the basis of treatment of early thrombi detected by the FUT. These results were reported in detail elsewhere by Kakkar and Corrigan in 1972 (27). From the findings of this study, it can be argued that thrombi which give rise to PE originate in the peripheral veins of the lower limbs, since early detection and treatment of those thrombi significantly reduce the incidence of fatal PE.

2.10. Clinical applications of FUT

The introduction of this relatively simple technique for the acccurate detection of DVT in the veins of the leg has provided an impetus to the study of the incidence, pathogenesis, prevention, and treatment of venous thrombosis.

phlebograms were not all of diagnostic quality in the iliac system.

Browse and Clemenson (23) found that 21% of patients with positive FUT had aches and pains in their legs and 23% had swelling when examined $3\frac{1}{2}$ years later. This suggests that chronic venous insufficiency is a common sequel of isotopically demonstrated deep venous thrombosis of the calf, since in 54 of the 61 limbs the isotopic abnormalities were confined to the calf.

The data in Table 3 clearly establish the association of pulmonary embolism and positive leg scans. This is to be expected based on the known propensity of iliofemoral venous thromboses, which are quite dangerous, to be associated with the generally benign calf vein thrombosis (15–17). The FUT is, therefore, quite sensitive (24/25 or 96%) but not highly specific (1350/1736 or 78%) for serious disease.

Undeniably, the wealth of information accumulated from the use of ^{125}I-fibrinogen scanning has contributed immensely to our understanding of venous disease, particularly in surgical patients. However, the relationship of the clots that appear within the first 24 h following operation to those that result in serious pulmonary emboli (most of which occur during or after the second week) has not been clearly established. Moreover, to conduct these studies routinely on 'high-risk' patients undergoing surgery would be prohibitively expensive, at least in the United States (21). Cranley (21) estimates a cost of $ 200 per patient screened, excluding any other test or therapy that might prove to be necessary. If we use the data in Table 3 as representative of the number of pulmonary emboli that could potentially be avoided by early detection of venous thrombi, the cost per pulmonary embolus would be approximately $ 15,000.

Hirsh and Hull (8) noted that 20% of all thrombi that develop following hip surgery are isolated to the femoral vein in the vicinity of the surgical wound. In patients undergoing hip replacement, they found that the FUT detected 20 of 43 (47%) of the popliteal or femoral vein thromboses and 33 of 40 (83%) of the calf vein thromboses. Harris et al. (13) found that the FUT detected only 16 of 40 (40%) fresh post-operative thrombi and only 25 of 43 (58%) of those developing away from the wound area. Moreover, they failed to detect 8 fresh thrombi forming in the wound area (none of which was associated with thrombi in the calf) and three distal thigh clots.
   Hume (9) used both FUT and IPG in a prospective study of patients undergoing hip reconstruction. In 56% of the patients, both tests were negative; and the incidence of pulmonary embolism was only 1%. When the FUT alone was positive (19% of the patients), pulmonary emboli occurred in 11%. Phlebography showed no clots in 67%, minute

2.10.1. *Value of FUT as a routine screening procedure in patients under-going general surgery.*   Using FUT as a routine screening procedure in a large number of 'high risk' nonorthopaedic surgical patients, a number of prospective studies have shown that the disease occurs quite frequently in older patients undergoing major abdominal or thoracic surgery (Table 4). The incidence of DVT has been reported to be in the ranges of 25–30%, and it has been found that about 50% of thrombosis became apparent within the first 24 h after surgery. Most scan abnormalities (approximately 89%) are limited to the calf region and are not associated with any clinical signs of thrombosis. Only infrequently (approximately 10%) are raised counts first detected in the popliteal fossa or over the lower thigh region in patients undergoing major elective abdominal or thoracic operations.
   The effects of various predisposing factors on the incidence of venous thrombosis, as diagnosed by the ^{125}I-fibrinogen technique, have been studied and have confirmed that advancing age, obesity, previous venous thrombo-embolism, varicose veins, and malignancy increase the likeli-hood of developing venous thrombosis (28). The other factors such as the type of operation, the use of prophylactic antibiotics, or the development of postoperative infection also affect the incidence of postoperative DVT (24).

2.10.2. *Patients undergoing hip surgery.*   These patients require special consideration for two main reasons: first, the counts are invariably raised over the surgical wound due to accumulation of radioactive fibrin and fibrinogen in the hematoma, the extent of which may vary considerably. Second, it has been shown recently (30, 31), that these patients have a very high incidence of isolated femoral vein thrombosis without concomitant calf vein thrombosis.
   However, the FUT is an accurate and reliable method for detecting thrombi in patients who are being operated for fractures of the neck of femur because these patients do not have a high incidence of proximal

Table 4. Incidence of DVT detected by ^{125}I-fibrinogen test in various groups of patients

Type of patients	No. studied	Developed DVT (%)
Surgical patients (over 40 years)	1084	25
Urologic (prostatectomy)	85	27
Gynecologic (hysterectomy)	126	22
Orthopedic (fracture of femoral neck)	150	50
Myocardial infarction	127	17
Geriatric	80	30
Obstetric (postpartum)	100	3
Total	1752	

femoral vein thrombosis. A comparison was made of FUT and phlebography in 50 consecutive patients who sustained subcapital or pertrochanteric fractures of the femoral neck (32). Twenty-seven (54%) developed DVT confirmed by phlebography; each of these was detected by FUT. Similar results have been reported by other workers (Table 5).

Table 5. Correlation of venographic findings with leg scanning in patients undergoing hip surgery.

| References | Thrombosis at venography if leg scan | | Overall agreement |
	Abnormal	Normal	
Field et al.	29/36	2/27	54/63 (86%)
Bergquist et al.	14/21	4/36	46/57 (81%)
Myrvoid et al.	25/29	3/53	75/82 (92%)
Harris et al.	25/29	26/51	67/88 (76%)

2.10.3. *Medical and postpartum patients.* FUT has also been used in medical and postpartum patients to detect the development of early and forming thrombi. The lowest incidence (3%) has been detected in postpartum women (18). Among medical patients, the incidence following myocardial infarction has been found to vary between 19% and 37% (33, 34). In paralysed legs of patients with recent cerebrovascular accidents, the incidence of DVT was found to be 60% (35).

2.10.4. *Natural history of DVT.* Few physicians would deny that venous thrombosis, difficult though it may be to diagnose, is also a common and benign disease. The extent to which intravascular thrombi may dissolve spontaneously is not yet known. Furthermore, information has not in the past been available regarding the types of thrombi that are safe and free of complications and those that may give rise to pulmonary emboli or are likely to damage valves and lead to the development of the postphlebitic syndrome. Using FUT and phlebography, it has been shown that, in surgical patients, the majority of thrombi form in the calf veins; a surprisingly high proportion of these remain confined to this region and undergo spontaneous lysis, and only in a small number do thrombi extend more proximally into the major veins. Of 667 surgical patients who were screened for the development of DVT, FUT detected thrombi in 164 (24.6%). In 47 patients the thrombi were bilateral and 38% of these developed within 48 hours of surgery. In a further 51% of patients thrombi developed between the third and sixth postoperative days, and in 9% after the seventh postoperative day. In 49 patients, the thrombus extended into the femoral vein (Fig. 4). It was difficult to accurately estimate the inci-

thrombi in 29%, and moderately extensive disease in 4%. When both the FUT and IPG were positive (25% of the patients), the incidence of pulmonary embolus was 20%. In these patients, the extent of thrombosis shown phlebographically was zero in 12%, minute in 15%, moderate in 30%, and extensive in 42%.

The observations of Morris and Mitchell (10) are consistent with those of Hume. Although they concluded that thigh scanning was not reliable either on the side of the fractured hip or on the non-injured side, thrombosis in the lower leg veins was invariably present in all patients with thrombi in the thigh. The disparity in these results is disturbing. While some investigators report good sensitivity and specificity with the FUT in patients undergoing hip surgery (Table 5), others clearly have not had such good fortune. At this point, it would be premature to predict what the potential role of FUT will be in screening this particular group of patients.

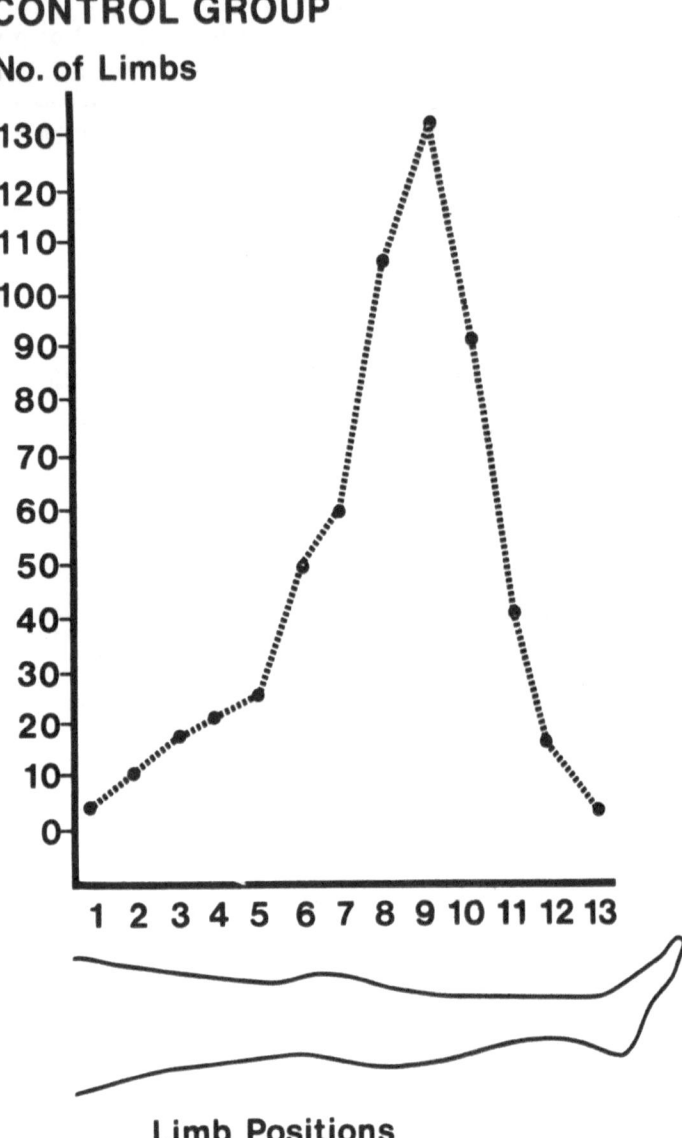

CONTROL GROUP

Fig. 4. Distribution and extent of isotopic thrombi in 164 patients with positive leg scans; in 49 patients, the thrombus extended into the proximal veins above the knee region.

dence of pulmonary embolism in this group of patients because all the patients with extending thrombi received full doses of heparin followed by oral anticoagulants. However, we have already shown (25) that, in a group of patients with extending thrombosis in the popliteal and femoral veins, minor pulmonary embolism occurs in approximately 50%, with only a small proportion proving fatal. Recent studies, using perfusion and ventilation lung scanning, have shown that minor pulmonary emboli may even occur in patients where the thrombotic process is confined to the calf veins only (25).

With regard to the long-term effects, i.e., the postphlebitic syndrome, the significance of isotopic thrombi has yet to be clearly demonstrated.

2.10.5. *Use of FUT in trials of prophylaxis of venous thrombosis.*   The FUT with its high diagnostic specificity and sensitivity has proved the most valuable tool in trials of prophylaxis of venous thrombosis.

The test has been used to evaluate the prophylactic effect of elastic stockings, leg elevation, and physiotherapy, electrical stimulation of the calf, intermittent calf compression, automatic foot movers, conventional anticoagulations, dextran, subcutaneous heparin and aspirin.

Although many of these trials have shown that the agent tested is effective in reducing the incidence of isotopic DVT, they provide no information of the important complications of pulmonary embolism. Furthermore, the reported incidence of fatal PE in surgical patients is approximately 1% (36), and there is no proof that these do not belong to 5–7% of patients who are not protected by a specific prophylactic agent.

Because of its extreme sensitivity to developing calf vein thrombi, the FUT permits prospective clinical studies of prophylactic measures to reach statistical significance in relatively small numbers of patients. This is perhaps the most important application of the ^{125}I-fibrinogen scan.

2.10.6. *Role in the detection of established venous thrombosis.*   The usefulness of the FUT in confirming the diagnosis of patients who present with suggestive symptoms and signs has also been investigated in two recent studies. In one study (37), 82 patients who presented with clinical DVT were arbitrarily classified into three groups with signs of minor, major or massive thrombosis. Diagnosis of venous thrombosis was confirmed by phlebography.

Of 102 limbs examined, there was concordance between the radioactive fibrinogen test and phlebography in 77 limbs (75.5%) while in 25 limbs (24.5%) the results did not agree. In 13 limbs, the radioactive fibrinogen test gave false-positive results; in these limbs, phlebograms were negative, and, subsequently, it was found that these patients suffered from conditions such as rupture of muscle fibers in the calf, hematoma within the calf, infection in that region, or arthritic knee joints. Two patients with signs of massive thrombosis were, in fact, in congestive cardiac failure, and exacerbation of symptoms in these was due to acute arterial thrombosis. In another 12 limbs, though phlebograms showed definite thrombi,

In comparison to other noninvasive testing procedures, the results with the FUT are not particularly encouraging. As reported by Kakkar (24), the sensitivity was fairly good, 84% (62/74); but the specificity was poor, 54% (15/28). The incidence of false-positive results was 17% (13/75) and of false-negative results, 44% (12/27). It is also important to re-examine the results reported by Browse et al. (11), which are quoted in this paragraph as indicating that 'only 10% of patients showed a venous thrombosis which was detected by phlebography and not by the FUT.' The 10% false-negative figure was calculated by dividing the number of false negative studies (19) by the total number of studies (195), a practice that tends to distort the true picture. A false-negative figure of 15% is more representative (19 false-negative results divided by 129 negative FUTs). The false-positive incidence was 30% (20/66). Browse and his colleagues (11) argue that 'it is very likely that the "false-positive" fibrinogen uptake tests are in fact true positives – that is, these are cases in which the thrombus was small and hidden within the muscle and so not detected by the phlebogram.' While this may be true, it is a very questionable way of assessing the results of a test. In fact, all other noninvasive tests discussed later in this chapter would benefit from this convenient assumption. The sensitivity in the series reported by Browse et al. (11) was only 71% (46/65) and the specificity, 85% (110/130). Moreover, when symptoms had been present for 0–5 days, the overall agreement between FUT and phlebography was only 59% and was even worse at 6–10 days, 48%. When the patients were on heparin, agreement was 50%; and when they were on warfarin for more than 6 days, it was only 40%. Finally, they found it necessary to exclude any patient with superficial thrombophlebitis, varicose ulceration, sepsis, hematoma, bruising, flesh wounds, active arthritis, or gross edema of the leg. These exclusions certainly constitute a severe deficit, since many patients with such conditions are suspected of having and indeed may have deep venous thrombosis.

The results reported by Mavor et al. (18) are even more discouraging. In patients who presented with pulmonary embolism and negative leg signs, the FUT was positive in only 11% (8/72). When compared with phlebography, the FUT detected only 2 of 40 thrombi (sensitivity 5%). The specificity was somewhat better, 81% (26/32). In another group of patients with signs of iliofemoral thrombosis, the FUT detected only 16 of 50 thrombi (32%) that were diagnosed phlebographically.

Based on these studies, one would be hesitant to institute, continue, withhold, or discontinue therapy in patients with suspected venous thrombosis on the

the radioactive fibrinogen test was negative. These findings indicate that a positive result will be obtained only if a thrombus is still forming; in fully established or old thrombi, the test may be negative, since the fibrinogen is not incorporated into a formed thrombus unless it is extending. However, in another study (36), it was surprising that only 10% of patients showed a venous thrombus which was detected by phlebography and not by the FUT, particularly considering that many of the 102 patients were receiving full doses of anticoagulants, administered to prevent extension of such thrombi.

In our studies (37), the FUT proved to be a valuable diagnostic tool, particularly in those patients with minor clinical signs, because it was in this group that clinical diagnosis was most fallible. There is a further advantage of using this test in such patients: whenever the test is positive, it provides a simple method of assessing the effectiveness of treatment. By observing the change in radioactivity at the site of a thrombus, it is possible to tell whether the thrombus is extending, remaining stationary, or being lysed.

2.10.7. *Role in the treatment of venous thrombosis.* The FUT has also been used to assess objectively the rate of dissolution of venous thrombi, either by natural or artificially induced fibrinolysis (39). Repeated measurements of surface radioactivity over the site of a thrombus, and over the areas where there is no thrombus, allow a quantitative assessment of the fate of the thrombi. The original differences between the radioactivity at the site of the thrombus and that of an adjacent site can be taken to present 100%. The percentage decline of this difference (thrombus radioacitvity) has been shown to represent the degree of dissolution as confirmed by phlebography (Fig. 5).

2.10.8. *Clinical management of isotopic thrombi.* Although the FUT is an accurate and reliable method for detecting thrombi in surgical, medical and postpartum patients, the method is less reliable in patients undergoing orthopedic procedures being performed on the limbs. In the nonorthopedic patients, the following three approaches can be used to select those patients who require anticoagulant therapy.

The first approach is to commence treatment only when the raised counts detected over the calf have extended to involve the lower thigh region. This approach is based on our earlier observations (23) that isotopic thrombi confined to the calf region are unlikely to produce significant pulmonary embolism because the majority of these thrombi undergo spontaneous lysis. In contrast, scan-detected popliteal or femoral vein thrombosis carries a high risk of embolism. Such an approach would result in treatment of approximately 5% of nonorthopedic high-risk patients and about 95% of patients with dangerous thrombi.

The second approach could be to treat all patients with isotopic thrombi, which are confirmed by venography. The rationale for treating such patients would be that, if left untreated, a proportion of calf thrombi may propagate into the popliteal and femoral vein where the risk of major embolism is high and may not be detected unless rigorous scanning programmes are being followed. However, the disadvantage of such an ap-

strength of the FUT alone. Some other diagnostic approach would have to be employed to confirm the diagnosis.

Hull et al. (25) used both the IPG and FUT to examine patients suspected of having deep venous thrombosis. They found that one or both of the tests were positive in 81 of 86 patients with positive phlebograms (sensitivity 94%). Both studies were negative in 104 of 114 patients (specificity 91%). The two tests detected all 60 patients with thrombi in the popliteal or more proximal veins. Because the IPG was positive in 59 of these 60 patients, they suggested that the FUT could be dispensed with when the IPG is positive.

Another problem with the FUT in diagnosing clinically suspected deep venous thrombosis is the fact that the scan may not become positive for 18–72 h (8, 11). This fact alone militates against its use in office or emergency room practice (21). However, DeNardo et al. (26) noted that 67% of the tests were positive at 3–4 h and 98% were positive at 24 h. Unfortunately, his figures were not corroborated by phlebography.

One area in which the ^{125}I scan can be useful is in the diagnosis of recurrent deep venous thrombosis in postphlebitic limbs. In these cases, most of the other noninvasive tests are not particularly helpful and even the phlebogram may be confusing. While a positive scan is indicative of an active process, a negative scan suggests that recurrent symptoms are due to the sequelae of chronic venous insufficiency rather than recurrent thrombosis. According to Barnes (27), only 20% of patients presenting with recurrent symptoms have positive scans.

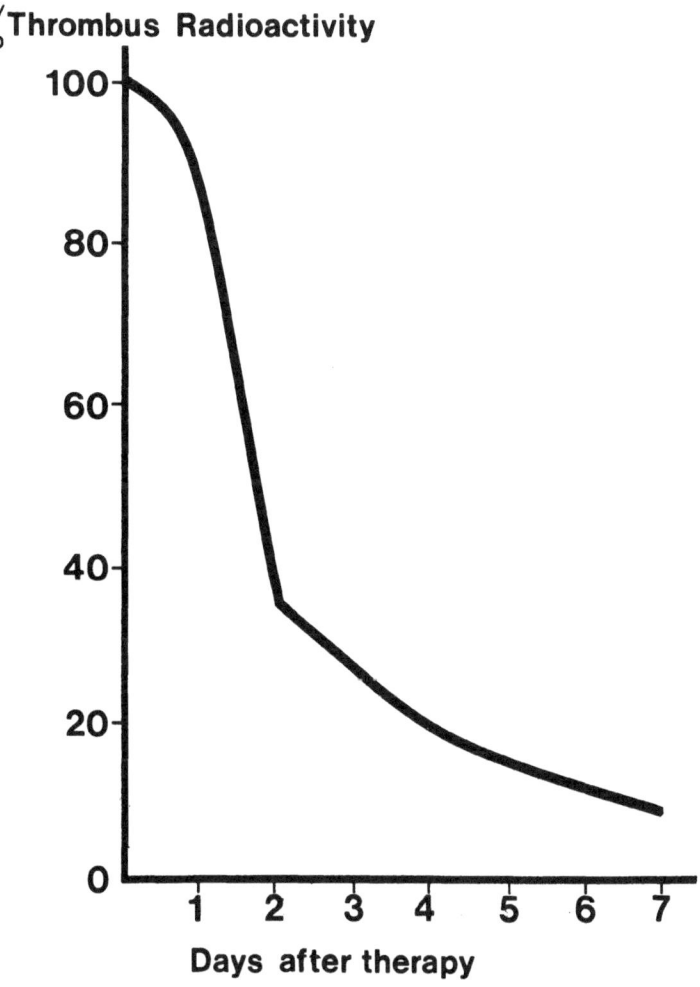

THROMBUS DISSOLUTION

%Thrombus Radioactivity

Days after therapy

Fig. 5. The rate of thrombus dissolution as judged by the FUT on the second day after treatment. The thrombus radioactivity had fallen to approximately 38% of the original, and at the end of 7 days, it was less than 10%, indicating that approximately 90% of the thrombus was dissolved during this period.

For the reasons outlined in the text, the treatment of all isotopically detected thrombi with anticoagulants, as proposed by Adar and Salzman (28), seems too radical. Hirsh and Hull (8) perform bilateral phlebograms on all patients with positive scans and treat only those individuals in whom the diagnosis is confirmed. When there is a relative contra-indication to anticoagulation in patients with small calf vein thrombi, they are followed with serial IPGs and FUTs. If no signs of proximal extension are detected, treatment is deferred until the risk of bleeding has decreased.

proach is that most postoperative scan-detected thrombi develop within the first 7 postoperative days, and full anticoagulant treatment of many patients at this stage is likely to be associated with high incidence of bleeding complications.

The third approach that has been suggested (40) is based on the fact that venography should be performed in all patients with a positive FUT. When the thrombi are confined to major veins proximal to the knee joints, patients should be treated with anticoagulants. The decison to treat calf vein thrombi could be based on their size, site, and extent.

3.   IMPEDANCE PLETHYSMOGRAPHY

For some time, plethysmography has been a standard method for investigating patients with arterial occlusive disease. Several workers (41–45) have documented the value of this method for investigating diseases of the venous system, particularly deep vein thrombosis.

3.1.   *Hemodynamic abnormalities caused by deep vein thrombosis*

The term maximum venous outflow (MVO) should be applied to the maximum rate at which the trapped blood leaves the calf once the congesting pressure is released. Thus MVO is calculated based on the tangent to the initial part of the outflow curve (29, 30). However, in practice it has proved to be more convenient to measure the volume decrease over a specified period of time, usually 2 or 3 sec. Since the slope of the outflow curve decreases rapidly during the first few seconds, venous outflow, measured by this technique, is less than the MVO.

Theoretically, MVO should depend only upon the pressure gradient from the calf veins to the central veins divided by the resistance imposed by the intervening venous channels. Three second venous outflow, on the other hand, is also a function of the changing elasticity of the veins and the maximum venous capacity (MVC) (30). Therefore, venous outflow is directly proportioned to venous capacity (31–33). This relationship is particularly evident when the veins are uninvolved with thrombi. Consequently, a low,

The two most important venous hemodynamic abnormalities resulting from deep vein thrombosis may be demonstrated by inflating a pressure cuff around the thigh and measuring the subsequent changes in calf blood volume with a plethysmograph (Fig. 6). The first abnormality is a reduction of the maximum venous volume of the calf. Thrombus in the veins and the pre-existing high venous pressure reduce the maximum volume capacity (MVC) of the deep veins. The second hemodynamic abnormality is seen after release of the cuff. The venous blood trapped in the calf drains from the leg more slowly because the blood must flow around partially

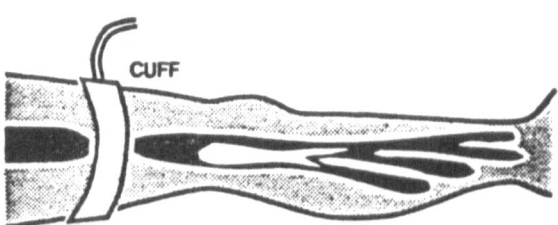

♦ MAX. VENOUS VOLUME

♦ MAX. RATE VENOUS EMPTYING

Fig. 6. The hemodynamic abnormalities produced by deep vein thrombosis can be measured by inflating a pressure cuff around the thigh and recording the maximum venous volume of the calf and the maximum rate of venous return emptying which occurs after cuff deflation.

occluding thrombi or, if the clot is completely obstructing, flow is through high resistance collateral vessels. The second abnormality, maximum rate of venous outflow)MVO), is a more sensitive hemodynamic index of deep vein thrombosis than MVC and this point is further illustrated in Fig. 7. In the normal person, calf blood volume quickly returns to the base line level after release of the thigh cuff. On the other hand, in patients with deep vein thrombosis, the blood drains from the calf at a slower rate. The maximum blood volume of the calf is also reduced, but Dahn and Eriksson (46) and Hallböök and Gothlin (47) have shown that this measurement is a less sensitive index of deep vein thrombosis.

apparently abnormal, venous outflow may be obtained in a normal extremity when the duration of venous congestion has been too brief to obtain maximum venous distention. By relating venous outflow to the venous capacity, many false-positive results can be eliminated (33). Methods for accomplishing this comparison may be graphical (32, 33) or may utilize an impedance ratio (34).

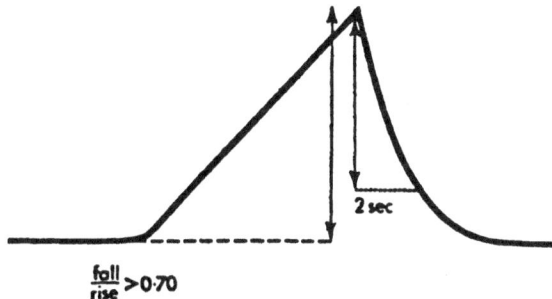

$$\frac{fall}{rise} > 0.70$$

Fig. 7. Calculation of impedance ratio. The impedance change occurring in the first 2 sec after cuff release is divided by the total impedance changes produced by cuff inflation. The ratio represents the fraction of the pooled blood emptying from the calf in 2 sec after release of the thigh cuff.

3.2. *Procedure of impedance plethysmography*

In earlier studies, Wheeler and his associates (42, 43) relied on sustained deep inspiration to impede venous return and trap blood in the calf. Unfortunately, this technique, though simple, gave a high false-positive and -negative result. The technique was further modified by using a thigh cuff to trap blood in the calf veins. The presently used technique has been described in detail by Wheeler et al. (48) and is as follows. The patient is placed in a supine position and the foot of the bed is elevated approximately 15°. This empties the normal venous system. A pillow is placed under the lower leg and foot for comfort. The knee is bent about 30–35°, and the hip is rotated externally. This position is usually facilitated by having the patient shift his weight onto the hip of the side being tested.

A conductive paste is then applied sparingly to 4 circumferential electrodes that are placed around the calf. The inner two electrodes should be approximately 10 cm apart. The electrodes should be in light contact around the calf. A 7 in. wide pneumatic cuff is placed around the lower thigh, with its lower edge at least 2 in. above the knee. The top and bottom

The rate of venous emptying increases with the degree of venous filling. This relationship is quite marked in normal limbs but is not so noticeable in limbs with proximal venous thrombosis. Hull and his colleagues (35) found that the sensitivity and specificity of impedance plethysmography rose significantly with increased venous filling produced by prolongation of the calf occlusion time from 45 sec to 120 sec and by repeated testing. The former was more effective than the latter. In their studies, a series of occlusions of 45, 45, 120, 45 and 120 sec were used on each limb separated by a 20–30 sec rest period. The sensitivity rose from 2% to 92% from the first to the last test and the specificity from 76% to 96%. It is probable that equal accuracy could be obtained with two 120 sec periods of occlusions.

'Phleborheography', the test described by Cranley and his associates (36), deserves further comment since it is based on a totally different concept from that employed by most other plethysmographic methods used to diagnose venous obstruction. to diagnose venous obstruction. In fact, the principle is not unlike Pneumatic cuffs designed to sense volume changes are placed around the thorax, mid-thigh, upper calf, mid-calf, lower calf, and foot. The two lower cuffs also serve as compression devices. In a normal limb, inspiration causes a temporary decrease in venous outflow and a rise in venous pressure. With expiration, the outflow increases and the pressure falls. As a result, phasic changes in limb volume produced by respiration are normally perceived in the recordings derived from the calf and thigh cuffs. Reduction or absence of these changes in limb volume are indicative of venous obstruction. Similar effects are important in the interpretation of flow patterns with the Doppler device.

In the first operational mode, the foot cuff is suddenly inflated (to 100 mm Hg) and deflated three times in rapid succession. In the absence of venous obstruction, there is no increase in limb volume detected by the thigh and calf cuffs. When, however, there is proximal venous obstruction, pumping of the foot results in an increase in limb volume. Again, this test is similar to the augmentation maneuvers applied in Doppler studies.

Finally, the cuff on the lower calf is inflated to 50 mm Hg and deflated rapidly. Normally, this pumping action serves to empty the veins within the foot, causing a decrease in foot volume but no increase in calf volume. In the presence of venous obstruction, the foot volume remains essentially unchanged, while the more proximal calf and thigh cuffs show an augmentation in limb volume.

edges of the cuff should have roughly the same snugness and should easily admit one finger when the cuff is deflated.

The thigh cuff is inflated to a pressure of 45 cm H_2O. This pressure is maintained for 45 sec in order to allow full distension of the venous system even in patients with reduced arterial input. The cuff pressure is then released. Since an important measurement is the rapidity of outflow in the first 3 sec, the cuff must deflate promptly.

The initial decrease in venous volume following inflation of the pneumatic cuff is recorded at a standard calibration (0.2% of resting base-line impedance/5 mm). The fall in venous volume within 3 sec after release of the tourniquet is similarly recorded. These two variables, reflecting MVC and MVO, are then plotted as a function of each other. If the test result appears normal, the procedure can be concluded at this point. If the result is abnormal, the examiner must exclude the possibility that the abnormal result is due to technical factors. Technical false-positives can occur with certain positions of the leg or with an external tourniquet effect due to the electrodes, the thigh cuff, the patient's clothing, or occlusive surgical dressings. The most common cause for a technical false-positive result is the position of the leg. If the knee is estended, the major veins may be under considerable longitudinal tension. There may also be compression of the popliteal vein by the posterior border of the tibia, as is sometimes seen on plebograms. If the leg is comfortably relaxed, with external rotation of the hig and slight flexion of the knee, venous outflow is usually unimpeded. If an abnormal test is obtained, the operator should first check the tightness of the electrodes, the pneumatic cuff, and the patient's clothing or bandages. The leg should then be repositioned. The test should not be called abnormal until the same result has been obtained with the leg repositioned in varying degrees of flexion of the knee, including flexion of the knee with the hip in neutral position, rather than external rotation.

In patients with very obese legs, an occasional artifact is introduced by skin movement when the thigh cuff is inflated. The artifact consists of a very rapid initial rise of the impedance tracing in the first 2–3 sec after inflation of the cuff followed by a levelling off after 3–5 sec. The rapid initial rise is usually free from the customary arterial pulsations. This artifact is more pronounced if the cuff is low on the thigh and the knee is flexed considerably. It can usually be eliminated by having the cuff higher on the thigh and decreasing the flexion of the knee. If the artifact cannot be prevented completely, the tracing should be scored by subtracting the initial sharp rise from both VC and MVO.

Another modification of this technique has been advocated by Cranley et al. (45) where two separate encircling cuffs are used – one for recording, the other for compressing. The recording cuff is placed in the mid-thigh region and the compressing cuff placed successively at different positions on the leg.

3.3. Calculation of results

The results may be analysed by using one of the following criteria.

3.3.1. The impedance ratio.

This represents the change in impedance occurring in the first 2 sec after cuff release divided by the total impedance change produced by cuff inflation (Fig. 7). The ratio represents the fraction of the pooled blood emptying from the calf in the 2 sec after release of the thigh cuff. This criteria was used by Johnston et al. (44) in 70 limbs and the presence of thrombosis was confirmed by venography. Venograms were normal in 38 limbs and in all but three of these the impedance ratio was greater than 0.70. Venography demonstrated thrombi in 32 limbs. Thirteen patients had recent thrombi (including two partially occluding small femoral clots) extending into the femoral or iliac veins and in each of these the impedance ratio was less than 0.65. In 4 patients with old femoral thrombi, the impedance ratio was also less than 0.65. One patient had thrombus extending into the popliteal vein and the impedance ratio was abnormal. In 12 limbs venography showed thrombi confined to the tibial or soleal veins. In only three of these was the impedance ratio less than 0.70.

3.3.2. Venous capacitance (VC)/maximum venous outflow rate (MVO).

Wheeler et al. (48) calculated their results by plotting the venous outflow (mm/sec) against venous capacitance (mm) as shown in Fig. 8. In 90 patients with normal venographs, the IPG was also interpreted as normal

A line of best discrimination between normal and abnormal impedance data has been identified by Hull and associates (32). With venous outflow on the ordinate and VC on the abscissa, this line intersects the ordinate slightly above the origin and slopes upward from left to right. When a point describing the coordinates of venous outflow and VC lies above the line, there is little likelihood that the limb harbors a proximal venous thrombosis. On the other hand, points below the line strongly suggest deep venous thrombosis in veins at or above popliteal level. However, as Wheeler et al. (33) observed: 'Common sense dictates that points close to the dividing line between normal and abnormal should be considered less reliable than those some distance away.' After analyzing their data, Wheeler et al. (33) developed a series of hyperbolic discriminate lines. These lines were labeled according to the 3 sec venous outflow rate at the point where they intersected the vertical axis. Of those limbs with

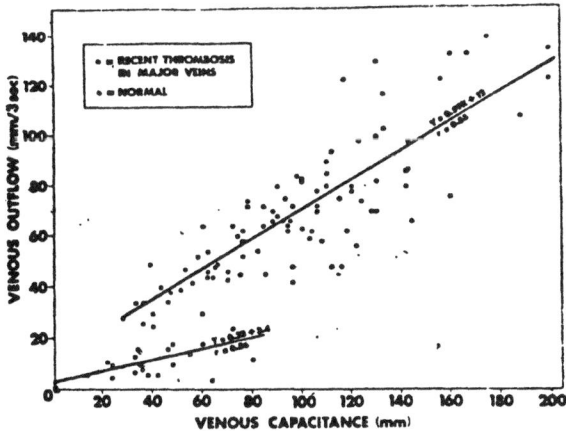

Fig. 8. Venous capacitance (VC) and maximum venous outflow rate (MVO) in 90 patients with normal phlebograms and 28 patients with recent thrombosis in the iliac, femoral or popliteal veins (Wheeler et al. 1974, reproduced by kind permission).

proximal deep venous thrombosis, 83% fell below line 15, 16% lay between 15 and 25, and only 1% were above 25. In contrast, 91% of values derived from normal limbs were above 25 and only 3% fell below 15. When the thrombosis was limited to the calf veins, half of the values were below 25 and half above. Use of these lines permits the physician to assess the reliability of individual reports. Obviously, if the points fall between 15 and 25, no clear diagnosis is possible, and other modalities are required to establish the presence or absence of venous thrombosis. In the series of Wheeler et al. (33) there was little likelihood of a major proximal deep venous thrombosis (1%) when the points lay above 25, but still a reasonable chance that the limb could be the site of calf vein thrombi (9%) or old venous disease (10%). Below 15, 79% of the limbs had major deep venous thrombosis, 11% old disease, and 4% calf vein thrombosis; only 6% were normal.

in 89 (99%). Recent thrombosis involving the popliteal, femoral or iliac veins was seen in 28 phlebograms. Twentyseven of those patients had abnormal IPG tests interpreted as consistent with recent venous thrombosis, an overall accuracy of 96%. IPG proved inadequate for the detection of early calf vein thrombosis. Small thrombi localized to one or more calf veins without any additional thrombi in the popliteal, femoral or iliac veins in 12 patients; only one of these patients had an abnormal IPG test. Similarly out of 20 patients who had old thrombi demonstrated by phlebography, the results of IPG were inconclusive.

3.4.   Accuracy of IPG

Several studies (45, 48, 49) have now shown that impedance plethysmography is a sensitive and specific method for the detection of proximal vein thrombosis. The largest experience has been reported by Hull et al. (50). Both phlebography and impedance plethysmography were performed in 346 consecutive patients with suspected venous thrombo-embolism. The limbs were classified according to the venographic results as no thrombosis, proximal (popliteal, femoral or iliac) vein thrombosis, and calf thrombosis. A discriminant analysis was performed. The impedance plethysmographic result was normal in 386 of 397 limbs which were normal on phlebography, a specificity of 97%, and abnormal in 124 of 135 limbs which showed proximal vein thrombosis, a sensitivity of 93%. Seventythree of 88 limbs with calf vein thrombi had a normal impedance result, i.e., a false negative result in 83% of limbs. Furthermore, 41 of the proximal thrombi were nonocclusive; 9 (22%) of these nonocclusive thrombi were also not detected. Thus the sensitivity of the IPG for nonocclusive thrombi in the popliteal and femoral veins was 78%.

The accuracy of IPG as a screening test for the detection of asymptomatic or subclinical thrombosis has also been assessed by the same authors (Hirsh and ref., Hull 51). In this study, 497 high-risk medical and general surgical patients and 219 patients who had elective hip surgery were included. The findings of IPG were compared with those of ^{125}I-fibrinogen uptake test. In general medical and surgical patients, IPG detected proximal vein thrombosis which was confirmed by venography in 23 patients and was falsely negative in 3. Of the 27 patients with calf vein thrombosis shown by venography, IPG detected only 5. In contrast, leg scanning was positive in 24 of the 26 patients with venographically proven proximal vein thrombosis and negative in only 2. In addition, leg scanning detected 25 of the 27 patients with calf vein thrombosis proven by venography. In 219 patients who had elective hip surgery, IPG detected 35 of 43 proximal thrombi and 6 of the 40 calf vein thrombi. The combination of the IPG and ^{125}I-fibrinogen scanning resulted in the detection of 41 of 43 proximal vein thrombi and 37 of 40 calf vein thrombi.

3.5. *Limitations and sources of errors*

As has been already mentioned, impedance plethysmography will detect thrombi that produce obstruction of venous outflow. Therefore the test will not detect most calf vein thrombi since they do not obstruct the main outflow tract. Similarly, small nonocclusive thrombi in the popliteal and femoral veins may also be missed. IPG may also be negative when proximal vein thrombosis is associated with well developed collaterals. The false-positive results may be obtained due to other conditions which also produce impairment to venous outflow, since the impedance test can not distinguish between thrombotic and nonthrombotic venous obstruction. Therefore the test is falsely positive if a patient is (a) positioned incorrectly or inadequately so that deep veins are constricted by contracting muscle, (b) the lower limb is not raised above the heart level, (c) if maximal filling of the limbs is not obtained; this may require 3 or 4 cycles of inflation and deflation (d) if the veins are compressed by extravascular mass, especially in the pelvic region (e) if venous outflow is also impaired by raised venous pressure, for example, congestive cardiac failure or constrictive pericarditis, and (f) if there is reduced arterial inflow to the limb due to severe obstructive arterial disease which can also lead to reduced outflow and have false-positive results.

4. ULTRASONIC TECHNIQUE

This technique has been used quite extensively for the diagnosis of venous thrombosis. The test has been described in detail by Strandness et al. (52), Sigel and others (53), and Evans and Cockett (54). The principle of the technique is that when a beam of ultrasound is reflected from a moving object, its frequency is altered according to the rate at which the object is moving due to the Doppler effect. In the blood stream, the particles act as reflectors, so that the frequency of an ultrasound beam, passing through a moving column of blood is altered according to the rate of the flow (Fig. 9). This changed frequency can either be recorded on paper or amplified into an audible signal. In a patent vein, the velocity of the venous flow can be briefly increased by compressing the extremity. In the presence of deep venous occlusion, such augmented flow signals (A wave) are dampened and may not be detectable (53).

4.1. *Procedure*

The Doppler ultrasound flow velocity detector contains an oscillator which activates a piezo-electric crystal in a handheld probe, so that it

If possible, the examination should be conducted in a warm room (25 °C) in order to ensure a rapid flow of blood in the veins, unimpeded by vasoconstriction. I prefer to have the legs slightly abducted, externally rotated, and flexed at the knee. If adequate venous flow is not detected in this position, the head of the bed may be elevated 30°, the legs extended at the hips and knee, or the feet exercised briefly. When the condition of the patient permits, the popliteal veins should be examined with the patient prone, the knees flexed, and the feet supported by pillows. Considerable pressure can be used when examining deep veins, but superficial veins must be examined with little or no pressure being applied to the skin, in order to avoid obliteration of the venous lumen.

The venous survey should always be complete and performed in a systematic fashion. Beginning with the common femoral vein, the examiner then moves down the leg to the superficial femoral, popliteal, and posterior tibial veins in that order. Following this, the saphenous veins at the ankle and mid-thigh are studied as well as any prominent superficial veins that may be functioning as collaterals. At each level, the signal from one limb is compared with that of the other to permit small differences in flow patterns to be recognized. The proper vein is best located by first identifying the adjacent artery and then shifting the probe slightly until the venous flow signal is optimized.

At each level, it is of utmost importance for the examiner to pause for a few moments to listen to the character of the spontaneous flow signal. The normal venous flow signal in the legs of a supine subject varies with respiration, decreasing with inspiration and increasing with expiration. When the probe is positioned distal to an obstruction, the flow signal loses its phasic character, becoming more continuous. Obviously, when the probe is over an occluded vein, no signal will be obtained. With care, a

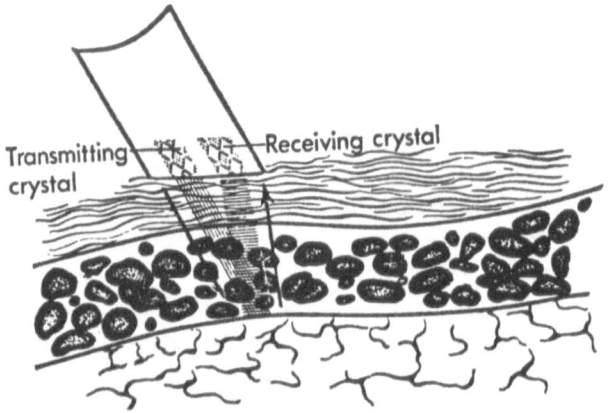

Fig. 9. Principle of the ultrasonic technique. The transducer is composed of two crystals: one crystal transmits the sound and the other receives back the scattered original at a different frequency.

emits an ultrasound beam. The second piezo-electric crystal in the probe acts as a receiving crystal for the reflected ultrasound beam. The difference in frequency of ultrasonic beams is within the available range and with suitable amplification can be transmitted as audible signals or flow sounds.

The patient is positioned carefully for examination, with the head slightly elevated, with the knees straight and the ankle supported to allow good filling of the calf veins. The transducer is applied to the skin overlying the vein to be studied using a suitable coupling medium. The transducer is applied to the common femoral vein, external iliac, popliteal and to the tibial veins at the ankle region. First of all, the thigh is gently squeezed by hand to produce alteration in the velocity of flow in the femoral vein. Distally the calf is lightly squeezed or a specially constructed calf squeezer may be applied to produce a similar effect (55). With the patient lying prone, the transducer is next applied to the popliteal vein and the distal calf is again squeezed gently. Absence of A-sounds represents occlusion of the deep venous system. It has been suggested that compression of the calf or thigh muscles may produce or detach a thrombus and thus produce pulmonary embolism. However, in practice, this has not been observed.

4.2. *Limitations and sources of error*

The Doppler flowmeter has many of the limitations of IPG. Although it is a quick and extremely simple way of detecting complete occlusion of the popliteal, femoral, or iliac veins, the test may be negative when recent small nonocclusive thrombi are present in the proximal veins. In addition, flow in large collaterals or in a very large superficial vein may produce a sound similar to that caused by flow in a patent major vein. Thrombi in the calf veins, the tributaries of the profunda, or the internal iliac veins cannot be detected because they do not cause major vein obstruction. Although the technique is simple, the interpretation of results is much more dependent on the experience of the examiner. False-positive results may be obtained if the underlying vein is obstructed by compressing it with the transducer or if compression over the femoral vein or calf is carried out when the limb is drained of blood.

4.3.   *Accuracy*

There have been several careful studies which have compared the results of Doppler flowmeter examination with venography in patients with clinically suspected venous thrombosis (55–58). The results of these studies show approximately 90–95% sensitivity to popliteal, femoral, or iliac vein thrombosis, a 15–20% sensitivity to calf vein thrombosis, and a low incidence of falsely abnormal results. Some workers have suggested that it is an ideal method for selecting patients who need phlebography. A normal or negative test can be taken to represent a patent vein or absence of a large thrombus in the iliofemoral venous segment. On the other hand, a positive test could be taken to indicate that phlebography should be performed to define the exact site and extent of thrombus.

It has also been suggested that the Doppler ultrasound technique could be used as a screening test to detect any thrombus as soon as it appears in the popliteal or femoral vein. In one study 322 legs were examined and 16 occluded veins were detected while in another study only 4 occluded veins were detected in 1717 examinations of patients, when examining patients twice a week. Thus the yield of the method when used as a screening technique is small and probably does not justify the time and expense. Neither of these studies was able to detect the number of false-negative results, because they were not controlled by phlebography.

5.   RADIONUCLIDE VENOGRAPHY

Radionuclide venography, introduced by Webber et al. (59) is a simple and comprehensive screening procedure for investigating the presence not only of thrombi in the deep veins of the lower limb but also for locating pulmonary emboli. It is based on the principle that macro-aggregation of albumin labelled with ^{99m}Tc when injected through a peripheral vein over the dorsum of the foot may be trapped below the site of an occluding thrombus or adhere to its surface, resulting in a hot spot which can be detected by a γ-camera.

spontaneous signal should be heard over all major veins of the legs except the posterior tibial vein and the saphenous veins. In my experience, if a 10 MHz probe is used, a spontaneous signal will be detected in 87% of normal posterior tibial veins and in 60% of normal saphenous veins at the ankle.

Compression maneuvers are used only after the examiner has had time to assess the character of the spontaneous signals. The extremity is gently but firmly squeezed at multiple levels both proximal and distal to the site of the probe. Pressure should be maintained for a few seconds before release. Compression collapses the underlying veins forcing blood to flow cephalad; retrograde flow is prohibited in normal limbs by closure of the valve cusps. Therefore, when the leg is compressed distal to the site of the Doppler probe, an augmented signal is detected. However, if there is obstruction of the vein between the probe and the point of compression, there will be little or no augmentation of the signal. When the probe is over a patent vein but located distal to an occlusion, compression of the limb below the probe may produce an augmented signal, but this signal will be low-pitched and abrupt, unlike the normal augmented signal, which is loud, high-pitched, and prolonged. Similar abnormal signals are detected when both the compression site and the obstruction are cephalad to the probe. Retrograde flow obtained during compression cephalad to the probe indicates venous incompetence and is usually diagnostic of chronic venous insufficiency.

Failure to detect nonocclusive thrombi in proximal veins is perhaps the most serious of the potential limitations of the Doppler method. Although some of these thrombi alter the venous flow pattern sufficiently to be recognized (37–39), undoubtedly many are missed since Doppler surveys are positive in only 48–61% percent of patients with pulmonary emboli (40. 41). Yet.

in defense of the Doppler technique, it must be pointed out that X-ray phlebography detects thrombi in leg veins of only 50–87% of patients with pulmonary emboli (3, 42–44).

The careful examiner should seldom confuse collateral venous signals for signals arising from major veins. Collateral veins are almost invariably located some distance away from the artery, they are often superficial and easily compressed, and they usually follow a circuitous course. Similarly, major superficial veins do not lie near a major artery; and they, also, are easily compressed with the probe.

While it is true that it is impossible to study those tributaries of major deep veins that have no superficial representation, clots are seldom isolated to these veins but exist in association with thrombi in veins that are accessible to ultrasound. For example, internal iliac thrombi are relatively rare, occurring in less than 6% of limbs with venous thrombosis (45) and only 3% of profunda femoris venous thrombi and 4% of calf muscle venous thrombi are isolated (15). On the other hand, clots in the posterior tibial vein can be recognized readily by the astute examiner. Since this vein is affected in 60% of limbs with calf vein thrombosis and since clots isolated to the below-knee region occur in about 20–46% of limbs with venous thrombosis (15, 16), the false-negative potential would be 8–18% (46, 47). However, our results suggest that the error rate is much less significant.

The major limitation to the use of the Doppler technique is that the examination requires experience (39). While many investigators have reported accuracies exceeding 90%, the beginning technicians and residents in our laboratory were wrong more often than they were right. Because many of the findings are subtle, a great deal of interpretive skill is required. The demands on the examiner are similar to those imposed by the stethoscope. However, the technique can be mastered if one learns to think

5.1. Procedure

The patient is examined supine; two specially designed narrow pneumatic cuffs are applied to each leg, one just above the ankle and the other just above the knee; these are inflated to 100 mm Hg. A cobalt spot marker is placed in the midline between legs at the level of the upper border of the patella, another just below the symphysis pubis and a third at the umbilicus. One mCi of ^{99m}Tc macro-aggregated albumin (MAA) is injected into each foot followed by approximately 20 ml saline flush. Imaging is carried out using a gamma camera fitted with a diverging collimator. The passage of isotope into the deep veins of the calf is followed on the persistance oscilloscope and the record is obtained on a polaroid film. Image is obtained of the femoral vein after a further injection into each foot of 1 mCi of MAA. Finally, the patient is positioned with the camera over the pelvis and lower abdomen. The cuffs are released and, with a further 10 ml of saline flush and active ankle exercising images of the iliac veins and inferior vena cava are obtained. At the end of the procedure, a lung scan is also obtained.

5.2. Limitations and sources of errors

The number of vessels imaged by radionuclide venography appear to be fewer than those filled by phlebography. In most cases, the individual vessels cannot be differentiated by radionuclide venography. Precise anatomic detail of thrombi is never demonstrated since tagging can only occur in partially occluded vessels or at the blood thrombus interface. Caution is also required with the interpretation of the hot spots. Hot spots do not necessarily mean the presence of thrombi, since particle entrapment is not a reliable factor in the diagnosis of thrombosis; the tag may remain in place due to venous stasis in addition to adhering tt the area of endothelial damage. False-positive results also occur when there are areas of inflammation or edema.

5.3. Accuracy

Although a number of studies have reported a correlation between phlebography and radionuclide venography, the number of patients investigated is rather small and their results do not permit any definite conclusions to be drawn. However, we have recently undertaken a study of 100 patients where the results of two methods were compared (60). There was a 72% overall correlation between the two methods with 16% false-positive and 12.5% false-negative results. In the calf, there was a correlation of 69% with 16% false-positive and 15% false-negative results. In the thig region, the results were more impressive with a correlation of 96%, 1% false-positive and 3% false-negative results. The iliac veins and inferior vena cava were invariably better demonstrated by radionuclide venography than by phlebography, even in the presence of almost complete occlusion of the femoral vein. The correlation between RNV and phlebographic findings was almost 100%.

5.4. Comments

Radionuclide venography is less invasive than phlebography and the radiation hazard is negligible. Little expertise is necessary and, apart from the insertion of a fine needle into a dorsal vein of each foot, both RNV and the subsequent lung scan may be performed by nonmedical personnel. The main disadvantages are that the patient must be examined by the γ-camera in the isotope department and such cameras are not available in all hospitals. In addition, it does not measure the true extent of the disease. At present, radionuclide venography must be considered as a clinical research tool for studies that require to know the incidence of peripheral thrombosis and pulmonary embolism.

6. THERMOGRAPHY

Thermography is a new, simple and truly noninvasive method which can be used for the detection of deep vein thrombosis. It is based on the principle that a leg containing thrombosed veins, particularly a thrombus that is obstructing the venous outflow of the limb, exhibits increased temperature and delayed cooling on exposure as compared to a normal limb. These abnormalities can be detected accurately with an aid of an infrared camera. A number of instruments are now available but most commonly used is an AGA Thermovision 680 medical system. This consists of a scanning camera and a display unit.

6.1. Procedure

The patients are examined in a supine position. Before recording the changes, the legs of the patient must be exposed to allow equilibration of the skin of the lower limbs at room temperature. The limbs are elevated to empty the superficial veins. The heat radiating from the legs is reflected on to an infrared camera by means of a heat-reflecting mirror placed at an angle of 45° over the legs. The pictures are taken of the front of the calves and thigh, a permanent record being obtained by taking a photograph of the display unit of the scanner. The thermographic appearance of normal

anatomically and physiologically, if spontaneous signals are emphasized, and if augmented signals are interpreted cautiously (46).

When compared to phlebography, Doppler venous studies at our institution proved to be 92% accurate for thrombi above the knee (47). The sensitivity was 97%; specificity, 88%; false-negative incidence, only 3%; and false-positive incidence, 12%. When the thrombi were confined to below-knee veins, the overall accuracy was 88% with a sensitivity of 95% and a specificity of 85%. The false-negative incidence was only 2%, but the false-positive incidence was 34%. These values are almost identical to those reported by Barnes et al. (48). The high false-positive incidence could be attributed to chronic disease, extrinsic compression, and to 'over-reading' minor changes in the venous flow pattern.

Based on these figures, if the Doppler study is negative, we feel safe in assuming that the patient does not have deep venous thrombosis. An exception to this would be the patient with pulmonary emboli and a negative Doppler, some of whom may have small nonocclusive thrombi. Treatment is instituted in the patient in whom the study is definitely positive; no other confirmation is required. A phlebogram is obtained in all positive studies when the possibility of extrinsic compression exists, when the presence of chronic disease confuses the picture, when the proximal extent of the thrombosis is uncertain, and when the examiner is unsure of the findings.

The major advantage of the Doppler technique in the diagnosis of deep venous thrombosis is its versatility. It can be used on practically any patient, under almost all clinical circumstances, and at any location – on the wards, in the emergency room, even within the patient's home. Results are available immediately; the test can be repeated as often as necessary; the study is safe and painless; and the equipment is inexpensive, rugged, and portable.

Other preparations such as ^{99m}Tc pertechnetate and ^{99m}Tc tagged human albumin microspheres (HAM) can be used also (49–51). Gamma-camera images obtained with these preparations resemble phlebograms but lack the definition of X-ray studies.

Suspicious findings include prolonged transit time in one limb and opacification of multiple venous channels. The latter can occur in the presence of venous valvular incompetency (52). Venous thrombosis is likely when there is nonvisualization of a venous segment or demonstration of venous collaterals in the thigh or pelvis. Retained hot spots or delayed imaging are less certain findings (53) and stasis of radioactivity in the calf alone is not indicative of venous thrombosis (54).

The relatively high incidence of false-positive hot spots with ^{99m}Tc MAA may be related to their irregular shape. Apparently, this is a less significant problem when 15–30 μm HAM is used (51, 55, 56). Unbound ^{99m}Tc pertechnetate produces no hot spots and provides a good image, but does not permit subsequent lung scanning (49, 50).

Radionuclide phlebography appears to be remarkably well adapted to the detection of thrombi in the thigh and pelvic region. Several groups of investigators report accuracies ranging from 97 to 100% (53, 56, 57). Collateral circulation in the pelvic area is often better demonstrated by the radionuclide study than it is by phlebography.

One major advantage of radionuclide venography is that it can be incorporated easily into the routine lung scanning procedure. Dean (52) reported pulmonary emboli in 17 of 28 patients with positive radionuclide venograms (61%). The technique is also quite helpful when ascending phlebography fails to opacify the pelvic veins adequately. Since radionuclide phlebography is quite accurate in the pelvic region, it can be used as a substitute for a phlebogram made through the femoral veins.

legs shows areas of pretibial and prepatellar cooling and even grey or mottled high picture: A decrease or absence of the pretibial and/or prepatellar cool areas and/or absence of the normal thigh pattern should be considered to be diagnostic of criteria of deep vein thrombosis (61, 62).

6.2. Limitations and sources of error

The important limitation of the technique is its inability to detect thrombi in the pelvic veins and inferior vena cava. The presence of extensive hematoma and other causes of inflammation such as arthritis, superficial thrombophlebitis and cellulitis will produce false-positive results. These must be excluded by clinical examination of the limbs before analyzing the results. Similarly the presence of extensive superficial varicosities must also be excluded.

6.3. Accuracy

The use of thermography in the diagnosis of DVT is comparatively new and the method has not been adopted widely for clinical use. The largest experience has been in patients who presented with clinical features suggestive of deep vein thrombosis (61, 63–65). A recent study has also assessed its value as a screening procedure for detecting early and forming thrombi in nonorthopedic patients during the postoperative period (64). The results were compared with those of the ^{125}I-fibrinogen uptake test. Three hundred and eighh patients (616 legs) were examined every day or every second day for 7–10 days postoperatively. The overall diagnostic agreement was 81.0%; the sensitivity was 62.1% and the specificity 90.3%. The agreement increased with proximal extension of the thrombi. Thermography became positive 0.26 days after the ^{125}I-fibrinogen test but in 19.8% thermography was positive before a positive fibrinogen test. In spite of these impressive results, its value as a screening procedure must be further investigated. The other disadvantage is that the apparatus is very expensive and many clinicians feel this factor outweighs the advantages of the technique; a simple, non-invasive test which can be repeated without discomfort to the patient.

REFERENCES TO MAIN TEXT

1. Ambrus JL, Ambrus CM, Back M et al: Radio-labelled thrombi. Ann. N.Y. Acad. Sci. 68: 97, 1957.
2. McFarlane AS: Labelling of plasma proteins with radioactive iodine. Biochem. J. 62: 135, 1956.
3. Hobb JT, Davies JWL: Detection of venous thrombosis with ^{131}I-labelled firbrinogen in the rabbit. Lancet 2: 134, 1960.

4. Palko PA, Mansen EM, Fedoruk SO: The early detection of deep vein thrombosis using ^{131}I-tagged human fibrinogen. Canad. J. Surg. 7: 215, 1964.
5. Nanson EM, Palko PD, Dick AA, Fedoruk SO: Detection of deep venous thrombosis using [131]tagged fibrinogen. Ann. of Surgery 162: 438, 1965.
6. Atkins P, Hawkins LA: Detection of venous thrombosis in legs. Lancet 2: 1217, 1965.
7. Flanc D, Kakkar VV, Clarke MB: The detection of venous thrombosis in the legs. Brit. J. Surg. 55: 742, 1968.
8. Negus D, Pinto DL, Lequesne LP et al: ^{125}I-labelled fibrinogen in the diagnosis of deep vein thrombosis and its correlation with phlebography. Brit. J. Surg. 58: 835, 1968.
9. Kakkar VV, Nicolaides AN, Renney JTG, et al: ^{125}I-labelled fibrinogen test adapted for routine screening for deep vein thrombosis. Lancet 1: 504, 1970.
10. McFarlane AS: In vivo behaviour of ^{131}I-fibrinogen. J. clin. Invest. 42: 346, 1963.
11. Rosa U, Scasselati GA, Pennisi F, et al: Labelling of human fibrinogen with ^{131}I by electrolytic oxidation. Biochem. Biophys. Acta (Amst.) 84: 519, 1964.
12. Katz J, Bonorris G: Electrolytic iodination of proteins with ^{125}I and [131]I. J. Lab. clin. Med. 72: 966, 1968.
13. Krohn KA, Welch MJ: Studies of radio-iodinated fibrinogen. II. Lactoproxidase iodination of fibrinogen and model compounds. Int. J. Radiol. Isot. (in press).
14. Coleman RE, Krohn KA, Metzger JM et al: An in vivo evalution of I-fibrinogen by four different methods. J. Lab. clin. Med. 83: 977, 1974.
15. Calculation: Courtesy of Dr. R. Edward Coleman. Division of Nuclear Medicine and Radiation Sciences, Edward Mallinckrodt Institute of Radiology, Washington University School of Medicine, St. Louis, MO.
16. National Council on Radiation Protection: Report No. 9, 1971.
17. Friend JR, Kakkar VV: The assessment of the risk of deep vein thrombosis in obstetric and gynaecological patients. 1979 (in press).
18. Friend JR, Kakkar VV: The diagnosis of deep vein thrombosis in puerperium. J. Obstet. Gynaecol. Brit. Comm. 77: 820, 1970.
19. McFarlane AS: Catabolism of iodine-labelled fibrinogen. Proc. roy. Soc. Med. 62: 1127, 1969.
20. Beaker J: The diagnosis of venous thrombosis in the legs using I-labelled fibrinogen. Acta chir. scand. 138: 667, 1972.
21. Browse NL, Clapham WF, Croft AN, et al: Diagnosis of established deep vein thrombosis with the ^{125}I-firbrinogen uptake test. Brit. Med. J. 4: 325, 1971.
22. Hickman J: Blood activity of ^{125}I-fibrinogen in venous thrombosis. Lancet 2: 469, 1970.
23. Kakkar VV, Howe CT, Flanc C, et al: Natural history of postoperative deep vein thrombosis. Lancet 2: 230, 1969.
24. Scottish Study: A multi-unit controlled trial: heparin versus dextran in the prevention of deep vein thrombosis. Lancet 2: 118, 1974.
25. Browse NL, Clemensen G, Croft DN: Fibrinogen detectable thrombosis in the legs and pulmonary embolism. Brit. Med. J. 1: 603, 1974.
26. Mavor GE, Mahafty RG, Walker MG, et al: Peripheral venous scanning with ^{125}I-fibrinogen. Lancet 1: 661, 1972.
27. Kakkar VV: Fibrinogen uptake test. Sem. Nuc. Med. 3: 229, 1977.
28. Kakkar VV, Howe CT, Nicolaides AN, et al: Deep vein thrombosis of the leg. Is there a 'high risk' group? Amer. J. Surg. 120: 527, 1970.
29. Nicolaides AN, Kakkar VV, Field ES, et al: Anti-biotics, post-operative infection and deep vein thrombosis. Brit. J. Surg. 59: 303, 1972.
30. Harris WM, Salzman EW, Athanasoulis C, et al: Comparison of ^{125}I-fibrinogen count scanning with phlebography for detection of venous thrombi after elective hip surgery. N. Engl. J. Med. 292: 665, 1975.
31. Stamatakis JD, Lawrence D, Nairn D, et al: Femoral vein thrombosis and total hip replacement arthroplasty. Brit. Med. J.
32. Field ES, Nicolaides AN, Kakkar VV, et al: Deep vein thrombosis with fractures of the femoral neck. Brit. J. Surg. 59: 377, 1972.
33. Murray TS, Lorimer AR, Cox FC, et al: Leg vein thrombosis following myocardial infarction. Lancet 2: 792, 1970.

The data in the paper of Bergquist and Halböök (58) deserves further scrutiny. Of 166 legs having positive thermograms, fully 40 were negative according to the ^{125}I-fibrinogen uptake test, indicating that 24% of all positive thermograms were falsely positive. Similarly, of 450 legs having negative thermograms, 77 (17%) were positive by ^{125}I-fibrinogen uptake. Based on this data, one would be hesitant to prescribe therapy when the thermogram is positive without confirming the diagnosis by some other test. Also, a negative thermogram would give only moderate assurance that no thrombi were present.

Henderson et al. (59) have used after exercise thermography to predict postoperative deep vein thrombosis. Prior to operation, the patients obtain a thermogram after they have exercised their legs for 3 min by walking in place. Hot spots appearing over the subcutaneous border of the tibia are considered abnormal and indicative of chronic venous insufficiency. The incidence of deep venous thrombosis detected postoperatively by the ^{125}I-fibrinogen uptake was greatly increased in those patients who had abnormal pre-operative thermographic studies. The authors conclude that an abnormal pre-operative after-exercise thermogram is an absolute indication for prophylaxis.

As Dr. Kakkar observes, thermography requires more investigation before its role is firmly established.

34. Maurer BJ, Wray R, Shillingford JP: Frequency of venous thrombosis after myocardial infarction. Lancet 2: 1385, 1972.

35. Warlow CP, Ogston D, Douglas AS: Venous thrombosis following strokes. Lancet 1: 1305, 1972.

36. Int. Multicentre Trial: Prevention of postoperative fatal pulmonary embolism. Lancet 2: 14, 1975.

37. Kakkar VV, The diagnosis of deep vein thrombosis using the ^{125}I-fibrinogen test. Arch. Surg. 104: 152, 1972.

38. Brose NL, Clapham WF, Croft DN, et al: The diagnosis of established deep vein thrombosis with the ^{125}I fibrinogen test. Brit. Med. J. 4: 325, 1971.

39. Kakkar VV, Flanc C, Howe CT, et al: Treatment of deep vein thrombosis. A trial of heparin, streptokinase and arvin. Brit. med. J. 1: 806, 1969.

40. Gallus AS: ^{125}I-fibrinogen leg scanning. Prophylactic therapy of deep vein thrombosis and pulmonary embolism. D.H.E.W. Publication no. (NIH) 76-866, 1975, p 77.

41. Boijsen F, Eriksson E: Plethysmographic and phlebographic findings in venous thrombosis of the leg. Acta chir. scand. 398: 43, 1968.

42. Mullick SC, Wheeler NB, Songster GF: Diagnosis of deep vein thrombosis by measurement of electrical impedance. Amer. J. Surg. 119: 417, 1970.

43. Wheeler, NB, Pearson D, O'Connell D, et al: Impedance phlebography. Arch. Surg. 104: 164, 1972.

44. Johnston KW, Kakkar VV, Corrigan TP, et al: An improved electrical impedance technique for the detection of deep vein thrombosis. Brit. J. Surg. 60: 313, 1973.

45. Cranley JJ, Gay AY, Grass AM, et al: A plethysmographic technique for the diagnosis of deep vein thrombosis of the lower extremities. Surg. Gynaecol. Obstet. 136: 358, 1973.

46. Dahn I, Eriksson E: Plethysmographic diagnosis of deep vein thrombosis of the leg. Acta. chir. scand. 398: 33, 1968.

47. Sumner DS, Lambeth A: Reliability of Doppler ultrasound in the diagnosis of acute venous thrombosis both above and below the knee. Amer. J. Surg. 138: 205, 1979.

48. Wheeler NB, O'Donnell JA, Anderson FA, et al: In: Occlusive impedance phlebography: A diagnostic procedure for venous thrombosis and pulmonary embolism. A progress in cariovasicular disaeases and pulmonary emboli. Ed. Sasahara AA, Sonnenglick EH, Lesch M, New York, Grune and Stratton, 1975, p 37.

49. Johnston KW, Kakkar VV: Plethysmographic diagnosis of deep vein thrombosis. Surg. Gynaecol. Obstet. 139: 41, 1974.

50. Hull R, Van Aken WG, Hirsh J, et al: Impedance plethysmography using the occlusive calf technique in the diagnosis of venous thrombosis. Circulation 53: 696, 1976.

51. Hirsh J, Hull R: Comparative value of tests for the diagnosis of venous thrombosis. Wld. J. Surg. 2: 27, 1978.

52. Strandness DE, Schultz RD, Sumner DS, et al: Ultra-sonic flow detection. A useful technique in the evaluation of peripheral vascular disease. Amer. J. Surg. 113: 311, 1967.

53. Sigel B, Pophy GL, Wagner DK, et al: Surg. Gynaecol. Obstet. 127: 339, 1968.

54. Evan DS, Cockett FB: Brit. med. J. 2: 802, 1969.

55. Yao JST, Henkin RE, Conn J, Jr., Quinn JL, III, Bergan JJ: Combined isotope venography and lung scanning. Arch. Surg. 107: 146, 1973.

56. Strandness DE, Sumner DS: Ultrasonic velocity detector in the diagnosis of thrombophlebitis. Arch. Surg. 104: 180, 1972.

57. Yao ST, Gourmos C, Hobbs JT: Detection of proximal vein thrombosis by Doppler ultrasound flow-detection method. Lancet 1: 1, 1972.

58. Sigel B, Felix NR, Pophy GL, et al: Diagnosis of lower limb venous thrombosis by Doppler ultrasound technique. Arch. Surg. 104: 174, 1972.

59. Webber MM, Bennett LR, Cragin M, et al: Thrombophlebitis – demonstration by scintiscanning. Radiology 92: 620, 1969.

60. Bentley PG, Hill P, de Haas H, Mistry F: Radionuclide venography – a comparison with contrast venography. Brit. J. Radiol. 1979 (in press).

61. Cooke ED, Pilcher MF: Deep vein thrombosis. Preclinical diagnosis by thermography. Brit. J. Surg. 61: 971, 1974.

62. Bergquist D, Hallböök T: Thermography in screening postoperative deep vein throm-

bosis. A comparison with the ^{125}I fibrinogen test. Brit. J. Surg. 65: 443, 1978.
63. Bergquist D, Dahlgren S, Efsing HO, et al: Thermographic diagnosis of deep vein thrombosis. Brit. med. J. 4: 684, 1975.
64. Bergquist D, Efsing HO, Hallbröök T: Thermography, a non-invasive method for diagnosis of deep vein thrombosis. Arch. Surg. 112: 600, 1977.
65. Leiviska T, Perttala Y: Thermography in diagnosing deep venous thrombosis in the lower limb. Radiologia Clin. 44: 417, 1975.

REFERENCES TO COMMENTARY

1. Haeger K: Problems of acute deep venous thrombosis. I. The interpretation of signs and symptoms. Angiology 20: 219, 1969.
2. Nicolaides AN, Kakkar VV, Field ES, Renney JTG: The origin of deep venous thrombosis: a venograhpic study. Brit. J. Radiol 44: 653, 1971.
3. Sanders RJ, Glaser JL: Clinical uses of venography. Angiology 20: 388, 1969.
4. Kakkar V: The diagnosis of deep vein thrombosis using the ^{125}I fibrinogen test. Arch. Surg. 104: 152, 1972.
5. Lambie JM, Mahaffy RG, Barber DC, Karmody AM, Scott MM, Matheson NA: Diagnostic accuracy in venous thrombosis. Brit. Med. J. 2: 142, 1970.
6. Coon WW, Willis PW: Deep venous thrombosis and pulmonary embolism. Prediction, prevention, and treatment. Amer. J. Cardiol. 4: 611, 1959.
7. Albrechtsson U, Olsson CG: Thrombotic side-effects of lower limb phlebography. Lancet 1: 723, 1976.
8. Hirsch J, Hull R: Comparative value of tests for the diagnosis of venous thrombosis. W. J. Surg. 2: 27, 1978.
9. Hume, M: Postoperative venous thrombosis – the dynamics of propagation, resolution, and embolism. In: Venous Problems, Bergan JJ, Yao JST (eds), Chicago, Ill. Year Book Medical Publishers, 1978, p 571–580, Ch. 38.
10. Morris GK, Mitchell JRA: Evaluation of ^{125}I fibrinogen test for venous thrombosis in patients with hip fractures: comparison between isotope scanning and necropsy findings. Brit. Med. J. 1: 264, 1977.
11. Browse NL, Clapham WF, Croft DN, Jones EJ, Thomas ML, Williams JO: Diagnosis of established deep vein thrombosis with the ^{125}I fibrinogen uptake test. Brit. med. J. 4: 325, 1971.
12. Kerrigan GNW, Buchanan MR, Cade JF, Regoeczi E, Hirsh J: Investigation of the mechanism of false positive ^{125}I labelled fibrinogen scans. Brit. J. Haematol. 26: 469, 1974.
13. Harris WH, Salzman EW, Athanasoulis C, Waltman A, Baum S, DeSanctis RW, Potsaid RW, Sise H: Comparison of ^{125}I fibrinogen count scanning with phlebography for detection of venous thrombi after elective hip surgery. N. Engl. J. Med. 292: 665, 1975.
14. Hume M, Sevitt S, Thomas DP: Venous Thrombosis and Pulmonary Embolism. Cambridge, Mass, Harvard University Press, Cambridge, 1970.
15. Diener L: Origin and distribution of venous thrombi studied by postmortem intraosseous phlebography. In: Thromboembolism, Etiology, Advances in Prevention and Management. Nicolaides AN (ed) Baltimore, University Park Press, 1975, p 149–166, ch. 10.
16. Nicolaides AN, O'Connell JD: Origin and distribution of thrombi in patients presenting with clinical deep venous thrombosis. In: Thromboembolism, Etiology, Advances in Prevention and Management. Nicolaides AN (ed) Baltimore, MD, University Park Press, 1975, p 167–180, ch. 11.
17. Stamatakis JD, Kakkar VV, Lawrence D, Bentley PG: The origin of thrombi in the deep veins of the lower limb: a venographic study. Brit. J. Surg. 65: 449, 1978.
18. Mavor GE, Mahaffy RG, Walker MG, Duthie JS, Dhall DP, Gaddie J, Reid GF: Peripheral venous canning with ^{125}I tagged fibrinogen. Lancet 1: 661, 1972.
19. Gruber UF, Duckert F, Fridrich R, Torhorst J, Rem J: Prevention of postoperative thromboembolism by Dextran 40, low doses of heparin, on xantinol nicotinate. Lancet 1:

207, 1977.

20. Doouss TW: The clinical significance of venous thrombosis of the calf. Brit. J. Surg. 63: 377, 1976.

21. Cranley JJ: Invited commentary of Hirsh J, Hull R: Comparative value or tests for the diagnosis of venous thrombosis. W. J. Surg. 2: 36, 1978.

22. Moreno-Cabral, R. Kistner RL, Nordyke RA: Importance of calf vein thrombophlebitis. Surgery 80: 735, 1976.

23. Browse NL, Clemenson G, Sequelae of an I^{125} fibrinogen detected thrombus. Brit. med. J. 2: 468, 1974.

24. Kakkar V: The diagnosis of deep vein thrombosis using ^{125}I fibrinogen. Arch. Surg. 104: 152, 1972.

25. Hull R, Hirsh J, Sackett DL, Powers P, Turpie AGG, Walker I: Combined uses of leg scanning and impedance plethymography in suspected venous thrombosis: an alternative to venography. N. Engl. J. Med. 296: 1497, 1977.

26. DeNardo GC, DeNardo SJ, Barnett CA, Newcomer KA, Jansholt A-L, Carretta RF, Rose AW: Assessment of conventional criteria for the early diagnosis of thrombophlebitis with the ^{125}I fibrinogen uptake test. Radiology 125: 765, 1977.

27. Barnes RW: Invited commentary of Hirsh J, Hull R: Comparative value of tests for the diagnosis of venous thrombosis. W. J. Surg. 2: 34, 1978.

28. Adar R, Salzman EW: Treatment of thrombosis of veins of the lower extremities. N. Engl. J. Med. 292: 348, 1975.

29. Barnes RW, Collicott PE, Mozersky DJ, Sumner DS, Strandness DE, Jr.: Noninvasive quantitation of maximum venous outflow in acute thrombophlebitis. Surgery 72: 971, 1972.

30. Strandness DE, Jr., Sumner DS: Hemodynamics for Surgeons. New York, Grune and Stratton, 1975.

31. Bygdeman S, Aschberg S, Hindmarsh T: Venous phlethysmography in the diagnosis of chronic venous insufficiency. Acta chir. scand. 137: 423, 1971.

32. Hull R, Van Aken WG, Hirsh J, Gallus AS, Hoicka G, Turpie AGG, Walker I, Gent M: Impedance plethysmography using the occlusive cuff technique in the diagnosis of venous thrombosis. Circulation 53: 696, 1976.

33. Wheeler HB, Anderson FA, Jr., Matesanz JM, Larsen JE: Impedance phlebography: the diagnosis of venous thrombosis by occlusive impedance plethysmography. In: Non-invasive Diagnostic Techniques in Vascular Disease. Bernstein EF (ed), Saint Louis, MD, Mosby, 1978, p 359–373, Ch. 34.

34. Johnston KW, Kakkar VV, Spindler JJ, Corrigan TP, Fossard DP: A simple method for detecting deep vein thrombosis. An improved electrical impedance technic. Amer. J. Surg. 127: 349, 1974.

35. Hull R, Taylor DW, Hirsh J, Sackett DL, Powers P, Turpie AGG, Walker I: Impedance plethysmography: the relationship between venous filling and sensitivity and specificity for proximal vein thrombosis. Circulation 58: 898, 1978.

36. Cranley JJ, Canos AJ, Sull WJ, Grass AM: Phleborheographic technique for diagnosing deep venous thrombosis of the lower extremities. Surg. Gynecol. Obstet. 141: 331, 1975.

37. Doig RL, Browse NL: Rapid propagation of thrombus in deep vein thrombosis. Brit. med. J. 4: 210, 1971.

38. Holmes MCG: Deep venous thrombosis of the lower limbs diagnosed by ultrasound. Med. J. Austr. 1: 427, 1973.

39. Barnes RW, Russell HE, Wilson MR: Doppler Ultrasonic Evaluation of Venous Disease, a Programmed Audiovisual Instruction. 2nd ed. Iowa City, Iowa, University of Iowa Press, 1975, p 1–251.

40. Alexander RH, Folse R, Pizzorno J, Conn R: Thrombophlebitis and thromboemolism: results of a prospective study. Ann. Surg. 180: 883, 1974.

41. Barnes RW, Kinkead LR, Wu KK, Hoak JC: Incidence of venous thrombosis in suspected pulmonary embolism: detection by Doppler. Circulation, 49–50 (Suppl. III): 299, 1974.

42. Browse NL, Thomas ML: Source of non-lethal pulmonary emboli. Lancet 1: 258, 1974.

43. Corrigan TP, Fossard DP, Spindler J, Armstrong P, Strachan CJL, Johnston KW,

Kakkar VV: Phlebography in the management of pulmonary embolism. Brit. J. Surg. 61: 484, 1974.

44. Walker MG: The natural history of venous thrombo-embolism. Brit. J. Surg. 59: 54, 1972.

45. Sevitt S, Gallagher N: Venous thrombosis and pulmonary embolism, a clinico-pathological study in injured and burned patients. Brit. J. Surg. 48: 475, 1971.

46. Sumner DS: Diagnosis of venous thrombosis by Doppler ultrasound. In: Venous Problems, Bergan JJ, Yao JST (eds), Chicago, Ill., Year Book Medical Publishers, 1978, p 159–185, Ch. 11.

47. Sumner DS, Lambeth A: Reliability of Doppler ultrasound in the diagnosis of acute venous thrombosis both above and below the knee. Amer. J. Surg. 138: 205, 1979.

48. Barnes RW, Russell HE, Wu KK, Hoak JC: Accuracy of Doppler ultrasound in clinically suspected venous thrombosis of the calf. Surg. Gynecol. Obstet. 143: 425, 1976.

49. Hobbs JT, Highman JM, Yao JST: The investigation of the iliac veins by an ultrasound technique and by radio-scanning with a gamma camera. J. Vasc. Dis. 1: 170, 1972.

50. Barnes RW, McDonald GB, Hamilton, GW, Rudd, TG, Nelp WB, Strandness DE, Jr.: Radionuclide venography for rapid dynamic evaluation of venous disease. Surgery 73: 706, 1973.

51. Henkin RE, Yao JST, Quinn JL, III, Bergan JJ: Radionuclide venography (RNV) in lower extrimity venous diases. J. nucl. Med. 15: 171, 1974.

52. Dean RH: Radionuclide venography and simultaneous lung scanning: evaluation of clinical application. In: Noninvasive Diagnostic Techniques in Vascular Disease. Bernstein EF (ed) Saint Louis MD, Mosby 1978, p 374–381.

53. Ennis JT, Elmes JT: Radionuclide venography in the diagnosis of deep vein thrombosis. Radiology 125: 441, 1977.

54. Ryo UY, Qazi M, Srikantaswamy S, Pinsky S: Radionuclide venography: correlation with contrast venography. J. nucl. Med. 18: 11, 1977.

55. Yao JST, Henkin RE, Conn J, Jr., Quinn JL, III, Bergan JJ: Combined isotope venography and lung scanning. Arch. Surg. 107: 146, 1973.

56. Vlahos L, MacDonald AF, Causer DA: Combination of isotope venography and lung scanning. Brit. J. Radiol. 49: 840, 1976.

57. Cordoba AS, Figueras NC, Garcia RF: Scintiscanning in venous thrombosis of the lower extremities. Surg. Gynecol. Obstet. 145: 533, 1977.

58. Bergquist D, Hallböök T: Thermography in screening postoperative deep vein thrombosis: a comparison with the ^{125}I fibrinogen test. Brit. J. Surg. 65: 443, 1978.

59. Barnes RW, Wu KK, Hoak JC: The fallibility of the clinical diagnosis of venous thrombosis. JAMA 234: 605, 1975.

10. Angiography in angiology

E. ZEITLER AND R. GROSSE-VORHOLT

Commentary by A.B. Crummy

1. INTRODUCTION

Recent years have seen remarkable advances in diagnostic angiography. Advances in equipment have enhanced the image quality and improvement in technique allows angiography of almost any vascular area with minimal risk and discomfort for the patient. The studies exquisitely delineate the nature, site and extent of anatomical defects (1–5). Though an angiogram may not be essential for the planning of every vascular operation, it is often the primary factor in determining whether surgery is feasible or appropriate.

2. EQUIPMENT FOR ANGIOGRAPHY

Detailed technical descriptions of the many types of radiographic equipment in general use are covered in specialized papers. Recent developments include large-field angiography with cassette changer (Pässler-Wenzlik, Gärtner-Reiser, etc.), rapid film changer (AOT, Franklin-changer, Puck-changer), image intensification cinematography, and spot film fluorography with 70 or 100 mm films. Cinematography and plain film changers, permitting exposure of 6 films per second (AOT) are essential for angiocardiography but are used for angiography of specific organs in the same fashion as the Puck plain film changer (2–4 exposures per second) or spot film fluorography.

The availability of diagnostic angiography has extended beyond centers possessing especially equipped angiography rooms by the use of TV-image intensifier fluorography coupled to any modern fluoroscope with image intensifier. The considerably lower radiation dose, which results in only minor loss of image quality, makes this the technique of choice for visceral angiography and for all procedures with children.

For peripheral angiography, the whole extremity can be completely documented on a single X-ray film (20 × 96 cm) using a long cassette changer and a greater focus-film distance or with larger cassettes (35 × 95 cm) and three single exposures (6). Often peripheral arteriography may be combined with an aorto-arteriogram when serial films can be exposed using a program-controlled table directed by punched-cards or a control unit (7). Four exposures are required for a peripheral abdominal leg antiogram, 3 for a bilateral leg angiogram, and 5 for a renal and abdominal leg angiogram.

2.1. Program selection

An individually adapted injection program allows a reduction in radiation dose, full utilization of the film, and complete visualization of the vascular area under examination. In choosing the appropriate injection program, test injections of contrast medium may give preliminary indications of the patient's vasculature; the regional circulation time, determined by prior injection of 1% fluorescein or a short-lived radionuclide (technetium 99m pertechnetate), is also valuable.

For abdominal and extremity arteriograms, an image selection with 10 serial exposures is adequate. Exposures distributed over a 19-sec period with two exposures per position are necessary to demonstrate a single arterial occlusion, but when occlusion at two levels is suspected, as in patients with gangrene, it is necessary to distribute the exposures over a longer period. The use of a special film foil system (rare earths; Medichrome films) and appropriate scanning patterns, can reduce exposure time and improve image quality.

Special problems and abnormal findings in limb and organ angiography are better visualized with a biplane technique especially when examining the abdominal aorta, pelvic vessels and the popliteal region. Simultaneous biplane angiography is only feasible with the abdominal aorta and popliteal region whereas anteroposterior, lateral films with tube angulation or oblique projections are necessary for the pelvic segment.

Improved results can be obtained with a magnified angiogram by increasing the object–film distance and reducing the focus–object distance (8, 9). This technique requires fine focus tubes (i.e., a focal spot size smaller than 0.2 mm) and a magnification factor of greater than 1/2.5; it is especially suited for visualization of the intracranial, foot and hand arteries as well as the renal, pancreatic and mesenteric vasculature.

Further improvement of results can be achieved by the use of electronic or photographic subtraction techniques (10). Here, a mask X-ray is taken before injection of the contrast medium to allow a true congruency of the anatomical detail. Though this technique is used mainly in cerebral angiog-

COMMENTARY

Since the renal arteries extend from the anterolateral aspect of the aorta posteriorly they are foreshortened in the frontal view. Therefore, a lateral view may be necessary to optimally evaluate the presence or extent of vascular disease of the dysplastic type. This is especially true when the dysplastic area involves the region of the renal artery bifurcation.

Similarly, oblique views are very helpful in the evaluation of stenoses with transplanted renal arteries. In the anteroposterior view, the anastomosis with the hypogastric or iliac artery may be obscured by opacification of the internal and external iliac vessel.

We believe that anteroposterior and lateral views are mandatory for the proper evaluation of the abdominal aorta and pelvic vessels and the origin of the profunda femoral as well as the popliteal artery and its bifurcation. We routinely film the vessels of the feet in patients with peripheral vascular disease. Generally, only the lateral projection is necessary for a satisfactory study of these vessels.

raphy, it can be applied to any vascular region as it is especially suited to resolving fine details.

2.2. *Puncture and catheterization technique*

Contrast medium can be injected directly into the vascular system at the site of a percutaneous puncture or through a catheter which may enter the vascular system remote from the site of the injection.

Direct needle angiography is applicable only to a limited number of sites: (1) carotid angiography with antegrade puncture direction; (2) brachial angiography with retrograde puncture direction in the angle of the elbow; (3) translumbar aortography with suprarenal or infrarenal puncture; (4) femoral angiography with retrograde puncture.

Puncture of the carotid artery is still performed in cases of suspected unilateral neurological diseases and after acute skull and brain trauma, but most prefer catheterization of the femoral artery.

Retrograde brachial angiography may be utilized to visualize the vertebral and right carotid arteries when the transfemoral approach is not feasible (11, 12). Only exceptionally should axillary and subclavian puncture be attempted (Fig. 1).

The percutaneous catheter replacement technique is now the most widely used angiographic method. The guidewire is advanced through the needle into the vessel, then the needle is removed and the catheter fed into the vessel over the guidewire (13, 14, 15). This method is safer and more flexible than the direct puncture technique. If an arterial puncture in the groin or axillae is not possible, the translumbar route can be used to introduce a catheter into the abdominal aorta and then it may be passed cranially into the thoracic aorta or caudally to the aortic bifurcation.

Direct puncture of the femoral artery is often suited for arteriography of the legs; however, since vascular disease is often generalized, an injection above the aortic bifurcation for visualization of the pelvic arteries and both extremities is desirable.

Direct puncture arteriography is also used for splenoportography. This technique was replaced for several years by indirect splenoportography where the contrast material was injected into the celiac or lienal artery. Recently, it has been shown that embolization of the puncture tract with autologous clot decreases the risk of bleeding from the splenic puncture site. This direct splenic puncture has regained some favor since opacification is greater than with indirect splenoportography.

Indirect angiographic techniques usually involve catheterization of the common femoral and occasionally the axillary artery. The introduction of a catheter into the brachial artery (for example, for coronary angiography after Sones) requires exposure of the vessel by cut-down as there is an increased incidence of thrombosis following percutaneous catheterization.

A large range of needles for arterial and venous puncture are commercially available; most of them having a sharp stylet with single or double mandrin (Seldinger needle (16, 17). For injection of the contrast medium, the needle is fitted with a connecting tube to a hand-drive or automatic injection syringe.

The catheters can be introduced either over a guidewire (Seldinger technique) or through Teflon sleeve cannulae previously inserted into the vessel with a needle combination (e.g., Cordis-Schleusse and Hettler's method). The catheterization instruments consist of a puncture needle, guidewires and catheters, a scalpel, a hemostat, and 1-way or 2-way adaptors.

Guidewires with various and variable rigidity, and tip configurations i.e., straight or curved, are used. Teflon-coating of guides aids in the

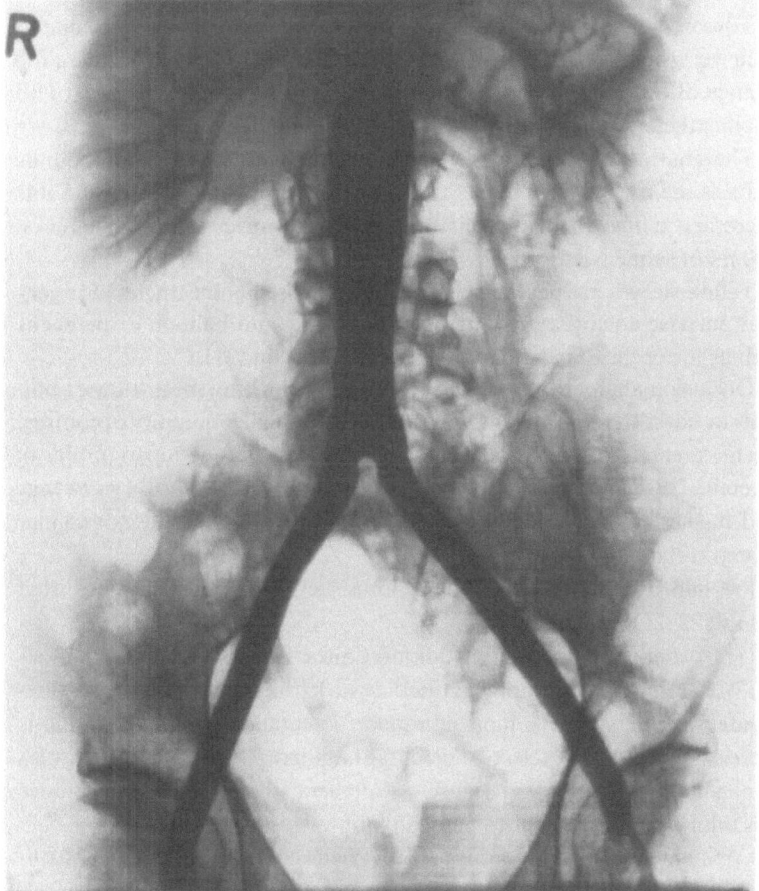

Fig. 1. Y-shaped prosthesis. Transaxillary peripheral arteriography.

prevention of platelet deposition on the guide surface. It is important that the guide be longer than the catheter; otherwise, neither safe catheter change nor safe catheterization can be performed.

Radiopaque polyethylene (Ödman catheter), Dacron, Teflon or polyurethane are all suitable materials for angiography. The tip of the polyethylene catheters can be tapered by hand, shaped on a wire in hot water or over a flame. For certain procedures, preshaping of the catheter is essential for entering branch vessels.

Teflon and polyurethane catheters are stiffer and are more stable in the vessel but shaping and tip tapering require high temperatures; therefore, they cannot be home-made and must be purchased in preshaped form. Teflon catheters are favored for aortography and selective cardio-angiography while for selective angiography of cerebral, coronary, and thoraco-abdominal vessels, home-made and commercially available polyethylene catheters with various curves are used.

Our experience has been that the polyurethane catheters have a greater propensity to clot than the polyethylene variety. In addition, they have more resistance in their passage through the soft tissues so that we feel that the polyethylene catheters are preferable.

Torcon control – polyurethane catheters are also suitable and, due to their very smooth surface with a low coefficient of friction, decrease the chance of initiating blood coagulation, an essential characteristic of all good catheters. These catheters are easily manipulated in situ.

The coating of Teflon-covered guidewires with heparin compounds reduces the risk of thrombus. Such is not the case with catheters, so it is necessary to flush them intermittently with heparinized saline (5000 IU vs. 500 ml of saline solution) (19, 20).

Teflon sleeves are necessary to introduce closed-end catheters for general purpose aortography, angio-cardiography and balloon catheters as well as for occlusion angiography or embolization (21).

Occlusion angiography can be achieved by blocking the in-flow or out-flow or both. Its main advantage is that, with a smaller quantity of contrast agent, greater opacification can be achieved. Selective angiography of cerebral, coronary, and abdominal vessels often requires a catheter change and in these circumstances, the use of a Teflon sleeve reduces vascular injury at the puncture site.

Preshaped commercial catheters for selective angiography are listed below (22–26).

(1) Coronary angiography (Judkins, Sones, Bourassa, Amplatz).

In most instances, a very small catheter will suffice for the transfemoral catheterization of the carotid vertebral system. It is our custom to use a 4.5 French radiopaque tubing such as that manufactured by Becton and Dickinson.

(2) Cerebral angiography (Hinck et al.): the head-hunter and side-winder catheters are the most common (percutaneous catheterization is increasingly used for selective cerebral angiography with catheters of a diameter of 7–5 Charriere because the smaller catheters which may induce less injury can be difficult to guide in long vessels).

(3) Splanchnic arteriography: polyethylene cobra- or side-winder catheters with steering aids (Cook deflectors and Medi-Tech control system) are advantageous for selective angiography, and specially shaped cathe-

ters for the splenic, hepatic, and gastroduodenal arteries can be self-manufactured.

(4) Renal and suprarenal arteriography: commercial catheters with and without side holes can be used for selective renal angiography though self-manufactured catheters with various shaped tips can be used effectively.

A number of other catheters have also been developed; for instance, co-axial catheters for embolization; simple and co-axial Teflon catheters and balloon catheters for percutaneous recanalization, and catheters with detachable balloons at the tip to occlude bleeding vessels or for embolization.

Further developments in this sector are to be expected, particularly with regard to the intra-arterial application of drugs and radioactive substances in the palliative cancer therapy (27, 28).

2.3. *Injectors*

A variety of automatic injection appliances are available for the rapid injection of contrast media. These injectors operate mechanically, hydraulically or hydropneumatically. There is also a mechanically geared hand injector which allows double the injection speed achieved by hand pressure.

Hydropneumatic injectors equipped with an ECG-controlled and ECG-pulsed injection device are to be used for intracardiac injections, particularly in children. Both pneumatic and mechanical injectors are well suited for aortography and selective arteriography. Most demands for optimal contrast media concentration will be met by the volume-controlled injection device with a set flow (ml/sec) at variable injection rise velocity (maximum flow being reached in 0–3 sec).

Though ECG-controlled and pulse-operated injectors are desirable for cardiography and coronography, they are not essential for most other examinations, although their use may reduce the total amount of contrast media required (2).

Automatic injectors for angiography should allow a choice of flow in ml/sec, a choice of the total volume of contrast media and the possibility to adapt the rise velocity with a possible delay before reaching the maximum flow in about 3 sec. The appliance must also keep the temperature of the contrast media at 37 °C and should have an automatic safety mechanism which interrupts the injection when too high a resistance is encountered.

2.4. *Contrast media*

The toxicity of the contrast media has been considerably reduced by the introduction of tri-iodinated materials. Further improvements of these contrast media have been in the use of pure sodium or methylglucamine salt or a combination of sodium and methylglucamine salt of tri-iodinated aromatic compounds. Depending on the field to be visualized, e.g., cerebral arteries, heart and coronary arteries or the remaining vascular system, mixed salts, pure sodium or meglumine salt contrast media are preferred according to their selective toxicity to various organs. The contrast media used mainly are either diatrizoates, iothalamates, iodamide, iositalmates, ioglicinates, ioxagline acid or metrizamide compounds.

The osmolarity of the contrast media is the decisive factor in causing pain. The new nonionic contrast media, metrizamide and the dimer ioxagline acid, induce less pain with comparable opacity and have very low toxicity compared to the tri-ioded diatrizoates and iothalamates (29). These improvements have contributed considerably to making angiography more comfortable (30).

The principal characteristics of currently-used contrast media are shown in Table 1.

Table 1.

	Numbers/molecule		Osmolality (mOsmol/kg)	
	Osmotic particles	*organically bound iodine atoms*	*280 mg iodine/ml*	*380 mg iodine/ml*
'Classic' contrast media	2 (1 anion + 1 cation)	3	1440	1960
Dimer-X ⊗	3 (1 anion + 2 cations)	6	930	1270
Amipaque ⊗	1 (nonionic)	3	470	630
Hexabrix ⊗	2 (1 canion + 1 cation)	6	490	655

2.5.   *Anesthesia*

Because of increased experience with better contrast media and radiographic techniques, arteriography is only performed under general anesthesia in very young children or uncooperative adults. Thus, the vast majority of the angiographic examinations are carried out under local anesthesia. General anesthesia, plexus anesthesia and spinal anesthesia are applied to reduce the peripheral arterioconstriction in hands and feet, though similar results can be obtained by injecting vasodilators (e.g., Priscoline, Bradicinin) (31) in the artery, by prewarming of the limb or by ingesting of alcohol (20 ml 35–45°/ml) or with reactive hyperemia before arteriography.

Local anesthesia should preferably be performed with anesthetics devoid of suprarenin (e.g., Lidocaine, Hostacaine, Xylocaine). An intracutaneous weal is first made followed by peri-arterial injection of the anesthetic agent.

Patients can be prepared for angiography with sedatives or tranquilizers (Valium 5 mg, Tranxilium 10 mg) given on the preceding evening and 0.5 h before the start of the examination. These measures, together with proper psychological guidance, result in an almost painless angiographic procedure, except for the unpleasant sensation of heat. Very anxious patients should best receive a premedication with a lytic (anxiolytic) cocktail (methadon, promethazin, chloropyramin, atropine 0.5 mg) which is also a prophylactic measure against hypersensitivity to the contrast medium, and the first treatment in case of complications. In patients with hypersensitivity to the contrast medium, desensitization can be tried with a high dose of glucocorticosteroid and antihistamine administered beforehand.

Before every angiogram, preparation must be made for the immediate treatment of complications. These include an oxygen apparatus and facilities for insufflation anesthesia and general anesthesia. Analeptics, noradrenalin infusions, barbiturates, antihistaminics and glucocorticosteroids must be at hand.

In view of the possible side-effects, arteriography should be carried out only in units where insufflation anesthesia is immediately available. This limitation does not exclude arteriography in outpatients as side-effects and complications are uncommon.

The use of lidocaine hydrochloride (the injectable variety without a preservative) mixed with 2 mg/ml of contrast agent will greatly reduce patient discomfort. We have used this in the aorta distal to the renal arteries and in both the upper and lower extremities in over 1000 patients with no significant problems. Patient comfort is greatly enhanced by this technique.

The use of premedication with antihistamines or corticosteroids is quite common. However, there is little evidence to indicate that these regimens are of any utility. The number of serious reactions is quite low and the chance of having a serious reaction if one has had one previously is only three times that of the general public. Therefore, it is very difficult to establish a protocol that would determine whether the use of such drugs is of use.

2.6. Complications

Complications of angiography can be classified as general or local. The general complications include hypersensitivity reaction to the contrast medium, cardiac arrhythmias and central nervous reactions. These general complications either occur as a consequence of contrast media incompatability or an exacerbation of the primary disease. The risk of cerebral arteriography correlates well with the underlying disease: the primary disease must be considered in assessing the overall risk of the procedure. A history of allergy does not preclude arteriographic examination. Some advocate premedication with corticosteroids or antihistamines, although the effectiveness of these measures has not been proved (Tables 2, 3).

Table 2. Serious complications in 4348 patients subjected to 8417 arteriographies (299 under general anesthesia and 4049 under local anesthesia).

Complications		
1. Complications of the central nervous system	15	0.34%
2. Cardiovascular complications	12	0.28%
3. Pulmonary complications	2	0.05%

Table 3. Number of reactions to contrast medium in 4348 patients subjected to 8417 arteriographies.

		% Total number of arteriographies	% Total number of reactions
Urticaria	49	0.58	38.6
Nausea	46	0.54	36.2
Vomiting	13	0.15	10.2
Pain	10	0.12	7.9
Sneezing reflex	2	0.2	1.6
Edema of the limb	1	0.01	0.8
Combinations	0	0.07	4.7

A prospective study has shown a low frequency of general complications in angiographic examinations.

Local complications are generally unrelated to the contrast media and include hematoma, hemorrhage, false aneurysm, thrombotic occlusion and peripheral embolism. Intramural or perivascular injection of contrast media and dissection of the vessel wall from subintimal passage of the guide or catheter may also occur (19, 20).

Fracture of the guide or catheter with embolism of the tip rarely occurs but embolism of cava-catheters during or after percutaneous introduction during re-animation or therapy may occur (Fig. 2). These catheters can be removed percutaneously with special devices (basket, pigtail, grip forceps). Percutaneous retrieval-techniques of foreign bodies are more common today.

Proper selection of catheter and guide, the use of heparinized rinsing fluid, atraumatic catheterization technique, and gentle compression of the puncture site, serve to reduce local complications. If thrombus formation on the catheter surface is suspected part of the thrombus can be removed by thrombosis suction, but if thrombosis of a stenotic pelvic artery occurs during angiography, dilatation of the stenosis with a balloon catheter (Grüntzig) (32) may be attempted. The puncture site must be compressed manually and then secured with a compression bandage applied firmly enough to avoid hemorrhage but not so tight as to produce vessel constriction. The patient should then remain under direct observation for 2 h. With high-risk patients or whenever there is good reason to suspect

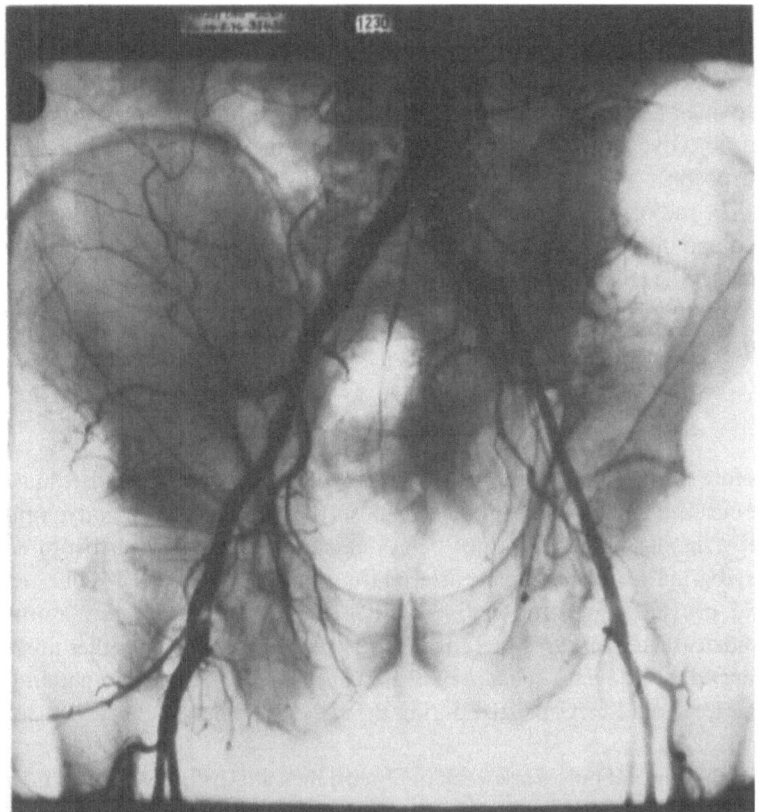

Fig. 2. Thrombus above the catheter in right groin. Stenosis in the left common iliac artery

possible complications, observation for 24 h is indicated. A brief examination some 2 h after arteriography will decide whether the patient can be
discharged or should remain in the hospital. If proper supervision at home
cannot be provided, then it is advisable that the patient spend the following
24 h in the hospital.

Since prevention is better than cure, it is recommended that all individual risk factors be considered before carrying out arteriography and
that adequate premedication and emergency facilities are available to cope
with possible complications.

3.   INDICATIONS FOR ANGIOGRAPHY

Because angiography is an invasive procedure carrying a certain element
of risk, noninvasive alternatives should be performed first. Frequently.
arteriography is performed with a view to immediate treatment, so the

specific aims of the investigation are (1) to confirm or exclude the suspected clinical diagnosis; (2) to assess the vascular system above and distal
to stenotic areas; (3) to assess the extent of pathological findings; (4) to
provide an overall picture of the state of the vasculature so as to aid in
an objective approach to subsequent treatment; and (5) for therapeutic
purposes.

The radiologist must be convinced that angiography is clinically justified and must take the final responsibility for making the decision for or
against the technique.

The following points must be taken into account when considering
angiography of specific regions.

3.1.   *Angiography of the limbs*

Before starting angiography, the inguinal, popliteal or axillary pulses must
be checked and, in the case of feeble pulse, the presence of a hemodynamically significant stenosis must be evaluated by auscultation. Most often
angiography of the complete arterial tree of both extremities is requested
and, provided a pelvic artery is patent at one side, the transfemoral retrograde catheterization is preferred. If vascular obliteration in other areas
(carotid, subclavian, celiac, renal) is suspected, then the corresponding
arteries should be visualized during the same examination (5, 22, 33, 34)
(Fig. 3, 4).

If the femoral pulses are weak or absent, then a translumbar aortogram
is indicated. As a routine, the radiologist should ensure that the patients

Evaluation of carotid, subclavian
and vertebral lesions should not
be undertaken unless one is
considering revascularization. In
these circumstances, we believe
that the extracranial
cerebrovascular lesions should be
studied first and correction
undertaken before peripheral
vascular arteriography and
possible surgery. There is
considerable controversy as to the
priority which should be accorded
to the evaluation and correction
of co-existent coronary artery and
extracranial cerebrovascular
disease. We do not have a set
protocol in our institution.

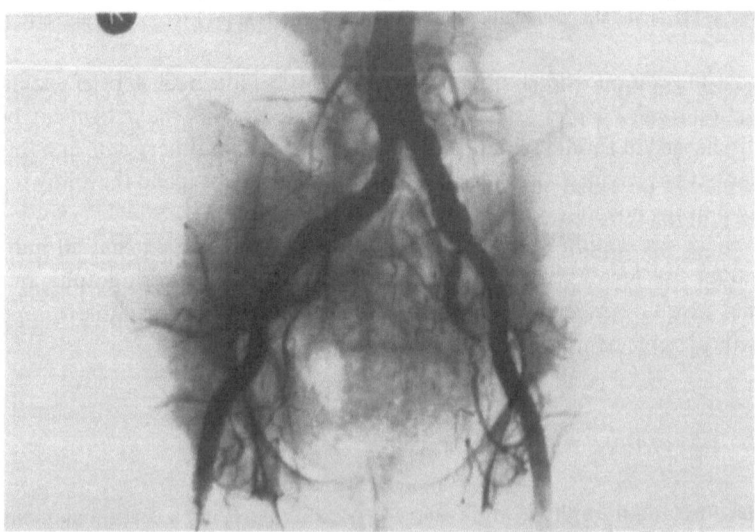

Fig. 3 *a-c.* **Peripheral arteriography.** Arteriosclerotic lesions in the pelvic arteries. Occlusion
of the left superficial femoral artery and right popliteal artery.

have undergone coagulation investigations and are not receiving anti-coagulants. If disease of the thoracic aorta is suspected, then it is possible to examine the area by retrograde, suprarenal translumbar passage of a Teflon catheter (6 or 7 Charriere). In emergencies, e.g., acute thrombosis or embolism in patients with inguinal pulses, a percutaneous, transaxillary catheterization is to be recommended if the coagulation values are abnormal or unknown (Fig. 5).

We use a no. 6 Teflon thin-wall catheter, 100 cm long, for thoracic aortography. Catheters which deliver 30 ml/sec for 2 sec may be obtained, and an injection at this rate is ample for opacification of the thoracic aorta and its major branches.

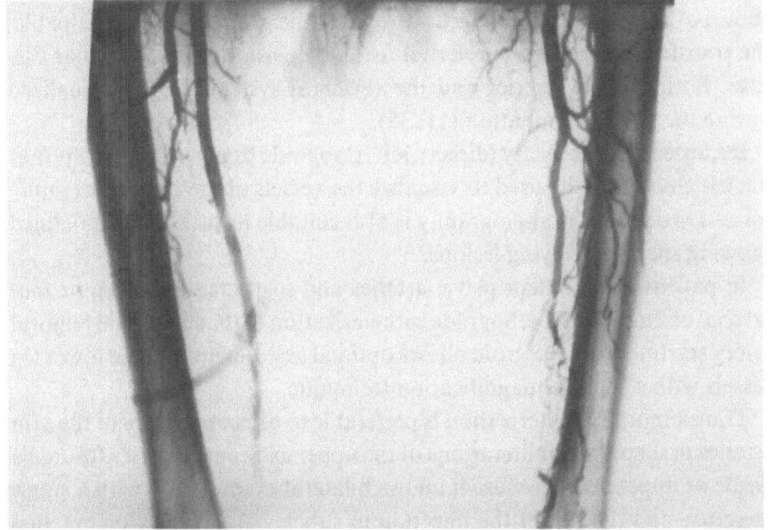

Fig. 3b.

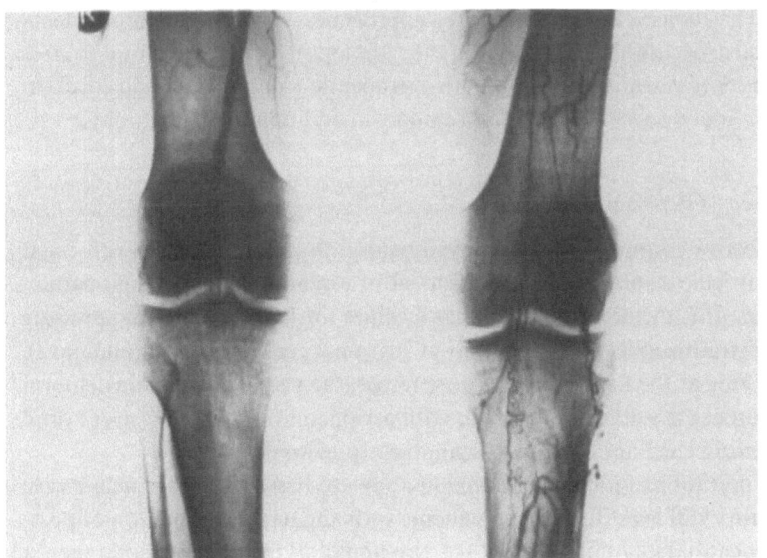

Fig. 3c.

In our hands, transfemoral catheterization of the subclavian, axillary, and brachial arteries is the preferred method. This technique allows more flexibility in positioning the catheter and is less likely to induce spasm. In addition, it is easier to puncture the femoral artery.

If the arteries of the thoracic girdle are clinically patent, then optimal documentation of the lower arm and hand can be achieved by direct brachial arteriography following a retrograde puncture in the angle of the elbow.

3.2.   Angiography of the cerebral supply arteries

The clinical state and clinically suspected diagnosis will determine the choice of angiographic technique. Provided the groin pulses are palpable, the transfemoral route is preferred for diagnosis of cerebrovascular disease. Both carotid arteries and the vertebral system may be visualized during the same examination (11, 35).

Left retrograde brachial arteriography of the posterior fossa is a suboptimal method of study and should only be used if the transfemoral approach is precluded. Direct carotid arteriography does not allow visualization of the opposite side of the vertebral artery without another puncture. It is also uncomfortable for the patient and increases the likelihood of a subintimal injection and should only be used when the transfemoral approach is not feasible.

Because of its simplicity (direct), left retrograde brachial angiography at the left elbow may be used to visualize the vessels of the posterior cranial fossa. Direct carotid angiography is also suitable in cases of well-defined growing space-occupying lesions.

In patients with patent pelvic arteries and suspected lower leg or foot arterial obliterations, orthograde catheterization of the superficial femoral artery starting from the groin allows optimal assessment of these lower leg vessels with a biplane magnification technique.

Transfemoral catheterization is preferable to direct puncture of the arm arteries in suspected obliterations of the upper extremity arteries (thoracic girdle or upper arm) because it allows bilateral examination with a single puncture and the site of the injection in subclavian, axillary or brachial artery can be selected according to the location of the abnormality.

The choice between these three approaches will depend upon the technical expertise and experience of the radiologist. The transfemoral route is the most versatile allowing both therapeutic embolization and local infusion of drugs in the region of tumors in addition to angiography.

3.3.   Coronary angiography

Selective coronary angiography should always be combined with a left ventriculography and the assessment of essential hemodynamic parameters. It is therefore assumed that facilities for ECG monitoring, pressure registration and cinematography at 50 frames per second are available (2). So long as the femoral pulses are present, the percutaneous transfemoral approach is suitable. In patients with peripheral vascular disease or aortic stenosis, the Sones brachial technique is preferred.

Indications for coronary angiography are based on: (1) patient's case history; (2) heart findings in patients with angina; (3) evaluation of post-myocardial infarction state; (4) arrhythmia; (5) pain on exertion relieved by nitropreparations; (6) differential diagnosis between coronary heart disease and myocardiopathy; (7) contemplated artificial value replacements; (8) correlation of physiological function with graft patency.

Coronary angiography should not be performed before 6 weeks following myocardial infarction since the mortality rate, depending on the general state of health of the patients, lies between 0.01 and 1%.

The transfemoral route can be used in anticoagulated patients, and

Coronary arteriography should be performed as close as is conveniently possible to the time of contemplated surgery. Therefore, if surgery, postmyocardial infarction, is to be delayed 6 weeks, so should the coronary arteriography. However, coronary arteriography can be undertaken in the acute phase if the patient's condition is not stable and one is contemplating emergent intervention.

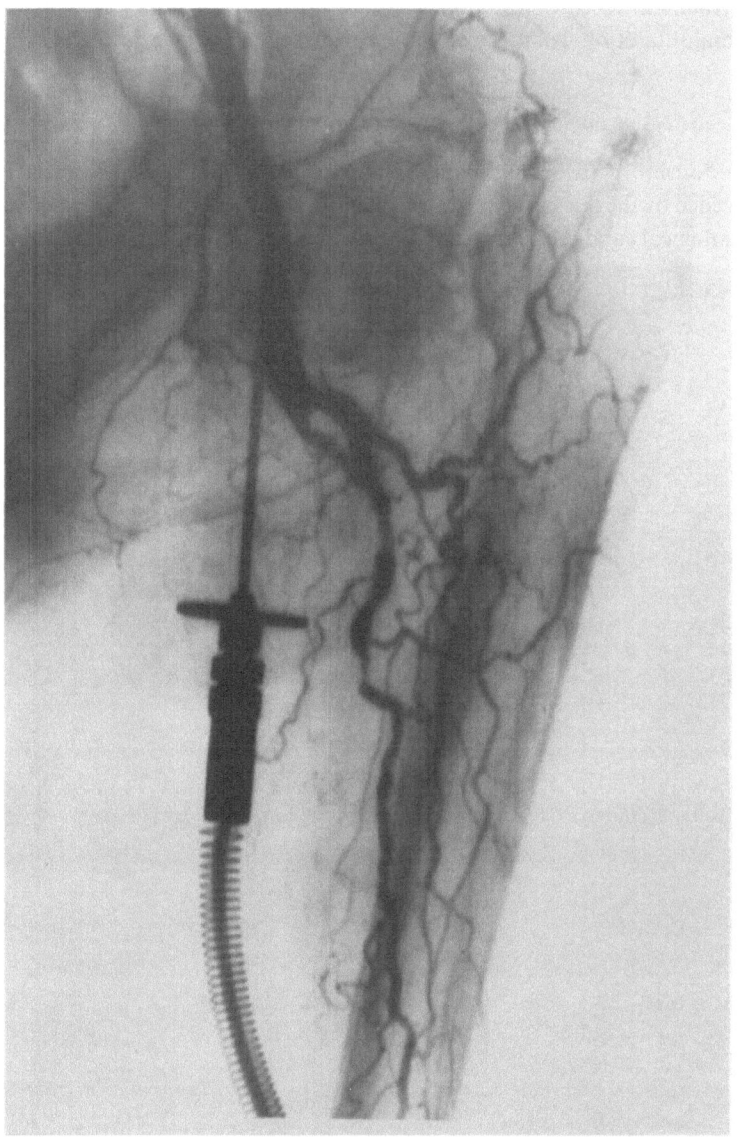

Fig. 4. Retrograde puncture of the left external iliac artery above the inguinal ligament in case of occlusion of the left superficial femoral artery.

it is recommended that 5000 IU heparin be administered prior to the procedure if the patient did not have anticoagulants.

Recent experience has demonstrated the possibility for recanalization of occluded coronary arteries after acute myocardial infarction, if at the time of coronary angiography an intracoronary infusion of streptokinase can be started or a guiding wire and catheter can be pushed easily through the obstruction. So coronary angiographies in the first 2 hours after myocardial sufarction will more often be performed in the near future (52).

3.4. *Selective angiography of organs*

The decision to proceed to angiography of abdominal organs must be preceded by the relevant clinical examinations including nuclear medicine, radiological and sonographic and, when available, CT-procedures.

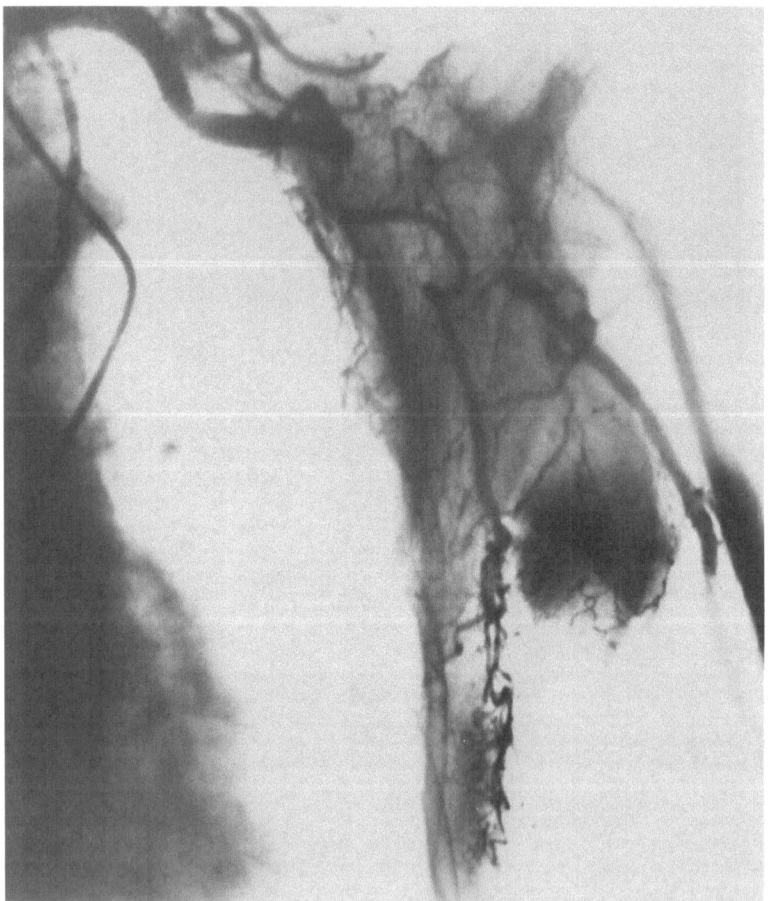

Fig. 5. Occlusion of the left axillary artery.

The decision must also be influenced by other factors such as the differential diagnosis and the possible treatment options. A poor clinical prognosis should exclude angiography, though, in certain inoperative cases, palliative treatment (e.g., embolization, vasoconstriction or the application of cytostatic drugs) by arterial catheterization may still be carried out.

General aortography may reveal gross or bilateral abnormalities as well as the vascular anatomy. Selective arteriography, especially of the abdominal organs and bronchial, cervical and spinal arteries, is always more informative than generalized angiography (24). The equipment should be at hand to proceed to selective arteriography as necessary so as not to subject the patient to an unnecessary second catheterization.

In emergency procedures, the simple technique of spot film angiography on an image intensifier, angiography during operation using an image intensifier spot film camera or memoscope, may yield valuable information on patients who cannot be immediately transferred to the X-ray department.

If the patient is to be subjected to the risk of arteriography, it is to be done under optimum circumstances. Makeshift studies should not be undertaken. To subject the patient to risk without the attendant diagnostic returns is not proper.

4. INTERPRETATION OF ANGIOGRAPHY

Possible pathomorphologic findings of an arteriogram are occlusion, stenosis, irregularity, aneurysm, single shunt, multiple shunts, vascular displacement, pathologic vascularization, vascular traumas (tear, laceration, rupture), vascular compression, function alterations (vasospasm, bead phenomenon, standing waves).

4.1. *Arterial obliterations*

The basic results of arterial obliteration are complete vascular occlusion, hemodynamically significant stenosis, and irregular changes of the arterial wall with loss of arterial tone. The presence of a well-developed collateral circulation indicates that the occlusion has been present for some time (37).

An acute occlusion frequently at an arterial bifurcation may be caused by thrombosis or the lodging of an embolus. The sites most often obliterated by embolism are aortic bifurcation, femoral bifurcation, arterial poplitea, brachial ramification, intracranial carotid bifurcation.

Vascular obstructions in the upper and lower extremities and major aortic branches and visceral arteries are readily demonstrated by angiography. The arteriographic approach is determined by the clinical circumstances.

Hemodynamically significant stenoses can be recognized angiographically if the diameter of the artery is reduced by more than half which corresponds to a 75% decrease in blood flow (36, 37).

In the differential diagnosis, consideration must be given to primary arterial changes, external compressions or displacements and tumor encasement. In view of therapeutic considerations, distinction between the following must be made: symmetrical stenoses; asymmetrical stenoses; stenoses with smooth surface; stenoses with an irregular surface.

Short membrane-like segmental stenoses up to 1 cm in length and elongated stenoses suggest more precise etiologies. A stenosis with a smooth vascular surface may be due to external compression or to an organized thrombus. Nonorganized thrombi are suggested by obliterations with a verrucous surface. These differences may be clinically important in view of possible thrombolytic therapy and the risk of embolism.

Stenotic changes, with or without hemodynamic changes, may be associated with atheromatous ulcerations of the intima as well as arterial dilatation or ectasia secondary to a degenerative process. Other forms of stenosis such as that due to congenital constriction of the aorta (aortic isthmus stenosis) or the arterial compression caused by abnormal insertion of muscles or tendons can also be recognized. Fibromuscular dysplasia causing the characteristic 'sausage chain' appearance is most frequently seen in the distal portion of the renal artery, but similar lesions occur in the internal carotid and external iliac arteries.

4.2. *Dilating arteriopathy*

Among the arteriopathies with dilatation are the true aneurysm, false aneurysm (pulsating hematoma) and the dissecting aneurysm (36).

The dissecting aneurysm may result from cystic medial necrosis (Erdheim-Gsell), arteriosclerosis or traumatic laceration of the intima. De Bakey distinguishes three general forms of dissecting aneursysm (ignoring the rare dissection of the abdominal aorta) according to the site of the lesion.

Infolding of the wall of the fractured aorta may occur following trauma,especially if the intima is separated from the media. The media is not diseased in the same manner that one would find in a true dissecting aneurysm. Therefore, to call this process a dissecting aneurysm adds confusion to the understanding of the pathology of the traumatic aneurysm.

It is important to assess the degree of distal extension and recognize simultaneous obliterations of lateral branches.

The radiographic criteria for a dissecting aneurysm are a band-like stripe (the intima) within the contrast media-filled aorta; step formation of the aorta at the beginning of the dissecting aneurysm; demonstration of two separate contrast-filled lumens; step formation at the peripheral end of the aneurysm; catheter position outside the contrast material column.

The true aneurysm is most often located in the infrarenal abdominal aorta. The exact size of the aneurysm may not be revealed by angiography due to the presence of a layer of thrombus along the wall. If the wall is calcified, films in antero posterior, lateral and left posterior oblique projections may allow measurement of the aneurysm. Ultrasound and computed tomography may give additional essential information.

Besides ectasia, the failure to opacify the lumbar arteries and mural calcification alongside the contrast column are useful criteria for the diagnosis of infrarenal abdominal aneurysm. Moreover, aneurysms are frequently localized in the popliteal artery; in the common femoral artery; in the renal and splanchnic arteries; in the intracerebral circulation.

The diffuse vascular ectasia seen in hypertension is often associated with elongation, curving or looping of the vessels and occasionally causes problems in angiographic opacification because of reduced blood flow. Arterial ectasis and elongation may produce difficulty with catheterization where kinked (arcus) aortae or loop formation in the pelvic arteries occurs. Kinking and loop formation may reduce the torque which can be applied to the distal end of the catheter.

A special form of degenerative vascular disease is the aneurysmatic arteriopathy where the pelvic and femoral arteries have segment-like dilatations and elongations producing constriction and even kink stenoses. Nearly always a second angiographic series is required to show defects of the popliteal and lower leg vessels and a certain diagnosis is only obtained by fluoroscopic spot film angiography or isotope-controlled release of the exposures.

A large-volume, slow injection (8–12 ml/sec for 7–10 sec, maximum volume 80 ml) with multiple exposures at 1–2 sec intervals over a period of 30–35 sec will solve the problem of timing.

Elongation, rotation, coiling and kinking of the internal carotid artery may be congenital or secondary to degenerative changes. These defects may produce neurological symptoms because of vascular obstruction when the head is in a particular position (38). These patients should first be studied in a neutral position and then in the position which results in the clinical symptoms.

Besides the degenerative diseases in which vascular dilatation or obliteration predominate, combination of both forms may appear, e.g., abdominal aortic or pelvic aneurysm associated with ischemic disease of the lower extremities.

4.3. *Special forms of arterial vascular disease*

4.3.1. *Thromboangiitis obliterans (Bürger's disease)* (Fig. 6). Clinically, Bürger's disease can be defined as an arteriopathy primarily seen in male smokers below the age of 40 years. It mainly affects the leg and foot and the forearm and hand arteries. The disease is characterized by a cutaneous phlebitis saltans or migrans. The histological changes are limited to signs of inflammation and proliferation of the small arteries and the dilating vasa vasorum and vasa nervorum (39).

The angiogram shows abrupt vascular occlusions in the tibial, radial or ulnar arteries. Furthermore, isolated and often asymmetric arcate-limited

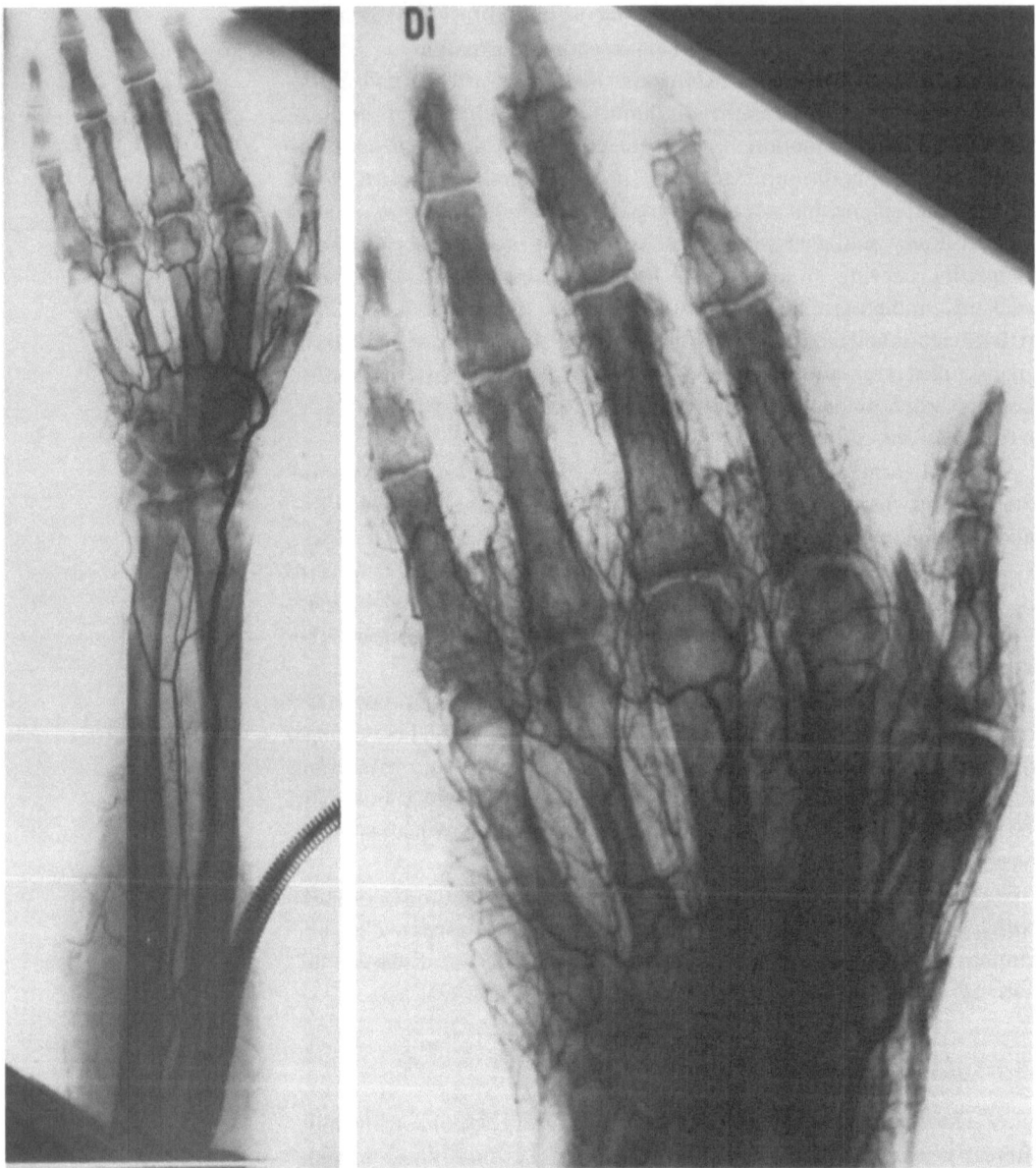

Fig. 6. Thromboangiitis obliterans with occlusions of the ulnar artery and of the interphalangeal arteries.

stenoses may occur in the popliteal artery. Occlusions in the femoral and pelvic arteries only occur in the advanced stage of the disease. The appearance of collateral vessels with heavy corkscrew-like meanders paralleling the occluded vessel is a characteristic feature of the disease.

Under general anesthesia, the femoral artery may take on a beaded appearance due to the formation of standing waves caused by peripheral occlusions. Similar beaded appearances occur in normal femoral arteries when the knee or hip joints are bent during angiography.

4.3.2. *Diabetic macroangiopathy.*   Diabetes is often accompanied by degenerative vascular changes such as vascular occlusion, multiple arcate-like narrowing of the extremity arteries and a relatively high incidence (40%) of multiple stenoses of the deep femoral arteries (40). Other common features are extensive collateral vessel formations which do not run parallel to the occluded main vessels and the formation of nongangrenous avascular areas of the feet caused by occlusions or stenoses of the small arteries of the feet or by arteriovenous shunt formation.

In diabetic angiopathy, one may see hypervascular areas in the interphalangeal folds, as a result of proliferation of a network of collateral arteries. In addition, areas of avascularity, vascular occlusion, stenoses or arteriovenous shunts occur. The digital arteries up to the tip of the toe usually appear normal. This condition can be seen with magnification arteriography in dorsoplantar projection after orthograde catheterization of the superficial femoral artery.

Our experience, which may reflect more advanced disease, is that the metatarsal and digital vessels have been obliterated, and we are unable in general to opacify them, in diabetic vascular disease.

4.3.3. *Hypertensive arteriopathy.*   Patients with a long-standing hypertension may display stenotic changes of the toe arteries distal to the metatarsophalangeal joints.

4.3.4. *Collagenoses.*   In patients with scleroderma, angiography reveals pointed and shrunken fingertips with narrowed or obstructed digital arteries. Poor collateral formation develops between occluded digital arteries; however, a collateral circulation extending from the second digital artery over the rami communicantes can be seen though the vascular network at the fingertips is very sparse. Stenotic changes of the branches of the arteries of the extremities as well as the pulmonary and renal arteries occur in other collagen diseases, e.g., lupus erythematosis.

In patients with primary chronic polyarthritis, displacement of the digital arteries secondary to joint swelling frequently results in external compression of the vessel in that region but, more distally, the arteries are normal.

In periarteritis nodosa, local lesions with small aneurysms and stenotic changes are seen in some 20–40% of patients. Selective renal, pancreatic and mesenteric angiography with magnification technique results in the best demonstration.

4.4. *Arteriovenous fistulae*

Abnormal communications between the venous and arterial systems may be either congenital or acquired.

Congenital arteriovenous fistulae may be either single or multiple, the latter being found in the soft parts of the extremities and in the skeleton. Among the congenital dysplastic angiopathies, distinction must be drawn between the F-P-Weber syndrome, where arteriovenous shunts are present, and the Klippel-Trenaunay syndrome where they are absent. Other abnormalities of the venous and arterial systems may also be present with changes in the lymphatic system.

In looking for arteriovenous fistulae, it is advisable to use TV control or tape-stored documentation followed by large-scale angiography. To quantitate the shunt volume and to exclude the possibility of missing arteriovenous shunts which are not identified during arteriography, examination with intra-arterially injected radioactive macro-aggregates (5–50 μm) is useful.

Posttraumatic arteriovenous fistulae are frequently single and are usually present in the same region as lesions in bones or soft parts of the extremities. After angiography in these patients, it is advisable to apply a pressure bandage to avoid postangiographic thrombosis in the venous system where the blood flow is reduced.

4.5. *Collateral circulation*

Collateral vessels bridging vascular obstructions can develop in the direct vascular path as well as a parallel arterial system. In general, the longer an obstruction has been present, the greater the collateral development. Stenosis of the collateral arteries above and below the occlusion can usually be seen and a sinusoidal dilatation – collateral sinus phenomenon – at the influx of the collateral vessel into the main vessel often occurs.

The important collateral arteries in the lower extremity are the deep femoral artery for bridging occlusions of the superficial femoral, the sural arteries for bridging the popliteal artery, and the fibular artery which usually remains patent and forms a collateral circulation for the foot and distal leg over the ramus communicans and ramus perforans respectively.

The internal iliac artery can bridge one side of the pelvic circulation to the other and the external iliac artery acts as a collateral for the common iliac artery connection to the deep femoral artery after one-sided occlusion of the pelvic arteries. In cases of occlusion of the abdominal aorta or

Arteriovenous malformations are also common in the bowel, central nervous system and the lung.

We have not encountered problems with thrombosis of veins where blood flow is reduced and therefore do not use pressure dressings.

stenosis of the pelvic arteries, the inferior mesenteric artery establishes an important collateral circulation to the two internal iliac arteries, and from there to the lower extremity arteries.

In the abdomen, the arch of Riolan may provide an extensive collateral circulation in the craniocaudal and caudocranial directions between the superior and inferior mesenteric arteries.

In complete aortic occlusion, a collateral circulation is established via the subclavian, internal thoracic and caudal epigastric arteries. This collateral system (Winslow's) can only be visualized by injection of contrast media into the ascending aorta respectively subclavian artery or retrograde in the common femoral artery behind the occlusion. In the presence of an aortic isthmus stenosis, the collateral circulation runs in the Winslow's collaterals and in the intercostal and lateral thoracic arteries in the craniocaudal direction. In aortic arch syndrome (Takayasu disease), the same collateral system operates only in the reverse direction. The mediastinal arteries may provide collaterals in the thoracic region. In the supra-aortic region, a collateral circulation can develop from one side to the other via the inferior thyroid external carotid and the vertebral arteries (subclavian steal syndrome).

Because of their complexity, the intracranial and extracranial collateral circulations to the brain are not discussed in this chapter.

The coronary circulation has both inter- and intracoronary collaterals. Intracoronary collaterals are those which arise from one coronary main branch while intercoronary collaterals are crossconnections from one main branch to another. In the coronary system, reverse flow and shuttle flow are clear demonstrations of hemodynamically significant obstructions; angiographic demonstration of coronary collaterals is an indirect gauge of the degree of arterial obliteration.

4.6. Posttraumatic vascular changes

Torn, lacerated or ruptured vessels and aneurysms can be well demonstrated angiographically. Their appearance at times may indicate the etiology. Historical data easily clarifies the situation.

4.7. Functional vascular changes

Local arterial spasm can be caused by external or internal trauma (Fig. 7). External trauma may be direct, such as knife wound or arterial puncture for diagnostic purposes, or indirect such as a deceleration injury. Internal trauma is most often caused by passage of guidewires or catheters. Mechanically induced vasospasm may give the vessel a spindle or anular shape. In order to exclude the presence of a functional vasoconstriction, it is recommended that the angiography be repeated after a brief interval or after intra-arterial injection of 1% Lidocaine.

Drug-induced arterial vasospasm may occur with oral or parenteral administration of ergotamine preparations. These drugs produce vaso-constriction of long segments of arteries, frequently the superficial femoral or brachial and occasionally the internal carotid arteries. Correlation with clinical history will usually clarify the situation. The arteries will usually regain their normal state within 6 weeks of discontinuation. Occasionally, vasospasm may be caused by drug-induced allergic hyperergic reactions (e.g., penicillins). In exceptional cases, drug-induced vasospasm may occur in other vessels. Mechanically induced spasm, especially during catheterization, can occur in any artery which has been catheterized.

4.8. *Displacement of vessels*

Displacement of a vessel may be the result of a contiguous mass.

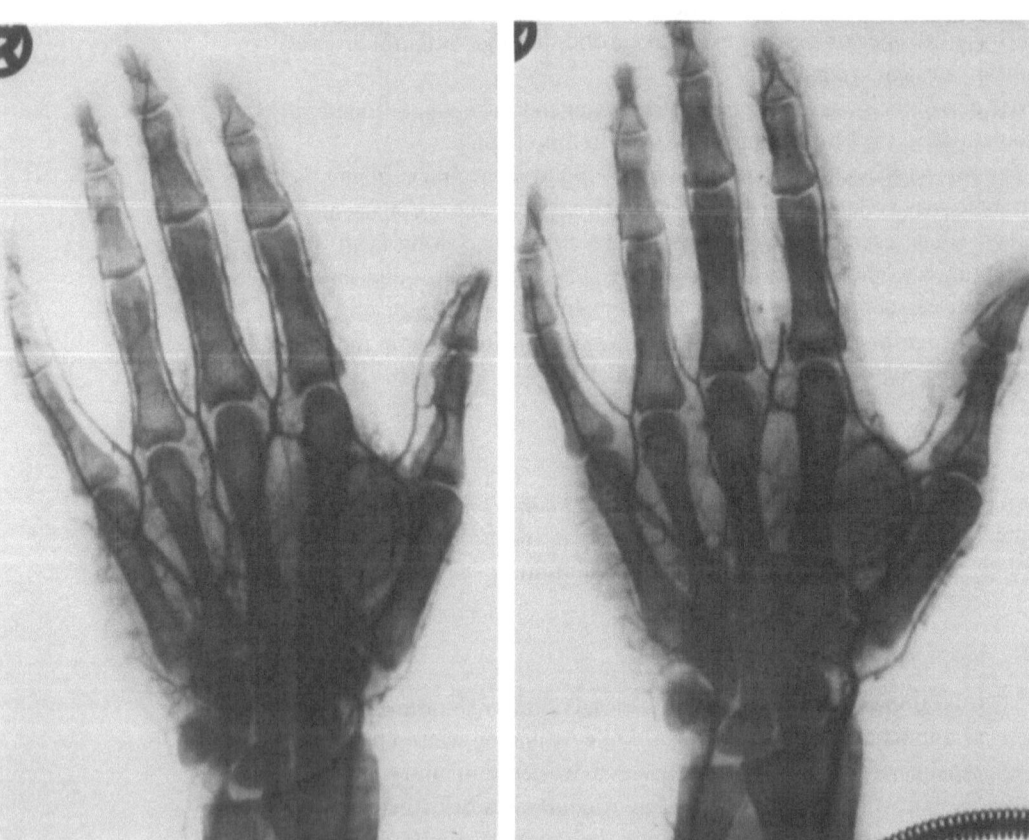

Fig. 7. M. Raynaud. Breakoff of the interdigital arteries before (a) and (b) after cooling.

4.9. *Abnormal patterns of vasculature*

The appearance of a tangled mass of vessels or the apparent flooding of contrast media is a characteristic pattern adapted by blood vessels within a space-occupying lesion and is often a sign of malignancy. This pattern is seen in areas of rapid malignant growth in parenchymatous organs and in bone sarcomas, whereas the benign tumors may displace existing vessels. A similar pattern, which may confuse the diagnosis, is mimicked by angiomatosis.

Abscesses, especially subacute ones, may have increased vascularity about the periphery and a dense capillary stain of the wall. It is frequently impossible to distinguish these angiographically from a malignant process. Historical data may be extremely helpful in this regard.

In the angiographic interpretation, the diagnosis must, however, be made in the context of the whole vascular system including the parenchyma (capillary phase) and of venous phases.

5. ANGIOGRAPHIC-THERAPEUTIC PROCEDURES

It has been shown that contrast material by itself has a vasodilating effect and a hemodynamical improvement in the collateral circulation of obliterated peripheral arteries (stage III and IV) has been measured. A brief vasodilatation can also be obtained after the intra-arterial injection of ATP, Priscoline and bradykinin, as well as reactive hyperemia just prior to the contrast material (32, 41–44).

Reactive hyperemia requires ischemia of at least 7 min. This may be uncomfortable for the patient, but if one has employed premedication and reassures the patient during this procedure, it is generally accepted well.

Drug-induced vasoconstriction can be useful in the control of hemorrhage. After selective catheterization and angiographic demonstration of a bleeding site, selective injection of vasopressin may result in hemostasis. Such treatment may obviate the need for surgery or allow surgery to be delayed until the condition of the patient is improved. Indications for this hemostatic approach after selective angiography include gastrointestinal hemorrhages and traumatic bleeding (e.g., in the pelvis and in limbs).

Once the diagnosis of a mesenteric thrombo-embolism is established by angiography, papaverin injected directly through a catheter which has been selectively placed in the mesenteric artery may be useful. The aim is to prevent the development of intestinal gangrene while the patient is prepared for surgery.

Cytotoxic drugs and radionuclides can be selectively injected following catheterization of the arterial supply of the tumor.

Catheterization and angiographic technique also offer the possibility of dilating vascular stenoses (Fig. 8), recanalizing vascular occlusions (Fig. 9) or conversely producing vascular obstructions, e.g., thrombosis or bleeding internal iliac vessels, preoperative occlusion of the renal artery prior to nephrectomy or closure of a patent ductus arteriosus.

Single Teflon catheters, co-axial Teflon catheters and balloon catheters are used for the percutaneous arterial dilatation, the so-called 'Dotter's

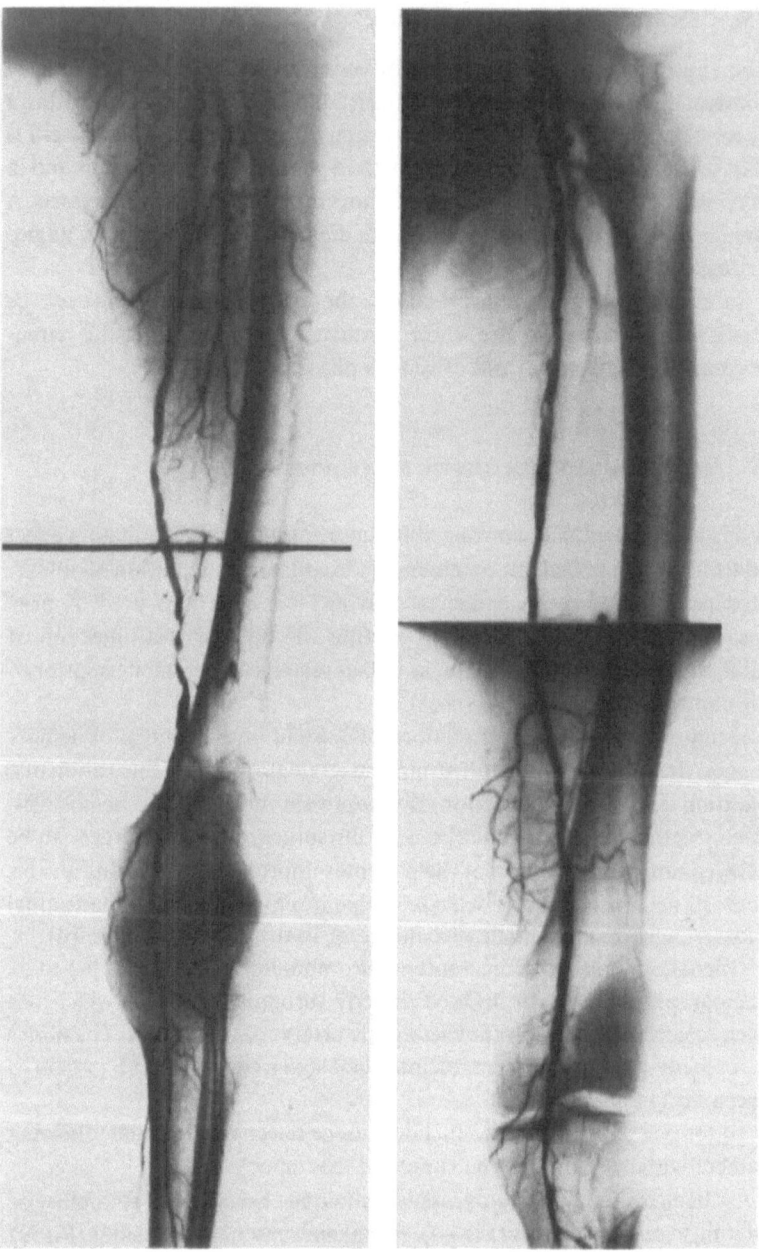

Fig. 8. Stenoses in the left superficial femoral artery before and after percutaneous trans-femoral dilation (Dotter's procedure) with Grüntzig-catheter.

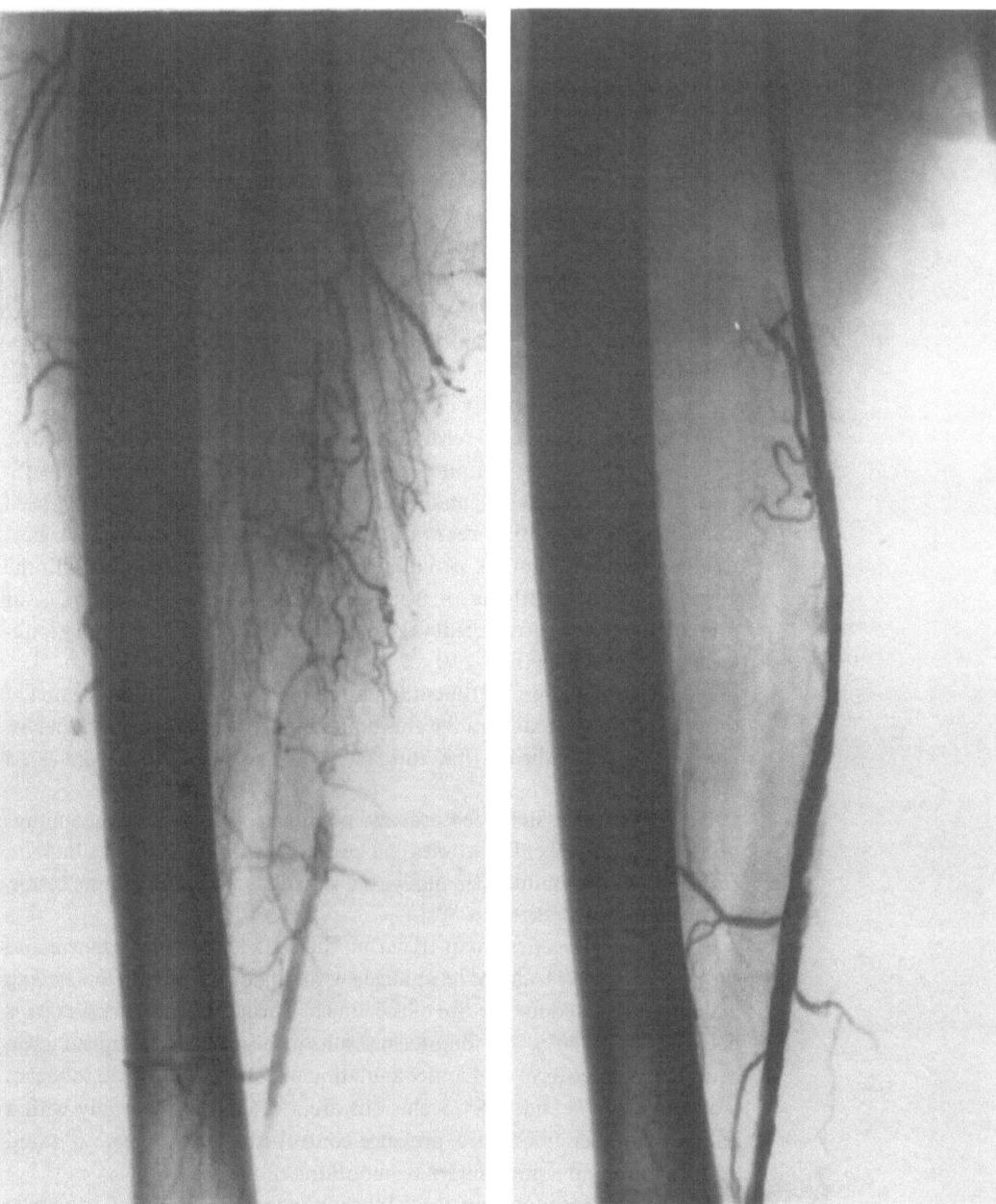

Fig. 9. Occlusion of the right superficial femoral artery. Percutaneous transfemoral recanalization of the occlusion (with single Teflon catheter French 10).

procedure'. Continuous control of the recanalization and dilatation with TV image intensifier is essential for this treatment. Drugs inhibiting platelet aggregation are administered before and after recanalization in an attempt to avoid rethrombosis.

The major indications for mechanical dilatation are (1) stenoses in the common and external iliac artery; (2) stenoses in the femoral and popliteal artery; (3) segmental occlusions not exceeding 10 cm in the femoral and popliteal artery; (4) stenoses in the renal artery; (5) stenoses and occlusions over a short distance in the proximal region of the leg arteries.

This approach is generally limited to patients in whom reconstructive arterial surgery is not feasible or at too great operative risk and should be tried before any amputation. Greater experience may broaden the application to patients currently considered candidates for surgery.

Percutaneous vascular recanalization often can be a real alternative treatment in patients with increased operative risk, e.g., cardiac insufficiency, renal insufficiency, malignancy, restricted mobility of the diseased limb because of another reason, and the patient's refusal of a surgical treatment. In our opinion, percutaneous transluminal dilatation with the Grüntzig balloon catheter of isolated stenoses of the iliac artery is, at present, the simplest treatment with the lowest risk and a satisfactory long-term prognoses (45) (Fig. 10).

A contra-indication for the catheter treatment is an occlusion located in the iliac arteries. Because of the anatomic course, often arcate in the pelvis, and our results indicate that surgery or fibrinolysis is to be preferred currently.

Isolated stenoses in the femoral and popliteal arteries with concomitant obliterations in lower leg arteries can be dilated with the Grüntzig balloon catheter without undue risk and with a satisfactory hemodynamic result. The primary success rate is 80%.

Short occlusions (less than 10 cm) in the distal superficial femoral and the popliteal arteries can be recanalized with single Teflon catheters having a diameter selected for the size of the lumen. The immediate success rate is between 70 and 80%. The long-term results in large measure depend upon satisfactory long-term oral anticoagulation and abstinence from tobacco. Isolated stenoses and short occlusions are recanalized preferably with a balloon catheter utilizing a pressure-controlled pump to permit rapid performance and a good internal smoothing of the artery.

Multiple stenoses or long occlusions in the femoral-popliteal artery are best dilated with a single Teflon catheter rather than with the balloon technique.

We have performed transluminal dilatation in over 1100 patients. There have been no deaths and only 2% required surgical intervention. The safe and satisfactory use of this method requires good technical facilities and extensive experience in selective angiography. Good cooperation between angiologists, vascular surgeons and radiologists will optimize treatment of these patients.

5.1. *Embolization*

Embolization with any of a variety of substances (autologous clot, synthetic material and spirals may be used to treat acute hemorrhage secondary to many conditions (46–49).

The most frequent indication for embolization is a renal carcinoma; embolization will decrease spontaneous bleeding or reduce blood loss during surgery. Each renal artery must be embolized (illustration) for an optimum embolization of the kidney. At present, the most suitable material is the Gianturco technique, whereby a metal spiral with woollen threads is introduced through a special applicator (Fig. 11).

Embolization with the Gianturco technique can also be applied in other

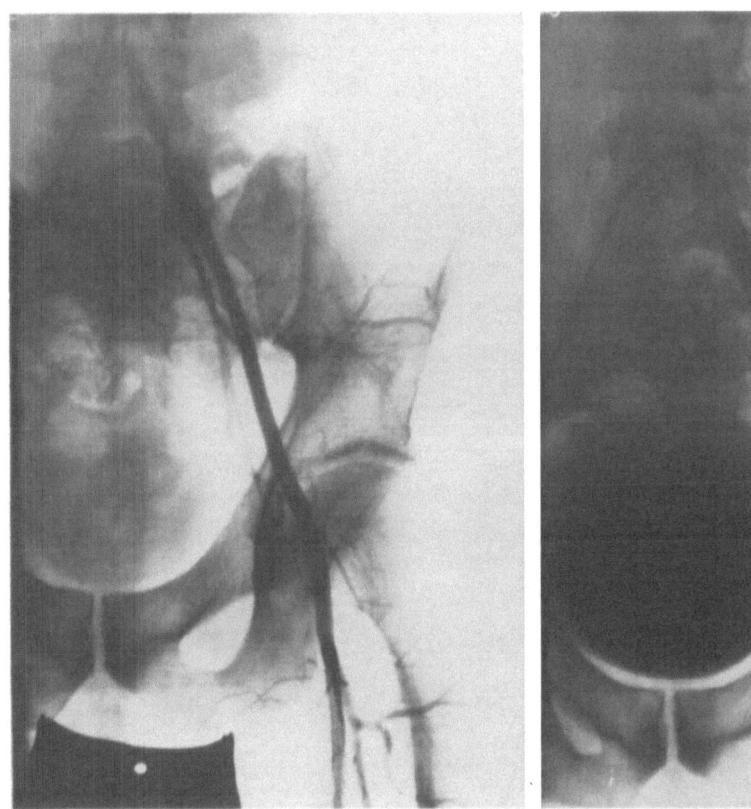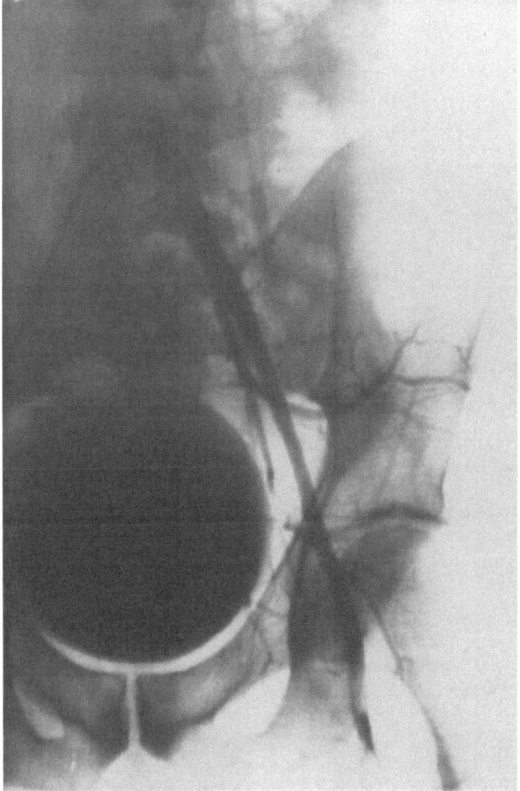

Fig. 10. High-grade stenosis in the left common iliac artery. Crossover percutaneous catheterization with Grüntzig-balloon-catheter, (a) before catheterization and (b) after catheterization.

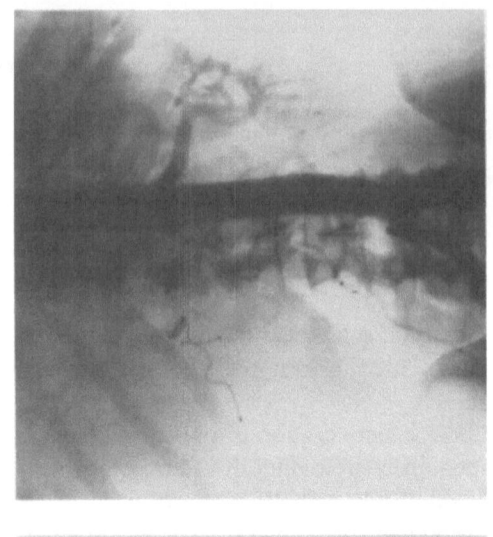

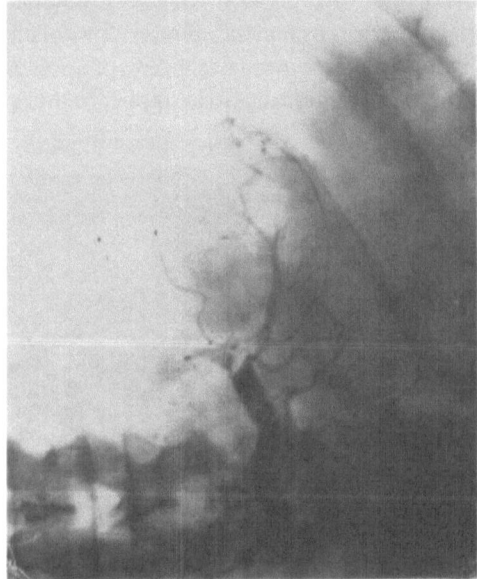

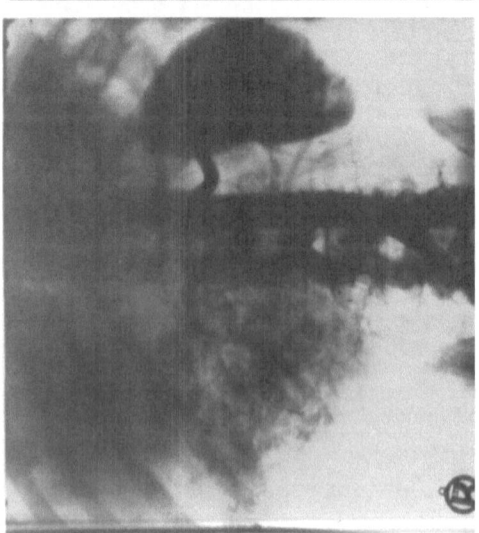

Fig. 11. Large hypernephroma in the right kidney (a and b): embolization with 3 Gianturco wires. Residual vascularization (c): control angiography two weeks later. Progression of the thrombosis of the renal artery.

arteries, e.g., the splenic or the internal iliac arteries. Further indications for the embolization are arteriovenous fistulae of the extremities, lung, face, neck, skull and brain. The use of a flow-guided catheter with detachable balloons is particularly recommended for the embolization of distally-located arteriovenous fistulae. The heavy flow in the shunt area helps to direct the balloon into proper position. This is especially true in intracerebral and pulmonary fistulae. A prerequisite is the radiologic control of the contrast-filled balloon during its progress to the proper position prior to obturation of the vessel.

Transhepatic catheterization and embolization for a bleeding coronary gastroesophageal varices is an alternative treatment to endoscopic hemostasis with a laser beam or sclerotherapy. The superiority of either method is still to be demonstrated.

For the occlusion of a patent ductus arteriosus, an individually adapted plastic plug may be applied over the catheter for obturation. This approach requires expertise in arterial and transvenous heart catheterization and is performed only in a few centers.

Percutaneous selective catheterization techniques have made possible the selective infusion of drugs into various organs. Transvascular biopsy of organs is under development.

REFERENCES TO MAIN TEXT

1. Abrams HL: Angiography, Boston, Little Brown, 1961.
2. Lichtlen PR: Koronarangiographie. Erlangen, Straube.
3. Loose KE: van Dongen RJAM: Atlas of Angiography, Stuttgart, Thieme, 1976.
4. Pässler HW: Die Angiographie zur Erkennung, Behandlung und Begutachtung peripherer Durchblutungsstörungen. Stuttgart, Thieme, 1958.
5 Wenz W, Beduhn D: Extremitätenarteriographie. Berlin, Springer, 1976.
6. Ludin H: Über einen neuen vollautomatischen angiographischen Groß-Kassettenwechsler. Radiol. Clin. 31: 78–84, 1962.
7. Wentzlik G: Beitrag zur Technik der Extremitätenarteriographie mit Serieangiogrammen. Röntgenblätter 4: 298–303.
8. Boijsen E: Vergrößerungstechnik in der abdominalen Angiographie. Radiologe 18: 167–171, 1978.
9. Wende S: Die cerebrale Vergrößerungsangiographie. Radiologe 18: 160–166, 1978.
10. Ziedses des Plantes BG: Subtraktion. Stuttgart, Thieme, 1961.
11. Hinck et al: Simplified selective femoro-cerebral angiography, an improved method. Radiology 89: 1048, 1967.
12. Olivecrona H: Complications of cerebral angiography. Neuroradiology 14: 175–181, 1977.
13. Amplatz K: Translumbar catheterization of the abdominal aorta. Radiology 81: 927, 1963.
14. Dembski JC, Zeitler E: Translumbale abdominale und thorakale Katheterangiographie. Fortschr. Röntgenstr. 120: 432–440, 1974.
15. McAffee JG: A review of the complications of translumbar aortography. Amer. J. Roentgenol. 75: 956, 1956.
16. Seldinger SJ: Catheter replacement of the needle in percutaneous arteriography. Acta Radiol. 39: 368–376, 1953.

17. Seldinger SJ: Visualization of aortic and arterial occlusion by percutaneous puncture or catheterization of peripheral arteries. Radiology 8: 73–86, 1957.

18. Hettler M: Angiographische Probleme und Möglichkeiten. I. Die sichere Arterienpunktion als Grundlage der Extremitätenangiographie und des Arterien-Katheterismus. II. Der perkutane Arterien-Katheterismus mit an der Spitze verschlossenem Katheter als Grundlage der Etagenaortographie. Fortschr. Röntgenstr. 92: 97 and 198, 1960.

19. Paulin SB, Jacobsson B: Thromboembolische Komplikationen bei perkutaner Katheterisierung. In: Angiographie und ihre Leistungen, Loose KE (ed), Stuttgart, Thieme, 1968.

20. Zeitler E: Die Gefäßthrombosen nach Katheterangiographie. Häufigkeit, Ursachen, Erkennung, Verhütung, Therapie. Bern, Huber, 1970.

21. Novak D, Weber J, Butzow GH: Okklusionsphlebographie. Technik und Anwendungsmöglichkeiten. Fortschr. Röntgenstr. 127: 222–231, 1977.

22. Dos Santos R: Sur l'artériographie. Bull. Soc. Chir. 61: 585–590, 1935.

23. Dos Santos R, Lamas A, Caldas J: L'artériographie des membres de l'aorta et de ses branches abdominales. Bull. Soc. nat. Chir. 55: 587–590, 1929.

24. Hanafee WN et al: Selektive Angiographie. Baltimore, William, Wilkins, 1972.

25. Luzsa G: Röntgenanatomie des Gefäßsystems. Barth, Johann Ambrosius, 1872.

26. Zeitler E: Aortoarteriographie in Angiologie, Heberer G, Rau G, Schoop W (eds), Stuttgart, Thieme. 1974, 243–298.

27. Debrun G, Lacour P, Caron JP, Hurth M, Comoy J, Keravel Y: Inflatable and released balloon technique experimentation in dog-application in man. Neuroradiology 9: 267–271, 1975.

28. Peeters F: Zur Methode des aufblasbaren und loszumachenden Ballons. Zur Behandlung von Karotis-Kavernosus-Fisteln. Fortschr. Röntgenstr. 129: 509–511, 1978.

29. Fromhold W, Hacker H, Schmirr HE, Vogelsang H: Amipaque workshop Berlin 1978. Klinische Erfahrungen mit dem ersten nichtionischen Röntgenkontrastmittel. Amsterdam, Excerpta Medica, 1978.

30. Zeitler E: Risiko der Arteriographie in Lokalanästhesie. Münch. med. Wschr. 120: 129–130, 1978.

31. Erikson U: Peripheral arteriography during bradykinin induced vasodilatation. Acta Radiol. (Stockh.) 3: 193, 1965.

32. Grüntzig A: Die percutane transluminale Rekanalisation chronischer Arterienverschlüsse mit einer neuen Dilatationstechnik. Baden-Baden, Witzstrock, 1977.

33. Dembski JC: Angiographische Befunde an den Extremitäten bei Hypertonie. In: Hypertonie, Zeitler E (ed), Baden-Baden, Witzstrock, 1976.

34. Lohmann FW: Chron. art. Durchblutungsstörungen der Extremitäten. Baden-Baden, Witzstrock, 1977.

35. Dembski JC: Detailangiographische Studien mit und ohne Vergrößerungstechnik an Carotisstenosen. VASA 277, 1974.

36. Zeitler E: Röntgenologische Diagnostik der dilatierenden Arteriopathie – Aneurysmen der Aorta und der Gliedmaßenarterien. In: Arteriovenöse-Fisteln – Dilatierende Arteriopathien (Aneurysmen), Vollmar JF, Nobbe FP (eds), Stuttgart, Thieme, 1976.

37. Zeitler E: Aspekte der Extremitätenangiographie. Bern, Huber, 1967.

38. Raithel D: Zerebrale Insuffizienz durch extrakranielle Gefäßverschlüsse. Erlangen, Straube, 1977.

39. Henniges D, Zeitler E: Angiographie der Füße. Fortschr. Röntgenstr. 118: 663–674, 1973.

40. Zeitler E: Angiographische Röntgendiagnose bei diabetischer Makroangiopathie. In: Diabetische Angiopathien, Alexander K, Cachovam A (eds), Baden-Baden, Witzstrock 1977.

41. Dotter CT: Transluminal Angioplasty – Pathologic Basis. In: Percutaneous Vascular Recanalization, Zeitler E, Grüntzig A, Schoop W (eds), Heidelberg, Springer, 1978.

42. Martin M, Schoop W, Zeitler E: Thrombolyse bei chronischer Arteriopathie. Bern, Huber, 1970.

43. Schmidtke I, Zeitler E, Schoop W: Spätergebnisse (5–8 Jahre) der perkutanen Katheterbehandlung (Dotter-Technik) bei femoro-poplitealen Arterienverschlüssen im Stadium

II. VASA 7: 4–15, 1978.

44. Zeitler E, Grüntzig A, Schoop W: Percutaneous Vascular Recanalization. Berlin, Springer (1978).

45. Zeitler E, Schmidtke I, Schoop W, Giessler R, Dembski J, Mansjour H: Ergebnisse nach perkutaner transluminaler Angioplastik bei über 700 Behandlungen. Röntgenpraxis 29: 78, 1976.

46. Boulas R, Kricheff H, Chase NE: Value of cerebral angiography in the embolization treatment of cerebral arteriovenous malformation. Radiology 97: 65–70. 1970.

47. Habighorst LV, Kreutz W, Eilers H, Sparwasser HH, Klug B: Katheterembolisation der Nierenarterie, eine Alternative zur präoperativen Radiotherapie bei Nierentumoren. Radiologe 17: 509–513, 1977.

48. Reissegger W, Stampfel G, Deocristoforo A: Präoperative Nierenarterienblockade mit Ballonkatheter. Fortschr. Röntgenstr. 126: 423, 1977.

49. Stanley RJ, Cubillo E: Nonsurgical treatment of arteriovenous malformation of the trunk and limb by transcatheter arterial embolization. Radiology 115: 604–612, 1975.

50. Moniz E: L'encéphalographie artérielle, son importance dans la localisation des tumeurs cérébrales. Rev. Neurol. 2: 2, 1927.

51. Zeitler E: Die perkutane Rekanalisation arterieller Obliterationen mit Kathetern nach Dotter (Dotter-Technik). Dtsch. med. Wschr. 97: 1392, 1972.

52. Rentrop P, Blanke H, Wiegand V, Karsch KR: Wiedereröffnung verschlossener Kranzgefäße im akuten Infarkt mit Hilfe von Kathetern. Dtsch. med. Wschr. 40: 1401–1405, 1979.

Some little-used and obsolete methods for studying peripheral circulation in patients with occlusive arterial disease

N.A. LASSEN

Commentary by D.E. Strandness

1. INTRODUCTION

The extremities being so readily accessible for study, it is not surprising that a multitude of methods have been described for measurement of peripheral circulation: plethysmographic methods of a wide variety, indicator methods, ultrasound, heat clearance, oxygen tension etc. Many of these have at one time been in clinical routine use, only to be superceded by more precise and simpler methods. This paper aims at discussing this topic. No attempt will be made, however, to list all the proposed methods and their variants. That would yield too kaleidoscopic a view and one would easily risk missing some of the variants.

Thus, deliberately omitting many details, the central theme will be that of affording a background for the choice of methods for routine use today. Quite another topic is that of scientific research of peripheral circulation. Here many of the 'obsolete' methods are of crucial importance!

2. THE BEST ROUTINE METHODS

The distal blood pressure, as measured by the ultrasound or strain-gauge technique, is easy to measure. And, the result, the distal arterial pressure in mm Hg, is immediately understandable for medical as well as lay people, including the patients. This advantage – the 'communicability' of the result – taken together with the reproducibility and diagnostic specificity is of cardinal importance. The result also is of great prognostic importance, since the lowest pressures (below 20 mm Hg) imply a grave risk that gangrene may result from even minor skin lesions.

There are a number of different methods for measurement of the distal blood pressure. Here shall only be mentioned, in addition to the two previously cited methods, the measurement of skin perfusion pressure by radioisotopes or by photo-electric techniques (of importance for assessment of the best level of amputation of a gangrenous extremity) and direct intra-arterial pressure measurement (of importance for evaluating the run-off in cases with multiple occlusions).

To this list of methods may be added a comment on methods used during or immediately after reconstructive vascular surgery. Here the best choice of techniques is not yet so easy in that angiography, electromagnetic flowmeters, direct and indirect pressure measurement and temperature recordings each offer some advantage.

3. SOME OBSOLETE METHODS

Despite the many clinicians that still use *oscillometry* routinely and with great diagnostic efficiency, this method must be termed obsolete. Efficient as it is, it suffers namely from the severe limitation that the results are not immediately understandable for the non-specialist. Another basic shortcoming is the fact that oscillations are often compared between the two legs as if one leg were 'diseased' and the other one 'healthy'. That is simply not correct. Usually both legs are somewhat diseased, but to a variable degree.

The *plethysmographic* methods for measurement of leg blood flow are also obsolete. There is no doubt that, when used after exercise (or after ischemia alone), they are very efficient for diagnosing occlusive arterial disease. Yet, the methods are rather time consuming and uncomfortable for the patient (ischemia cannot be used even after certain types of reconstructive surgery). Moreover, and perhaps most importantly, the results are *not* immediately understandable for the non-specialist and can *not* be compared from one laboratory to another except when – as is rarely the case – precisely the same instruments and procedures are used.

Many *radioisotopic* methods based on the arrival and distribution of tracers in the leg are also obsolete. This is the case for the measurement of the arrival time on the foot of ^{24}Na or ^{99m}Tc injected in an arm vein. The methods are certainly able to show abnormalities in severe cases. But they are semiquantitative in nature. Other indicator methods based on radio-isotopes or heat (actually cold in most cases) are designed for flow measurement. But this is of limited value clinically, in particular in relation to more distal occlusions. And again the results are impossible to understand without special knowledge. Yet, as commented on in the previous section (and as we shall return to below) radioisotopes can be used in other ways that one cannot term obsolete in relation to clinical problems.

Before leaving the 'graveyard' of obsolete methods some words may be said about a few more. Heat clearance by skin or muscle is difficult to render into a truly quantitative technique. Thermography also suffers from the ubiquitous nature of the tracer – heat, respectively cold. However elegant, the new thermocameras cannot be of much use for routine diagnosis of occlusive arterial disease.

4.   SOME LITTLE-USED METHODS

In some special and rather uncommon clinical situations, it is of value to use some little-used methods in routine cases.

Occlusions of the digital arteries of fingers or toes are in some cases best diagnosed by pulse plethysmography. Digital arterial blood pressure, as measured by a cuff around the digit and a sensor at fingertip, cannot in all cases be relied upon to reveal the severity of the lesion, because it may be situated distal to the cuff. Pulse plethysmography of the fingertip, as carried out with the mercury strain-gauge used for distal pressure recordings, will show the diminution and damping of the pulse.

Branch thrombosis, e.g., occlusion of the peroneal artery, the anterior tibial artery or the hypogastric artery, may result in typical symptoms of intermittent claudication and yet the distal blood pressures and blood flow can be normal. In this case a method is needed that assesses flow in the critical muscle, when symptoms are present (during walking). We use ^{133}Xenon injected locally but ^{201}Thallium injected intravenously should also be of use (cf. Section 1).

Arterial occlusion combined with signs of high vasomotor tone is another example. In a small number of patients obstructive and vasospastic symptoms appear to coexist. Typically the distal blood pressure is reduced to 60 or 50 mm Hg, a level that normally suffices to ensure completely adequate flow at rest. Yet, occasionally such patients may suffer quite badly from cold feet. In such patients a lumbar sympathetic blockade with measurement of the temperature response should be used before sympathectomy is considered. Only if a clearcut temperature rise of more than 2 °C is observed do we recommend sympathectomy.

COMMENTARY

The author makes a proper and appropriate separation between methods that are obsolete for clinical purposes but still may be useful in research in a host of peripheral vascular disorders.

Hopefully, few would disagree with the comments relative to oscillometry. The results are not quantitative and of little value in assessing the degree of functional impairment.

5.   COMMENTS ON ONE METHOD THAT WE NEED TO DEVELOP

In ending this discussion we would like to take a look at techniques currently proposed or actually being tried out. Clearly, the subjective nature of this survey escalates one order of magnitude when we try to foresee the developments in the near future.

The main routine method for diagnosing the presence and severity of arterial occlusions will probably remain that of measuring the distal systolic blood pressure with a cuff (ankle and toe) and a sensor placed below the cuff. It also will remain the main method for objectively assessing the results of medical and surgical therapy. But as a sensor the mercury-in-silastic straing-gauge may yield place to other receptors that do not break so easily or are more practical to put in place. Photo-electric devices sensing the arrival of blood to the toe might also be used, but only in the CD (direct current) mode as the signal cannot depend on detecting pulsations in low pressure legs.

Ultrasound mapping of the arteries, a noninvasive form of arteriography, can undoubtedly be developed further. It can best be applied to the groin and perhaps to the poples too. As the equipment should also be usable in other sites, in particular to map the carotid bifurcation and the abdominal aorta, the costs may not be prohibitive.

Multiple level arterial occlusions remain a most real clinical challenge. Arteriography will remain the best way of diagnosing the condition (in our experience segmental blood pressure recordings are simply not reliable enough). Having thus seen the multilevel nature of the disease, how does one diagnose the relative severity of the proximal and distal obstructions? Will the run-off be adequate for a partial (proximal) reconstruction to remain patent and be of value? We currently make simultaneous pressure recordings of systemic arterial pressure (the arm) between occlusions (direct puncture of the intermediary arterial segment, usually the common femoral artery) and distally (at the ankle). Thus, measuring the step-down in pressure over the two most important levels, a prediction of the effect of partial reconstruction can be made. This procedure is rather time consuming and might be facilitated if one could develop a technique (photo-electric measurements on the skin?) for indirect blood pressure recording *without* occluding limb circulation by a cuff.

This comment leads up to the final one regarding measurement of skin perfusion pressure. A small sensor of the type one uses to measure the pressure in an automobile tyre and that accurately (and rapidly) could measure the blood pressure in any small skin area would be most welcome. It would render the cumbersome isotope measurements of these pressures obsolete, and, by rendering this type of information readily available, constitute an important aid in evaluating the prognosis of ischemic ulcers and in selecting the proper level of amputation.

While there may be some argument relative to the use of plethysmography in measuring flow for clinical purposes, the author's points are well taken. Even if used more widely the significance of the numbers provided have little meaning to those physicians not familiar with the methods. This is in contrast to pressures which are readily understood even by the non-specialist and can be obtained much more quickly and simply with a variety of methods. The same reasoning would appear to apply to the isotope methods which have been used to measure skin and muscle flow.

I would agree with the comments relative to heat clearance from skin and muscle. While they may be of use in detecting deep vein thrombosis, they would appear to be of little use in the case of peripheral arterial disorders.

I would disagree with the concept that branch occlusions (not involving the main arterial trunks) can be assessed by isotope clearance methods. Such lesions are exceedingly rare and it is doubtful whether the lesions mentioned in and of themselves are capable of producing intermittent claudication.

It is correct that multiple level arterial disease remains a serious problem, particularly with regard to the significance of incomplete stenoses. There is little doubt that the use of intra-arterial pressure particularly in the femoral artery combined with vasodilatation remains the best method of assessing the significance of the proximal lesion. In fact, it is my belief that it remains the best method of identifying the degree of stenosis from a functional standpoint. It should be used much more widely in this particular situation. It is likely, with developments in real time, spectral analysis of femoral arterial velocity patterns may prove to be as accurate and certainly less difficult for the patient.

12. Venous pressure measurement and foot volumetry in venous disease

DAVID LAWRENCE AND V.V. KAKKAR

Commentary by O. Thulesius

COMMENTARY

The chapter gives a nice summary of the noninvasive possibilities to investigate the venous circulation with regard to the existence and degree of chronic venous insufficiency.

Venous pressure measurements in a superficial foot vein actually reflect both the superficial and deep venous system. Due to absence of valves of the outward-pointing valves of the perforating veins of the foot (below the malleolus) (1) it is possible to assess the function of the deep venous system by tourniquet-occlusion of the saphenous veins. It is true that we are primarily concerned with the function of the *deep venous system* since abnormalities have serious clinical consequences. I agree if we refer all communicating veins between the superficial and deep venous system (e.g., perforators) to the deep venous system.

1. INTRODUCTION

The development of techniques for the investigation of the venous system of the leg has been hampered by the nonavailability of suitable noninvasive methods, particularly when compared to the ever-expanding technology available for the study of the peripheral arterial system. Consequently, the study of the venous system has, until recently, relied extensively upon venous pressure measurement since the earlier publications relating to its use (1-5).

Although Bjordal (6) has placed electromagnetic flowmeters around the veins in volunteers, this technique does not lend itself to widespread use in the clinical field, and must remain a research method. However, Thulesius (7) in 1973 gave some encouragement to workers studying the venous circulation when he reported the use of a volumetric device, the foot volumeter, and its use in the study of the venous system.

The aim of this review is to discuss the techniques of venous pressure measurement and foot volumetry; to report upon a comparative clinical study between the two techniques, and finally to discuss the possible use of foot volumetry in the long term follow-up of patients who have recently sustained a significant deep venous thrombosis.

2. VENOUS PRESSURE MEASUREMENT

Any movement of blood (and therefore change in pressure) within the venous system of the lower limb relies upon several factors, the more important of which are the 'vis a tergo' or entry of blood from the arterial circulation; the activity of the calf muscle pump and the functional capabilities of the venous valves.

Unlike the arterial circulation, the venous circulation is extremely susceptible to external factors, notably the effects of gravity. Pollack and Wood (3), in their detailed study, showed that the venous pressure at the foot in the normal supine patient averaged almost 12 mm Hg and that on quiet standing this rose to almost 90 mm Hg. They attributed this rise to the pressure which would be exerted by a column of blood extending from the right side of the heart to the foot.

Simple, static measurements of venous pressure, though helpful, give no information regarding the underlying pathophysiology of the venous system, and it is therefore necessary to perform measurements in a dynamic situation.

Although earlier workers measured venous pressure in the I.V.C., the common femoral vein and the popliteal vein (8), the detailed studies on the anatomy (9) and the physiology (10) of the venous networks of the foot by Pegum and Fegan have made it apparent that the insertion of a cannula into a superficial dorsal foot vein, preferably on the medial aspect, would give reliable information concerning the deep venous system. It is worth making the point that, although functional assessments of the superficial venous system can be made, it is with the deep venous system, and its capabilities, that we are primarily concerned as clinicians, for it is generally agreed that defects in this system can lead to some of the most intractable clinical problems which have to be dealt with.

2.1. *Method*

Although earlier workers have developed slight modifications of the basic system of measurement, I propose to describe the essentials of the system as used in our unit.

A 21-G scalp vein cannula (siliconised needle, 20-G bore) is inserted into a distal vein on the dorsum of the medial aspect of the foot. We have found that the more distal the position, the less likelihood there is for either obstruction to the needle, or its actual dislodgement from the vein. The needle is connected to a Bell and Howell pressure transducer (type 4-327-L220) by means of a 25 cm length of soft polythene tubing filled with heparinised saline, and then to a chart recorder.

The transducer should bear a constant relationship to the end of the catheter and our practice is either to strap the transducer to the leg, or to mount it on some foam rubber on the floor.

Before proceeding to study any patient the system must be calibrated. The simplest method is to open the system to the atmosphere for the zero reading and then to calibrate to 100 mm Hg by means of a sphygmomanometer. The system should be recalibrated at the conclusion of any individual set of measurements.

Venous pressure is recorded with the patient standing quietly. When the

As stated, it is important that the transducer bears a constant relationship to the end of the catheter (or rather: tip of the needle). If true absolute pressure measurements are to be performed, the level of the transducer-diaphragm must be equal to the intravenous measuring site. Therefore it is astonishing that this cannot have been the case in the present study, since the author states: 'the transducer was either strapped to the leg or mounted on the floor'. This must give rise to variations of the recorded venous pressure due to inconstant hydrostatic pressure levels, especially with exercise, if the foot is elevated above the floor (transducer). This may also be the reason for the observed poor reproducibility of pressure amplitudes with stepping.

The authors use tourniquet occlusion of the superficial veins by applying a pressure of 120 mm

Hg. This pressure level seems somewhat high and it cannot be excluded that this pressure level also affects the deep venous system, especially in short persons. Norgren (2) used 80 mm Hg. The right compression pressure can be checked with ascending phlebography after injection of contrast media on the foot.

pressure is seen to stabilise, the patient is instructed to perform a standard exercise. Our own practice is for the patient to perform 20 steps, at the rate of one per 2 sec in time to a metronome. On completion of the exercise, the patient stands still, until it can be seen that the pressure has returned to the pre-exercise level. Each measurement is repeated three times and between each the system is flushed through with heparinised saline.

There is one modification to the test as described which is used when studying patients with superficial varicose veins. Following the standard measurement as described, a 4 cm wide pneumatic cuff is placed around the leg, immediately above the malleoli, and inflated to 120 mm Hg. This has the effect of occluding the superficial venous system but not the deep veins. In this way it becomes possible to obtain a truer indication of the capability of the deep venous system, free of any distorting effect due to reflux of blood (and therefore higher pressure) from the incompetent superficial venous system.

Essentially there are three measurable parameters to be derived from the test: (1) the resting pressure; (2) the end exercise pressure – or 'pressure drop'; (3) the time taken for pressure to return to the pre-exercise level – 'the return time'.

Other authors (11, 12) have measured the amplitude of pressure for each step, but we have not found this to be a useful or reliable index, and have found it to have poor reproducibility.

A representative tracing from a patient with a normal venous system is shown in Fig. 1. Resting pressure is of the order of 90 mm Hg, and at the end of exercise this has fallen to about 20 mm Hg. The majority of this reduction occurs during the first few steps taken. When exercise is complete there is a gradual return to pre-exercise pressure levels.

Fig. 2a shows the record from a patient with uncomplicated varicose veins. The resting pressure is of a similar level, but the reduction in pressure during exercise is somewhat less marked and less rapid, and the 'return time' is somewhat quicker.

Fig. 2b represents the same patient, but with an ankle tourniquet in place. It is apparent that the patient has a normal deep venous system.

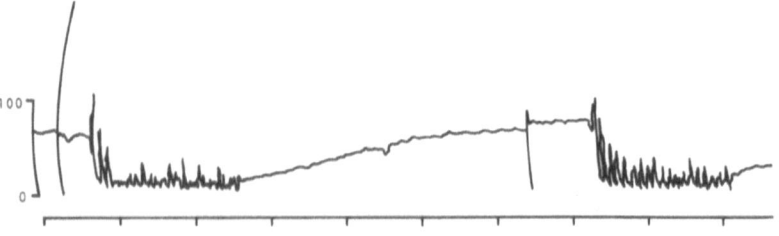

Fig. 1. Venous pressure in normal patient.

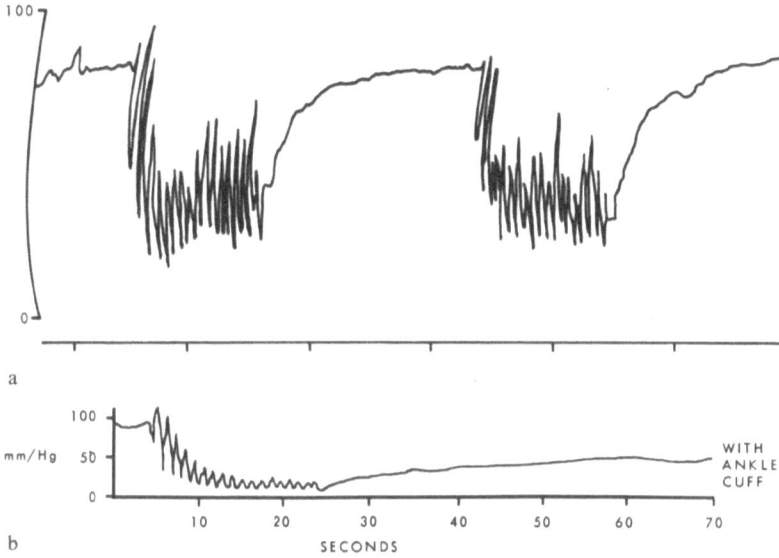

a

b

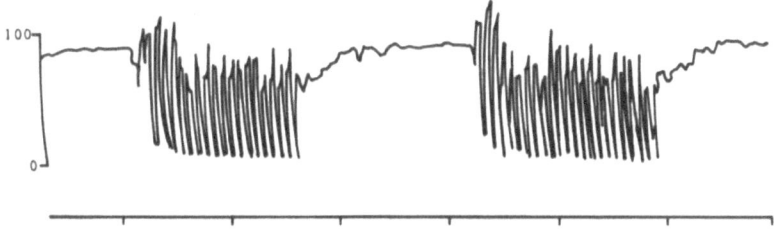

Fig. 2. (a) Venous pressure in patient with superficial venous incompetence. (b) Same patient as (a) but with ankle cuff.

Lofgren (13) has reported similar findings using a slightly different technique.

Fig. 3 illustrates a typical tracing from a patient with an established postphlebitic syndrome. The pressure fall during exercise is smaller, the amplitude of the tracing is larger and the 'return time' is very short. The application of a tourniquet does not alter the appearances of the trace.

There is general agreement in the literature regarding the pressure values for the varying groups of patients and this is summarised in Table 1. It should be noted that, although the mean values are reasonably consistent, there is a substantial degree of scatter. This indicates that in any individual patient the measurement of venous pressure may not yield conclusive data.

Some patients who have an acute or residual degree of obstruction to the major deep veins, without adequate collateral circulation, may demonstrate an actual rise in pressure during exercise (14).

Fig. 3. Venous pressure in patient with deep venous incompetence.

Reference should also be made to the extensive studies with venous pressure measurements obtained by German and Swiss authors such as Nachbuhr (3) and Kriessmann (4).

Other researchers, notably Arnoldi (11) and Bjordal (6, 15), by using double cannulation techniques and additional electromagnetic flowmeters have used venous pressure measurement to gain a greater degree of understanding regarding the direction and flow of blood in and between the deep and the superficial venous systems. These techniques are, however, not suited to widespread clinical use.

The measurement of venous pressure has, therefore, proved to be a very informative method for the assessment of the venous system in both health and disease. However, one should not lose sight of the fact that any type of measurement in thin-walled, readily collapsible, low pressure venous systems is very likely to result in artifacts due to instrumentation. This was particularly true when manometers with a low frequency response were used. In addition, the inertia in the column of fluid in cannulae adds to the inaccuracy. The use of short lengths of narrow bore polythene tubes has lessened this and it appears to not be of critical importance.

Currently, with the increasing development of catheter-tip micromanometers, with high frequency response, these limitations will be largely overcome.

3. FOOT VOLUMETRY

The attractions of a simple, noninvasive technique for the functional evaluation of the venous system are obvious. Venous pressure measurement, although able to give worthwhile information, has several disadvantages, not least of which is that it is uncomfortable for the patient, and this necessarily reduces its usefulness, since it is impractical to use it more than once or twice.

Reference should be made to the study by Aschberg (5) using strain-gauge plethysmography.

The ulitisation of noninvasive techniques such as plethysmography in the measurement of volume changes of parts of the lower limb, in response to position or exercise, is well documented (21, 22). However, almost without exception they have remained largely research procedures. Essentially this is because the instruments tend to be rather cumbersome and there are considerable built-in sources of error associated. Some of these

Table 1. Normal patients.

Author	Number	Resting pressure (mm Hg)	Pressure reduction on exercise (mm Hg)	Return time (sec)
Pollàk 1949	11	86.6 (79–92)	64.3 (—)	31 (8–57)
Pegum 1967	10	90.0 (70–130)	65.0 (35.0–130.)	—
Hjelmstedt 1968	45	—	61.5 (46.0–80.6)	—
Corrigan 1973	20	85.0 (75.0–95.0)	69.0 (60.0–80.0)	45.0 (24.0–80.0)
Lawrence 1977	10	87.0 (76.0–86.0)	49.0 (42.0–60.0)	23.0 (17.0–30.0)

criticisms have been overcome with impedance plethysmography but this too has yet to become a standard clinical technique.

More encouraging, however, was the report by Thulesius and his colleagues (23) of the use of a compact water-plethysmographic technique with which very small changes of foot volume could be determined. Gauer and Thron (24) had earlier shown that the volume of the foot was smaller after exercise than during standing.

Essentially the foot volumeter, as its name implies, is designed to measure these changes of volume during exercise. It is an open-water bath incorporating a critically damped photo-electric float sensor (Fig. 4) which operates an optical wedge, and is connected to a suitable chart recorder. In this way, a continuous, accurate, record of small variations in foot volume ($\pm$ 1 ml), both at rest and during exercise, can be achieved.

In a normal limb with a competent venous system, the volume of the foot falls during exercise (24) due to the effects of the foot and calf muscle pump propelling blood towards the right side of the heart. If either the deep or the superficial venous sytems are incompetent, then not only will less blood be moved proximally, but also there will be a rapid reflux of blood in a distal direction.

3.1. *Method*

The patient's foot is placed in the water-bath which is then filled with

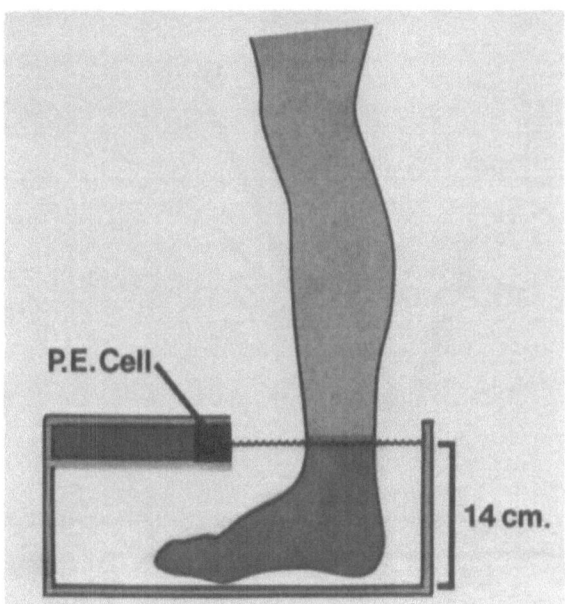

Fig. 4. Diagrammatic representation of apparatus.

water at 37 °C to a constant depth of 14 cm. This level is determined by the photo-electric sensor operating a magnetic cut-off valve. Because of the increase in the volume of the foot on assuming the upright position (25) it is necessary, before conducting any measurements, to allow a period of time for equilibration to take place. This usually takes between 2 and 4 min. At this point the system is calibrated by means of a 5 ml syringe.

A standard exercise is performed which comprises 20 knee bends, to an angle at the knee of approximately 45°, at the rate of one every two seconds, in time to a metronome. It is important that the heel of the foot stays in contact with the bottom of the water-bath, otherwise troublesome turbulence will be set up. On completion of the exercise, the patient stands still until it can be seen from the chart recorder that the foot volume has returned to the pre-exercise level. The rate at which this happens will be determined by the arterial inflow and by the reflux of venous blood, if any. The volume of the foot is determined by pumping the contents of the water-bath into a calibrated reservoir, having the same capacity.

Typical tracings obtained with this apparatus are illustrated (Figs. 5–7). In the normal individual (Fig. 5) there is a progressive fall in the foot volume during exercise (in this example, almost 30 ml), followed by a slow return to the pre-exercise level. A patient with severe deep venous incompetence (Fig. 6) has a much smaller reduction in foot volume, with a rapid return to the pre-exercise level. Fig. 7 illustrates a typical tracing from a patient with superficial venous incompetence.

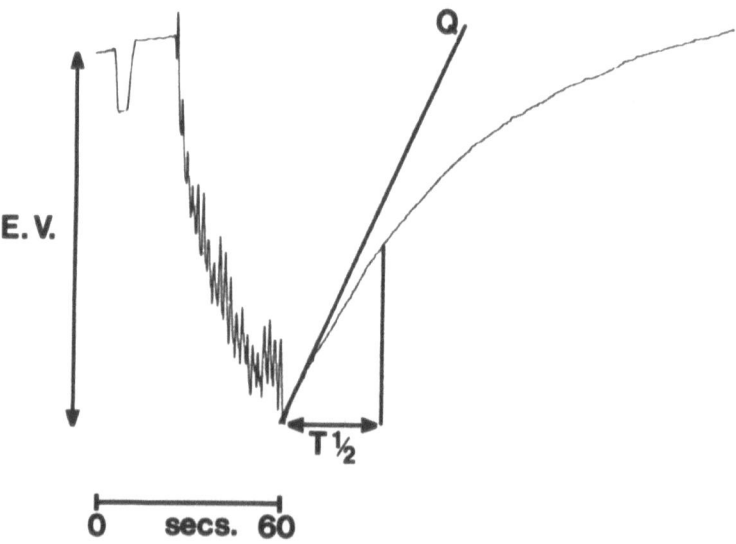

Fig. 5. Tracing from patient with normal venous system.

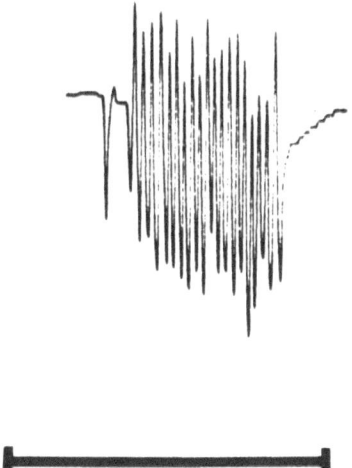

Fig. 6. Tracing from patient with incompetent
deep venous system.

Several parameters are determined by foot volumetry (Fig. 5). The
expelled volume (E.V.) is readily calculated, and this is related to the foot
volume (E.V.R.). The maximum rate of refilling of the foot volume, 'Q',
is determined by calculating the slope of the first part of the refilling
curve. A quotient Q/E.V.R. is used for comparative analysis and $T\frac{1}{2}$ is the
time taken for refilling of half the expelled volume.

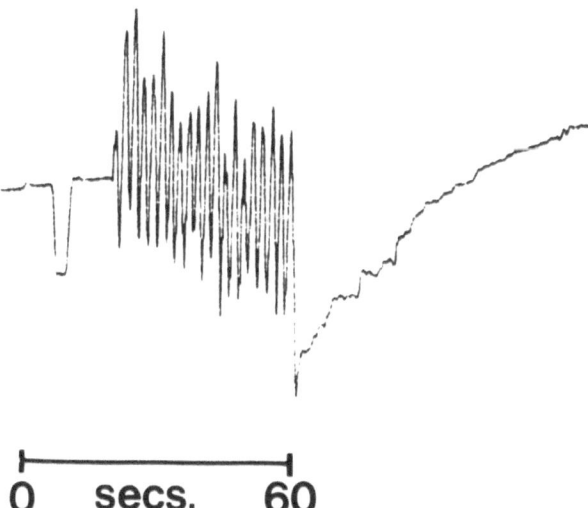

Fig. 7. Tracing from patient with incompetent superficial venous system.

Thulesius has calculated the experimental error to be 1.1% of the mean foot volume (1112.7 ml).

The results obtained by Thulesius in Sweden and in our Unit using this technique are summarised in Table 4. On average, the patient with a postphlebitic limb reduces his foot volume by only half of normal. However, of possibly greater significance is the fact that the foot volume returns to pre-exercise levels about 5 times more rapidly than normal. This rapid return represents the distal reflux of blood within the incompetent deep venous system. These findings are similar qualitatively to those reported by Sakaguchi (22).

In order to compare the accuracy of this technique with that of venous pressure measurement, a study was performed in which 28 patients referred to our Unit were investigated by means of both venous pressure measurement and foot volumetry. After careful clinical examination and ascending phlebography, they were allocated to one of three groups: (1) normal, (2) uncomplicated superficial venous incompetence, (3) deep venous incompetence.

Table 2. Uncomplicated superficial varicosities.

Author	Patients	Resting pressure (mm Hg)	Pressure reduction on exercise (mm Hg)	Return time (sec)
Pollack 1949	7	81.1 (71.0–85.5)	37.4 (29.5–47.4)	2.8 (1.2–5.5)
Hjelmstedt 1968	12	—	52.3 (31.1–74.3)	—
Corrigan 1973		84.0±5.0 (±1 SD)	40.0±20.0 (± 1 D)	11.0±7.0 (± 1 SD)
Lawre.ce 1977	10	84.0 (71.0–94.0)	39.0 (22.056.0)	16.0 (3.0–22.0)

Table 3. Patients with deep venous insufficiency.

Author	Patients	Resting pressure (mm Hg)	Pressure reduction on exercise (mm Hg)	Return time (sec)
Pollack 1949	6	87.7 (62.0–102.0)	11.1 (6.0–19.0)	1.0 (—)
Hjelmstedt 1968	4	—	27.3 (22.0–68.0)	—
Corrigan 1973	6	80.0 (75.0–95.0)	24.0 (0.0–30.0)	8.0 (0–18.0)
Lawrence 1977	11	86.0 (72.0–100.0)	28.0 (8.0–48.0)	5.0 (2.0–8.0)

Table 4. Comparison of results obtained by foot volumetry.

Group	Study	Patients	Expelled volume (ml)	'Flow' – Q/EVR	$T\frac{1}{2}$ (sec)
Normal	Sweden	29	17.0±7.0	1.6±0.8	25.9±12.0
	U.K.	14	21.2±4.8	2.1±0.9	19.8±8.3
Varicose veins	Sweden	29	12.8±5.1	5.7±4.1	10.3±5.1
	U.K.	23	13.0±4.9	5.3±2.5	6.5±2.6
Postphlebitic	Sweden	11	9.8±4.9	13.4±8.6	4.6±3.4
	U.K.	16	9.2±4.7	15.9±6.2	3.8±2.5

Two parameters obtained by venous pressure measurement were analysed: pressure reduction, and return time. Table 5 gives the results obtained from venous pressure measurement. Student's unpaired t-test was used for statistical analysis. In this group of patients, venous pressure measurement was able to differentiate only between groups 1 and 3 ($p < 0.001$) but was unable to separate groups 1 and 2 or groups 2 and 3.

The results from foot volumetry are summarised in Table 6. Three parameters were used – E.V.R.; Q/E.V.R.; and $T\frac{1}{2}$. Foot volumetry was able to differentiate between all three groups ($p < 0.025$–0.001), Q/E.V.R. being the most sensitive factor.

Table 5. Results of venous pressure measurement.

Group	Patients	Pressure reduction (min/Hg)	Return time (sec)
Normal	7	48.5 ± 5.5	22.6 ± 7.7
Superficial varicose veins	11	38.8 ± 18.3	15.6 ± 14.6
Deep venous incompetence	10	27.8 ± 20.1	5.2 ± 2.5

Foot volumetry appears to be a simple, readily reproducible technique which is ideally suited to repeated analyses on individual patients. Patient compliance with the exercise is also much greater than with venous pressure measurement. There were, however, some minor difficulties. Occasionally a result would appear which would be almost impossible to evaluate. It would also be an advantage if a small ankle tourniquet, such as used with venous pressure measurement, could be incorporated.

It would appear that, of the techniques available, foot volumetry would be the most suitable for widespread clinical use. Norgren has already reported (26) upon its use in the reassessment of patients who have had superficial varicose veins treated. This technique was able to give objective evidence of the improvement in the functioning of the venous systems of these patients.

3.2. Foot volumetry and the natural history of deep venous thrombosis

Despite the very high incidence of the postphlebitic limb (estimates vary from 0.5% (27) to 2.2% (28)) the precise aetiology remains obscure, although there are some general areas of agreement which have been well reviewed by Strandness and Sumner (29).

Edwards and Edwards showed experimentally (30) that, within a few days of a deep venous thrombosis, the delicate venous valves became irreparably damaged, and rendered incompetent. However, Bauer (31) in his very detailed study reported that one year after the thrombotic episode only 3 out of 99 patients had any induration and none had ulceration. At

With regard to foot volumetry it is interesting to note the good correspondence between our Swedish results and the study from King's College Hospital, both with regard to normal control subjects and cases with superficial and deep venous insufficiency. For the evaluation of the deep venous system and for the location of perforators we always use tourniquet occlusion below knee and above ankle with a pressure of 80 mm Hg.

5 years under half had induration and only one-fifth had ulceration, but at 10 years, 90% of his patients had induration and 80% had ulceration. Bauer's work first demonstrated the apparent inevitability of these sequelae following a significant deep venous thrombosis.

Not all patients suffering from deep venous thrombosis (DVT) develop these problems and, in an attempt to determine which patients may be at future risk, a prospective study was designed, using the foot volumeter for objective assessment.

Patients with a venographically proven acute DVT were divided into two groups. Group A were those having thrombosis in the calf veins alone, and group B having thrombosis in the whole of the deep venous system. Some preliminary results are shown in Table 7. Results were classified as 'normal', 'intermediate' and 'severe'. A criticism of this data is that the length of follow-up is longer in the group having the major thromboses. However, this does not appear to be significant, since the majority of patients show no conversion from one result to another after the initial 3-month period.

It is apparent that about one-half of patients sustaining a calf vein thrombosis (no attempt has yet been made to subdivide this group, according to the number of calf veins involved) show no functional evidence of insufficiency. Of probably greater significance is, however, that within 9 months of suffering a major deep venous thrombosis, half the patients already showed evidence of 'severe' functional derangement. Four patients in this group demonstrated a 'normal' response. All of these patients had had almost complete lysis of their thrombus by thrombolytic therapy.

The implications from these very early results are that although it may be many years before the clinical manifestations of the postphlebitic syn-

Table 6. Results from foot volumetry (means $\pm$ 1 S.D.).

Group	Patients	EVR (ml/100 ml foot vol.)	Q/EVR	$T\frac{1}{2}$ (sec)
Normal	7	1.9±0.4	1.9±0.8	20.9±10.1
Superficial varicose veins	11	1.2±0.3	5.1±2.1	5.9±2.0
Deep venous incompetence	10	0.7±0.4	16.9±6.9	3.6±2.6

Table 7. Follow-up of patients.

Thrombus	Patients	Follow-up (months)	Normal	Intermediate	'Severe'
Calf vein	36	6.6	17	16	3
Calf and femoral veins	32	9.6	4*	12	16

* Indicates successful thrombolytic therapy.

drome become obvious, it appears that there is evidence of deep venous insufficiency within the first few *months* after the DVT.

The suggestion is therefore that foot volumetry may be able to select these highly 'at-risk' patients at an early stage and they can be offered the benefits of effective, long-term supportive therapy.

It may be worthwhile mentioning that other groups, working with a foot volumeter, have also reported similar results. Partsch in Vienna (6) has done extensive studies with volumetry and compared them with other noninvasive and invasive tests. Foot volumetry is not only a very suitable noninvasive method for the assessment of the degree of superficial or deep venous insufficiency but is also quite suitable for the evaluation of the effect of treatment such as stripping-operations or compression treatment (cf. Gjöres and Thulesius, ref. 7).

REFERENCES TO MAIN TEXT

1. Smirk FH: Observations on the causes of oedema in congestive heart failure. Clin. Sci. 2: 317–335, 1936.
2. Burch GE, Winsor T: The phlebomanometer. A new apparatus for direct measurement of venous pressure in large and small veins. Amer. med. Assoc. 123: 91–92, 1943.
3. Pollack AA, Wood EH: Venous pressure in the saphenous vein at the ankle in man during exercise and changes in posture. J. appl. Physiol. 1: 649–662, 1949.
4. White EA, Warren R: The walking venous pressure test as a method of evaluation of varicose veins. Surgery 26: 987–1002, 1949.
5. DeCamp PT, Ward JA, Oschner A: Ambulatory venous pressure studies in postphlebitic and other disease states. Surgery 29: 365–380, 1951.
6. Björdal RI: Simultaneous pressure and flow recordings in varicose veins of the lower extremity. A hemodynamic study of venous dysfunction. Acta chir. scand. 136: 309–317, 1970.
7. Thulesius O, Norgren L, Gjores JE: Foot volumetry, a new method for objective assessment of oedema and venous function. VASA 2: 325–329, 1973.
8. Stegall HF: Muscle pumping in the dependent leg. Circulat. Res. 19: 180–190, 1966.
9. Pegum JM, Fegan WG: Anatomy of venous return from the foot. Cardiovasc. Res. 1: 241–248, 1967.
10. Pegum JM, Fegan WG: Physiology of venous return from the foot. Cardiovasc. Res. 1: 249–254, 1967.
11. Arnoldi CC: Venous pressure in patients with valvular incompetence of the veins of the lower limb. Acta. chir. scand. 132: 628–645, 1966.
12. Hjelmstedt A: Pressure decrease in the dorsal pedal veins on walking in persons with and without thrombosis. Acta. chir. scand. 134: 531–539, 1968.
13. Lofgren KA: Measurement of ambulatory venous pressure in the lower extremity. Surg. Forum 5: 163–168, 1954.
14. Walker AJ, Longland CJ: Venous pressure measurement in the foot in exercise as an aid to investigation of venous disease in the leg. Clin. Sci. 9: 101–114, 1950.
15. Bjordal RI: Circulation patterns in incompetent perforating veins in the calf and in the saphenous system in primary varicose veins. Acta chir. scand. 138: 251–261, 1972.
16. Pollack AA, Taylor BE, Myers TT, Wood EH: The effect of exercise and body position on the venous pressures at the ankle in patients having venous valvular defects. J. Clin. Invest. 28: 559–563, 1949.
17. Warren R, White EA, Belcher CD: Venous pressures in the saphenous system in normal, varicose and postphlebitic extremities. Surgery 26: 435–445, 1949.
18. Bjordal RI: Pressure patterns in the saphenous systems in patients with venous leg ulcers. Acta. chir. scand. 137: 495–501, 1971.
19. Corrigan TP, Kakkar VV: Early changes in the post-phlebitic limb: their clinical significance. Brit. J. Surg. 60: 808–813, 1973.
20. Lawrence D, Kakkar VV: Foot volumetry – a technique for the functional assessment of the leg. Brit. J. Surg. 64: 298, 1977.
21. Ludbrook J, Loughlin J: Regulation of volume in postarteriolar vessels of the lower limb. Amer. Heart J. 67: 493–507, 1964.
22. Sakaguchi S, Ishitobi K, Kameda T: Functional segmented plethysmography with mercury strain gauge. Angiology 23: 127–135, 1972.

23. Thulesius O, Norgren L, Gjores JE: Foot volumetry, a new method for objective assessment of oedema and venous function. VASA 2: 325–329, 1973.
24. Gauer OH, Thron HL: Postural changes in the circulation. In: Handbook of Physiology, Sec. 2, Circulation, Vol. III, Hamilton WF, Dow F (eds), 1965, p 2409–2439.
25. Henry JP, Slaughter OL, Greiner T: A medical massage suit for continuous wear. Angiology 6: 482–494, 1955.
26. Norgren L: Foot volumetry before and after surgical treatment of patients with varicose veins. Acta. chir. scand. 141: 129–134, 1975.
27. Boyd AM, Jepson PR, Rathcliffe AH, Rose SS: The logical management of ulcers of the leg. Angiology 3: 207–215, 1959.
28. Gjores JE: The incidence of venous thrombosis and its sequelae in certain districts in Sweden. Acta chir. scand. Suppl. 206, 1956.
29. Strandness DE, Sumner DS: Haemodynamics of chronic venous insufficiency. In: Haemodynamics for Surgeons, New York, Grune and Stratton, 1975, p 445–462.
30. Edwards EA, Edwards JE: The effect of thrombophlebitis on the venous valve. Surg. Gynaecol. Obstet. 65: 310–320, 1937.
31. Bauer G: A roentgenological and clinical study of the sequels of thrombosis. Acta chir. scand. 86: Suppl. 74, 1942.

REFERENCES TO COMMENTARY

1. Lofgren EP, Myers TT, Lofgren KA, Kuster G: The venous valves of the foot and ankle. Surg. Gynaecol. Obstet. 127: 289, 1968.
2. See ref. 26 in main text.
3. Nachbuhr B: Die periphere Venendruckmessung. Zbl. Phlebol. 10: 224, 1971.
4. Kriessman A: Periphere Phlebodynamometrie. VASA Suppl. 4, 1975.
5. Aschberg S: Crural venous obstruction or incompetence. Acta chir. scand. Suppl. 436, 1973.
6. Partsch H: Verbesserte Förderleistung der Wadenmuskelpumpe unter Kompressionsstrümpfen bei Varizen und venöser Insuffizienz. Phlebol. und Proctol. 7: 58, 1978.
7. Gjöres JE, Thulesius O: Compression treatment in venous insufficiency evaluated with foot volumetry. VASA 6: 364, 1977.

13. Phlebography and cinephlebography

VIJAY V. KAKKAR

Commentary by H.L. Neiman

1. INTRODUCTION

Phlebography was first introduced by Dos Santos in 1937 (1), and later, in 1940, Bauer (2) advocated its routine use in the management of deep vein thrombosis. Unfortunately its value as a diagnostic tool was not appreciated by clinicans, mainly because of the lack of a simple technique which would consistently produce good quality X-rays. The method employed consisted of injecting large amounts of contrast medium through a vein on the dorsum of the foot in an attempt to completely fill the deep and superficial venous systems of the leg, and taking exposures at set times after the injection. This technique often produced unsatisfactory films and 'false-positive' results because of streamline flow and poor mixing of the contrast medium. The introduction of modern X-ray diagnostic equipment, including the image intensifier and television monitor screen, has enabled venographic techniques to be developed to a point where they may now be relied upon as an effective method for demonstrating most venous thrombi that are of clinical interest.

A number of improved venographic techniques have recently been described by several authors (3–7). Although each of these has been claimed by its exponents to be superior, they are in essence all based on a similar principle of watching almost continuously the filling of the deep veins of the legs with contrast medium, exposing films at the correct time and thus allowing more precise diagnosis than ever before as to whether a thrombus is present or not. The technique of ascending functional cinephlebography (8) has the added advantage that it not only provides information concerning the patency of the deep veins but also demonstrates valvular function with the patient in an almost upright position.

COMMENTARY

Contrast phlebography is the standard by which other diagnostic techniques for evaluation of lower extremity venous diseases are assessed. Contrast venography is the only examination which provides direct evidence of the presence of deep vein thrombosis, the extent of the pathologic process and chronicity.

As Dr. Kakkar states, there are numerous techniques for performing ascending phlebography, each with supposed advantages. The salient point, however, is that any technique is satisfactory when performed in a conscientious fashion. We prefer a modification of the Rabinov and Paulin technique which utilizes non-weight-bearing of the examined leg and no tourniquet (1).

2.   ASCENDING FUNCTIONAL PHLEBOGRAPHY

The main features of this technique of phlebography are as follows. The patient lies supine on a horizontal mobile table. A specially constructed pneumatic tourniquet is placed just above the ankle and another in the midthigh region (Fig. 1). The distal tourniquet is distended to a pressure of 80–100 mm/Hg to prevent filling of the superficial veins of the leg and to direct the contrast medium into the deep veins. A scalp vein 21G thin wall (20G bore) infusion cannula is introduced into a vein on the dorsum of the great toe; this vein is selected because it is easy to cannulate and directly joins the plantar plexus through the first intra-osseous space. Therefore, any contast medium injected into this vein flow directly to the deep veins (Fig. 2). In grossly swollen limbs, the vein can be visualized by gently massaging the edema fluid away from such a site. The cannula is attached to a 50 ml syringe containing 30–40 ml of contrast medium that has been warmed to body temperature. The tourniquet at the thigh is now distended to just above systolic pressure; this ensures adequate filling of all the deep distal veins. The contrast medium is injected slowly and its progress in the

With our technique the patient is examined in a semi-upright position which allows for maximal filling without flow artifacts (2). As noted in the adjacent manuscript, it is usually helpful to fluoroscopically visualize the contrast material ascending in the veins. Filming in an anterior-posterior, externally rotated oblique and a lateral view of the leg are obtained after the injection of 50 ml of contrast material. The lateral view of the

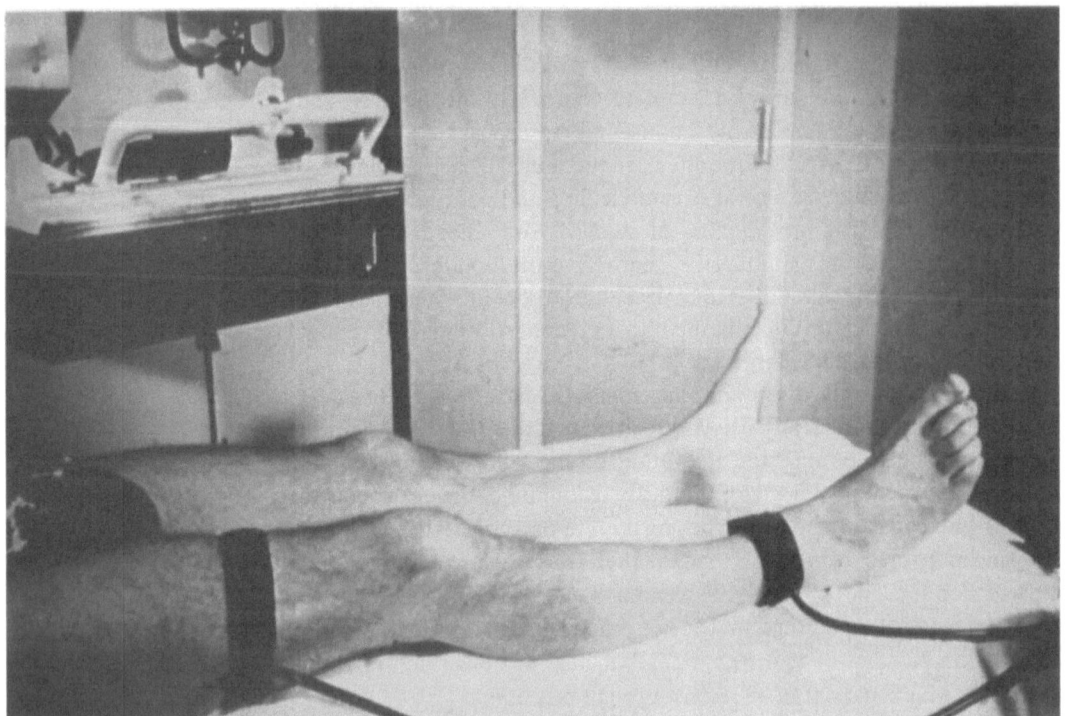

Fig. 1. Position of pneumatic cuffs which are applied to (a) direct the contrast medium into the deep venous system (ankle cuff). and (b) create a pressure zone in the popliteal vein to ensure adequate filling of tibial veins (midthigh cuff).

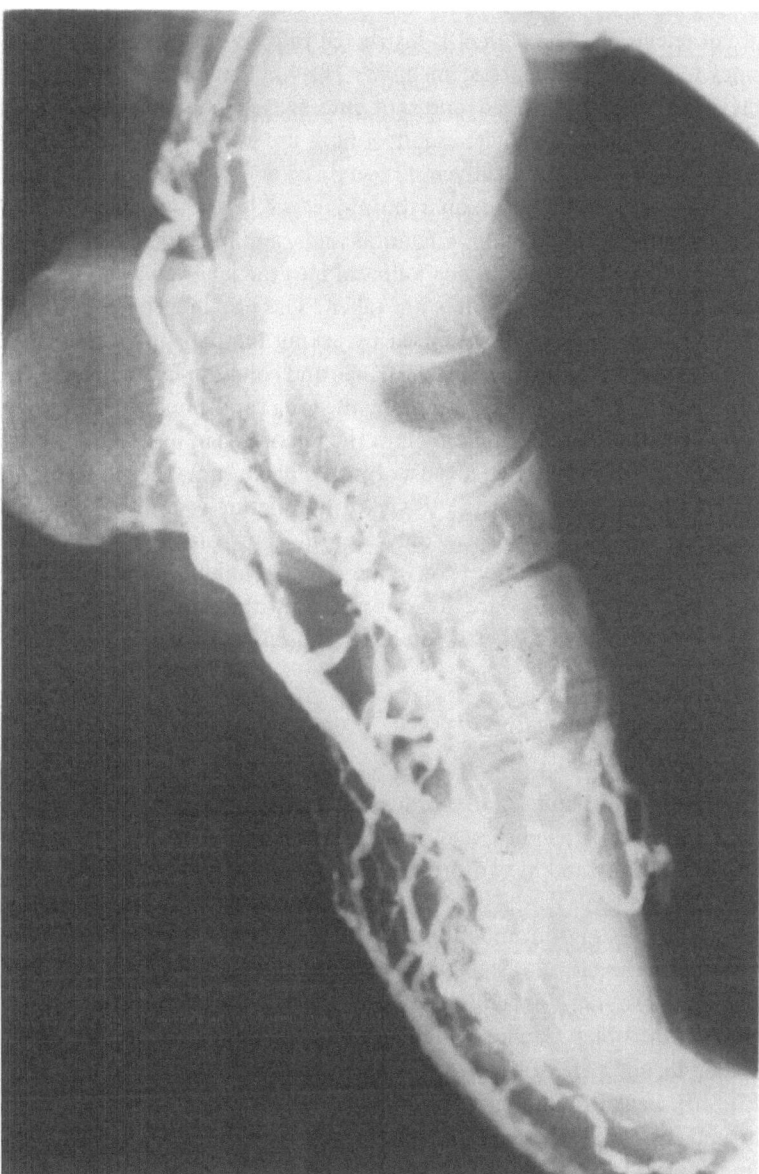

Fig. 2. Lateral X-ray of the foor showing selective filling of the planter plexus, and the contrast medium flowing directly in the tibial veins.

leg is particularly important to demonstrate the posterior tibial and soleal veins (3, 4). Radiographic exposures should be made in the range of 70 kV. Additional contrast material is then injected and anterior-posterior and externally rotated oblique views of the popliteal region are obtained. Positioning the knee slightly flexed often results in better popliteal vein filling (5).

The upper femoral and iliac veins are visualized by gentle application of pressure to the calf or rapid flexion of the foot 5 or 6 times. This allows for a surge of contrast material into the desired areas. A Valsalva maneuver during this time may help to visualize the proximal portion of the profunda femoris and internal iliac veins. This latter technique demonstrates the profunda femoris vein in approximately 50% of cases (1). In the remainder, a flow defect from the profunda femoris vein is usually seen as a secondary sign of patency.

Occasionally, there is poor preferential filling of the superficial venous system with poor visualization of either part, or all of the deep venous systems by this technique. In this situation, a tourniquet is applied at the ankle and a repeat injection of approximately 50 ml of contrast material is made. This technique forces contrast material into the deep venous system as in a standard tourniquet type examination and allows for visualization of intraluminal thrombus. Diversion of flow into the superficial venous system without the use of a tourniquet is strong circumstantial evidence of deep venous thrombosis. The additional use of the tourniquet, however, absolutely confirms the diagnosis and excludes the possibility of faulty needle placement.

The described technique has the advantages of producing excellent filling of the deep venous system, including the soleal veins as well as the femoral and iliac veins. Multiple views of each of these veins also reduce the possibility of missing a small thrombus. The main advantage, however, is that the technique is easily performed and has a high patient acceptability. As such, the technique can be advocated for widespread use for the previously noted indications. The procedure can be performed quickly and is applicable to any radiologic facility.

The technique, as advocated by Dr. Kakkar on the other hand, probably is more sensitive in detecting thrombi, particularly in the small soleal branches and is the definitive method for performing venography. The disadvantage, however, is that it is somewhat more time consuming and it requires more highly trained personnel to produce an adequate study.

Finally, the widely used technique of Rogoff and DeWeese (6) has the advantage of allowing for examination of both legs simultaneously. The technique also utilizes smaller amounts of contrast material. The disadvantages, however, are that the anterior tibial veins and soleal sinusoids are often poorly visualized. The femoral vein and iliac veins may also be seen poorly. If significant deep vein thrombosis is present, the application of the tourniquet with associated injection of contrast material may cause significant patient discomfort as there is a stripping effect by the contrast material between the thrombus and vein intima producing the characteristic railroad track sign of deep vein disease. This obviously decreases patient acceptance of the procedure.

tibial veins is observed with the aid of an image intensifier and closed-circuit television. The patient is instructed to plantar flex the foot 5 or 6 times to propel the contrast medium. The tibial veins are seen on the television screen to be filled, and spot films are taken in both the anterio-posterior and lateral planes; usually 4 films are exposed over this region (Fig. 3). Next, the popliteal vein is visualized and two films are exposed over this area. Now the proximal tourniquet is released; this allows filling of the superficial and common femoral veins, and films are taken (Fig. 4 and 5). The contrast medium is followed into the iliac veins and inferior vena cava and again two films are taken. The proximal portion of the profunda femoris vein is visualized by asking the patient to perform a Valsalva maneuver once the external iliac and common femoral veins are filled. The examiner hand is run along the long saphenous vein in the leg and thigh emptying the contents into the femoral vein just before a film is taken. By this technique, it is usually possible to show the whole of the deep venous system from the tibial to the inferior vena cava (Fig. 6). However, the soleal veins are only seen in approximately 85% of the patients. Recently, a modification of the above technique has been devised whereby the soleal veins are invariably filled with contrast medium and thrombi starting there (Fig. 7) can be diagnosed with greater confidence.

2.1. Criteria for diagnosis of venous thrombosis

There seems to be fairly general agreement concerning the venographic criteria for the diagnosis of venous thrombosis. When a filling defect persists in a well-opacified vein, remains unchanged in shape or location during screening and in two subsequent radiographs, then a diagnosis of venous thrombosis can be accepted with reasonable confidence (Fig. 8). Partially occluding thrombi are usually seen as well-defined translucent areas with a rim of contrast medium surrounding them. Their extent varies from small, solitary thrombi to extensive, serpiginous clots involving the whole of the tibial, popliteal, and femoral veins (Fig. 9). Completely oc-cluding thrombi are of two types: with and without collateral circulation (Fig. 10). Lack of filling in veins or segments of veins as an indication of thrombosis should be accepted with great caution. Artefacts having a similar appearance can occasionally be produced by sudden muscular contraction and spasm. Similarly, other ancillary radiographic evidence, such as 'reversed flow' and 'knot whole' filling defects, should be viewed with suspicion.

2.2. Complications of ascending venography

Many patients complain of discomfort in the heel during injection of the

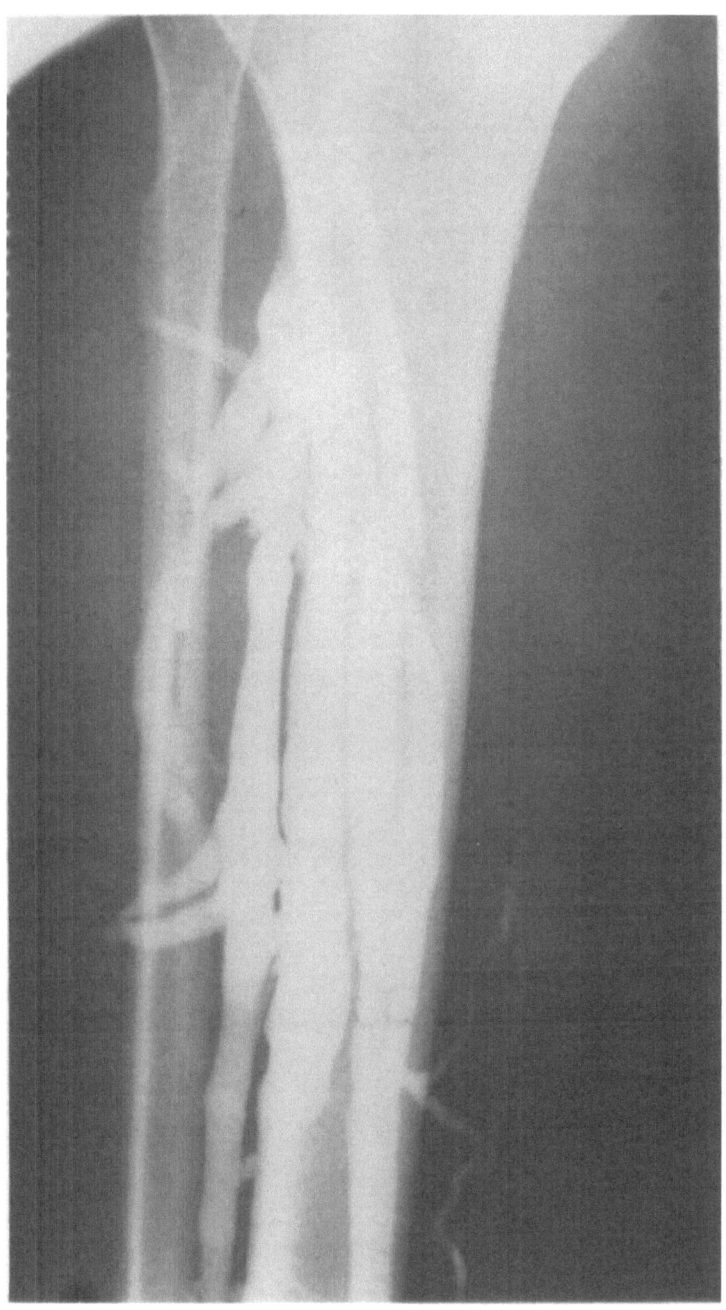

Fig. 3. Normal appearance of the tibial veins.

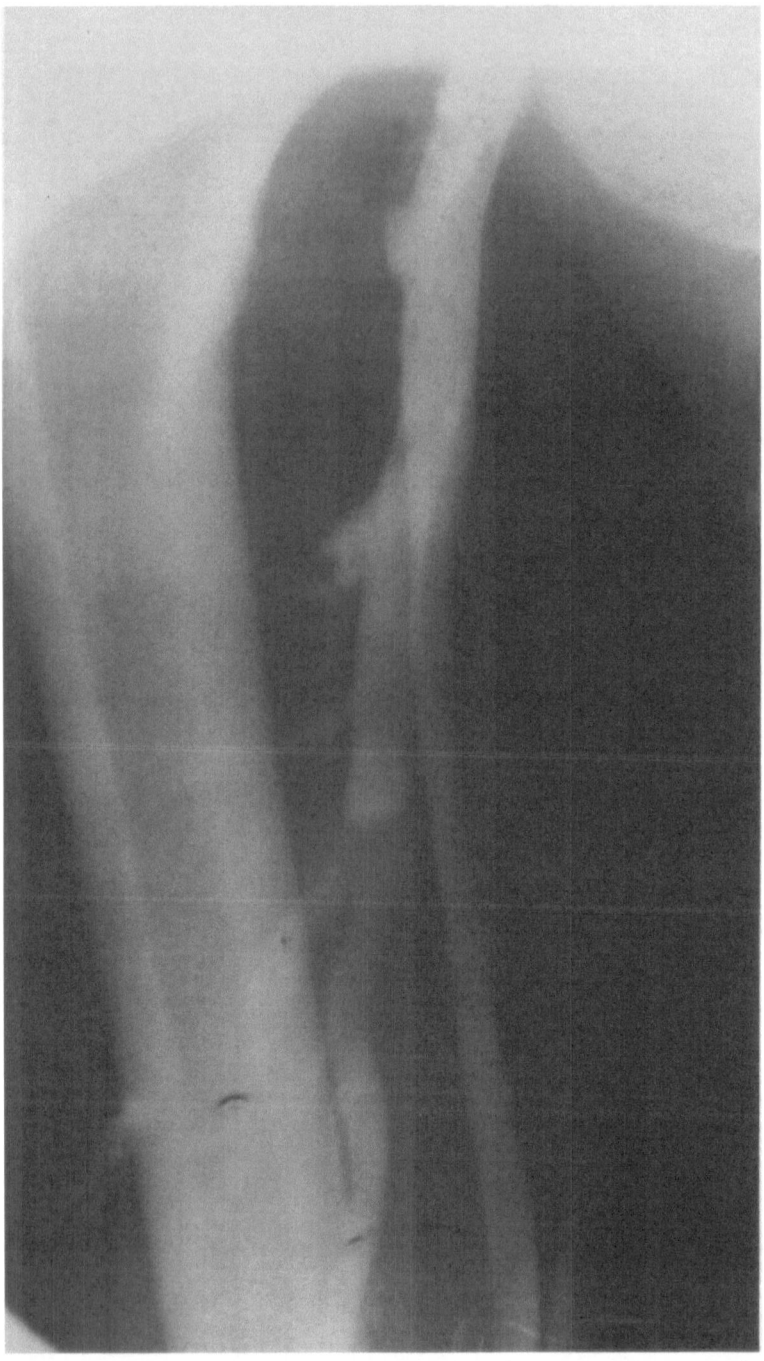

Fig. 4. Normal appearance of the femoral vein; profunda femoral vein is also visualized.

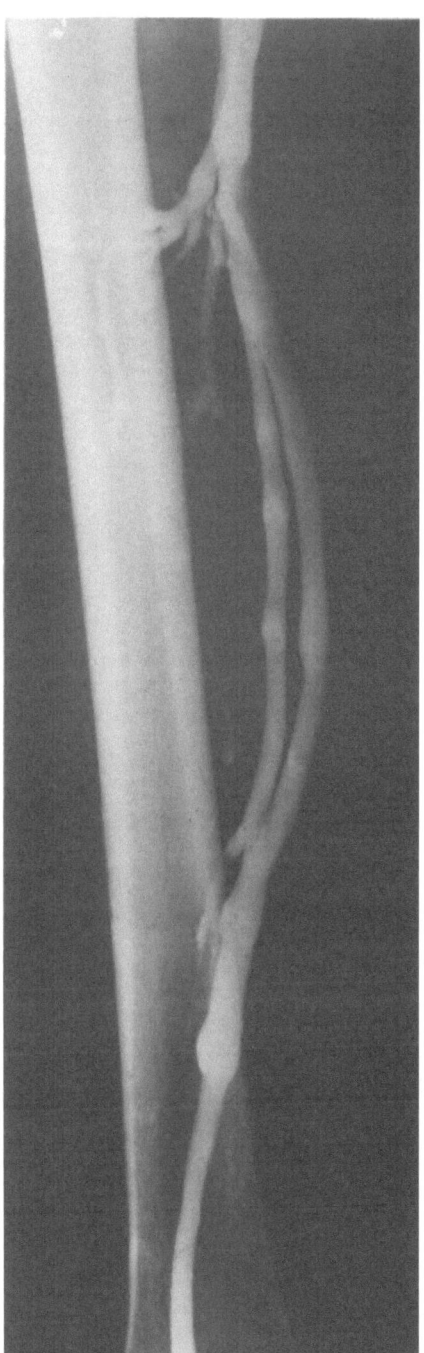

Fig. 5. Bifid femoral vein with filling of the proximal profunda vein. The appearance of this femoral vein is seen in approximately 10% of healthy individuals.

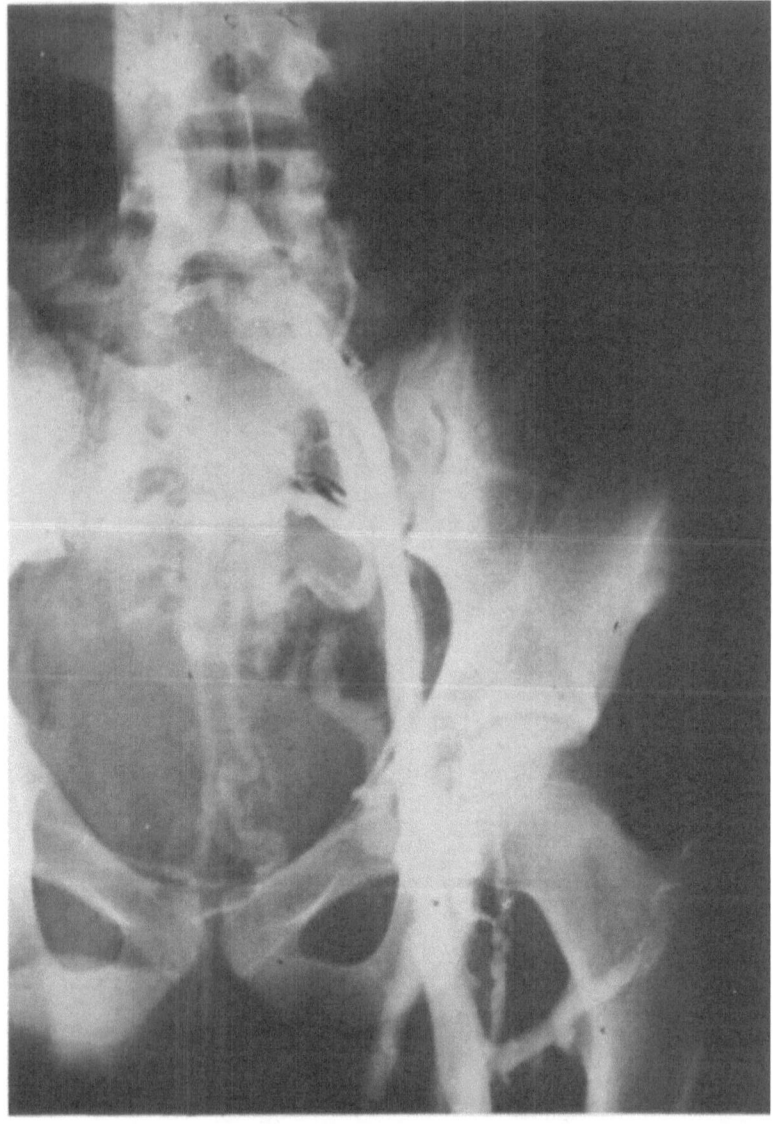

Fig. 6. Phlebogram showing the common appearance of the common and internal iliac veins.

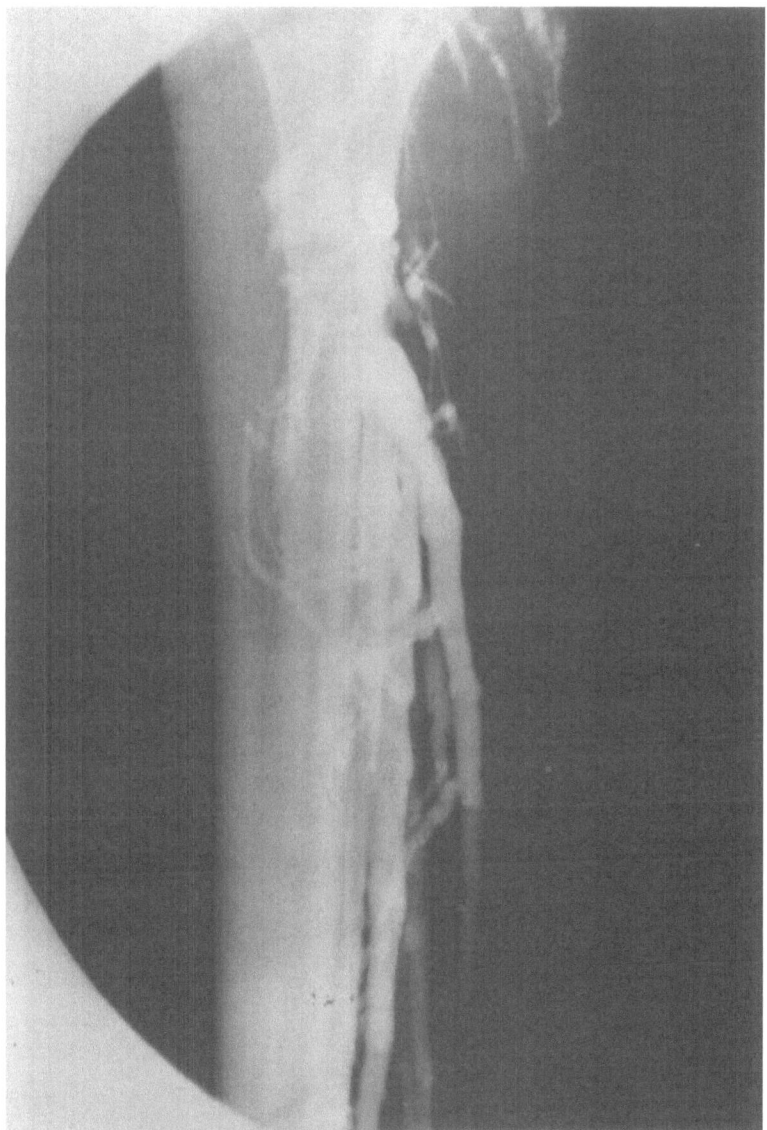

Fig. 7. Lateral X-ray of the calf region showing tibial and soleal veins. Soleal veins containing valves communicating with the tibial veins.

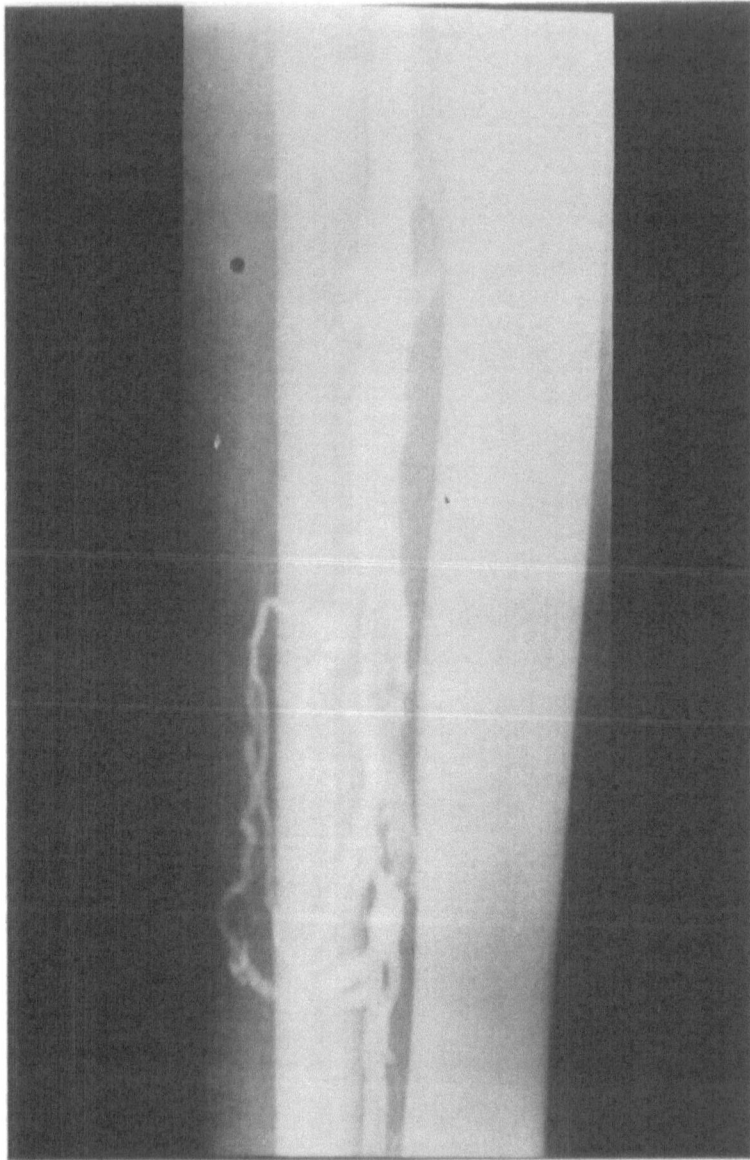

Fig. 8. Phlebogram showing a thrombus in the tibial vein. The thrombus is represented on a filling defect surrounded by a rim of contrast medium, and evidence of a collateral circulation. ,

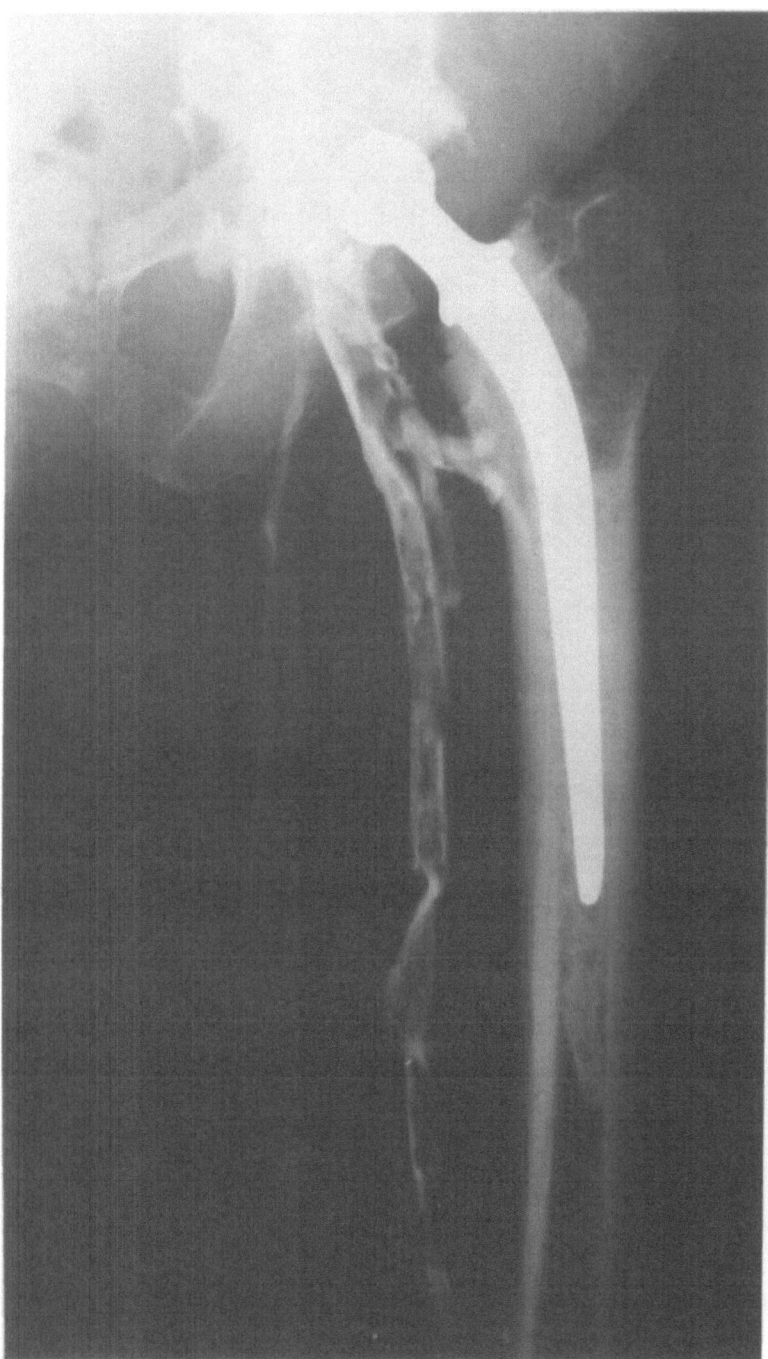

Fig. 9. Phlebogram showing a large serpiginous clot involving the whole of the femoral vein.

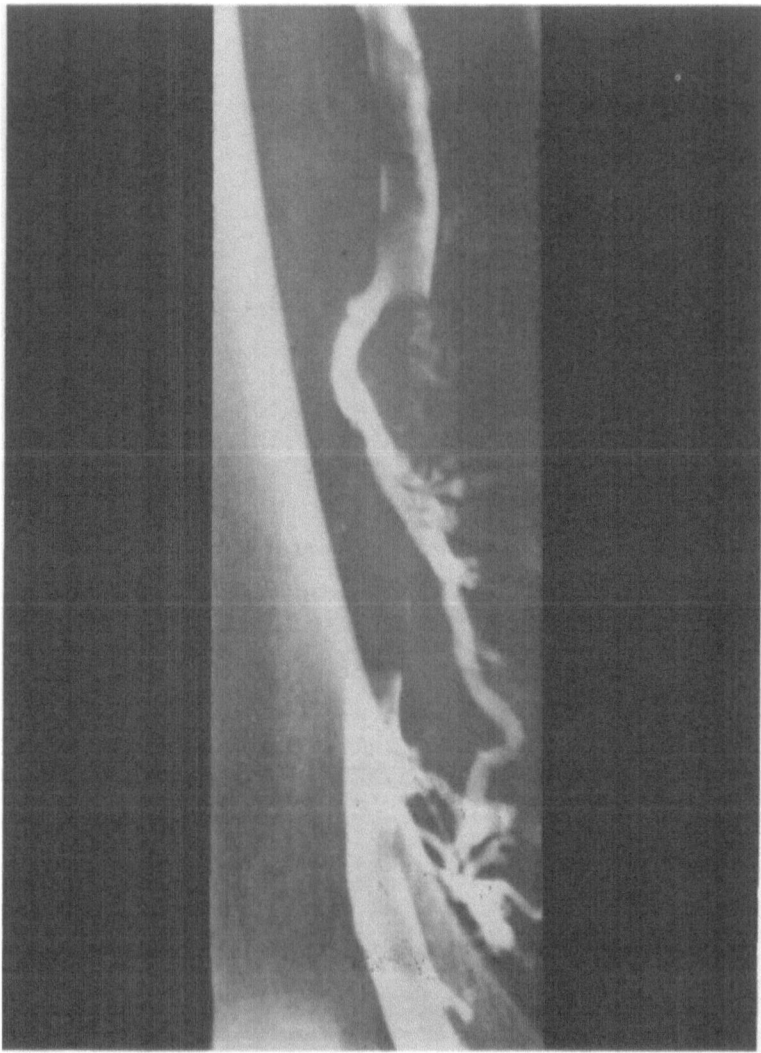

Fig. 10. **Phlebogram showing a thrombus which has produced complete occlusion of a** segment of the femoral vein. There is also evidence of well developed collateral circulation.

contrast medium, but this is never severe enough to warrant abandoning the examination or administering general anesthesia. In very apprehensive patients, an analgesic such as pertazocine or omnapass may be given 1 h prior to the examination. Other complications include extravasation of the contrast medium at the injection site, superficial thrombophlebitis and postphlebography thrombosis. Extravasation can result in extensive inflammation, blistering of the involved skin and in a few patients this may lead even to sloughing of the skin. The frequency of this complication can be minimized by exerting a gentle pressure during injection of the contrast medium. Pain in the calf has been reported to be a frequent complication – it has been suggested that thrombosis may in fact be initiated by phlebography; the reported incidence has varied between 3 and 33% (9–11). To some extent, the incidence of postphlebography thrombosis is related to the nature and time of contrast medium: a prolonged contact between the medium and vascular endothelium may cause damage and thus initiate thrombosis. These side-effects, which are presumably due to chemical irritation, can be minimized by restricting the amount of medium which is injected. A total of 60–80 ml of contrast medium is usually sufficient to ensure adequate filling of the whole of the deep venous system. Furthermore, at the end of the procedure, the veins are cleared of contrast medium by elevating the leg and by injecting 150 ml of normal saline containing 2500 units of heparin. Complete clearance of the contrast medium from the deep veins should be confirmed by fluoroscopy of the leg. In few patients, pulmonary embolism has also been observed when phlebography has been performed in the presence of thrombi in the deep veins. The exact frequency of this complication is again difficult to define because of the difficulty in diagnosing subclinical pulmonary embolism.

We strongly concur with Dr. Kakkar on the use of heparinized saline following venography. We place the patient in a slight Trendelenburg position and infuse 100–200 ml of heparinized saline. With this technique there has been a paucity of postvenography complications.

3.   OTHER TECHNIQUES OF PHLEBOGRAPHY

Deep veins of the lower limbs and pelvis can also be visualized by intra-osseous phlebography; the contrast medium being injected either in the medullary cavity of tibia or in the greater trochanter. However, this technique has now been largely abandoned because it requires general anesthesia, is frequently associated with local bony complications and has also been reported to cause death from fat embolism (9). The inferior vena cava and the iliac veins can be visualized by injecting contrast medium directly into the common femoral vein or by retrograde injection through a catheter passed via the right atrium and inferior vena cava (12). Retrograde catheterization is more complex than the percutaneous puncture of the femoral vein. The advantage of the retrograde technique is that it allows the internal iliac system to be examined and is frequently combined with

The method of ascending functional cinephlebography as described is exciting in that the majority of phlebographic techniques do not concern themselves with normal lower extremity venous hemodynamics. The technique of Dr. Kakkar allows for a functional assessment of the state of the lower extremity venous valves. This may potentially indicate a site for surgical correction of incompetent valves or placement of grafts. The disadvantages are that it requires cine-equipment which may not be readily available on a tilting X-ray table in many departments. Perhaps the use of rapid sequence 100 mm spot films can be substituted for the cine camera.

We have recently begun using descending phlebography to evaluate valve competence. This technique is carried out by placing a short 6.5 French catheter in the common femoral vein by standard percutaneous techniques. The patient is elevated to a 60° semi-upright position. Contrast material is slowly injected through the catheter in 15 ml aliquots under fluoroscopic observation (7). The patient is first instructed to perform a strong Valsalva maneuver at which time visualization of the common femoral vein, superficial femoral vein, and profunda femoris vein is often well demonstrated. Additional contrast material is then injected during quiet respiration and the flow of contrast material is observed. Valve function is classified in the following manner: (1) No reflux of contrast material is seen, indicating competent valves. (2) Leakage of a minimal amount of the contrast material through the proximal valve, but with the majority of flow being in an antegrade fashion. This indicates minimal incompetence. (3) Leakage of much of the contrast material through the valve and to the level of the knee but significant central flow remaining, indicating moderate incompetence. (4) Leakage of most or all of the contrast

pulmonary angiography. In 80–90% of patients, the iliac veins can be adequately visualized by the technique of ascending phlebography. However, in the presence of the complete occlusion of the femoral vein, iliac venography may be the only method for defining the upper extent of a thrombus in such veins.

3.1. *Ascending functional cinephlebography*

When deep vein thrombosis has occurred it seems likely that prevention of late sequelae can best be brought about by the rapid and complete dissolution of thrombus with the preservation of valvular function. In the past valvular function has been assessed by ascending phlebography (13) or by retrograde phlebography (14–16). These methods demonstrated only the presence or absence of valves, but not their function. A technique was developed which assessed the function of valves, with patient in an almost upright position (8).

The patient lies on a fluoroscopic X-ray table which is tilted to an angle of 60° to the horizontal. A pneumatic cuff is placed just above the ankle, and is distended to a pressure of 100 mm Hg in order to prevent filling of the superficial veins of the leg and to direct the contrast medium into the deep venous system. A scalp vein 21G thin-wall (20G bore) infusion cannula is introduced into a vein on the dorsum of the great toe; this vein is selected because it is easy to cannulate and directly joins the plantar plexus through the first interosseous space. Therefore any contrast medium which is injected through this vein flows directly into the deep veins. The cannula is attached to a 50 ml syringe filled with 45% sodium diatriozate which has been warmed to body temperature, and the contrast medium is injected slowly. The patient is instructed to plantar flex and dorsiflex the foot in order to propel the contrast medium. As the contrast medium progresses in the tibial veins, continuous observations are made on the television monitor. The function of the valves, seen on the television monitor, is recorded on both cine and static films (Fig. 11). The contrast medium is now followed into the popliteal and femoral veins and the function of their valves is assessed. The effect of the Valsalva maneuver on these valves is also recorded. Lastly, the contrast medium is followed into the iliac veins to confirm their patency. At the end of the examination the contrast medium is washed out of the deep veins by 150 ml of normal saline containing 2500 units of heparin. Clearance is confirmed by screening the leg.

The valvular function was considered to be normal when both the valve cusps were seen to open and close with onward flow of blood and no retrograde flow occurred (Fig. 12). It was considered that function was poor when the valve cusps were present but did not open and close and

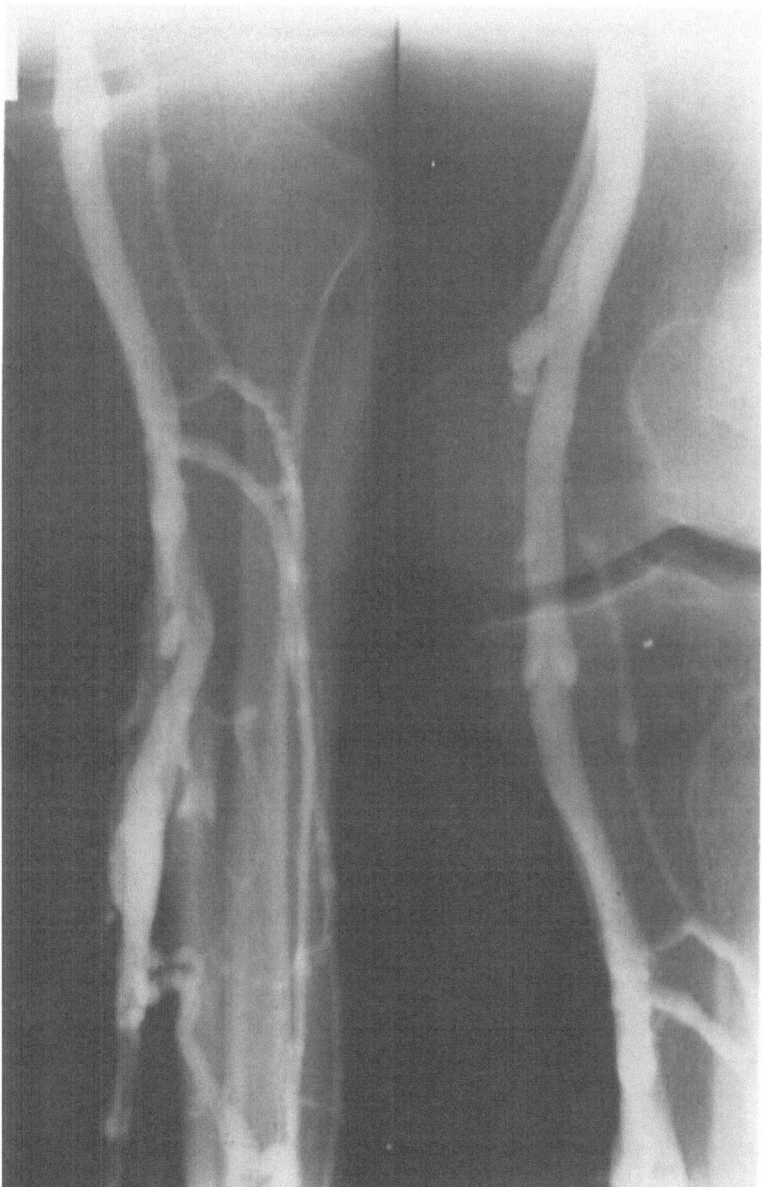

Fig. 11. Later X-ray of the popliteal vein shows a normal popliteal valve which is closed (a) and the same valve when open to allow onward flow of blood.

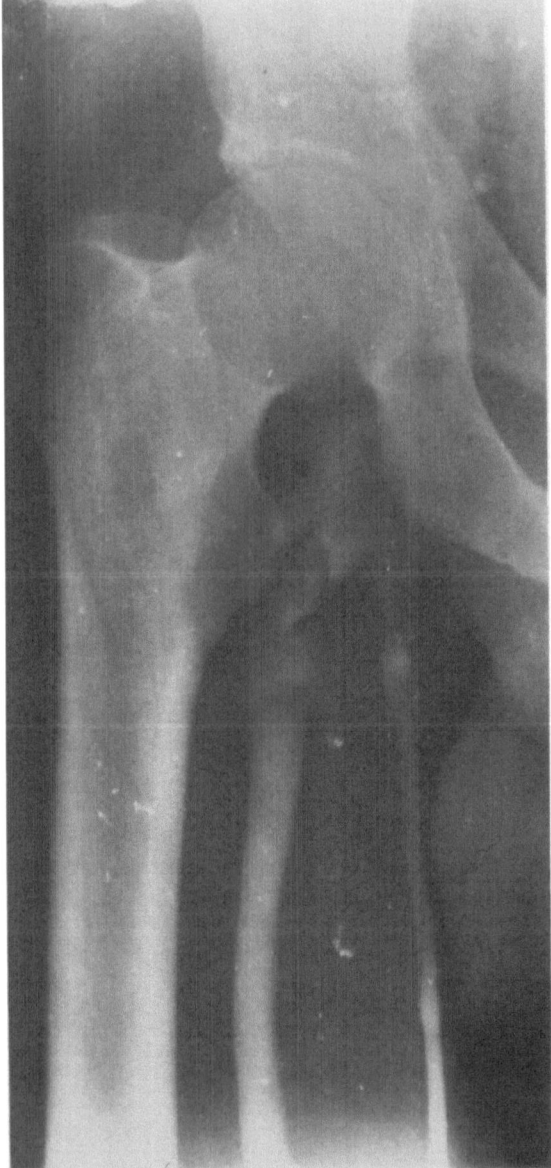

Fig. 12. Phlebogram showing a competent valve in the femoral vein. Both cusps of the valve can be seen without in retrograde flow of the contrast medium.

retrograde flow occurred (Fig. 13). A completely recanalized vein was evenly filled with contrast medium and had a smooth lumen. Recanalization was considered to be incomplete when filling of the vein was constantly uneven with an irregular lumen.

4. COMMENTS

Even with the recent modifications in technique, it is doubtful if phlebography will ever become widely used as a screening procedure to investigate a large number of 'high risk' patients. The techniques are cumbersome, time-consuming, involve a modest radiation, can at times cause considerable discomfort to the patient, and require specifically trained personnel to produce good quality X-rays. Despite these disadvantages, it is the single most useful investigation available for confirming the diagnosis in a patient suspected of having this disease. It not only confirms the diagnosis, it also provides valuable information as to the exact site, extent, and nature of the thrombus, which can be of considerable help in deciding the best possible treatment. Such information is absolutely essential in deciding whether a particular patient is suitable for thrombolytic therapy. Phlebography has also proved to be useful in the management of patients who present with features suggestive of major or minor pulmonary embolism (17). In this study, 102 patients presenting with clinical features suggestive of pulmonary embolism were investigated. Ascending phlebograms, chest X-rays and pulmonary perfusion scans were performed in all the cases. Of 33 patients with a high probability of pulmonary embolism, 29 (87%) had thrombi in the peripheral veins shown by phlebography of 45 patients with no evidence of pulmonary emboli on lung scan, the deep veins were normal in 30, while in the remaining 15 (33%) phlebogram showed the presence of thrombi. In all 7 patients where pulmonary angiography confirmed the presence of extensive emboli the phlebogram showed thrombi in the peripheral veins. Phlebography was of considerable help in deciding whether to give anticoagulant therapy. Fifity-eight patients in whom phlebograms showed the presence of major or minor thrombi in the deep veins received a continuous infusion (30,000–40,000 units per day) and oral anticoagulants were started at the same time and continued for a period of at least 12 weeks. The dose of heparin was increased to prolong the thrombin clotting time by the normal control by 20–25 sec, but reduced if the time exceeded 120 sec. For oral anticoagulant therapy, the dosage of warfarin sodium was so adjusted as to maintain the prothrombin time between one and a half and two times the control value. The 44 patients with normal phlebograms were not given anticoagulants. During the follow-up period 5 patients had recurrence of symptoms of

material with little or no evidence of central flow, indicating severe incompetence.

Normal valve function probably consists of a valve which is either completely competent or allows for leakage of a minimal amount of the contrast material. Leakage of a small or moderate amount of blood through a valve is a normal variant and apparently causes no symptoms. Usually, this retrograde flow is trapped by a lower valve in the thigh (7, 8).

This technique has correlated well with noninvasive flow studies in the small group of patients that we have studied and has not been associated with any complications (9).

In our institution, the indications for phlebography are: (1) clinical findings and noninvasive tests in variance with each other, (2) definite evidence of pulmonary emboli but negative noninvasive studies, suggesting the presence of deep vein thrombosis, (3) chronic venous disease with a suspected new thrombotic event, (4) failure to respond to heparin therapy or previous surgical treatment, (5) lower extremity swelling in which the etiology is obscure, (6) prior to venacaval interruption, (7) recurrent pulmonary emboli after venacaval interruption.

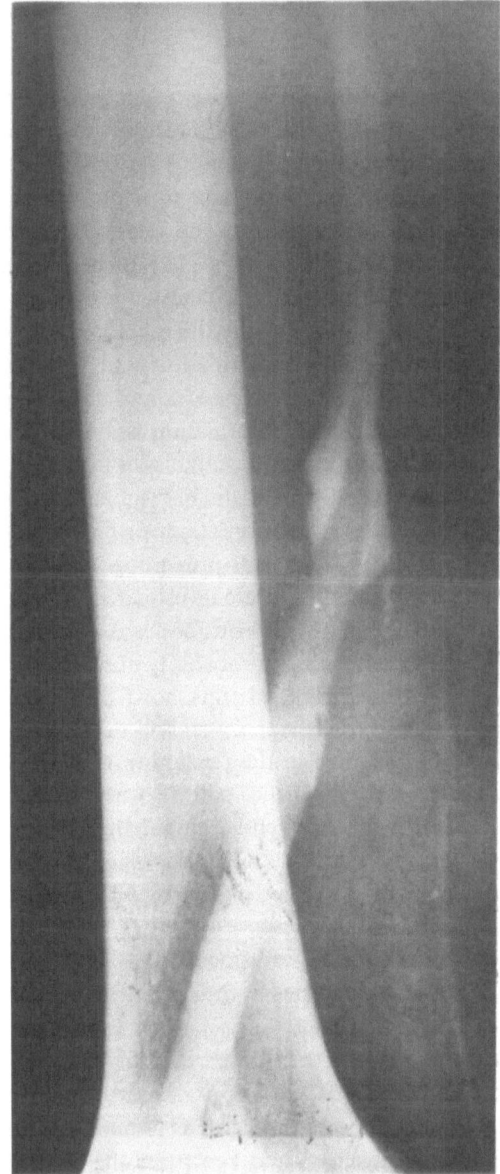

Fig. 13. X-ray showing an incompetent valve in the femoral vein.
Both cusps of the valve fail to approximate and there is evidence of
this retrograde flow of the contrast medium.

pulmonary embolism. All 5 were from the group of patients in whom phlebograms had confirmed the presence of major deep vein thrombosis. None of the patients who had normal phlebograms and did not receive anticoagulants had evidence of recurrent pulmonary embolism. Eight patients died; all came to autopsy. In 3 autopsy confirmed the presence of pulmonary emboli, and all had phlebographic evidence of deep vein thrombosis. Two patients died as a result of myocardial infarction and 1 from carcinoma of the bronchus. In these patients phlebograms had shown a normal deep venous system during life and this was confirmed at autopsy examination. The other indications for phlebography include assessment of deep venous system before surgery on the superficial veins of the lower limbs or before reconstructive surgery for occlusion of the iliac veins. There can be no doubt that phlebography provides the only available baseline which can be used to validate other noninvasive diagnostic tools now being developed as screening tests.

In contrast, the cinephlebography has very limited clinical application and at this stage must remain an investigational research tool, especially to determine what are the critical factors involved in the preservation of function of venous valves and what form of initial treatment is likely to be most successful in the eventual return of the veins to normal.

REFERENCES TO MAIN TEXT

1. Dos Santos JC: Phlébographie directe: conception, technique, premiers résultats. J. int. Chir. 3: 625, 1938.
2. Bauer G: A venographic study of thromboembolic problems. Acta. chir. scand. Suppl. 84: 5, 1940.
3. Craig JO: Practical Procedures in Diagnostic Radiology. Oxford, Blackwall, 1965, Ch. 27.
4. Thomas ML, Fletcher EWL: The technique of pelvic phlebography. Clin. Radiol. 18: 399, 1967.
5. Kakkar VV: The I^{125} labelled fibrinogen test and phlebography in the diagnosis of deep vein thrombosis. Milbank Memorial Quart. 1,2: 206-229, 1972.
6. Nicolaides AN, Kakkar VV, Field ES et al: The origin of deep vein thrombosis: a venographic study. Brit. J. Radiol. 44: 653, 1971.
7. Rabinov K, Paulin S: Roentgen diagnosis of venous thrombosis in the leg. Arch. Surg. (Chic.) 104: 134, 1972
8. Kakkar VV, Howe CT, Laws JW et al: Late results of treatment of deep vein thrombosis. Brit. med. J. 1: 810, 1969.
9. Thomas L: Phlebography. Arch. Surg. (Chic.) 104: 145, 1972.
10. Harris WH, Salzman EW, Anthamasoulis C et al: Comparison of ^{125}I fibrinogen scanning with phlebography for the detection of venous thrombi. New Engl. J. Med. 292: 665, 1975.
11. Albrechtsson U, Olsson CG: Thrombotic side effects of lower limb phlebography. Lancet 1: 273, 1976.
12. Dow JD: Retrograde phlebography in major pulmonary embolism. Lancet 2: 1107, 1973.
13. Scott NW, Roach JF: Phlebography of the leg in the erect position. Ann.Surg. 134: 104, 1951.

14. Lukes JC: The diagnosis of the chronic enlargement of the leg with description of new syndrome. Surg. Gynaecol. Obstet. 73: 472, 1941.
15. Bauer G: The aetiology of leg ulcers and their treatment by resection of the popliteal vein. J. int. Chir. 8: 937, 1948.
16. Shumacker HB, Jun Moore TC, Campbelll JA: Functional venography of the lower extremeties. Surg. Gynaecol. Obstet. 98: 257, 0000.
17. Corrigan TP, Fossard DP, Spindler J et al: Phlebography in the management of pulmonary embolism. Brit. J. Surg. 61: 484-488, 1974.

References to Commentary

1. Rabinov K, Paulin S: Roentgen diagnosis of venous thrombosis in the leg. Arch. Surg. 104: 134, 1972.
2. Neiman HL: Phlebography in the diagnosis of venous thrombosis. Venous problems, Bergan JJ, Yao JST (eds) Chicago, Year Book Medical Publishers, 1978.
3. Thomas ML, Carty H: The value of the lateral projection in the diagnosis of venous thrombosis of the calf. Clin. Radiol. 25: 459, 1974.
4. Nicolaides AN, Kakkar VV, Renney JTG: The soleal sinuses: Origin of deep vein thrombosis. Brit. J. Surg. 87: 860, 1970.
5. Arkoff RS, Gilfillan RS, Burhenne HJ: A simple method for lower extremity phlebography–pseudoobstruction of the popliteal vein. Radiology 90: 66, 1968.
6. Rogoff SM, DeWeese JA: Phlebography of the lower extremity. JAMA 172: 1599, 1960.
7. Kistner RL: Transvenous repair of the incompetent femoral vein valve. Venous Problems, Bergan JJ, Yao JST (eds), Chicago, Year Book Medical Publishers, 1978.
8. Kistner RL: Surgical repair of the incompetent femoral vein valve. Arch. Surg. 110: 1336, 1975.
9. Neiman HL, Herman RJ, Yao JS, Malave SR: Descending venography: A method of evaluating lower extremity valvular function. Radiology (in press).

14. Lymphography

R. MAYALL

Commentary by M. Elke

1. DEFINITIONS

Lymphography is the method used to visualize the lymphatic system. Lymphangiography is the method for roentgenographic visualizing the lymph vessels. Lymphoadenography is the method for the roentgenographic delineation of the lymph nodes.

Visual lymphography is the method whereby local lymphvessels are made visible to the naked eye by intradermal injection of a suitable dye which then enters the lymphatic system (1). Normally this is the first step of a radiological lymphography, followed by direct injection into a visible lymph vessel of some radiopaque fluid (2, 3). Lymphangioadenography is the method for visualizing simultaneously the lymph vessels and the lymph nodes. Presently, lymphography is often used as a diagnostic aid in leg edema and in many lymphatic diseases.

2. HISTORICAL REVIEW

Following the development of techniques for arteriography and phlebography, work on the radiological visualization of the lymphatic system in man began. The Portugese Rodrigues, Pereira and Carvalho (4–6), presented their first papers in 1930 and Funaoka (7) simultaneously published a similar method. Hudack and McMaster (8) (in 1933) injected an 11% aqueous solution of Patent-blue-violet into the skin to study the superficial collecting ducts of the limbs. This technique was called lymphatochromy by Seabra in his thesis of 1943 (9) whereby he was able to inject the contrast dye into the testis albuginea membrane to obtain a satisfactory lymphogram. At the same time, the Brazilians Marques and de Barros (10) injected the inguinal lymph nodes with hydrosoluble and other contrast solutions (Per-abrodil, Thorotrast, Iodipina, Diodrast) with excellent visualization of the lymphatic system. Servelle (11) was able to get excellent lymphog-

COMMENTARY

Besides lymphangiography (filling phase) and lymphadenography (storage phase) the control X-rays (periodic longitudinal section) taken over a period of a few months up to 1 or 2 years give information on the position, shape, contour, structure and volume of lymph nodes without control-lymphography (1–13). As a rule only after this period may a second lymphography be required.

The ideal, nonmicroembolizing contrast media with storage power has not yet been found. Therefore, the intensive research for new contrast media or preparations of contrast media is still proceeding. But despite the research for better contrast media, the perspectives of the modern ultrasonic and X-ray computer-tomography for clinical lymphography must not be forgotten (8, 14–24).

raphy of the leg, by injecting Thorotrast into a lymph blister after aspiration of 1500 ml of lymph. Using a vital dye method, Kinmonth (3) proposed in 1951 at the Medical Research Society of London his technique of direct intralymphatic injection. This simple method closed the experimental phase of lymphography.

Another important step forward was the discovery of an oily medium which does not diffuse into the tissues and therefore allows visualization of the retroperitoneal lymphatics and lymph nodes and even the thoracic duct (12).

Lymphography is now used routinely; and many investigators have introduced minor modifications improving the original technique (13–39).

3.   TECHNIQUES

The technique for lymphography may vary slightly according to the area to be visualized, but includes the visualization of the superficial lymphatics, the dissection and catheterization of a lymphatic vessel and the injection of a radiopaque substance.

3.1.   *Visualization of superficial lymph vessels*

There are many dyes with affinity for the lymphatic vessels, of which some are liposoluble (Sudan Blue, Sharbach Red, Aniline Blue) and others are hydrosoluble (Congo Red, Lithate Carmin, Direct Sky Blue, Trypan Blue, Methylene Blue, Pontamine Sky Blue, India Ink and Patent-blue-violet, Blue Evans and Prontosil). Our preference is a 2.5% solution of patent-blue-violet, because of its low toxicity, promptness and intensity with which the dye stains the collecting trunks. The dye is injected alone or mixed with 1% procaine.

For the staining of the lymphatic vessels we are exclusively using an isotonic watery solution of 2.5% Patent-blue-violet injected into the first interdigital fold of the foot. In very sensitive patients, the solution is mixed with the same amount of a 1% procaine solution. Only in the presence of disturbed lymphatic drainage (lymphatic edema) or when a second lymphography has to be performed do we inject a second vital dye depot into the 4th interdigital (21, 25–28) fold of the foot. The patient is informed beforehand that the urine will be

In the absence of edema, 0.5 ml of Patent-blue-violet is mixed with the same volume of anesthetic and injected intradermally into the 1st metatarsal webspace of the foot or into the 2nd interdigital space of the hand. When there is congenital lymphedema or fibredema, it is advisable to inject a more concentrated solution of up to 11% Patent-blue-violet, because in these cases the lymphatics are sometimes difficult to visualize. In a few cases it is necessary to inject the dye into the fourth interdigital cleft to visualize the lymph pathway of the medial and lateral region of the foot or hand. When there is aplasia of the trunks, the dye diffuses as a blue spot in the skin without showing any blue channels. To visualize the deep lymphatic system of the leg, it is necessary to inject the dye at the inner side of the foot over the periosteum of the os calcaneum or on the sole of the foot; 1–2 ml of the dye are often required and can, for instance, be injected beneath the medial malleolus.

A few seconds after the injection of the dye the normal lymph trunks stain as blue streaks, when the patient is not melanodermic. The reticulated patches of the dye in the skin, called 'dermal back flow' (2) have a different meaning. Although obstruction of the lymphatic vessel is not rare, the diagnosis of aplasia or hypoplasia cannot be made without a complete dissection of different parts of the extremity in search of the normal trunks. I agree with Pflug and Johnson (40) that 'the more experienced the operators are, the less often the diagnosis of aplasia is made'.

Abnormal dermal back flow without edema of the extremity may also be due to the presence of functioning lymphatic-venous communications (15). Dermal back flow is not specific for lymphedema but, suggests an anomaly of the lymphatic circulation. If this method is performed under general anesthesia it is advisable to be aware of a blue-greyish coloration of the patient's skin which varies in degree according to the quantity of the dye injected and is not to be confused with cyanosis. The blue dye is eliminated in the urine and within one or two days the blue skin coloration disappears.

colored greenish for some hours, the complexion may become greyish for perhaps 1 or 2 days and at the site of the injection itself a circumscribed blue staining of the skin may occur for some weeks. The experienced examiner is able to find unstained superficial lymphatic vessels on the back of the foot after preparation. They are recognized by a transparent reflecting wall with a water-clear content, valves and branching of about the same caliber. In contrast, fine subcutaneous veins have an opalescent wall and a minute blood hairline in the lumen (obstruction and dilatation of the vessel with silk-loop). The visibility of blue-stained lymph vessels through the skin varies individually. It depends on the position of the lymph vessels in the subcutaneous tissue and the thickness of the skin.

3.2. *Dissection and catheterization of the lymphatic vessel*

3.2.1. *Material.*

To carry out a routine superficial lymphography it is necessary to have available the following sterile equipment.

(1) Strong syringes of 2 ml, 5 ml and 20 ml made of polypropylene are desirable to prevent refluxes, breakages and leaks, mainly during the injection of Patent-blue-violet or when using the high pressure injectors.

(2) Needles no. 19 or 21 for local anesthesia and the injection of the dye.

(3) Sterile lymphangiography sets with needles of different sizes (BD 27 or 30 with short level) and medical grading tubes for differing calibers of the lymphatic vessels, supple polyvinyl tubing is preferred to stop the needle springing out. Catheters can be easily home made. Polythylene tubing with a fine beveled point can be used.

(4) Skin antiseptics.

(5) Local anesthetic solution of 1% procaine or similar drugs without vasoconstrictors.

(6) Sterile towels, gauze swabs, adhesive tape.

(7) Saline solution, to be used during the catheterization of the lymphatic vessel because some of the iodinated contrast materials used for X-ray lymphography upon mixing with procaine are agglutinated within the plastic tubing, therefore impeding flow.

(8) Scalpel and blades, preferably with a sharp point and not curved.

(9) Two straight and 2 curved mosquito clamp forceps, 1 pair of dissecting forceps.

The material on our sterile trolley corresponds in general to former lay-outs. In 1964-65 we were mainly using the trocar needle designed by Rüttimann and DelBuono with a calibre of 35-55/100 mm. Since 1966 we have preferred the trocar needle (stylet and blunt needle) with a spiral spring designed by De Roo. This needle has the advantage that the length of the protruding stylet tip can be varied by finger-pressure (21, 25, 26). In addition we use also a U-shaped preparation table developed by us (25, 26) which can be fixed to the foot-end of the examination table. This small table can be adjusted horizontally and vertically and enables a firm position of the hands during preparation and lymph vessel puncture. Because of this comfortable position the hands tire less and the puncture will be easier (Fig. 1a–f, see p. 389-390).

(10) Two toothed forceps, mosquito size, and a pair of small sized skin retractors or skin hooks.

(11) Surgical needles with holders for skin suture.

(12) Mononylon and skin sewing threads.

(13) Portable magnifying lens or a surgical dissecting microscope for difficult dissection of the hypoplastic lymphatics which are very common on the hand and in patients with congenital lymphedemas.

(14) An automatic injector with constant pressure and weight or electrically weight driven motor and warming system (Fig. 1a and b).

(15) Ampoules of water-soluble and oil-soluble contrast medium. Lipiodol-UF is in our experience the best oil-soluble medium.

(16) Ampoules of 2 ml of Patent-blue-violet, 2.5% and 11%.

(17) An adjustable lamp.

A silk loop is placed around the prepared lymph vessel and by pulling it slightly the vessel is obstructed and dilated. Then, after puncture of the vessel, the needle is fixed with this silk into the vessel. A second thread is needed to improve fixation and seal the puncture. We also prefer the transverse incision because further lymph vessels can easily be found with only a slight enlargement of the incision. The incision can be slightly more stretched by using small hooks.

3.2.2. *Dissection of the lymphatic vessel.*   After the injection of the dye, massage and movements of the fingers and foot are not recommended as they increase the diffusion of the blue color through the walls of the lymph pathways which then become blurred, and complicate their dissection. Immediately, after the injection of the dye, using skin antisepsis and under careful local anesthesia, a small transverse incision is made on the dorsum of the foot just over the visible lymph trunk. A longitudinal incision is

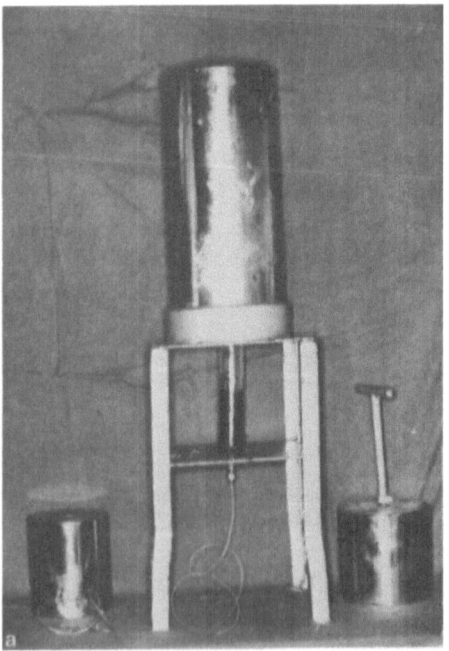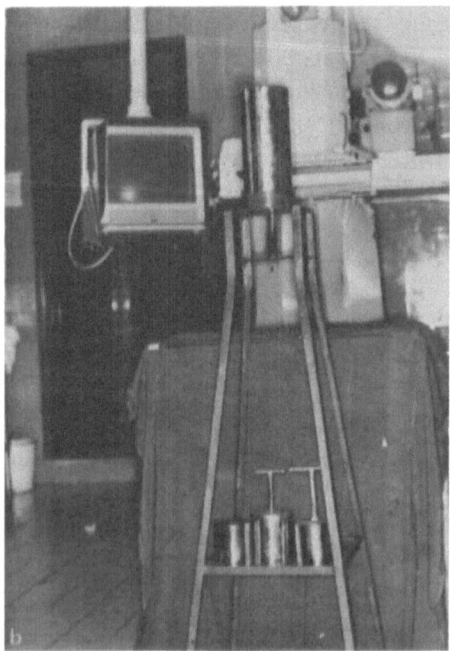

Fig. 1. (a and b) Simple gravity injectors for lymphography as used at Gamboa Hospital.

recommended when the visible lymphatic has a straight direction; it is easier to dissect the lymph trunk and to lay bare a longer portion of the lymphatic. When the patient is melanodermic or there are no visible lymphatics, a transverse incision is made and if necessary enlarged at both sides. To prevent bleeding, a small elevation of the foot is sometimes necessary to enhance hemostasis.

After careful dissection of the cellular subcutaneous tissue, the lymphatic vessel appears as a blue trunk which is isolated between two threads. By blocking the proximal thread and milking the distal part of the foot, the lymphatic vessel distends which facilitates the clearing up of advencial fat tissues around the trunk for a distance of about 6–10 mm. It is advisable to dissect a long lymphatic segment which is blocked between two separate threads during the filling phase that precedes the introduction of the needle into the best selected trunk. The insertion of the needle within the lymphatic lumen, kept stretched by the distal thread and blocked by the proximal thread, can be made by hand or with the help of specially designed needle holders (1). Reflux of the blue colored lymph is the best sign that the needle is within the vessel. The needle is then gradually further advanced with gentle pressure of a syringe filled with saline and should pass a visible valve of the dilated lymph vessel, in order to prevent leakage of the contrast medium during injection under pressure and to avoid the need to fix the needle to the lymphatic by a fine thread. The needle and the tubing are then fixed to the skin with adhesive tape and, to prevent the dislodgment of the needle, the distal thread of the lymphatic trunk is also fixed with a separate adhesive tape to the skin, avoiding any traction on the lymphatic trunk. If there are no signs of leaks or dislodgment of the needle, the injection of the contrast medium can start. The patient must be warned to remain quiet while the contrast medium is injected. It is advisable to fix the hallux of nervous patients with adhesive tape to the table. For small children and non-cooperative patients, the precedure is carried out under general anesthesia.

After insertion of the needle, it is recommended to frequently monitor the progress of the dye by taking serial radiographs or by using an image amplifier and television fluoroscopic control to avoid unintentional injection of oil-soluble contrast medium into a small vein. Experience shows that this may happen even in expert hands. When using a water-soluble contrast medium, roentgenograms are taken during the injection to avoid the mohair-yarn shape produced by the diffusion of the contrast medium around the vessel (41). When oil-soluble contrast medium is injected, the extravasation takes a ragged appearance as the result of a fast injection under too high a pressure.

The volume of the contrast medium to be injected depends on the age and the disease to be studied and on the quality of the contrast oil- or

The position of the needle is then checked with an injection of a small amount of sodium chloride. Should the situation not be clear, an injection of a minute air-bubble out of the cone of the 2 ml syringe is of great help. If the needle is in the right position, the small air-bubble, which floats away, can be seen through a binocular magnifying eye glass. In none of our 2000 patients was general anesthesia needed. For small children we ask for sedation and supervision during the procedure by a pediatrician. Only in exceptional cases was premedication (5–10 mg Valium i.v.) for adults required. After checking on the test-film of both legs, made after preliminary injection of 0.3 ml Lipoidol-UF, if the lymph vessels are unmistakably visible, the physician is then allowed to administer the total amount of Lipoidol-UF contrast medium. Beginners have to show this test-film to the authorized chief physician. We think this control to be the best protection against inadequate injection. At the same time it serves as a documentary picture for correct injection. The total amount of contrast medium is determined on basis of weight, age and general status of the patient and by the examination purpose. After injection of 4 ml per lower extremity in an adult person of average size, we take a first plain abdominal supine view. When at that time the contrast media has reached the third lumbar vertebral body, the injection is completed with the slow injection automatic injector.

Otherwise a maximum of 1–2 ml up to the total amount of 6 ml per extremity will be reinjected. Only in exceptional cases should a maximum of 7 ml per lower extremity be injected. Generally, lumbar tracks fill up well if the patient is made to move the legs after injection of 5–6 ml per extremity (muscular pump!) and 20–40 min later films of retroperitoneal lymph vessels are taken. The risk of pulmonary micro-oil-embolization after intralymphatic injection of Lipoidol-UF can only be decreased by a reduction of the amount of injection fluid. We have tested in a double-blind trial the prophylactic effect of phospholipid 'EPL' (Nattermann AG, Cologne, Germany) in 97 patients. In a control group 34 patients received no infusions and another 31 patients only 5% glucose infusions. The result was definitively disappointing concerning the claimed prophylactic effect of phospholipid infusions against micro-oil-emboli of the lungs after lymphography (29).

water-soluble medium. For an average sized adult, 7 ml per lower limb and 4 ml per upper limb are often required, but this dose can be reduced by monitoring the injection. One- to two-thirds of this volume suffice in children according to their age. When using oil-soluble contrast, it is essential to decrease the volume of the injected material in order to minimize the danger of pulmonary oil embolism. In old patients with a poor general condition or with emphysema, heart failure or chronic pulmonary disease and in children, smaller doses of oil contrast medium are used and, if possible, the progress of the injection should be monitored.

For the visualization of the giant lymphangiectases in filariotric patients much larger volumes of contrast medium are required; we have encountered no complications even after administration of up to 30 ml of oil-soluble contrast medium. A water-soluble contrast medium is presently used only for the study of the morphology and function of the lymph pathways of the limbs. The high viscosity of the oil-soluble contrast medium requires more time and a higher pressure to inject. To speed its injection without the risk of extravasation or rupture of the lymphatic wall, we recommend the lymphatic injection of a benzopyrone compound (coumarin-rutin), commercially available in ampoules of 2 ml with 50 mg active drug. This drug has no toxicity and considerably shortens the time required to perform the lymphadenography due to its accelerating effect on lymph-flow.

The injection rate of water-soluble contrast medium is from 2 to 4 ml per minute when using the smallest needles and plastic tubes. The injection rate of an oil-soluble medium is slow, about 1 ml in 10 min. Some authors recommend warming the contrast medium to body temperature to facilitate its injection.

For the preparation of the lymph vessels, the injection and X-ray exposures, examination cubicles in a quiet section of the radiological department should be available. With an adjustable ceiling appliance, the exposures can be taken in any of the chosen cubicles without moving the patient. We use an automatic injector with a friction coupling. The principles of wound treatment correspond to the ones already mentioned. Tests with tissue glue for needle fixation and wound-closure gave unsatisfactory results and were therefore abandoned.

4.   INJECTORS

For the injection of a water-soluble contrast medium, no special instrument is required; however, for an oil-soluble contrast medium, it is advisable to use a high pressure injector, with constant pressure and speed, automatically operated, either by gravity or another device. We recommend a simple gravity injector with three different iron weights of 5, 6 and 14 kg, easily changable to vary the pressure and the speed (Fig. 1) (42). Normally, 5 kg are sufficient for lymphography with water-soluble contrast medium and a maximum of 11 kg for oil-soluble contrast medium.

Immediately after the end of the injection, particularly of an oil-soluble contrast medium, the surgical wound must be carefully washed with saline to prevent the formation of lipophagic granulomas or a local inflammatory process. When the skin is normal, the incision can be closed by interrupted sutures with mononylon, depending on the length of the incision. When there is elephantiasis with fibredema we prefer the wound to close spontaneously, avoiding any suppurative or inflammatory process. Adhesive tape, in a cross position, results in a satisfactory fixation of the wound margins provided the foot is immobilized. The use of an oral broad spectrum antibiotic is recommended. The wound is covered with a dry sterile gauze dressing and the patient should stay in bed to avoid foot edema. The stitches in normal skin can be removed after 6 or 7 days and in lymphedematous patients after 10 or 12 days.

5. COMPLICATIONS FROM LYMPHOGRAPHY

Lymphography may be considered a safe procedure but nevertheless minor incidents and major accidents have been reported in the literature. These complications are produced by the dye, by the contrast medium or as a result of local surgical trauma.

5.1. Minor complications related to the injection site

Delayed healing, aseptic inflammation or infection of the incision at the dorsum of the foot are common. Delayed reabsorption of the dye is caused by poor local lymphatic flow conditions and is not due to the physicochemical composition of the dye. The same interpretation is valid for the dystrophic skin changes at the site of injection. Lymphorrhea at the site of surgical incision with fistula formation has been reported (15, 43, 44), but, in our experience, subsides spontaneously after gentle local compression and elevation of the extremity.

Lymphangitis, beginning at the site of injection, is caused either by extravasation of the contrast medium or by infection at the injection site, followed by satellite adenitis, which responds well to antibiotic therapy. Droplets of oil-soluble contrast medium or its extravasation around the lymphatic vessel due to excessive pressure during injection can be responsible for formation of lipophagic granulomas (15). To prevent this extravasation, Collard (45–47) developed a new injector apparatus with modulated pressure, decreased from 30 mm Hg after a set time to 5 mm Hg and returning to 30 mm Hg 10 minutes later.

Parethesias or a slight pain in the foot may follow the procedure and even last a few months.

General hypersensitive reactions are produced by the dye or by the contrast medium. Giant urticaria of the total body was observed once in our experience and occurred after the injection of 1 ml of 2.5% Patent-blue-violet but subsided rapidly after administration of antihistamines and corticosteroids.

The frequency of complications after lymphography varies considerably in the literature (14, 17, 21, 25, 26, 30–39). They depend on: (1) the amount and type of injected contrast medium; (2) the mode of injection (velocity, site of injection etc.); (3) previous damage and therapeutic influence; (4) the basic disease and its stage; (5) the way of registration of side-effects (prospectively or retrospectively, check-list with registration of minimal side-effects etc.). We recorded during a decade, with the aid of a questionnaire, prospectively minimal and also clinically not relevant side-effects in 1,243 patients. Following information was documented: the injected amount of contrast medium; standard chest films before lymphography and 4 h and 20 h after completion of the injection (to compare the intensity of pulmonary micro-oil-embolization); temperature; evolution of the blood pressure; frequency of respiration; subjective symptoms, such as nausea, retrosternal pain, irritation to cough, itching and detectable symptoms such as dyspnea, skin and mucous membrane reaction, circulatory collapse, delayed wound healing etc. (Elke M, Willi RW, 1977, unpublished controls). Micro-oil-emboli of the lungs are of special interest because of their frequency and transient disturbance of lung function (17, 29, 30, 31, 33, 38–42). According to the total amount of injected contrast medium, two groups were formed. In group (a) 1087 patients were given less than 16 ml Lipoidol-UF (average total 11 ml for both legs); in group (b) 156 patients were given more than a total of 16 ml Lipoidol-UF (average total 20 ml for both legs).

Considering minute subjective and objective symptoms (e.g., minimal micro-oil-embolization on standard chest-films without subjective or otherwise detectable symptoms) we registered in group (a) in a total of 38% and in group (b) in a total of 50% of the examined patients, some side-effects noted on our check-lists. The presence of discrete micro-oil-emboli on the standard chest films without any clinical symptoms, was in both groups by far the most common complication and accounts for over 90% of all registered side-effects (see Fig. 2a/b and p. 392). Clinically relevant side-effects (urticaria, edema, collapse, vomiting, delayed wound-healing, micro-oil-embolization with subjective, resp. clinical or functional symptoms) were only found in 1.7% of group (a) and in 3% of group (b). Out of 1243 registered examinations the following are especially worth mentioning: Seven patients had an immediate reaction to Patent-blue-violet, beginning 5–20 min. after injection and characterized by urticaria, itching, symptoms of the mucous membranes or circulatory collapse (Fig. 2c). One patient had a delayed reaction 1.5 h after injection of Patent-blue-violet with urticaria, dyspnea, cyanosis and signs of collapse.
A delayed reaction to Lipoidol-UF occurred in 2 patients. One had urticaria, blotchy skin, mucous membrane edema and arthralgia with a positive epicutan test to Lipoidol-UF 2 weeks after the second lymphography. The other patient experienced 3 days after lymphography severe erythrodermia, edema and

Sialorrhea, nausea and vomiting are not uncommon after administration of a large dose of water-soluble contrast medium and are possibly related to hypersensitivity to iodine.

Cardiovascular complications such as hypertension or hypertensive crises were surprisingly rare in a report based on 32,000 lymphographies (48). There is a slight elevation of the skin temperature in about 20% of patients over a 24–48 h period after the procedure which subsides spontaneously (43).

6. ACCIDENTS

6.1. *Fatalities*

A fatility rate of 1/1,800 has been reported in a total of 32,000 lymphographic examinations; death was attributed to cardiac failures in 2 cases, to respiratory failure in 7 cases, to cerebral complications in 2 cases, and no precise cause of death was given in 6 cases (48).

6.2. *Pulmonary complications*

The incidence of pulmonary oil-embolism or venous thrombo-embolism, pulmonary edema, pneumonia and haemoptysis was 1/4,000, 1/32,000, 1/2,500 and 1/320, respectively, in the last report of Koehler (48). These complications can be of a minor nature but are sometimes fatal; it is therefore essential to tailor the dose of the oil-soluble contrast medium to each particular situation and to monitor its inflow with image intensified fluoroscopy (49). Hemoptysis probably results from break-down of oil and release of fatty acids in the lungs. A better fixation in the lymph nodes of the oil-soluble contrast medium can be obtained after the intravenous injection of benzopyrones (coumarin-rutin) which prevents a fast flow to the lung, reducing the risk of pulmonary complications (47).

6.3. *Cerebral complications*

Cerebral embolization is the most serious, but an uncommon complication which is only observed after the injection of oil-soluble contrast medium (50); 9 cases were reported by Koehler (51) from which 6 recovered.

6.4. *Anaphylactic shock*

This complication is exceptional and due to iodism and was reported to respond to vasopressors and corticosteroids (50). *Acute renal failure, hemolytic crises, inflammatory goiter and worsening of the lymphedema* have also been reported but are very rare.

6.5.   *Dissemination of tumor cells*

It has been suggested that any intralymphatic injection could increase the number of tumor cells in the thoracic duct with major risk of metastasis. However, Battezzati and Donini stated that 'opinions still differ widely as regards the incidence of circulating tumor cells and the exact relationship between circulating tumor cells and metastases' (43). These authors recommended administering prophylactically cytostatic drugs when performing lymphography in patients with neoplastic diseases.

7.   CLINICAL APPLICATION

Fig. 2 gives the normal appearance of the afferent and efferent lymph vessels of the deep lymphatic system when the contrast medium is injected in the posterior tibial lymphatic vessel at the inner border of the ankle (a), with the filling phase of thigh lymph vessels (b) and the inguinal lymphangioadenogram (c). Simple congenital lymphedema is limited to one member of the family and hereditary congenital lymphedema or Milroy's disease affects several members of the family suggesting a genetic defect. Fig. 3a shows hypoplasia of the superficial and deep lymph circulation (lower arrow) with distal back-flow in a patient with *congenital lymphedema*. There are some tortuous and dilated lymphatics with dermal backflow (skin lymphatics) as seen in (b). There are also communications between the superficial and deep lymphatic system in congenital lymphedema (upper arrow, Fig. 3c). There is dermal backflow, a well developed collateral circulation and lymphovenous shunts. When there are hypoplastic lymph vessels in the iliac region and visible lymph nodes are small and fewer than normal then primary lymphedema is almost certain.

We have often observed *lymphovenous anastomoses* and communications with the superficial lymphatic system of the lower leg which were unknown to the anatomist (52). Such anastomoses between the superficial lymph system and the posterior tibial deep lymphatic system are shown in Fig. 4. When there is a complete superficial block, the lymphatic circulation shows drainage to the deep lymphatic system. If this deep pathway is also blocked, there is drainage along the venous wall lymphatic chain, the so-called 'manchettes perivasculaires' (53–55).

Lymphedema praecox is an idiopathic but frequent form of lymphedema affecting primarily females, which begins between the age of 10 and 20

inguinal pain. Four patients had clinical and roentgenological symptoms of pulmonary infarction exclusively in the group with the higher dose of contrast media. Two patients developed small lymphatic cysts at the puncture site, which healed after excision (Fig. 2d). One patient developed a lymph fistula and lymphangiitis at the site of injection starting 10 days after lymphography (Elke M, Willi RW, 1977, unpublished controls) (17, 21, 35, 43). It is to be stressed that patients' age, pre-existing damage and an aggressive oncologic therapy, e.g., radiotherapy, increase the risk of side-effects, especially of micro-oil-embolization of the lungs (31, 32, 36–39, 44). Comparing the X-rays and histological examinations of lymph nodes at different intervals after lymphography we noted a certain parallelism between the extent of the sinus dilatation and foreign body reaction. Fibrotic changes of the lymph nodes after lymphography cannot be distinguished from pre-existing fibrotic alterations. Up to two years after lymphography there was no certain increase of fibrosis when perfused and non-perfused lymph nodes were compared. Some small lymph nodes can fill poorly or not at all with Lipoidol-UF and still be normal (34, 45). A remarkable observation is the accumulation of Lipoidol-UF in pulmonary metastases of hypernephromas. Fine droplets of the contrast medium are seen throughout the metastases, frequently in a ring shape. Using I^{131}-tagged Lipoidol-UF, histochemical and autoradiographic investigations demonstrated the intracellular storage of the iodine-lipid in pulmonary metastases (46, 47).

With raised lymphatic pressure, biogenetic pre-existent but normally closed lymphovenous anastomoses (LVA) can be opened. LVA connect with a shunt lymph vessel and a vein, lymph node and a vein respectively. Such LVA's were

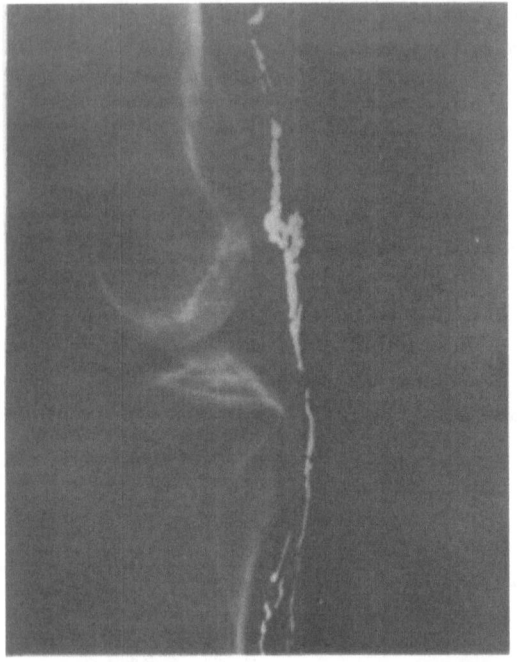

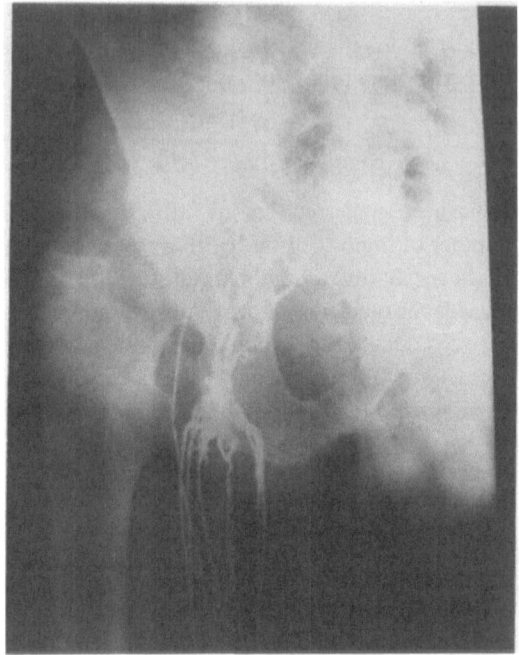

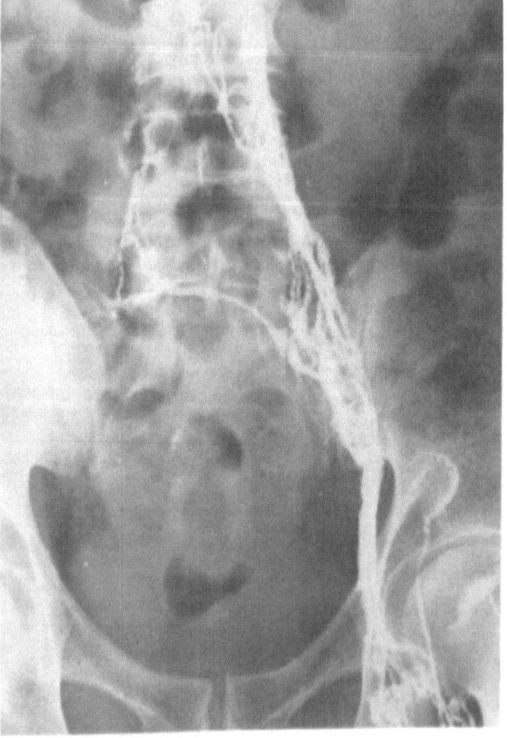

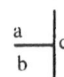

Fig. 2. (a) Normal view of the afferent and efferent lymph pathways of deep system when the contrast medium is injected on the posterior tibial lymphatic on the inner border of the ankle. (b) Normal filling phase of a thigh lymphangio-adenogram. (c) Filling phase of a normal inguinal lymphangioadenogram.

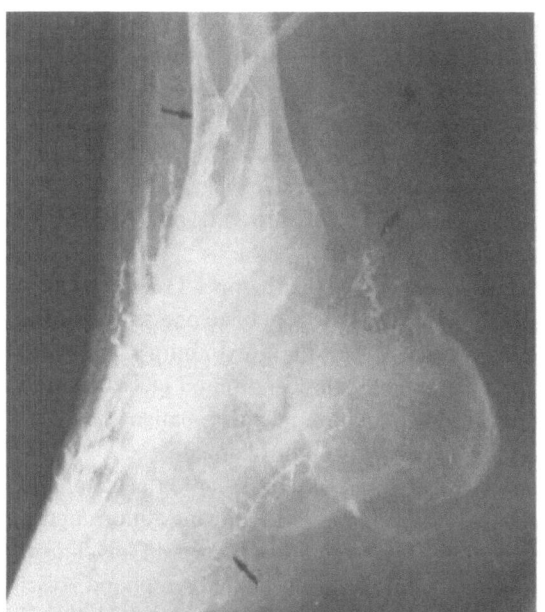

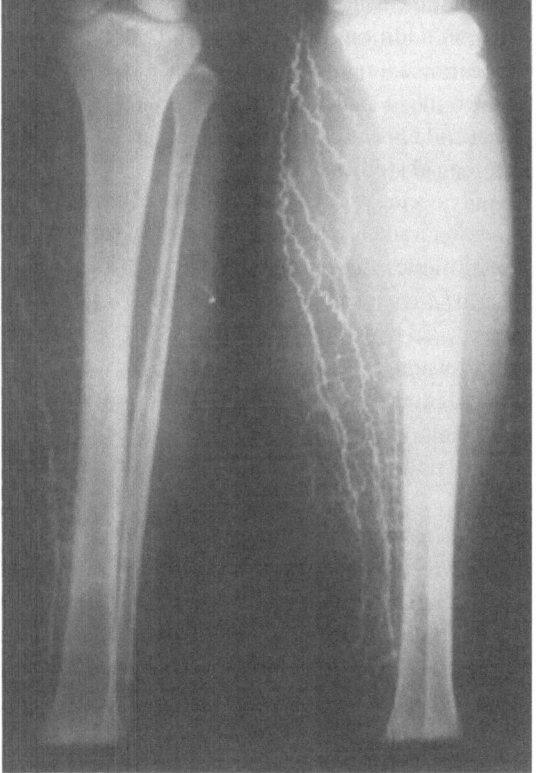

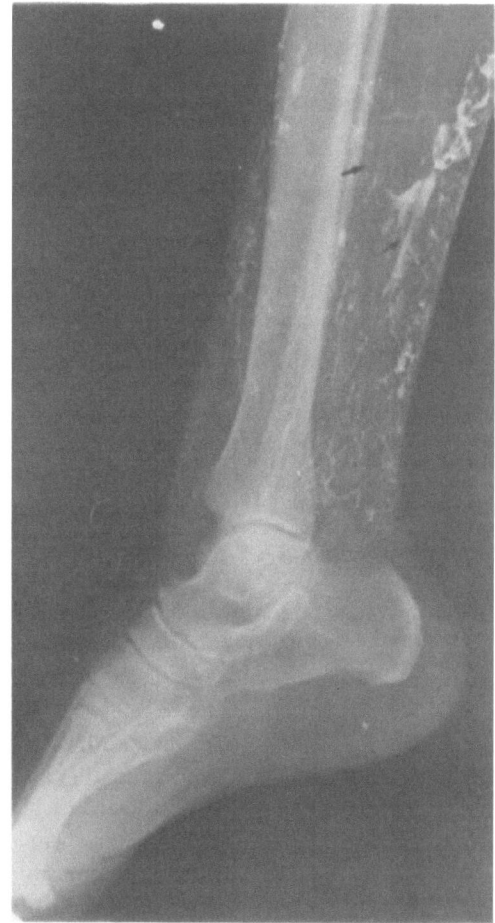

a | c
b |

Fig. 3. (a) Congenital lymphedema of the leg. Perivenous lymphatics (upper arrow). Delayed film. Obstruction of superficial and deep lymph circulation (lower arrow). Distal back flow. Tortuosity below obliterans lymphangiopathy. (b) Congenital lymphedema. Lymphangiectasis. Tortuous and dilated lymphatics. Dermal backflow. Numerical hyperplasia. Collateral circulation with rectification of the direction. (c) Congenital lymphedema. Communications between the superficial and deep lymphatic system (upper arrow). Dermal backflow. Bore differences, intensive collateral circulation and atypical visualization of the lymph pathways. Lymphovenous shunts.

found so far between the lymphatic system, and in leg veins, femoral veins, external iliac veins and common iliac veins, renal veins, inferior vena cava and branches of the portal vein. With such shunts the normally interposed groups of lymph nodes can be bypassed and the oily-contrast medium can embolize directly and in a higher concentration in the capillary system of the lungs or in the intrahepatic portal system. The same holds for small corpuscular elements, such as, for example, tumour cells (21, 32, 44, 48) (Fig. 3a, b) (see p. 392). Besides an increase in intralymphatic pressure (e.g., with extended tumour infiltration), inflammations, phlebothrombosis, injuries, and operations can also open LVAs. There are methodical limits in the detection of LVAs by intralymphatic administered contrast medium. Sequence pictures reveal LVAs often only by chance and their direct cinematographic demonstration is time consuming, expensive and exposes the patient to further irradiation. Indirect markers of open LVAs are a rapid and unusually strong embolization of lung capillaries, a reticular concentration of contrast medium in the liver (portal drainage) or a disproportionate dose of contrast medium required to fill the lymphatic system ('thinking' of intralymphatically administered contrast medium). It is obvious that, in case of suspected LVAs, the dose of contrast medium has to be limited and the injection of oily-contrast medium stopped.

years. As shown in Fig. 5a, there is numerical hyperplasia of the lymph vessels (black stars) with distal reflux, varicous and tortuous lymphatics and dermal back-flow around the foot. Fig. 5b shows blocked lymphatics below the knee with intense dermal backflow, lymphangiectasy, tortuosities and visualization of extensive precapillaries and capillaries. A third case of lymphedema praecox is shown in (c) where megalymphatic, varicose and tortuous hyperplasia vessels with intense dermal and distal back-flow are present.

In the *congenital dysplastic angiopathy* called Klippel-Trenaunay syndrome there is a hemangioma with overgrowth of bone and soft tissue in the same region and extensive varicose veins in the extremity. Lymphatic aplasia or hyperplasia is not uncommon in this condition. Fig. 6 shows the intense distal reflux and collateral circulation in such a patient with evidence of lymphangiectasis and varicose tortuous lymphatics.

Also in the *postphlebitic syndrome* there is involvement of the lymphatic vessels which is often underrated (52, 56–59). The following abnormalities of the superficial and deep lymphatic vessels can be observed in this clinical condition: (a) limitation to one major tortuous, dilated lymphatic vessel around the vena saphena magna (Fig. 7a); (b) increased permeability of the superficial and deep lymphatic vessels located near the ulceration as can be seen in Fig. 7b where, in addition, lymph vessels are abnormally large and have a beaded appearance; (c) intense dermal backflow around the ankle with even backflow to the os calcaneum (Fig. 7c, black star) due to inflammatory lymphedema and fibrous chronic lymphangiitis, as can be demonstrated by histopathological studies.

Obstructive lymphedema may occur, for instance, in cases of Hodgkin's disease, lymphosarcoma or after radical amputation of the breast with removal of the axillary lymph nodes for carcinoma. The arm begins to swell on resumption of physical activity, sometimes only after several years if chronic fibrosis has been induced by irradiation therapy. Fig. 8a shows the marked perilymphatic diffusion in the arm following mastectomy. There are numerous varicose dilatations and tortuous lymphatics in the entire extremity with dermal pools of contrast medium. Filling defects and enlargement of the first axillary nodes are often caused by metastases of a breast carcinoma (Fig. 8b).

A complication of vena saphena magna stripping is *iatrogenic lymphedema* as shown in Fig. 9a and b. Only one section of a lymphatic vessel is visible around the ankle and has a tortuous appearance (a). In some circumstances leaking lymphatic vessels (lymphatica porosa) lead to extravasation during the injection of hydrosoluble contrast medium at normal pressure (Fig. 10).

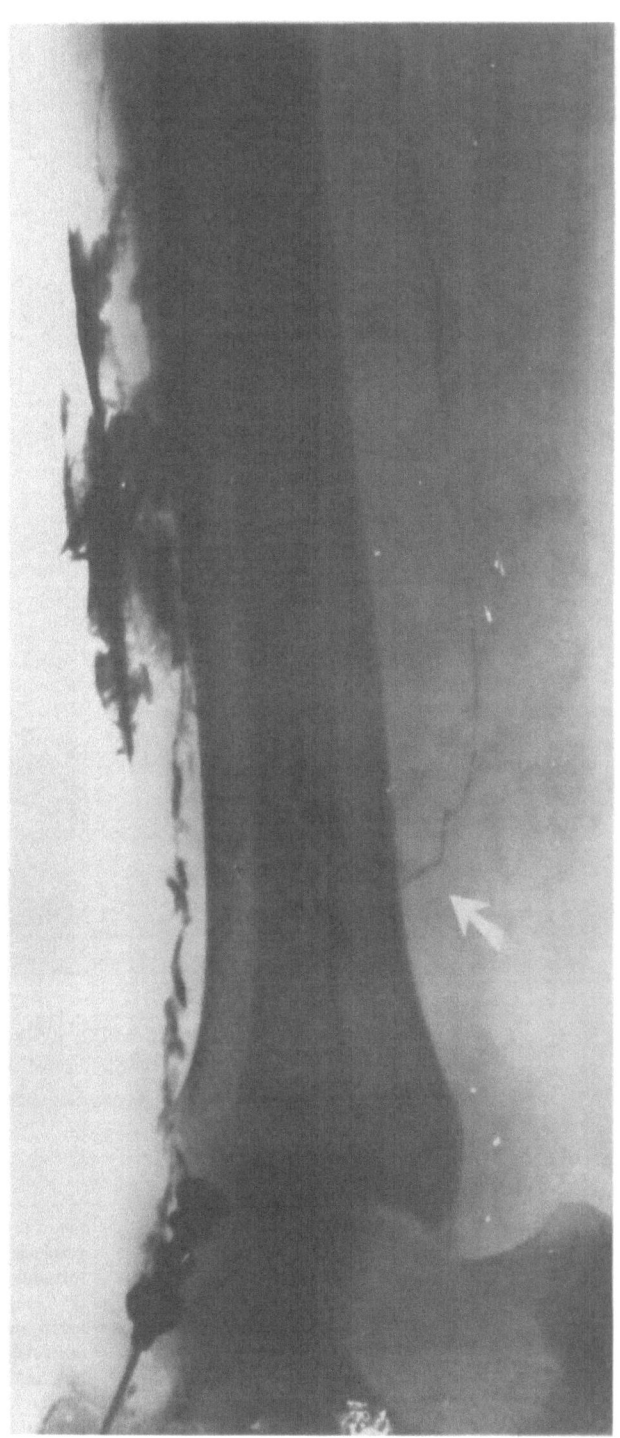

Fig. 4. Posttrauma lymphedema of the leg. Anastomosis between the superficial lymph system to the posterior tibial deep lymphatic (white arrow).

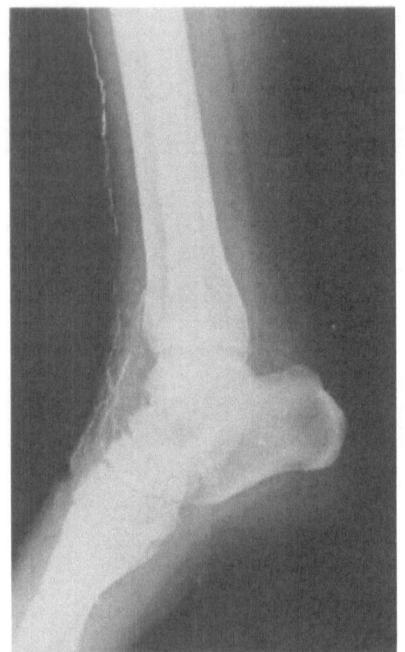

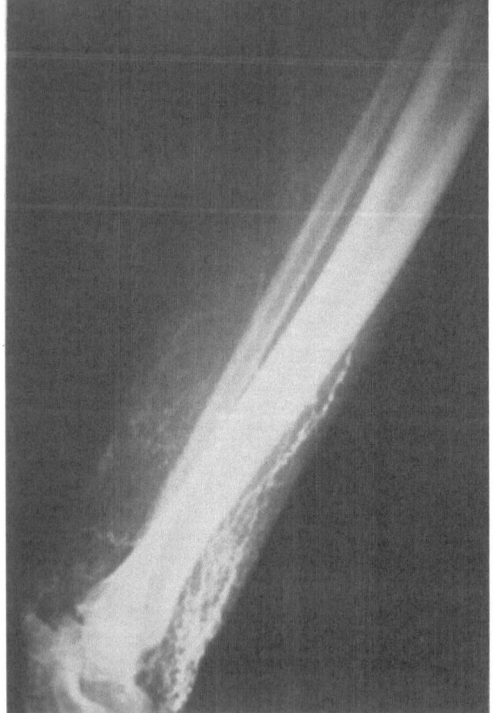

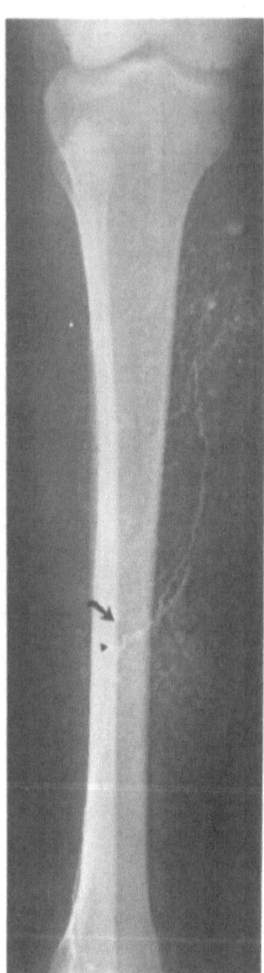

$\dfrac{a}{c}\Big|\,b$

Fig. 5 (a) Congenital praecox lymphoedema: numerical hyperplasia in the leg (black stars), with distal reflux, varicous, tortuous lymphatics and dermal back flow around the foot. (b) Congenital praecox lymphedema. Blocked lymphatics below the knee showing intense dermal backflow, lymphangiectasy and tortuosity, visualization of extensive precapillary and capillary networks. (c) Congenital praecox lymphedema. Megalymphatic, varicous hyperplasia, tortuosity and intense dermal and distal backflow.

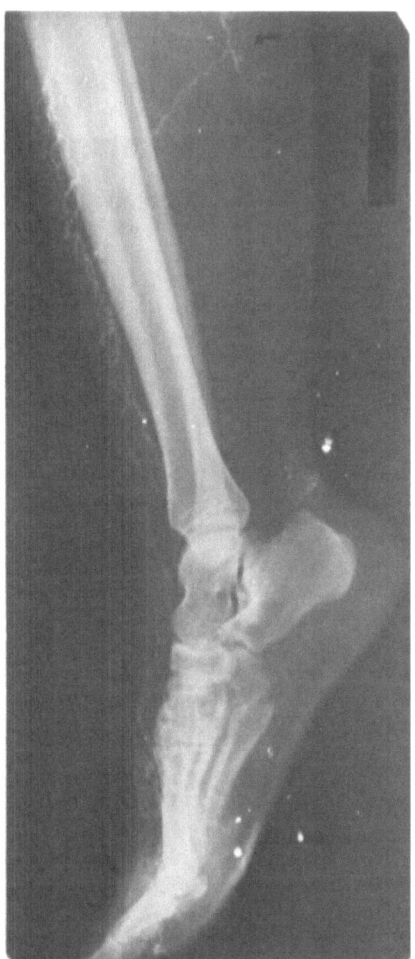

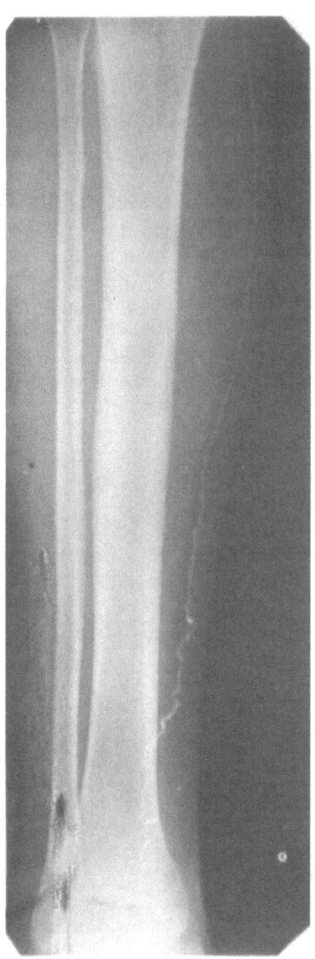

Fig. 6. **Klipperl-Trenaunay** Syndrome. Intense distal reflux and collateral circulation. Lymphangiectasis and varicose tortuous lymphatics.

Fig. 7a (a) Chronic postphlebitic syndrome with severe edema. Lymphography shows only one tortuous, dilated and varicous vessel.

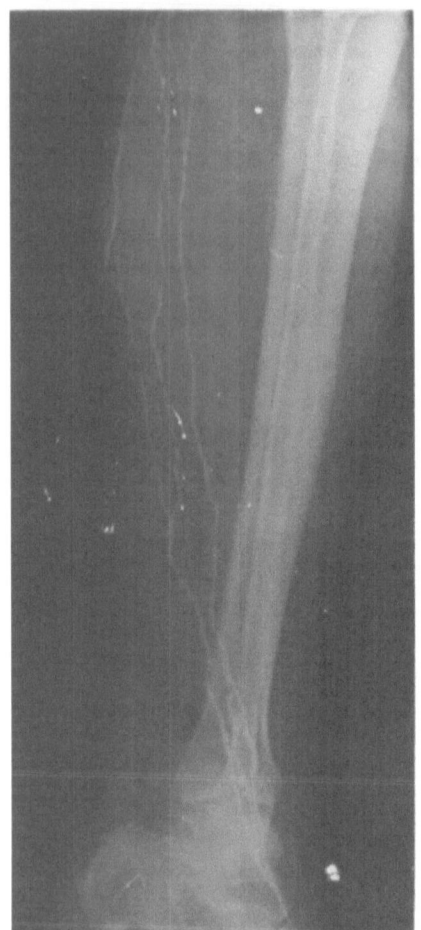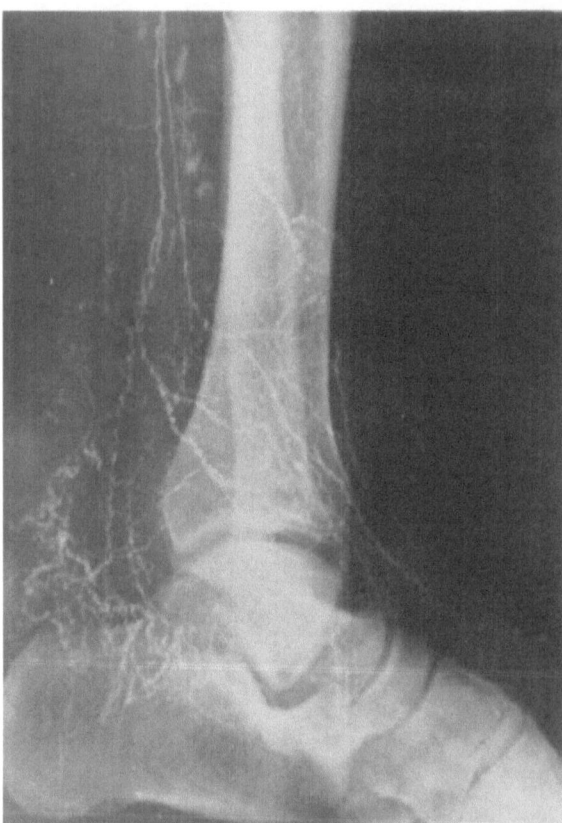

Fig. 7b, c.(b) Chronic postphlebitic syndrome: lymphography on the filling phase showing pronounced lymphangiectasy, enlarged lymphatic on the mid-leg with beaded appearance and increased permeability. (c) Inflammatory lymphedema, secondary to postphlebitic syndrome. Numerical hyperplasia of lymph trunks with tortuosity, distension, dermal back flow and distal reflux to the calcaneous (black star).

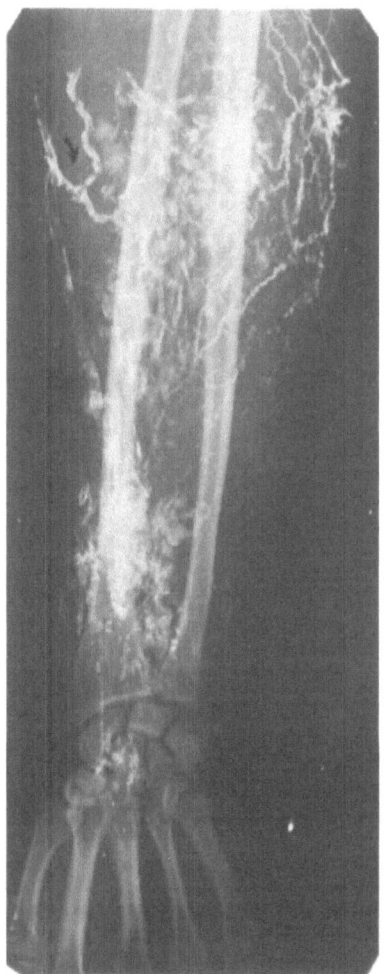

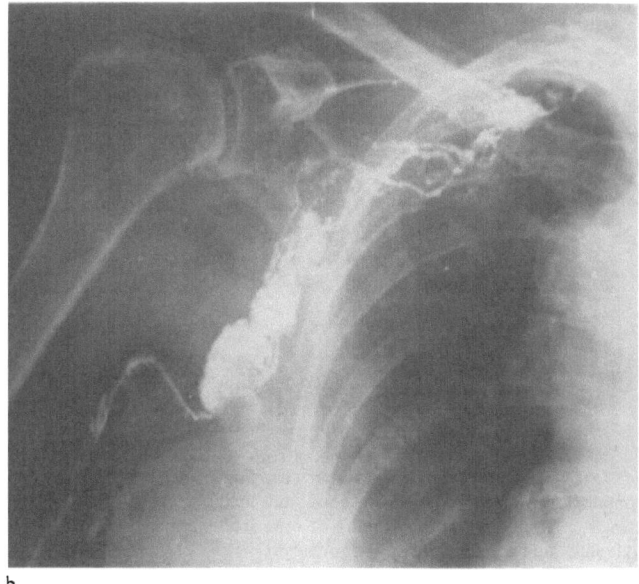

a
b

Fig. 8. (a) Postmastectomy lymphedema of the upper limb. Marked perilymphatic diffusion. Varicosities and tortuosity of the lymphatics. Intense perivenous injection in areolar tissue after extravasation. (b) Breast carcinoma: upper limb lymphoadenography showing filling defects and big enlargement of the first axillary nodes caused by metastasis confirmed by histopathology.

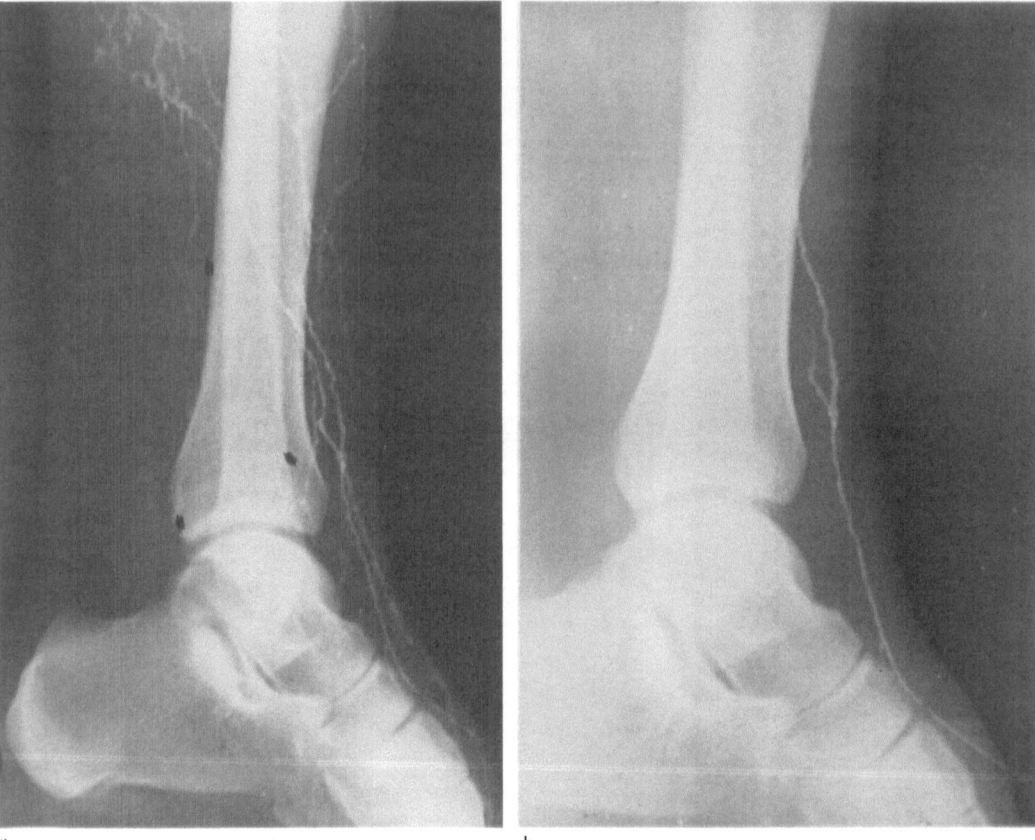

a   b

Fig. 9. (a) Iatrogenic lymphedema after stripping of vena saphena magna. Occlusion of the lymph trunks in the groin. Lymphography shows dilated varicous and tortuous trunks with moderate backflow and numerical hyperplasia. (b) Iatrogenic lymphedema poststripping of vena saphena magna. Only one part of the lymphatic trunk is visible around the ankle showing lymphangiectasy and tortuosity.

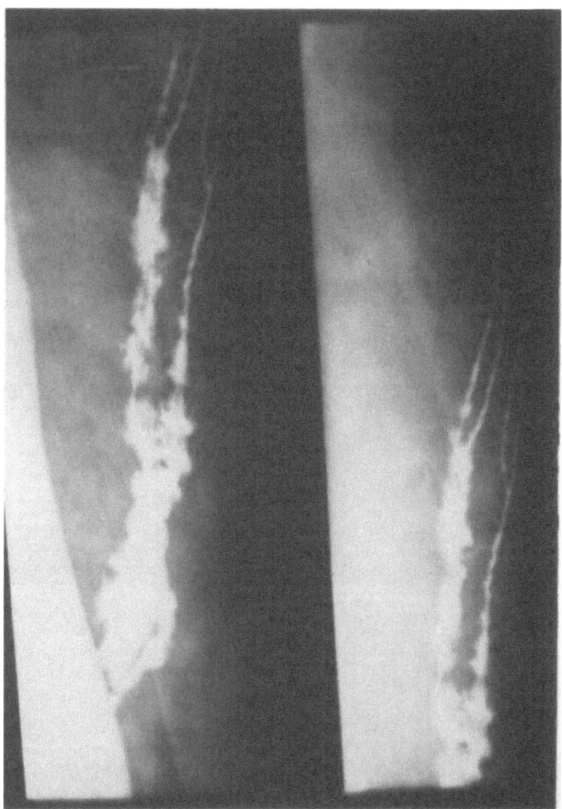

Fig. 10. 'Lymphatica porosa' due to leaky lymphatic wall, leading to extravasation, during the moment of injection of hydrosoluble contrast medium, with normal pressure.

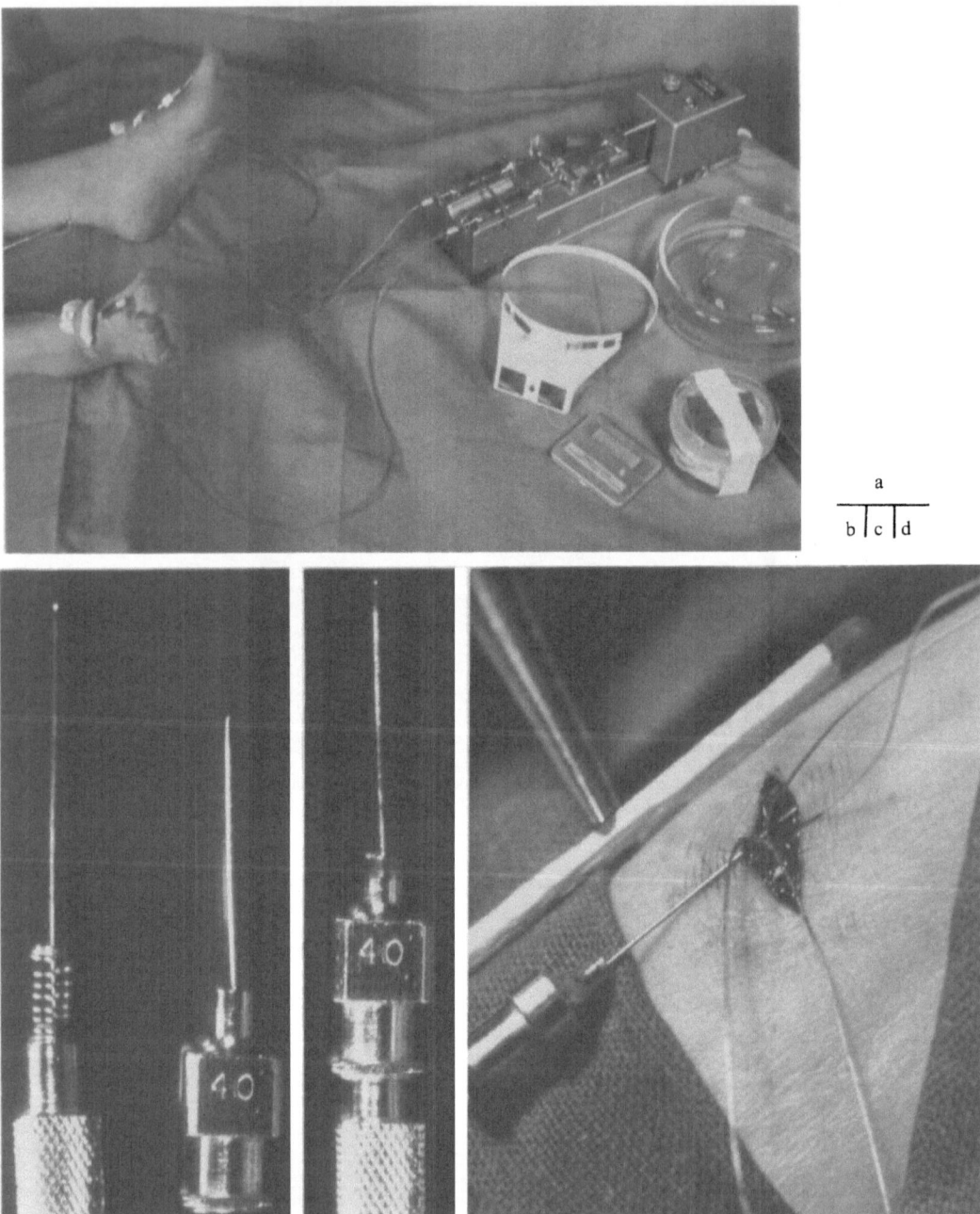

Fig. 1 *to commentary.* (a) Automatic injector with 10 ml syringes and special lymphography needles (Roo T, de: Medica mundi 10: 101, 1965; Amer. J. Roentgenol. 98: 948, 1966), ready for injection. Binocular magnifying eye glass. (b) The two parts of the De Roo-needle, stylet with a small spring and 40/100 mm needle. (c) For punction the stylet will be pushed forwards. (d) De Roo-needle in situ.

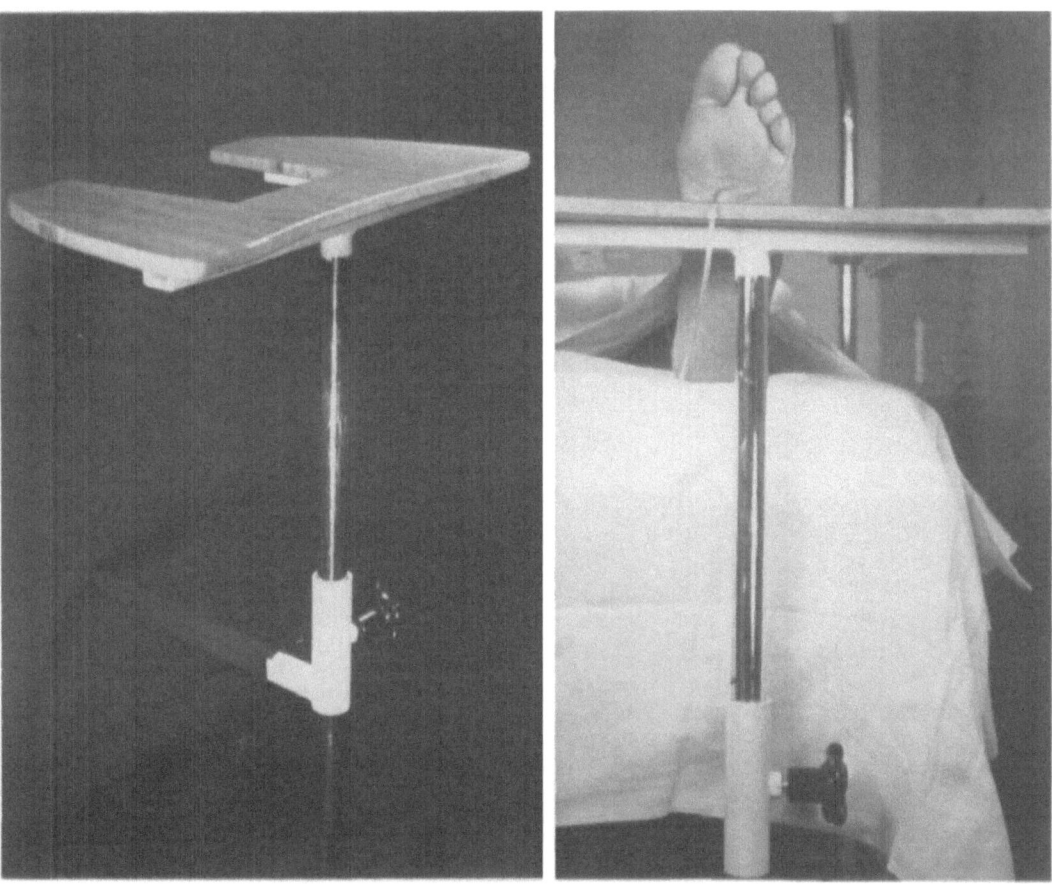

e

Fig. 1 *to commentary*. (e and f) Small desk with horizontal and vertical adjustment.

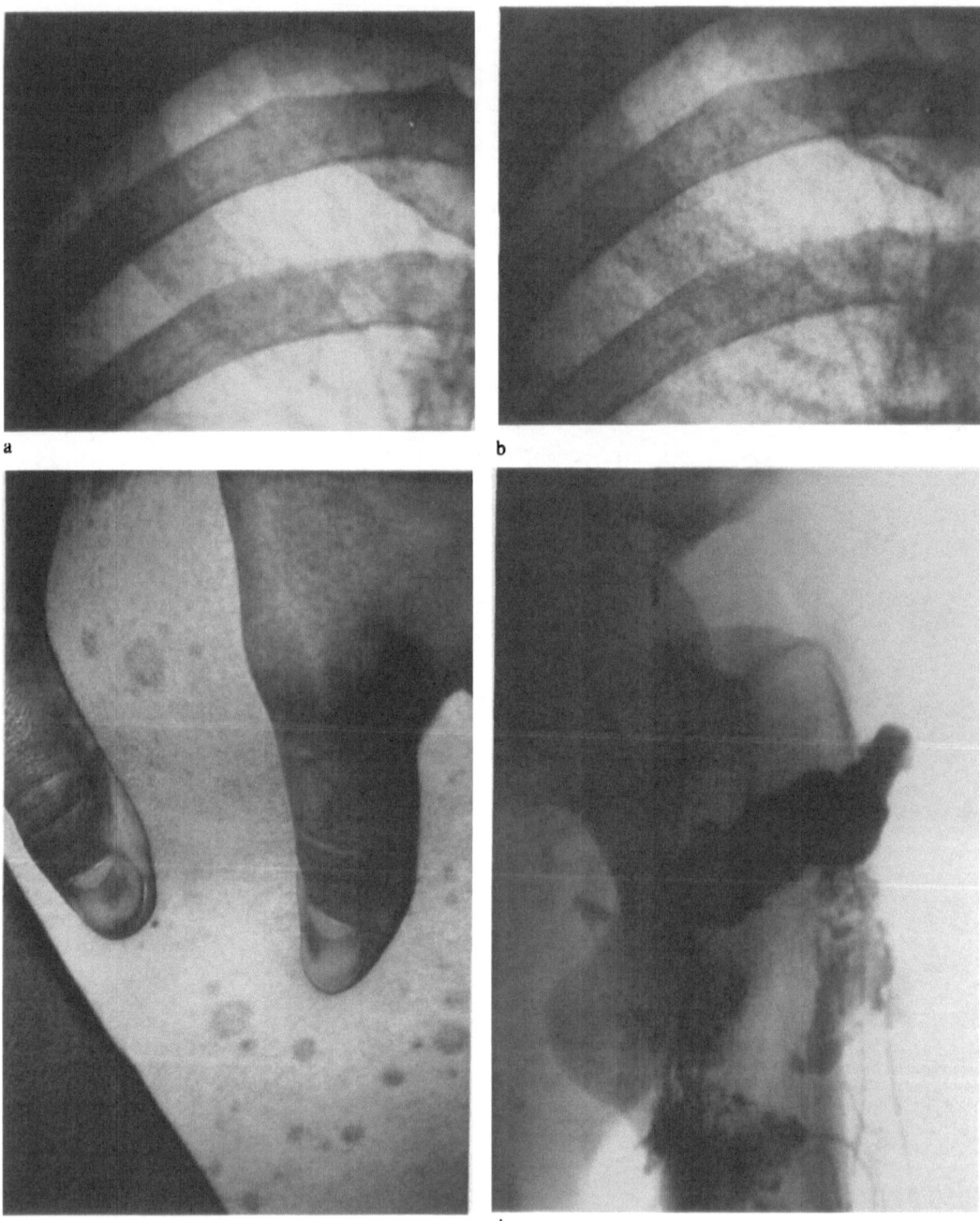

Fig. 2 *to commentary.* (a) Part of the thorax X-ray before Lipoidol-UF injection and (b) 20 h after injection of totally 18 ml (in the early times of clinical lymphography 1964) with massive micro-oil-emboli in the lungs. (c) Exanthema involving the skin of the whole body with wheals and pruritus 40 min after s.c. injection of Patent-blue-violet. (d) Lymph-cyst. Lymphography 12 days after lymph node dissection.

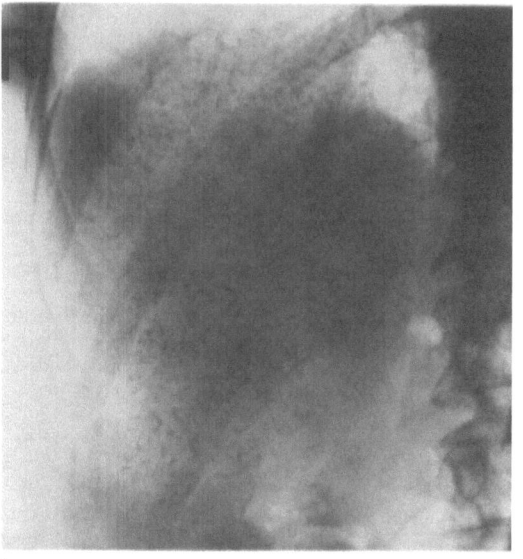
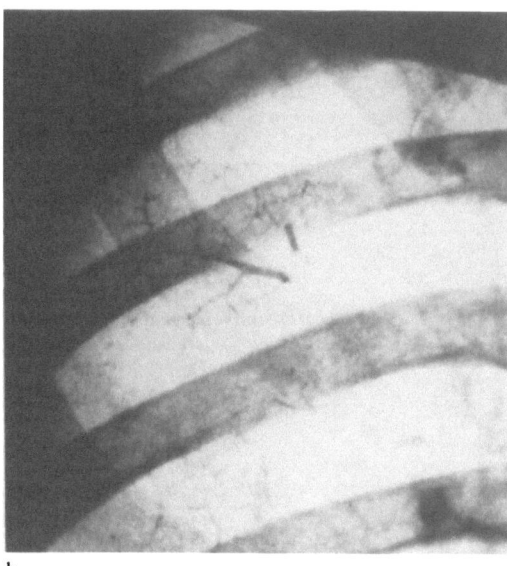

a   b

Fig. 3 to commentary.(a) Massive oil emboli in the lungs in a case with LVA. (b) Oil embolization with striated-spotted contrast media depots in the liver in a case with LVA.

REFERENCES TO MAIN TEXT

1. Kinmonth JB: The Lymphatic Diseases – Lymphography and Surgery, London, Edward Arnold, 1972, 1-19.
2. Kinmonth JB: Radiologic visualisation of the lymph system. Anatomic considerations and some primary anomalies. In: Lymph and the Lymphatic System, Springfield III, Thomas, 1968, p 3-10.
3. Kinmonth JB, Rob CG, Simeone FA: Vascular Surgery, London, Edward Arnold, 1962, p 345-352.
4. Carvalho R, Rodrigues A, Souza Pereira A: La mise en évidence par la radiographie du système lymphatique chez le vivant. Ann. Anat. Path. Anat. norm. Méd.-chir. VIII (2): 193, 1931.
5. Rodriguez A, Carvalho R, Souza Pereira A: Sur une nouvelle méthode de mise en évidence des lymphatiques sur le vivant. In: XXVIe Réunion de l'association des anatomistes, Varsovie, 1931.
6. Rodriguez A, Carvalho R, Souza Pereira A: Le thorotrast dans la mise en évidence radiographique des lymphatiques sur le vivant. In: C.R. Assoc. Anat. 1933.
7. Fumaoka S: Untersuchungen über die Physiologie der Lymphbewegung. Die Röentgenographie des Lymphgefasses, Arbeiten aus der dritten Abteilung des Anatomischen Institutes der Kaiserlichen Universität Kyoto. Fasc. 1, 1930, Cit. par Carvalho R, Rodrigues A, Souza Pereira A: XXVIe Réunion de l'Association des Anatomistes, Varsovie, 1931.
8. Hudack SS, Mc.Master PD: The lymphatic participation in human cutaneous phenomena, study of the minute lymphatic, in living skin. J. exp. Med. 57: 751, 1933.
9. Seabra JJ: Linfatografia. Bahia, Brasil, Tese, 1943. Seid ME, Burihan E, Neme F: Quilotorax. Uma complicação rara da aortografia translombar com comprovação linfográfica. Rev. Bras. Cardiovasc.1 (11): 50, 1975.
10. Marques R, Caetano de Barros M: Linfografia (Nota Prévia). In: Revista Médica Panamericana, I, Vol. 1, 3, Pernambuco, Brasil, Recife, p 334-339, 1945.
11. Servelle M: Pathologie Vasculaire Médicale et Chirurgicale, Paris, Masson and Cie, 1952.

12. Wallace S, Jackson L, Schaffer B, Gould RJ, Greening RR, Weiss A, Kramer S: Lymph-angiograms: their diagnostic and therapeutic potential. Radiology 76: 179–199, 1961.

13. Abrams HL: Lymphography in lymphoma. In: Angiography, Abrams HL (ed), second ed. Vol. II, Boston, Little Brown, 1971, p 1389–1420.

14. Arnulf G: Practical value of lymphography of the extremities. Angiology (1) 9: 1–6, 1958.

15. Arvay N, Picard JB: La lymphographie, Paris, Masson and Cie, 1963, 24–27.

16. Averette HE, Hudson RC, Viamonte M, Parks RE, Ferguson JH: Lymphoadenography in the study of female genital cancer. 15(4): 769–775, 1962.

17. Bélanger RMD, Harel C, Quimet, Oliva D, Katz L: Technique de lymphographie per catheter. J. Canad. Assoc. Radiol. XVI: 237–239, 1965.

18. Braga Lopes F, Mayall RC: Cancer Vulva e Linfoadenografia. Diagnóstico e Trata-mento. Rev.Bras.Cir., 51 (3): 137–143, 1958.

19. Caetano de Barros M: Fisiopatologia das vias linfáticas periféricas – Tentativas de terapeutica. Agosto, Publicações Médicas, Ano XVI, no. 1, 1944, 3–19.

20. Desprez-Curely JP, Bismuth V, Langin A, Descamps J: Accidents et incidents de la lymphographie. Ann. Radiol. 7: 577, 1962.

21. Ducros R: L'épreuve au bleu. Phlébologie 19 (2): 129–132, 1966.

22. Edwards JM, Kinmonth JB: Lymphovenous shunts in man. Brit.med.J. 4: 579–581, 1969.

23. Flores Izquierdo G, Paparelli H, Ramirez Espinosa F, Fabela CS: Linfografias. In: Memorias del VIIe Congreso Latino-americano de Angiologia, Mexico, 1964, p 533–539.

24. Földi M: Erkrankungen des Lymphsystems – Chylöser Reflux. Baden-Baden. Verlag Gerhard Witztrock, 1971, p 128, 217, 223.

25. Gooneratne BWM: Lymphography Clinical and Experimental, London, Butterworths, 1974, p 18–19.

26. Gregl A: Arm Lymphographie – Technik Indikation und Ergebnisse Nebenerschei-nungen. Folia Angiologica, XXIV: 30–34, 1976.

27. Gruart FJ: Progress on the lymphographic study of the Head and Neck – Progress in Lymphology, Mayall RC, Marlys H Witte (eds) London, Plenum Press, 1977, p 145–146.

28. Kuisk H, Blackard CE, Schenk DC: Technique of funicular lymphography without the use of indicator dyes. In: Progress in Lymphology, Mayall RC, Marlys H Witte (çds) New York, Plenum Press, 1977, p 197–208.

29. Marques MSB: A propos d'une nouvelle technique pour la lymphoadénographie des membres inférieurs, Angéiologie XXVIII: 109–115, 1976.

30. Masselot J, Bergiron C, Markovits P: Valeurs comparées de la lymphographie, de la cavographie et de l'urographie intraveineuse dans l'étude des métastases de testicule – A propos de 60 cas. J. Radiol. 52 (11): 653–662, 1971.

31. Mayall RC: Phlebolymphographic documentation – Progrès cliniques et thérapeutiques dans le domaine de la phlébologie, Rapport du IIIe Congrès International de Phlébo-logie. Apeldoorn, Stenvert and Zoon, 1970, p 136.

32. Mayall RC: Técnicas de Linfografias superficiais e profundas dos membros inferiores. Rev.Med. Sul de Minas, 7 (11): 86–89, 1961.

33. Mayall RC: Lymphography of deep trunks of the legs, Bull.Soc. int.chir. 21 (5): 486–499, 1962.

34. Ottaviani G: El Sistema linfatico en biologia y en clinica. In: Forum Médica no. 12. La Linfologia, un nuevo ramo de la Medicina, p 5–7 (undated).

35. Praderi LA, Curuchet E: La linfografia del Conducto Toraxico en el estudio de la ex-tension lesional del cancer de esofago. In: Memorias del 7e Congreso Latino Americano de Angiologia, Mexico, 1964, 529–531.

36. Rodriguez-Azpurua: El valor e importancia de la linfangiografia en las enfermedades vasculares de los miembros inferiores. Angiologia XII (4): 210–230, 1960.

37. Severo Marques M, Degni M: Exploração radiológica dos linfáticos dos membros inferiores (sistema profundo). In: Abstracts Vth International Congress of Lymphology, Buenos Aires, Rio de Janeiro, March 23–29, 1975, 251.

38. Tossati E: Lymphatiques profonds et lymphoédèmes chroniques des membres. Paris, Masson and Cie, 1974, 73–76.

39. Totti A, Fabi M: Esplorazione radiologica del Sistema Linfatico. Torino, Minerva medica, 1961.

40. Daintree Johnson H, Pflug J: The Swollen Leg, William Heinemann Medical Books, p 82–86, 1974, London.
41. Kaindl F, Manheimer E, Pfleger-Schwarz L, Thurnher B: Lymphangiographie und Lymphoadenographie der Extremitäten. Stuttgart, Thieme, 1960, p 30.
42. Kitainik E, Swiatlo MR, Villa JJ: Linfografia y Linfoadenografia – Tecnica y Instrumental Simplificado. In: Publicaciones del I Congreso Argentino de Angiologia, Buenos Aires, 1966, p 32–33.
43. Battezzati J, Donini I: The Lymphatic System. Padua and London, Piccin Medical Books, 1972, p 100–110.
44. Battezzati M, Tagliaferro A, Donini I, Rossi L: La Linfoadenografia. Torino, Pan Minerva Medica, 1961.
45. Collard M: La perméabilité lymphatique anormale et l'effet des avitaminoses sur le coeur in Basic Lymphology. Földi M (ed) (Second Ringelheim Symposium) Folia Angiologica Supplementa, Berlin, Verlag Haupt and Koska, 1974, p 66 and 115.
46. Collard M: In: Folia Angiologica, Suppl. Vol. III, Földi M (ed), Basic Lymphology, Berlin, Verlag Haupt and Koska, 1974, p 66.
47. Collard M: In: Diskussion Folia Angiologica, Suppl. Vol. III, Földi M (ed), Basic Lymphology, Berlin, Verlag Haupt and Koska, 1974, p 114–115.
48. Koehler PR: Complications of lymphography. In: Progress in Lymphology, Mayall RC, Marlys H Witte (eds) New York, Plenum Press, 1977, p 209–213.
49. Weissleder H: Lymphography – Endolymphatic Radionuclide Therapy – das Medizinische. Sohn, Ingelheim am Rhein, Prisma, 1977, p 4–17.
50. Gruwez JA: La lymphographie, Acta chir. belg. Suppl. II, 1–250: 167–195, 1968.
51. Koehler PR: Injuries and complications of the lymphatic system following renal transplantation, Lymphology 5: 61, 1972.
52. Mayall RC: Linfoadenografias. Rev. Bras. Cardiovasc. 7 (4): 333–338, 1971.
53. Collete JM: Les lymphatiques des parois veineuses et les fistules lymphoveineuses périphériques. In: Progrès Cliniques et Thérapeutiques dans le domaine de la phlébologie, Van der Molen HR, Van Limborgh J, Boersma W (eds), Apeldoorn, Stenvert and Zoon, 1978, p 344.
54. Collete JM, Picard JD, Collard M, Godard S: Contribuiçâo clinica da linfografia no conhecimento das linfangiopatias superficiais e viscerais e das alterações ganglionares, Rev. Bras. Cardiovasc. 1: 148–171, 1965.
55. Collete JM: New trends in Basic Lymphology. Experientia Suppl. 14, Basel, Birkhäuser, 1967, p 48 and 221.
56. Mayal RC, Barbosa C: Lymphographie après Saphénectontes et dans les séquelles de thrombophlébite. Corrélations thérapeutiques. Phlébologie (2) XXI: 175–178, 1968.
57. Mayal RC: Edemas linfáticos e venosos dos membros inferiores. Rio de Janeiro, Gráfica Villani Filhos, 1970, p 37–46.
58. Mayall RC: Panel Discussion, XI Congresso Brasileiro de Angiologia, Rio de Janeiro, 1962, Angiopatias, Brasil, Vol. 3, no 2, 1963, p 114–129.
58. Mayall RC: Importancia de la Linfografia en Patologia Venosa. In: Memorias del VII Congreso Latinoamericano de Angiologia, Mexico, 1964, p 541.

ADDITIONAL BIBLIOGRAPHY TO MAIN TEXT

Bruun S, Engeset A: Lymphoadenography: A new method for the visualisation of enlarged lymphnodes and lymphatic vessels (preliminary report). Acta Radiol. 45: 389–395, 1956.
Cançado JC: Contribuições para a aplicação clínica de linfografia – Tese. Belo Horizonte (MG) Brasil, 1965, Publ. 352 Imprensa da Universidade de Minas Gerais.
Castelino RA, Bergiron C, Markovits P: Repeat lymphography in children with Hodgkin's Disease. Cancer 38: (7) 90–95, 1976.
Chavez CM, Berrong LG, Evers CG: Hepatic oil embolism after lymphangiography. Amer. J. Surg. 110 (3): 456–460, 1956.
Chavez CM: Visceral Lymphography. Publicaciones del I Congreso Argentino de Angiologia, 4–8 Sept, 53–54, 1966.

Fracchia RC: Linfografias, Rev. Med. (Rosario) 53: 17–36, 1963.

Fuchs WA: Other complications of lymphangiography. In: Angiography, (Ed) Adams H, second edition, Vol. II, Boston, Little Brown, 1971, p 1436–1440.

Fuchs WA: Lymphographie und Tumor Diagnostik, New York, Springer, 1965, p 101.

Godart S, Collette J, Dalem J: Pathologie chirurgicale des vaisseaux lymphatiques, Acta chir. belg. Suppl. I: 1–116, 1964.

Hidden G: Abdominal Lymphnodes – Lymphadenographic Representation and reality. In: Abstracts V International Congress of Lymphology, March 23–29, Buenos Aires, Rio de Janeiro, 1975.

Lucas HS: Revisão do estudo do sistema linfático – Algumas complicações na cancerologia, (Reprints) Rev. Bras. Cancerol. 24: (38) (39) 90, 1968.

Mariano da Rocha Neto J, Chagas Gama GS: Tomografia no estudo radiológico de linfonodos normais e patológicos. Rev. Fac. Med. U.F.S.M. 3 (1): 61–67, 1971.

Marques R: Limites e Alcances de Linfografia. Rev. Bras. Cardiovasc. 6 (4) 323–340, 1970.

Mayal RC: Lymphography in postphlebitic syndrome. J. Cardiovasc. Surg. 1, 2: 176–179, 1960.

Picard JD, Ducros R: La diachromophanie en l'étude de la résorption d'un colorant dans les oedèmes. In: Radiographie et Photographie Médicales. Suresnes, France, Kodak-Pathé.

Picard JD, Delouche 6: La diachromophanie en Pathologie Mammaire. In: Radiographie et Photographie Médicales, Suresnes, France, Kodak Pathé.

Roo T de: Additional examination in lymphography: a radiological surgical-pathological correlation. Lymphology 7: 45–49, 1974.

Roo T de: Lymphography. In: Atlas of Angiography, Loose KE, van Dongen RJAM, Thieme, Stuttgart, 1976, p 383–429.

Rusznyak I, Foldi M, Szabó G: Lymphatics and lymph circulation. Oxford, Pergamon Press, 1960, p 635.

Shanbrom E, Zheutlin N: Radiographic studies of the lymphatic system. Arch int. Med. 104: 589–593, 1959.

Souza Pereira JMM, Souza Pereira A: A linfografia no estudo do sistema linfático normal. Rev. Bras. Cardiovasc. 1 (4): 223–252, 1965.

Souza Pereira JMM: Linfografia – Anatomia Radiológica e Fisiopatologia do Sistema Linfático (Estudo Experimental), Porto, Portugal Bloco gráfico, 1964.

Tallroth K, Wiljasalo M, Wiljasalo S: Lymphography in bone soft tissues sarcomas. Rev. Bras. Cardiovasc., 1 (11): 61, 1975.

Yamauchi S: Treatment of filarial chyluria. In: Progress in Lymphology, Mayall RC, Witte MH (eds), New York, Plenum Press, 1977, p 363–369.

Teixeira J: Personal information.

Winkel K, Schertel L: Lymphography with xeroradiography. Rev. Bras. Cardiovasc. 1 (11): 60, 1975.

Webster AM: New Collegiate Dictionary, Springfield, Mass., Merriam, 1975, p 201.

REFERENCES TO COMMENTARY

1. Elke M: Angenäherte Bestimmung des Lymphknotenvolumens nach dem Lymphogramm und seiner prozentualen Volumenveränderung bei Verlaufskontrollen. 1. Mitteilung: Theoretische Voraussetzungen. Fortschr. Röntgenstr. 112: 398, 1970.

2. Elke M, Schmid P: Vorschlag zur angenäherten Bestimmung des Lymphknotenvolumens nach dem Lymphogramm. 2. Mitteilung: Statistischer Vergleich der prozentualen Volumenänderung lymphographisch normaler und pathologisch veränderter Lymphknoten mit und ohne Behandlung. Fortschr. Röntgenstr. 112: 591, 1970.

3. Elke M, Rutishauser G, Renner KH: Die Bewertung des Lymphogramms und seiner Verlaufs-Kontrollen für die Metastasendiagnostik und Indikationsstellung zur operativen bzw. Strahlentherapie des Blasenkarzinoms. In: Glauner R (ed) Radiologische Diagnostik u. Therapie bei malignen Tumoren im Becken. Stuttgart, Thieme, 1970.

4. Elke M: Vorschlag zur angenäherten Bestimmung des Lymphknotenvolumens nach dem Lymphogramm. 3. Mitteilung: Nomogramme zur Bestimmung von Lymphknotenvolumen und deren prozentuale Aenderung bei Verlaufskontrollen. Fortschr. Röntgenstr. 115: 631, 1971.

5. Elke M, Hug I, Schmid P: Volumetrische Verlaufskontrollen an normalen Lymphknoten. Radiol. diagn. 13: 614, 1972.

6. Elke M, Kolakowski L: Elements of lymphographic analysis. (Elementy analizy limfograficznej). Pol. Przeg. Radiol. i. Med. Nukl. 37: 267, 1973.

7. Elke M, Ferstl A, Hug I: Lymphographie maligner Primärtumoren. Radiol. clin. biol. 42: 258, 1973.

8. Elke M, Ferstl A, Schwegler N: Aussagewert und -grenzen verschiedener Untersuchungsmethoden bei der Diagnose und Differentialdiagnose im Lymphsystem entwickelter retroperitonealer Tumoren. Radiologe 15: 377, 1975.

9. Hug I, Elke M: Vorschlag zur angenäherten Bestimmung des Lymphknotenvolumens. 4. Mitteilung: Bestimmung der Messgenauigkeit im Modellversuch. Fortschr. Röntgenstr. 116: 786, 1972.

10. Hug I, Elke M, Sauer R, Schmid P: Volumetrische Verlaufsmessungen an normalen und pathologischen Lymphknoten. Radiologie 15: 390, 1975.

11. Ludvik W, Wachtler F, Zaunbauer W: Veränderungen am Lymphogramm durch Operation und ionisierende Strahlen. Fortschr. Röntgenstr. 110: 307, 1969.

12. Röder K, Lüning M, Zyb AF: Verlaufskontrollaufnahmen und Wiederholungslymphographien. In: Lymphographie bei malignen Tumoren, Lüning M, Wiljasalo M, Weissleden H (eds), Stuttgart, Thieme, 1976, p 270 (new edition in prep., in Engl.).

13. Sauer R, Elke M, Hug I, Schmid P: Volumenänderung normaler Lymphknoten nach Strahlen- und Chemotherapie. Strahlenther. 147: 82, 1974.

14. Barke R, Elke M: Kontrastmittel. Kapitel 5. In: Lymphographie bei malignen Tumoren. Lüning M, Wiljasalo M, Weissleder H (eds), Leipzig, Georg Thieme Verlag, 1976, p 33–39 (new ed. in prep., in Engl.).

15. Breiman RS, Castellino RA, Harell GS, Marshall WH, Glatstein E, Kaplan HS: CT-pathologic correlations in Hodgkin's disease and non-Hodgkin's lymphoma. Radiology 126: 159, 1978.

16. Elke M, Wolff G, Hartmann G: Experiments with an emulsion of Lipiodol-UF (Guerbet) to avoid pulmonary embolization. In: Progress in Lymphology, Rüttimann A (ed), Stuttgart, Thieme, 1967, p 336.

17. Fischer HW: Complications in Lymphography. In: Lymphography in cancer. Fuchs, Davidson, Fischer (eds), Berlin, Springer, 1969.

18. Harell GS, Breiman RS, Glatstein EJ, Marshall WH, Castellino RA: Computed tomography of the abdomen in the malignant lymphomas. Radiol. Clin. N.A. 15: 391, 1977.

19. Jentsch F, Stringaris K, Kaiser G, Kirschner H: Computertomographie des kleinen Beckens als Grundlage für strahlentherapeutisches Vorgehen. Lokalisation und Bestrahlungsplanung beim Prostata-Carcinom. Radiologe 17: 268, 1977.

20. Kreel L: The EMI whole body scanner in the demonstration of lymph node enlargement. Clin. Radiol. 27: 421 1976.

21. Lüning M, Wiljasalo M, Weissleder H: Lymphographie bei malignen Tumoren. Leipzig, Thieme, 1976 (new edition in prep., in Engl.).

22. Maklad NF, Chuang VP, Doust BD, Cho KJ, Curran JE: Ultrasonic characterization of solid renal lesions: echographic, angiographic and pathologic correlation. Radiology 123: 733, 1977.

23. Marchal G, Coenen Y, Wilms G, Baert AL: The accuracy of CT-Scan in the diagnosis of retroperitoneal metastases of malignant testicular tumours. Fortschr. Röntgenstr. 128: 746, 1978.

24. Sagel SS, Stanley RJ, Levitt RG, Geisse G: Computed tomography of the kidney. Radiology 124: 359, 1977.

25. Elke M, Hug I: Erprobte Modifikationen der lymphographischen Untersuchungstechnik. Röntgenpraxis 2: 37, 1971.

26. Elke M, Hug I, Kolakowski L: Modern methods and techniques of lymphography with special references to a personal modification. Pol. Rev. Rad. Nucl. Med. 36: 93, 1972.

27. Rauste J: Lymphographic findings in granulomatous inflammations and connective tissue diseases. Acta radiol. Suppl. 317: 1972.
28. Tallroth K: Lymphatic dissemination of bone and soft tissue sarcomas. Acta radiol. Suppl. 349: 1976.
29. Elke M, Hartmann G: Prophylaktische Versuche am Modell einer Fettembolie mittels Phosphatid-Infusionen. Dtsch. med. Wschr. 95: 1012, 1970.
30. Brunner P: Beitrag zur Frage ölhaltiger Kontrastmittelembolien. Fortschr. Röntgenstr. 121: 49, 1974.
31. Elke M, Kolakowski L, Hug I: Observations on side effects of contrast media used in lymphography. Pol. Rev. Rad. Nucl. Med. 34: 535 1972.
32. Elke M, Ferstl A: Lymphovenöse Anastomosen: Diagnose, Differentialdiagnose und Abflusswege. Fortschr. Röntgenstr. 119: 43, 1973.
33. Fraimow W, Wallace S, Lewis P, Greening RR, Cathcart RT: Changes in pulmonary function due to lymphangiography. Radiology 85: 231, 1965.
34. Hodel C, Elke M: Vergleichende röntgenologische und histologische Befunde zur Kontrastmittelspeicherung nach Lymphographie. Fortschr. Röntgenstr. 107: 765, 1967.
35. Kelly JF: A complication of skin testing with iodinated radiographic contrast medium. Radiology 110: 353, 1974.
36. Sauer R, Elke M: Häufigkeit und Intensität pulmonaler Mikroölembolien nach Erst- und Wiederholungslymphographien bei Patienten vor und nach Bestrahlung abdomineller Lymphknotengruppen. Radiol. clin. biol. 42: 403, 1973.
37. Sauer R, Elke M: Der Kontrastmittelgehalt retroperitonealer Lymphknoten nach Lymphographie und seine Beeinflussung durch Lymphknoten-Pathologie, Strahlentherapie und Kontrastmittelmenge. Fortschr. Röntgenstr. 122: 10, 1975.
38. Sokol GH, Clouse ME, Kotner LM, Sewell JB: Complications of lymphangiography in patients of advanced age. Amer. J. Roentgenol. 43: 128, 1977.
39. Vahrson H: Lymphographie und massive Oelembolie. Strahlentherapie 140: 651, 1970.
40. Elke M: Vergleichende Versuche mit Lipiodol-UF und 20%iger Lipiodol-Emulsion beim Tier. Radiol. diagn. 13: 690, 1972.
41. Fernholz H-J: Szintigraphische Untersuchungen über Aenderung der Lungenperfusion nach Lymphographie mit öligen Kontrastmitteln. Fortschr. Röntgenstr. 114: 526, 1971.
42. Koenig H: Zur Dosisabhängigkeit der Nebenwirkungen durch Lipoidol-UF bei der Lymphographie. Radiol. diagn. 18: 29, 1977.
43. Redman HC: Dermatitis as complication of lymphography. Radiology 86: 323, 1966.
44. Malek P: Pathophysiological and radiological aspects of lympho-venous anastomoses. Experentia (Basel) Suppl. 14: 167, 1967.
45. Ravel R: Histopathology of lymph nodes after lymphangiography. Amer. J. clin. Path. 46: 335, 1966.
46. Elke M: Speicherung von öligem Kontrastmittel in Lungenmetastasen eines hypernephroiden Karzinoms nach Lymphographie. Fortschr. Röntgenstr. 103: 625, 1965.
47. Elke M, Hodel C: Lipidspeicherung in Hypernephrommetastasen der Lunge nach Lymphographie. Z. Krebsforsch. 69: 253, 1967.
48. Malek P: In vivo evidence of lympho-venous communications in the popliteal region. Acta radiol. 3: 344, 1965.

ADDITIONAL BIBILIOGRAPHY TO COMMENTARY

Bergiron C, Markovits P, Allal M, Pickarski JD, Vanel D: Value of lymphography in the work-up of prostatic carcinoma. In: 6th International Congress of Lymphology 20–25 June, 1977. Prague, Book of Abstracts, 1977, p 7.22.
Castellino RA, Ray G, Blank N, Govan D, Bagshaw M: Lymphangiography in prostatic carcinoma. Preliminary observations. J. Amer. med. Assoc. 223: 877, 1973.
Castellino RA: The role of lymphography in 'apparently localized' prostatic carcinoma. Lymphology 8: 16, 1975.
Cerny JC, Farah R, Rian R, Weckstein ML: An evaluation of lymphangiography in staging

carcinoma of the prostate. J. Urol. 113: 367, 1975.

Chiappa S, Uslenghi C, Bonadonna G, Marano P, Ravasi G: Combined testicular and foot lymphangiography in testicular carcinomas. Surg. Gynecol. Obstet. 123: 10, 1966.

Elke M: Die unspezifisch-reaktive Lymphknotenhyperplasie. Dtsch. Röntgenkongress, Hamburg, 1968. Beiheft Fortschr. Röntgenstr., 1969.

Elke M, Nidecker A: Metastasierungswege von Hodentumoren und lymphographische Metastasenmorphologie. Radiol. diagn. 13: 660, 1972.

Elke M, Rutishauser G: Die Lymphographie als Zusatzuntersuchung bei urologischen Tumoren. Fortschr. Röntgenstr. 107: 224, 1967.

Fuchs WA, Girod M: Lymphography as a guide to prognosis in malignant testicular tumors. Acta Radiol. Diagn. 16: 305, 1975.

Hulten L, Kingblom L-G, Linghagen J, Rosencrantz M, Seeman T, Wahlqvist L: Funicular and pedal lymphography in testicular tumors. Acta chir. scand. 139: 746, 1973.

Jewett HJ: Cancer of the bladder. Diagnosis and staging. Cancer 32: 1072, 1973.

Johnson DE, Kaesler KE, Kaminsky S, Jing BS, Wallace S: Lymphography as an aid in staging bladder carcinoma. Sth. Med. J. 69: 28, 1976.

Jonsson K, Ingemansson S, Ling L: Lymphography in patients with testicular tumours. Brit. J. Urol. 45: 548, 1973.

Lüning M, Tietz M: Wertbestimmung lymphographischer Metastasenkriterien bei malignen Ovarialtumoren. Radiol. Diagn. 18: 325, 1977.

Maier JG, Schamber DT: The role of lymphangiography in the diagnosis and treatment of malignant testicular tumours. Amer. J. Roentgenol. 114: 482, 1972.

Nakanishi S: Die Passage der Lymphflüssigkeit in einer Lymphdrüse. Lymphologia (Kyoto) 1: 49, 1951.

Prout Jr, GR: Diagnosis and staging of prostatic carcinoma. Cancer 32: 1096, 1973.

Safer ML, Green JP, Crews Jr, QE, Hill DR: Lymphangiographic accuracy in the staging of testicular tumors. Cancer 35: 1603, 1975.

Soimakallio S: Lymphography in urological Oncology. Univ. Kuopio (Finland). Medicine, Ser. Orig. Rep. 2, 1978.

UICC: TNM classification of malignant tumours. Union internationale Contre le Cancer, Geneva, 1978.

Wajsman Z, Baumgartner G, Murphy GP, Merrin C: Evaluation of lymphangiography for clinical staging of bladder tumors. J. Urol. 114: 712, 1975.

15. Guidelines for clinical trials set up to determine the usefulness of drugs in patients with symptoms ascribed to decreased flow in a particular vascular area

M. VERSTRAETE

Commentary by J.D. Coffman

COMMENTARY

Rest pain is considered by some specialists as unusual in muscle but common secondary to decreased nutritive flow to the skin and nerves.

1. INTRODUCTION

The causal relationship between decreased nutritive blood flow* in the muscle circulation and intermittent claudication and rest pain, and between decreased nutritive flow in the skin circulation and the development of skin defects, is well established.

Data pertaining to clinical pharmacology of agents used in patients with peripheral arterial insufficiency are only relevant at the clinical level if they do favourably affect the patient's symptoms. Minimum requirements for avoiding common pitfalls in the clinical evaluation of these agents are desirable and described in these guidelines (1).

Since, in most instances, the mode of action of 'vasodilatatory agents' remains unclear, it is recommended that this misleading general term should be abandoned in favour of a more restricted and specific descriptive term such as 'agent reducing intermittent claudication' or an 'agent healing skin defects' (2). Indeed a therapeutically active drug can have vasodilatatory properties or act on the microcirculation or derive its beneficial action from other properties.

2. MINIMUM REQUIREMENTS FOR THERAPEUTIC EFFICACY IN CLINICAL TRIALS WITH AGENTS IMPROVING MUSCLE AND/OR SKIN FLOW

(1) *Definition and appropriate selection of patients admitted to the trial:* All inclusion and exclusion criteria used to select patients must be mentioned in detail. In addition, the sites, extent and duration of the main arterial obliterations and their clinical symptoms must be mentioned. It is also important to know of certain habits (e.g., smoking, physical exercise, diet,

---

* In using the term blood flow, it is volume flow (cm^3/sec) that is generally understood rather than flow velocity (cm/sec).

intake of alcohol and certain drugs...) or the presence of associated diseases which may influence the course of the vascular condition (e.g., hypertension, diabetes, abnormal lipid spectrum, etc.). The protocol has to mention all factors which in addition to the experimental drug may influence the course of the vascular disease.

(2) Once included in the trial, patients may only be withdrawn on the basis of *strict criteria for withdrawal which have been defined in advance*. Nevertheless the first analysis of the results should preferably be based on the intention of treatment, including the withdrawals.

(3) *Due recognition of the natural course of the disease and of the placebo effect* also in the absence of any drug on the spontaneous evolution may compensate an arterial obliteration, e.g., by developing a collateral circulation. It is therefore essential to follow a contemperaneous control group. To ensure that the trial drug and placebo are allocated to patients of the same risk groups, randomisation of preselected and in some instances stratified patients must be used. When analysing the results one still has to demonstrate that the two groups were equal at the start in respect of factors relevant to the basic disorder and the sites of the arterial occlusions.

(4) *Necessity of a long observation period in order to reach stable base line values for the various parameters assessed:* a long single-blind run-in phase is considered essential; a placebo is given to all patients in addition to routine treatment such as physical training, abstinence from smoking tobacco, weight reduction, appropriate diet, intake of alcohol, etc. Other drugs used are carefully listed. During this run-in period the various parameters to be used in the following double-blind period are assessed at regular intervals (e.g., monthly). Experience has learned that approximately 3 months are required to reach a stabile baseline.

It is preferable to study patients with intermittent claudication present for a prolonged time before the run-in period. Patients with a recent onset of symptoms often improve or deteriorate during the following several months. Therefore, patient selection should also be based on duration of symptoms.
To expect a large group of patients to physically train, abstain from tobacco, lose weight, follow a diet, and change alcohol intake is probably unrealistic and often leads to a mixed group of patients for final analysis. A test of a therapeutic agent can be performed on patients stratified to include some of these variables.

(5) *Prudent interpretation of subjective findings:* one of the problems in assessing the course of patients with occlusive arterial disease is documentation of improvement. Purely subjective factors (e.g., intermittent claudication) should preferably not be the only criteria for judging the clinical effect of an agent recommended for claudication. Quantitative methods are to be used, e.g., exercise tolerance tests which should in any case be standardised (e.g., on a treadmill, ergograph, etc.). Even when standardised these methods still maintain a subjective endpoint and therefore a double-blind technique is essential to avoid a subconscious bias on the part of the investigators and patient. It is also highly recommended that a third, independent agent should distribute the materials (placebo and experimental drugs) to the investigator, prepare the randomisation tables, collect and analyse the data which will subsequently be given to the interested parties after completion of the trial. This is so that neither the manufacturer nor the investigator knows the code before the completion of the trial *and* analysis of the results. One should avoid converting sub-

Quantitative tests are necessary that do not use a subjective endpoint. At the present time, objective tests are the measurements of indices comparing pedal with brachial artery systolic blood pressures using the Doppler and disappearance rates of isotopes from muscles during exercise or following ischemic exercise in patients with intermittent claudication. Foot or digit blood flow can be measured by plethysmography in rest pain or vasospastic diseases.

It is often very difficult to compare therapeutic agents with placebo because of the side effects of the active agents such as flushing, headaches, etc. Placebos cannot duplicate these effects. Placebo controlled, double-blind cross-over studies cannot overcome this problem.

jective findings which cannot be measured objectively (e.g., decrease in rest pain) into scores which are then considered as if they were objective, digital data and have to be treated by the appropriate statistical methods. Whenever possible, subjective data should be correlated with objective quantitative parameters.

(6) *Necessity of pursuing the double-blind trial for an adequate length of time:* both treatment groups should be followed long enough to detect the bias of seasonal changes, the development of gross tolerance, or major side-effects of the drug. Most often this requires a treatment period of 5–6 months of double-blind phase. Too long a period will need to take into account the spontaneous evolution of the disease which would, however, also become apparent in the control group. On the other hand the proposed period may be too brief to show up any development of tolerance or late side-effects. If, at the end of this double-blind period, drug administration is suspended, one should also study if and when the improved parameters return to the original values reached at the end of the run-in phase. One can also consider a placebo-controlled, double-blind cross-over study with, for example, a 1 month interruption period (single-blind placebo) to avoid a possible carry-over effect from the previous span of 2 months. To avoid observer bias, half of the patients should receive their treatments in one order (say A, then B) and the other half in the reverse order (B, then A) and each treatment period should not be less than 3 months.

(7) *On the importance of frequent recording of the systemic blood pressure in patients admitted to the trial:* Distal to an arterial occlusion, there is a low perfusion pressure which the local circulation tends to circumvent by vasodilation, at least during exercise. This autoregulation operates down to a maximal dilation, at which point the flow passively follows fluctuation of infusion pressure. In an advanced stage of occlusive arterial disease collaterals may already in rest have reached their maximal dilatation. In these circumstances, drugs which decrease the mean systemic pressure, even to a minor extent, may produce a major reduction in blood flow.

Systemic blood pressure should, therefore, be measured not only at rest but also during exercise.

(8) *In which subgroups of patients with a peripheral arterial disease is the proposed agent clinically useful?* In demonstrations of the effectiveness of a drug, the proponent is expected to define the clinical candidates and not to draw conclusions which may be valid for one subgroup of patients but do not hold for a broader group (e.g., single arterial occlusion versus diffuse vascular alterations or single occlusions but at different levels of the arterial tree). More particularly, the proponent has to prove in appropriate clinical trials that a given drug is clinically useful in patients with vasospastic conditions, with organic disease of medium size arteries (atherosclerosis, Buerger's disease), smaller arteries or skin vessels in order to avoid indiscriminate recommendations.

(10) *Clear distinction between the therapeutic and prophylactic value of a*

drug: a drug may be useful in the treatment of a given symptom(s) but this does not necessarily imply that the progression of the underlying disease can be prevented or halted. Appropriate trials must be devised to prove either the prophylactic or the therapeutic value of the new drug.

Objective tests are necessary for this reason. Analgesics or even Achilles tendon severance will relieve intermittent claudication but are neither of therapeutic nor prophylactic value.

(10) *Importance of the route drug administration:* clinical trials performed with the experimental drug given simultaneously or subsequently by parenteral and oral routes do *not* prove the efficacy of oral treatment alone.

(11) *Dose prediction and clinical trials:* appropriate clinical trials have to be set up so that the optimal dose of a given substance can be determined. Too often a higher dose of a substance is being recommended than the one which at the beginning gave satisfactory clinical results.

(12) *Interaction with other drugs:* as the agents under discussion are for long-term use, their interaction with other drugs, commonly used in the same patients, is to be studied.

REFERENCES TO MAIN TEXT

1. Verstraete M: Critères d'appréciation de l'utilité clinique de médicaments recommandés pour le traitement de l'insuffisance artérielle chronique des membres. Considérations critiques. Acta Clin. Belg. 32: 8–14, 1977.
2. Verstraete M: Peripheral vasodilator drugs: a misnomer. Drugs 19: 81–83, 1980.

Index